Advances in Neurology
Volume 55

Advances in Neurology

INTERNATIONAL ADVISORY BOARD

Advances in Neurology
Volume 55

Neurobehavioral Problems in Epilepsy

Editors

Dennis B. Smith,M.D.
*Oregon Comprehensive Epilepsy Program
Good Samaritan Hospital and
Medical Center;
Department of Neurology
Oregon Health Sciences University
Portland, Oregon*

David M. Treiman,M.D.
*Neurology and Research Services
West Los Angeles VA Medical Center;
Department of Neurology
UCLA School of Medicine
Los Angeles, California*

Michael R. Trimble,F.R.C.P., F.R.C.Psych.
*Consultant Physician in
Psychological Medicine
and Raymond Way Lecturer in
Behavioural Therapy
Department of Psychological Medicine
The National Hospital for Neurology
London, England*

Raven Press ✳ New York

Library of Congress Cataloging in Publication Data

Neurobehavioral problems in epilepsy / editors, Dennis B. Smith, David
M. Treiman, Michael R. Trimble.
    p.   cm.—(Advances in neurology ; v. 55)
  ISBN 0-88167-714-0
  1. Epilepsy—Psychological aspects. 2. Neuropsychiatry.
I. Smith, Dennis B. II. Treiman, David M. III. Trimble, Michael R.
IV. Series.
  [DNLM: 1. Behavior. 2. Epilepsy. W1 AD684H v. 55 / WL 385
N4933]
RC321.A276 vol. 55
[RC372.5]
616.8 s—dc20
[616.8'53]
DNLM/DLC
for Library of Congress   90-9111
                                              CIP

To Bonnie, Lucy, and Jenny

Advances in Neurology Series

Vol. 55: Neurobehavioral Problems in Epilepsy: *D. B. Smith, D. M. Treiman, and M. R. Trimble, editors.* 485 pp., 1991.

Vol. 54: Magnetoencephalography: *S. Sato, editor.* 284 pp., 1990.

Vol. 53: Parkinson's Disease: Anatomy, Pathology, and Therapy: *M. B. Streifler, A. D. Korczyn, E. Melamed, and M. B. H. Youdim, editors.* 624 pp., 1990.

Vol. 52: Brain Edema: Pathogenesis, Imaging, and Therapy: *D. Long, editor.* 640 pp., 1990.

Vol. 51: Alzheimer's Disease: *R. J. Wurtman, S. Corkin, J. H. Growdon, and E. Ritter-Walker, editors.* 308 pp., 1990.

Vol. 50: Dystonia 2: *S. Fahn, C. D. Marsden, and D. B. Calne, editors.* 688 pp., 1988.

Vol. 49: Facial Dyskinesias: *J. Jankovic and E. Tolosa, editors.* 560 pp., 1988.

Vol. 48: Molecular Genetics of Neurological Neuromuscular Disease: *S. DiDonato, S. DiMauro, A. Mamoli, and L. P. Rowland, editors.* 288 pp., 1987.

Vol. 47: Functional Recovery in Neurological Disease: *S. G. Waxman, editor.* 640 pp., 1987.

Vol. 46: Intensive Neurodiagnostic Monitoring: *R. J. Gumnit, editor.* 336 pp., 1987.

Vol. 45: Parkinson's Disease: *M. D. Yahr and K. J. Bergmann, editors.* 640 pp., 1986.

Vol. 44: Basic Mechanisms of the Epilepsies: Molecular and Cellular Approaches: *A. V. Delgado-Escucta, A. A. Ward, Jr., D. M. Woodbury, and R. J. Porter, editors.* 1,120 pp., 1986.

Vol. 43: Myoclonus: *S. Fahn, C. D. Marsden, and M. H. Van Woert, editors.* 752 pp., 1986.

Vol. 42: Progress in Aphasiology: *F. Clifford Rose, editor.* 384 pp., 1984.

Vol. 41: The Olivopontocerebellar Atrophies: *R. C. Duvoisin and A. Plaitakis, editors.* 304 pp., 1984.

Vol. 40: Parkinson-Specific Motor and Mental Disorders, Role of Pallidum: Pathophysiological, Biochemical, and Therapeutic Aspects: *R. G. Hassler and J. F. Christ, editors.* 601 pp., 1984.

*Vol. 39: Motor Control Mechanisms in Health and Disease: *J. E. Desmedt, editor.* 1,224 pp., 1983.

Vol. 38: The Dementias: *R. Mayeux and W. G. Rosen, editors.* 288 pp., 1983.

Vol. 37: Experimental Therapeutics of Movement Disorders: *S. Fahn, D. B. Calne, and I. Shoulson, editors.* 339 pp., 1983.

Vol. 36: Human Motor Neuron Diseases: *L. P. Rowland, editor.* 592 pp., 1982.

Vol. 35: Gilles de la Tourette Syndrome: *A. J. Friedhoff and T. N. Chase, editors.* 476 pp., 1982.

Vol. 34: Status Epilepticus: Mechanisms of Brain Damage and Treatment: *A. V. Delgado-Escueta, C. G. Wasterlain, D. M. Treiman, and R. J. Porter, editors.* 579 pp., 1983.

*Vol. 33: Headache: Physiopathological and Clinical Concepts: *M. Critchley, A. Friedman, S. Gorini, and F. Sicuteri, editors.* 417 pp., 1982.

*Vol. 32: Clinical Applications of Evoked Potentials in Neurology: *J. Courjon, F. Mauguiere, and M. Revol, editors.* 592 pp., 1982.

Vol. 31: Demyelinating Diseases: Basic and Clinical Electrophysiology: *S. Waxman and J. Murdoch Ritchie, editors.* 544 pp., 1981.

Vol. 30: Diagnosis and Treatment of Brain Ischemia: *A. L. Carney and E. M. Anderson, editors.* 424 pp., 1981.

*Vol. 29: Neurofibromatosis: *V. M. Riccardi and J. J. Mulvihill, editors.* 288 pp., 1981.

Vol. 28: Brain Edema: *J. Cervós-Navarro and R. Ferszt, editors.* 539 pp., 1980.

Vol. 27: Antiepileptic Drugs: Mechanisms of Action: *G. H. Glaser, J. K. Penry, and D. M. Woodbury, editors.* 728 pp., 1980.

Vol. 26: Cerebral Hypoxia and Its Consequences: *S. Fahn, J. N. Davis, and L. P. Rowland, editors.* 454 pp., 1979.

*Vol. 25: Cerebrovascular Disorders and Strokes: *M. Goldstein, L. Bolis, C. Fieschi, S. Gorini, and C. H. Millikan, editors. 412 pp., 1979.*

Vol. 24: The Extrapyramidal System and Its Disorders: *L. J. Poirier, T. L. Sourkes, and P. Bédard, editors. 552 pp., 1979.*

*Vol. 23: Huntington's Chorea: *T. N. Chase, N. S. Wexler, and A. Barbeau, editors. 864 pp., 1979.*

Vol. 22: Complications of Nervous System Trauma: *R. A. Thompson and J. R. Green, editors. 454 pp., 1979.*

*Vol. 21: The Inherited Ataxia: Biochemical, Viral, and Pathological Studies: *R. A. Kark, R. Rosenberg, and L. Schut, editors. 450 pp., 1978.*

Vol. 20: Pathology of Cerebrospinal Microcirculation: *J. Cervós-Navarro, E. Betz, G. Ebhardt, R. Ferszt, and R. Wüllenweber, editors. 636 pp., 1978.*

*Vol. 19: Neurological Epidemiology: Principles and Clinical Applications: *B. S. Schoenberg, editor. 672 pp., 1978.*

*Vol. 18: Hemi-Inattention and Hemisphere Specialization: *E. A. Weinstein and R. P. Friedland, editors. 176 pp., 1977.*

*Vol. 17: Treatment of Neuromuscular Diseases: *R. C. Griggs and R. T. Moxley, editors. 370 pp., 1977.*

Vol. 16: Stroke: *R. A. Thompson and J. R. Green, editors. 250 pp., 1977.*

*Vol. 15: Neoplasia in the Central Nervous System: *R. A. Thompson and J. R. Green, editors. 394 pp., 1976.*

Vol. 14: Dystonia: *R. Eldridge and S. Fahn, editors. 510 pp., 1976.*

Vol. 13: Current Reviews: *W. J. Friedlander, editor. 400 pp., 1975.*

Vol. 12: Physiology and Pathology of Dendrites: *G. W. Kreutzberg, editor. 524 pp., 1975.*

*Vol. 11: Complex Partial Seizures and Their Treatment: *J. K. Penry and D. D. Daly, editors. 486 pp., 1975.*

Vol. 10: Private Models of Neurological Disorders: *B. S. Meldrum and C. D. Marsden, editors. 270 pp., 1975.*

*Vol. 9: Dopaminergic Mechanisms: *D. B. Calne, T. N. Chase, and A. Barbeau, editors. 452 pp., 1975.*

*Vol. 8: Neurosurgical Management of Epilepsies: *D. P. Purpura, J. K. Penry, and R. D. Walter, editors. 370 pp., 1975.*

Vol. 7: Current Reviews of Higher Nervous System Dysfunction: *W. J. Friedlander, editor. 202 pp., 1975.*

Vol. 6: Infectious Diseases of the Central Nervous System: *R. A. Thompson and J. R. Green, editors. 402 pp., 1974.*

*Vol. 5: Second Canadian-American Conference on Parkinson's Disease: *F. McDowell and A. Barbeau, editors. 526 pp., 1974.*

*Vol. 4: International Symposium on Pain: *J. J. Bonica, editor. 858 pp., 1974.*

*Vol. 3: Progress in the Treatment of Parkinsonism: *D. B. Calne, editor. 402 pp., 1973.*

*Vol. 2: The Treatment of Parkinsonism—The Role of DOPA Decarboxylase Inhibitors: *M. D. Yahr, editor. 304 pp., 1973.*

Vol. 1: Huntington's Chorea, 1872–1972: *A. Barbeau, T. N. Chase, and G. W. Paulson, editors. 902 pp., 1973.*

---

*Out of print.

Preface

Misconceptions about behavioral change in epilepsy have existed throughout written history and persist today. The following quotation is from *The New York Times Book Review*, January 14, 1990:

> Malfunctioning in a small area of the brain can not only cause epilepsy but can render someone highly religious and make him give up all addictions, such as drink and tobacco; it also takes away sexual desire. (It may be that the form Christianity took was the result of an epileptic attack suffered by St. Paul on the road to Damascus.) When the epileptic focus is removed, the person returns to normality: he gives up religion, enjoys a drink and takes an interest in sex.
>
> Stuart Sutherland

While it is shocking to find statements such as this today, it should come as no surprise. Controversy is no stranger to either the lay or the medical literature on epilepsy and behavior.

The association between epilepsy and disturbed behavior has a long history going back to the earliest medical writings on epilepsy (Temkin*). Over time such links were rarely questioned, until, in the mid-nineteenth century, several workers, namely Falret† and Morel‡, developed theories that not only implied associations between epilepsy and certain behavioral or personality profiles, but also that some cyclical behaviors themselves could be evidence of an epileptic process, even in the absence of seizures. There followed a considerable literature on both ictal and interictal problems of patients with epilepsy, and controversies emerged, with various antithetical views being expressed. For some, interictal behaviors and changes were inevitable, for others rare.

Based largely on clinical observations, fairly elaborate hypotheses have been developed linking psychoses, violence, and epilepsy, and a variety of explanations for behavioral change in epilepsy have been proposed. The effects of recurrent head injury, the influence of adverse social forces and stigmatization, and more recently the effects of long-term anticonvulsant therapy have all been implicated. The idea that the seizure process itself may be the important variable was revived by the late Normal Geschwind and colleagues, especially with the concept that identifiable personality changes resulted from specific temporal lobe lesions (Waxman and Geschwind). These hypotheses have spurred healthy debate, but the frequent lack of sound scientific methodology in behavioral research (especially in behavioral studies in epilepsy) has led to skepticism in the rest of the scientific community. This skepticism affects the acceptance of current investigations in behavioral aspects of epilepsy. Behavioral research has been further hampered by misguided individuals and organizations who, in an effort to protect people with epilepsy from the stigma of broad associations with cognitive deficits, behavioral syndromes, and psychoses, downplay suggestions that specific behaviors and cognitive change may be associated with epilepsy.

---

*Temkin O. *The falling sickness*. Baltimore: Johns Hopkins, 1945.

†Falret J. De l'etat mental des epileptiques. *Arch Gen Med* 1860;16:661–679.

‡Morel BA. Traite des dequerescences physiques, intellectuelles et morales de l'espece humans et des causes que produiscent ses varietes maladaptires. *Bailliere* 1857;Vol. 1, Paris.

The behavioral sciences are still in their infancy, and some investigations of behavioral change in epilepsy still suffer from a lack of scientific rigor. Nonetheless, many good studies have been completed, and many more are in progress. New understandings of some of the basic mechanisms underlying behavior, and behavioral change and its relationship to epilepsy and its treatment, are emerging. The existence of behavioral and cognitive changes associated with epilepsy is now well documented and the relative contribution of factors such as antiepileptic drugs, seizure type and duration, interpersonal and environmental effects, and underlying cerebral pathology are being better defined. A whole new range of behavioral, neuropsychological, physiological, chemical, anatomical, and imaging techniques are being used to explore these problems.

Partly because of the increasing sophistication of the methodologies which can now be brought to bear on these problems, there has been a tremendous surge of interest in behavioral aspects of epilepsy within the last decade. Debates about the nature and even existence of specific behavioral syndromes associated with epilepsy have been entered into with renewed vigor. The results of well-controlled studies have been reported and a better understanding of the basic neurochemical, physiologic, and anatomic substrates of behavioral change has evolved. Nonetheless, misconceptions about the relationship of epilepsy and specific behavioral syndromes, psychoses, and violence continue, and at times tend to obfuscate rational discussion and impair objective analysis of the neurobehavior literature. It is in the setting of these continuing controversies and new available data that we decided the time was right to produce a multiauthored book summarizing the "state of the art" in behavioral epilepsy research. An international group of contributors has been selected, all of whom have clinical and research interests in epilepsy and its behavioral expressions.

This book presents what is currently known about the anatomic, pathologic, physiologic, and neurochemical substrates of behavior, and relates this knowledge to specific ictal and interictal behavior, as well as to cognitive changes described in patients with epilepsy. Psychosocial factors affecting behavior are not ignored, but this book emphasizes a review of the latest information available regarding basic mechanisms that may be common to both epileptogenesis and behavioral and cognitive changes associated with epilepsy.

The Editors

Acknowledgments

The editors wish to thank Ms. Bonnie Becker for her invaluable organizational skills and for her editing support. We also gratefully acknowledge the American Epilepsy Society, which sponsored the symposium from which this work was derived.

Contents

Neurological Substrates of Behavioral Change

1. Neurobiological Substrates of Ictal Behavioral Changes 1
   Pierre Gloor

2. Neurochemical Substrates of Ictal Behavior 35
   Brian S. Meldrum

3. Interictal Psychiatric Disorders: Neurochemical Aspects 47
   E. H. Reynolds

4. Are Complex Partial Seizures a Sequela of Temporal
   Lobe Dysgenesis? 59
   Arnold B. Scheibel

5. Psychosis and the Temporal Lobe 79
   Janice R. Stevens

The Effect of Epilepsy and Seizures on Behavior

6. Neurobiological Evidence for Epilepsy-Induced
   Interictal Disturbances 97
   *Jerome Engel, Jr., Richard Bandler, Neil C. Griffith, and
   Sally Caldecott-Hazard*

7. Behavioral Correlates of Interictal Spikes 113
   C. D. Binnie, S. Channon, and D. L. Marston

8. Acute Behavioral Symptomatology at Disappearance of Epileptiform
   EEG Abnormality: Paradoxical or
   "Forced" Normalization 127
   Peter Wolf

9. Interictal Psychoses of Epilepsy 143
   Michael R. Trimble

10. Behavioral Consequences of Epilepsy in Children: Developing a
    Psychosocial Vocabulary 153
    David C. Taylor and Moira Lochery

11. Evocation and Inhibition of Seizures: Behavioral Treatment 163
    Peter Fenwick

12. Epilepsy and Disorders of Mood 185
    Dietrich Blumer

The Effects of Treatment on Behavior

13. Cognitive Effects of Antiepileptic Drugs 197
     Dennis B. Smith

14. Behavioral Effects of Antiepileptic Drugs 213
     Carl B. Dodrill

15. Effects of Antiepileptic Drugs on the Developing Central
     Nervous System 225
     Bruce R. Ransom and Joann G. Elmore

16. Antiepileptic Drugs in Affective Illness: Clinical and
     Theoretical Implications 239
     *Robert M. Post, Lori L. Altshuler, Terrence A. Ketter, Kirk Denicoff,
     and Susan R. B. Weiss*

17. Effects of Temporal Lobe Surgery on Behavior 279
     Rebecca Rausch

18. Behavioral Changes Following Corpus Callosotomy 293
     Alexander G. Reeves

Ictal and Interictal Behavioral Syndromes

19. Ictal Manifestations of Temporal Lobe Seizures......................... 301
     Heinz-Gregor Wieser

20. Frontal Lobe Seizures and Epilepsies in
     Neurobehavioral Disorders.. 317
     *Antonio V. Delgado-Escueta, Barbara E. Swartz, Gregory O. Walsh,
     Patrick Chauvel, Jean Bancaud, and Dominique Broglin*

21. Psychobiology of Ictal Aggression 341
     David M. Treiman

22. Ictal Amnesia and Fugue States... 357
     A. James Rowan and David H. Rosenbaum

23. Memory Function in Patients with Epilepsy 369
     Pamela J. Thompson

24. Memory Dysfunction in Epilepsy Patients as a Derangement of
     Normal Physiology 385
     *Eric Halgren, June Stapleton, Patricia Domalski, Barbara E.
     Swartz, Antonio V. Delgado-Escueta, Gregory O. Walsh, Mark
     Mandelkern, William Blahd, and Jim Ropchan*

25. The Geschwind Syndrome 411
     D. Frank Benson

Environmental and Psychosocial Issues

26. Modern Approaches to Neuropsychological Testing 423
Stanley Berent

27. Neurobiological, Psychosocial, and Pharmacological Factors
Underlying Interictal Psychopathology in Epilepsy 439
Bruce P. Hermann and Steve Whitman

28. Emotional Effects on Seizure Occurrence 453
Richard H. Mattson

29. Legal Implications of Behavioral Changes in Epilepsy 461
John Gunn

Subject Index 473

Contributors

Lori M. Altshuler, M.D.
Biological Psychiatry Branch
National Institute of Mental Health
National Institutes of Health
Bethesda, Maryland 20892

Jean Bancaud, M.D.
INSERM Unit 97, Epilepsy Research Unit
  and the Neurosurgical Department
Centre Paul Broca
75014 Paris, France

Richard Bandler, Ph.D.
Department of Anatomy
University of Sydney
N.S.W., Australia

D. Frank Benson, M.D.
Department of Neurology
UCLA School of Medicine
Los Angeles, California 90024

Stanley Berent, Ph.D.
Neuropsychology Program
University of Michigan Hospitals
Ann Arbor, Michigan 48109

C. D. Binnie, M.D.
Department of Clinical Neurology
The Maudsley Hospital
London SE5 8AZ, England

William Blahd, M.D.
Department of Medicine
University of California, Los Angeles
Los Angeles, California 90024;
Nuclear Medicine Services
Wadsworth VA Medical Center
West Los Angeles, California 90073

Dietrich Blumer, M.D.
Director, Neuropsychiatry Program
Epicare Center
Baptist Memorial Hospital
Memphis, Tennessee 38104;
Department of Psychiatry
University of Tennessee, Memphis
Memphis, Tennessee 38146

Dominique Broglin, M.D.
INSERM Unit 97, Epilepsy Research
  Unit, and the Neurosurgical
  Department
Centre Paul Broca
75014 Paris, France

Sally Caldecott-Hazard, Ph.D.
Department of Neurology
UCLA School of Medicine
Los Angeles, California 90024

S. Channon, M.D.
The Middlesex Hospital
London WC1, England

Patrick Chauvel, M.D.
INSERM Unit 97, Epilepsy Research
  Unit, and the Neurosurgical
  Department
Centre Paul Broca
75014 Paris, France

Antonio V. Delgado-Escueta, M.D.
Department of Neurology, Brain Research
  Institute, and California Comprehensive
  Epilepsy Program
UCLA School of Medicine
Los Angeles, California 90024;
West Los Angeles VA Medical Center
West Los Angeles, California 90073

Kirk Denicoff, M.D.
Biological Psychiatry Branch
National Institute of Mental Health
National Institutes of Health
Bethesda, Maryland 20892

Carl B. Dodrill, Ph.D.
Regional Epilepsy Center
Harborview Hospital
Seattle, Washington 98104;
Department of Neurological Surgery
University of Washington School of
*   Medicine*
Seattle, Washington 98104

Patricia Domalski, M.A.
Department of Psychology and California
*   Comprehensive Epilepsy Center*
University of California, Los Angeles
Los Angeles, California 90024;
Southwest Regional Epilepsy Center/
*   Neurology*
West Los Angeles, California 90073

Joann G. Elmore, M.D.
Department of Internal Medicine
Yale University School of Medicine
New Haven, Connecticut 06510

Jerome Engel, Jr., M.D., Ph.D.
Department of Neurology
UCLA School of Medicine
Los Angeles, California 90024

Peter Fenwick, M.D.
The Maudsley Hospital
London SE5 8AZ, England

Pierre Gloor, M.D., Ph.D.
Department of Neurology and
*   Neurosurgery*
Montreal Neurological Institute
Montreal, Quebec, Canada H3A 2B4

Neil C. Griffith, M.D.
Department of Neurology
Westmead Hospital
Westmead, N.S.W., Australia

John Gunn, M.D.
Department of Forensic Psychiatry
Institute of Psychiatry
London SE5 8AF, England

Eric Halgren, M.D., Ph.D.
Department of Psychiatry, Brain Research
*   Institute and California Comprehensive*
*   Epilepsy Center*
University of California, Los Angeles
Los Angeles, California 90024;
Southwest Regional Epilepsy Center/
*   Neurology*
West Los Angeles, California 90073

Bruce P. Hermann, Ph.D.
Epicare Center
Baptist Memorial Hospital
Memphis, Tennessee 38103;
Departments of Psychiatry and
*   Neurosurgery*
University of Tennessee, Memphis
Memphis, Tennessee 38146

Terrence A. Ketter, M.D.
Biological Psychiatry Branch
National Institute of Mental Health
National Institutes of Health
Bethesda, Maryland 20892

Moira Lochery, M.D.
Department of Child and Adolescent
*   Psychiatry*
University of Manchester
Swinton M27 1FG, England

Mark Mandelkern, M.D., Ph.D.
Department of Medicine
University of California, Los Angeles
Los Angeles, California 90024;
Nuclear Medicine Services
Wadsworth VA Medical Center
West Los Angeles, California 90073

D. L. Marston, M.D.
The Maudsley Hospital
London SE5 8AZ, England

Richard H. Mattson, M.D.
Department of Veterans Affairs
VA Medical Center
West Haven, Connecticut 06516;
Department of Neurology
Yale University Medical School
New Haven, Connecticut 06510

Brian S. Meldrum, M.D.
Department of Neurology
Institute of Psychiatry
London SE5 8AF, England

Robert M. Post, M.D.
Chief, Biological Psychiatry Branch
National Institute of Mental Health
National Institutes of Health
Bethesda, Maryland 20892

Bruce R. Ransom, M.D., Ph.D.
Department of Neurology
Yale University School of Medicine
New Haven, Connecticut 06510

Rebecca Rausch, Ph.D.
Department of Psychiatry and
Biobehavioral Sciences, and
Department of Neurology
Reed Neurological Research Center
University of California, Los Angeles
Los Angeles, California 90024

Alexander G. Reeves, M.D.
Chairman, Section of Neurology
Dartmouth Medical School
Hanover, New Hampshire 03756

E. H. Reynolds, M.D., F.R.C.P.,
F.R.C.Psych.
Department of Neurology
Maudsley and King's College Hospitals
London SE5 8AZ, England

Jim Ropchan, Ph.D.
Nuclear Medicine Services
Wadsworth VA Medical Center
West Los Angeles, California 90073

David II. Rosenbaum, M.D.
Department of Neurology
Mt. Sinai School of Medicine
New York, New York 10029

A. James Rowan, M.D.
Department of Neurology
Mt. Sinai School of Medicine
New York, New York 10029;
The Bronx VA Medical Center
The Bronx, New York 10468

Arnold B. Scheibel, M.D.
Departments of Anatomy and Cell
Biology, Psychiatry, and Behavioral
Sciences, and Brain Research Institute
UCLA Medical Center
Los Angeles, California 90024

Dennis B. Smith, M.D.
Oregon Comprehensive Epilepsy Program
Good Samaritan Hospital and Medical
Center;
Department of Neurology
Oregon Health Sciences University
Portland, Oregon 97210

June Stapleton, Ph.D.
Department of Psychology and California
Comprehensive Epilepsy Center
University of California, Los Angeles
Los Angeles, California 90024;
Southwest Regional Epilepsy Center/
Neurology
West Los Angeles, California 90073

Janice R. Stevens, M.D.
Neuropsychiatry Branch
NIMH Clinical Research Unit
National Institutes of Health
St. Elizabeth's Hospital
Washington, D.C. 20032

Barbara E. Swartz, M.D., Ph.D.
Department of Neurology and California
Comprehensive Epilepsy Center
University of California, Los Angeles
Los Angeles, California 90024;
Southwest Regional Epilepsy Center/
Neurology
West Los Angeles, California 90073

David C. Taylor, M.D.
Department of Child and Adolescent
Psychiatry
University of Manchester
Swinton M27 1FG, England

Pamela J. Thompson, Ph.D.
Department of Psychology
Chalfont Centre for Epilepsy
Chalfont St. Peter
Buckinghamshire SL9 ORJ, England

David M. Treiman, M.D.
Neurology and Research Services
West Los Angeles VA Medical Center
Los Angeles, California 90073;
Department of Neurology
UCLA School of Medicine
Los Angeles, California 90024

Michael R. Trimble. F.R.C.P.,
  F.R.C.Psych.
Consultant Physician in Psychological
  Medicine and Raymond Way Lecturer in
  Behavioural Therapy
Department of Psychological Medicine
The National Hospital for Neurology
London WC1N 3BG, England

Susan R. B. Weiss, Ph.D.
Biological Psychiatry Branch
National Institute of Mental Health
National Institutes of Health
Bethesda, Maryland 20892

Steve Whitman, Ph.D.
Center for Urban Affairs and Policy
  Research
Northwestern University
Evanston, Illinois 60201

Gregory O. Walsh, M.D.
Department of Neurology and California
  Comprehensive Epilepsy Center
University of California, Los Angeles
Los Angeles, California 90024;
Southwest Regional Epilepsy Center/
  Neurology
West Los Angeles, California 90073

Heinz-Gregor Wieser, M.D.
Department of Neurology
University Hospital Zurich
CH-8031 Zurich, Switzerland

Peter Wolf, M.D.
Epilepsy-Centre Bethel
4800 Bielefeld 13
Federal Republic of Germany

Advances in Neurology
Volume 55

Advances in Neurology, Vol. 55, edited by
D. Smith, D. Treiman, and M. Trimble,
Raven Press, Ltd., New York © 1991.

1

Neurobiological Substrates of Ictal Behavioral Changes

Pierre Gloor

*Montreal Neurological Institute and Department of Neurology and Neurosurgery,
McGill University, Montreal, Quebec H3A 2B4, Canada*

Behavioral changes related to epilepsy are numerous, and their causes are varied: Some represent psychological reactions to the debilitating social consequences of recurrent seizures, some that are usually enduring are the expression of the underlying brain pathology related to the seizures, and, finally, some transient behavioral changes result directly from the seizure discharge itself. It is with the latter problem that the present review is concerned. When considering this issue there are two aspects that need to be distinguished: The first is that of the neuroanatomical substrate of ictal behavioral changes, and the second is that of the neurophysiological substrate of such changes. Behavioral changes that result from ictal discharge reflect the role of the brain structures affected by the discharge; this represents the neuroanatomical aspect of the problem. Furthermore, the ictal discharge involving such an anatomical substrate can produce ictal behavioral changes in one of two ways: Either it can activate the function that is "represented" there, or it can, on account of its unphysiological nature, interfere with it to the extent that the functions depending on the involved area become paralyzed. This represents the neurophysiological aspect of the problem.

Before going further into this topic, however, it is necessary to delineate the scope of this review. We must first define what we mean by "behavior" in the present context. A case could be made that any ictal sign or symptom involves or reveals a facet of behav-

ior; for instance, "motor" or "sensory" functions which are mediated by the motor cortex or primary sensory areas certainly are important components of behavior. When we speak of "behavior" (e.g., in the context of "behavioral neurology"), we do not, however, usually take such an all-encompassing view and restrict its meaning to what is often called "higher nervous functions." In this review I shall confine myself to this more restrictive definition. Without this list being necessarily exhaustive, we can include under this rubric functions such as perception, memory, affect, speech (expressive and receptive), social behavior, goal-directed and skilled motor behavior (to avoid the philosophically slippery term of "voluntary motor behavior"), and, finally (and unavoidably), "consciousness," even though this is philosophically as well as scientifically the most slippery and most unwieldy of all terms.

ANATOMICAL SUBSTRATES OF ICTAL BEHAVIORAL CHANGES

In the second half of the last century, Hughlings Jackson (1) recognized that the signs and symptoms exhibited by patients during epileptic seizures reflect the functional role of the area in which such discharge takes place. Ever since, attempts have been made to relate the various forms of behavior displayed by patients during the ictus to specific functions "represented" in specific areas of the cerebrum (2). Hughlings Jackson was indeed the first to use this approach not only to identify the site of onset of seizures, but also to clarify the functions of the areas thus affected.

Seizure discharges are known to cause ictal alterations of behavior, particularly when the following structures are involved: the association areas of the isocortex, the limbic structures of the temporal lobe, and, finally, the cerebral cortex as a whole when it is subjected to the relatively mild form of seizure activity represented by generalized spike-and-wave discharge. Apart from this situation seen in absence attacks and petit mal status, the majority of ictal behavioral changes result from seizure discharge involving the temporal lobe, both in its limbic and isocortical components.

NEUROPHYSIOLOGICAL MECHANISMS INVOLVED IN THE ICTAL ELICITATION OF BEHAVIORAL PHENOMENA

Two mechanisms must be distinguished that may, in the course of seizures, lead to behavioral changes: One is a positive effect of seizure discharge (i.e., epileptic activation of a behavioral mechanism represented in the area subject to ictal discharge), and the other is a negative effect of the seizure discharge (i.e., epileptic interference with the normal function of a region upon which a given behavioral mechanism depends) (2). The negative effect exerted on behavioral mechanisms in these circumstances can assume one of two forms: It may cause an inability to engage in a certain form of behavior (such as uttering or understanding words) because the substrate sustaining this function has become paralyzed by ictal discharge, or it may release behavioral mechanisms normally suppressed by structures rendered nonfunctional by the ictal discharge. It is often assumed that behavioral changes resulting from ictal discharge must all be attributable to epileptic interference (3). The assumption is based on the belief that the underlying physiology of any behavioral mechanism is "too complex" to be susceptible to activation by the crude type of unphysiological activity represented by seizure discharge or induced by electrical stimulation. True activation of mechanisms represented in

an area of cortex is therefore thought to be essentially restricted to elementary motor and sensory functions, such as (a) the contraction of certain muscles in response to discharge involving the motor cortex or (b) the elicitation of phosphenes or other elementary sensory manifestations in response to discharge involving the striate or other sensory cortices. When, in the course of a seizure, complex behavioral manifestations such as experiential phenomena or automatic behavior appear which on first impression seem to indicate that some brain mechanism has become activated by the ictal discharge, it is assumed that these manifestations nevertheless must reflect negative effects of that discharge. It may be argued that their apparently positive nature can be attributed to a release phenomenon which becomes manifest, because a mechanism which normally restrains these behavioral mechanisms has become inactivated by seizure discharge. The logical conclusion to be drawn from this view is that the behavioral mechanisms that are "released" during a seizure and that manifest themselves in the form of either subjective experiences or outward behavior must have their neural substrate in parts of the brain that are not involved in the seizure discharge. This interpretation is likely to be applicable to some apparently positive ictal phenomena such as automatism; however, as will be argued later, it cannot readily account for experiential phenomena.

PERCEPTION

Are true perceptual phenomena ever elicited by seizure discharge? The answer is "yes," if one accepts that perceptual illusions and hallucinations are to be included under this rubric. As we shall see, however, determining the true nature of a presumed hallucinatory experience is not easy.

In the case of illusions, we are dealing with a distortion of actual experience. The object of perception actually exists within the sensory environment of the patient as he is subject to an illusion, but what he perceives deviates from what one would expect he should perceive at that time. Illusions of this kind in the visual sphere include (a) macropsia or micropsia, (b) the illusion of motion (i.e., objects coming nearer or moving farther away), (c) distortion of the shape of objects seen, (d) a change in the intensity of color perception (i.e., colors fading or becoming more intense), or (e) increased vividness of stereoscopic vision. There is evidence that such changes occur because one or another of the visual association areas becomes affected by the seizure discharge (2,4–6). The term "affected" (rather than "involved") is used advisedly here, because it is not at all certain whether actual seizure discharge in visual association cortex is the only possible electrophysiological substrate of such illusions. Mullan and Penfield (4) found that stimulation of the nondominant temporal lobe isocortex as far rostral as the temporal polar region could elicit visual illusions. Curiously, they report no such illusions from dominant temporal cortical stimulation; this suggests that visual illusions in temporal lobe seizures, as opposed to hallucinations, may have some lateralizing significance. Visual illusions may even be elicited by discharge or electrical stimulation of the amygdala and perhaps of other limbic structures in the mesial temporal region as well (7). For instance, one of our patients, E.A., had an illusion of increased vividness of stereoscopic vision with ictal discharge or electrical stimulation involving the amygdala. He described his experience as follows: "I felt as if I were looking through a Viewmaster." The illusion could be reproduced by amygdaloid stimulation without eliciting an electrical afterdischarge. With more intense stimulation, a small habitual seizure was evoked which was ushered in by the same visual illusion associated with a chest sensation. The seizure discharge involved only the mesial structures of the right temporal lobe. At first glance, it appears incongruous that such a visual illusion which most likely is indicative of involvement of visual association cortex can be elicited by amygdaloid stimulation. How this can tentatively be explained will be discussed later when considering a possible mechanism for the elicitation of experiential phenomena.

Perceptual illusions can also occur in the auditory sphere with temporal lobe discharge; for instance, sounds may sound louder or fainter (2,4,6). In Mullan and Penfield's (4) study, points which on stimulation yielded auditory illusions were about equally represented in both temporal lobes and were located almost exclusively in the first temporal convolution, a localization confirmed by Bancaud (6).

Hallucinations represent the second type of perceptual phenomena that may be induced by seizure discharge. In this case the sensory environment does not contain a source of sensory signals related to the experience the patient has. The latter is entirely generated within his own brain. In this context I shall not discuss elementary hallucinations such as phosphenes or paresthesiae, since they do not possess the perceptual and experiential qualities characteristic for complex hallucinations, most of which involve the visual modality, the auditory modality, or both modalities combined. Hallucinations of this type are true experiential phenomena, because they have subjective qualities normally associated with experiences of everyday living (2,3,5–10). In the visual sphere they may consist of seeing a place, a person, or a face; in the auditory modality they may involve hearing a voice or a piece of music being played. As is the case in everyday living, however, perceptual features are often only one aspect of these hallucinatory phenomena, since they are frequently associated with mnemonic and affective features. It is for this reason that describing them as "experiential" seems to be a most appropriate terminology. The anatomical substrate of these phenomena and their possible pathophysiological mechanism will be dealt with later when discussing experiential phenomena in general.

Before discussing their possible substrates and mechanisms, it may be opportune to describe the subjectively experienced phenomenology of these hallucinations. There is no doubt that in certain instances the patient may indeed have the experience of seeing or hearing something that has qualities which normally are those of visual or auditory perceptions emanating from the environment in everyday life. Thus, a patient may be able to describe some perceptual details of a hallucination or may be able to locate a hallucinated object in his extrapersonal space. The object of the hallucination may be identifiable as a specific person or locale known to him. One of our patients (C.G.), for instance, said that the voice he heard in some of his seizures or in response to amygdaloid stimulation was that of his wife. Another may be able to describe some specific visual features of the hallucination. To illustrate this, it may be useful to describe in some detail a combined visual–auditory hallucination experienced by one of our patients (G.B.). His seizures were ushered in by a stereotyped aura: He saw in front of him a human face that looked familiar to him, yet he was never able to tell whose it was. The face sometimes spoke, and the patient thought that he heard what it said but could not remember it. The main feature of this hallucination was visual rather than auditory. Depth electrode recordings showed that the seizure discharge involved the right temporal lobe and maximally involved its limbic structures (Fig. 1). The patient's habitual aura of seeing a face was reproduced by electrical stimulation of the right amygdala without elicitation of an afterdischarge. The stimulation was then repeated, and the current was left on while the patient was asked to describe the hallucination in detail during the ongoing electrical stimulation. While he was being tested in this fashion he was looking straight ahead, and no person was standing within his range of vision. Immediately upon the start of electrical stimulation the patient told us that he saw the face. It remained visible to him throughout the entire duration of stimulation (56 sec). When asked to point to the face, he pointed right in front of him. While still seeing the face during continued stimulation, he was questioned about its perceptual attributes. It was that of a man, but the patient was unable to tell us whether the hair was long or short. When asked whether he saw the face in color or in black and white, he failed to reply, looked pale, and seemed to suffer some sort of discomfort (later described by him as a malaise in his stomach). Stimulation was therefore stopped at this point. Immediately afterwards upon questioning, he told us that the face had moved as if speaking and that he thought he had heard something, like someone speaking. He had the feeling it was a voice he knew, but he could not say whose voice it was. He also believed that at the time he understood what the voice had said, but he could not repeat it because, he thought, he had forgotten it. He believed the face was that of someone he knew, but he could not identify it. There was no afterdischarge.

In this instance there seems to be no doubt that the patient had a true visual hallucination. He could localize the hallucinated face in his extrapersonal space and partially describe its features. However, it is also important to stress that perceptual details remained incomplete. Nevertheless, there was the conviction that the face he had seen and the voice he had heard were those of someone he knew, but he could not identify the person. This observation exemplifies the fragmentary nature of many of the perceptual hallucinations occurring during temporal lobe seizures or stimulations. Yet in spite of this, these patients do have experiential qualities similar to those of normal life experiences, since they somehow relate to aspects of the patient's personal life: In this case the hallucinated face struck the patient as being familiar.

In other instances it is difficult to determine whether a hallucination the patient describes is truly a perceptual phenomenon rather than a vivid thought or a vivid memory. This was the case for a patient (N.L.) who at the beginning of her attacks always had the experience of seeing or thinking of two comic strip characters she had often looked at with her mother when she was a child. She was never able to tell us clearly whether she actually saw these figures or only had a very vivid thought of them. The hallucination came on when seizure discharges were confined to the limbic structures of the left temporal lobe (Fig. 2), and it was readily reproduced by left amygdaloid stimulation without eliciting an afterdischarge.

In some other instances the sensory aspect of a hallucination may not be present or is very crude, and yet the experience is very compelling to the patient who can identify a specific event in his personal life as its source. What is fascinating in these instances is that the patient is capable of identifying the specific content of the experience, even though he may admit (when prompted) that the perceptual details are partially or even totally lacking. An example of this is an observation made on a young patient with epilepsy (A.M.) in whom right amygdaloid stimulation, when first performed, evoked an immediate re-

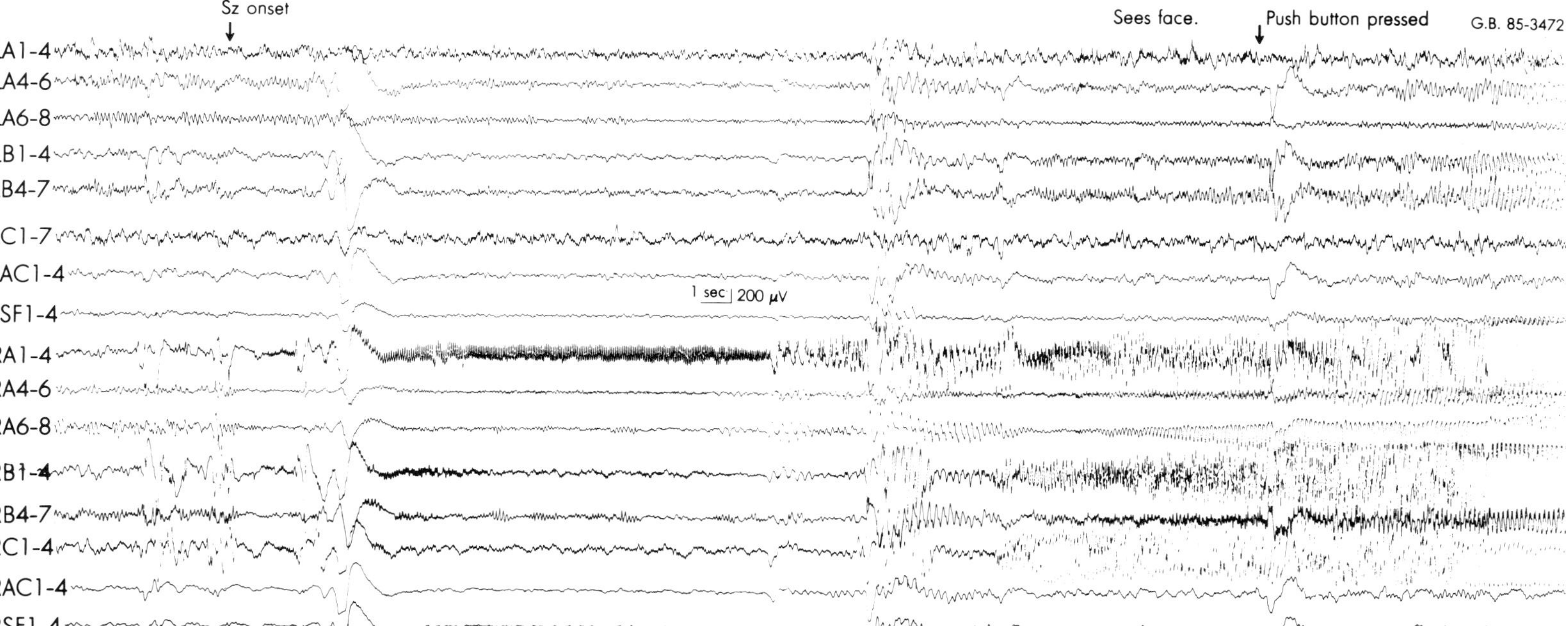

FIG. 1. Patient G.B. Visual hallucination during spontaneous right-sided temporal lobe seizure recorded with depth electrodes. LA and RA: Left and right anterior temporal depth electrode strands with 10 contacts spaced 5 mm apart. Contacts numbered 1 and 2 are in the amygdala (the others are in increasingly more superficial portions of the temporal lobe), recording from deep sulcal and superficial temporal isocortex. LB and RB: Left and right intermediate temporal depth electrode strands with contacts 1 and 2 in the anterior hippocampus; the others are the same as in LA and LB. LC and RC: Left and right posterior temporal depth electrode strands with contacts 1, 2, 3 in parahippocampal gyrus and hippocampus; the others are the same as in LA and LB. LAC1–4 and RAC1–4: Left and right mesial frontal electrodes with contacts 1 in left and right cingulate gyrus. LSF1–4 and RSF1–4: Left and right superior frontal electrodes with contact 1 in left and right supplementary motor cortex.

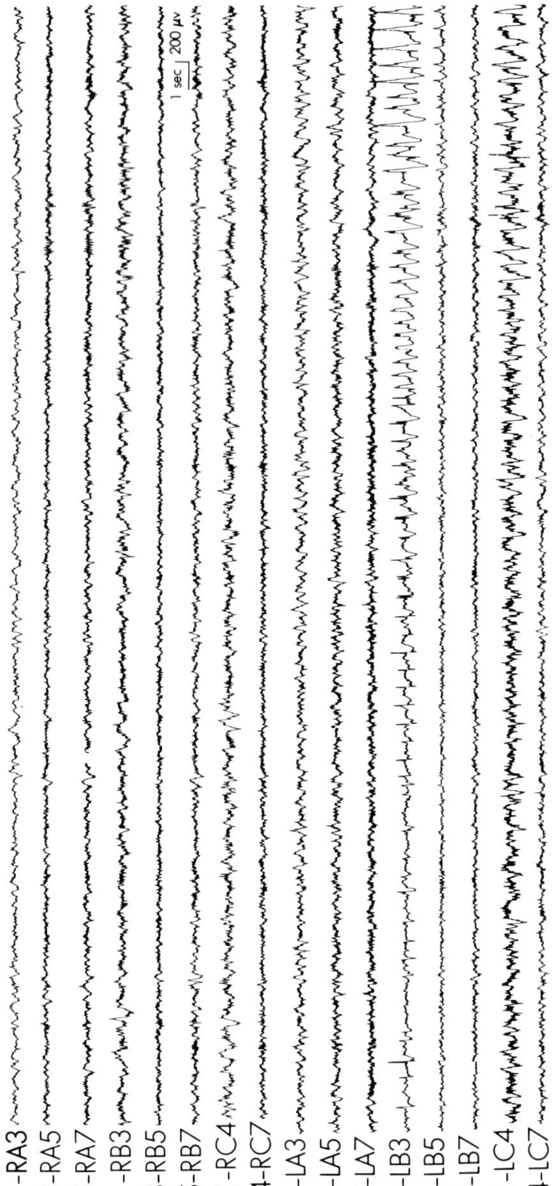

N.L. 77-1083-1
RA1-RA3
RA3-RA5
RA5-RA7
RB1-RB3
RB3-RB5
RB5-RB7
RC1-RC4
RC4-RC7
LA1-LA3
LA3-LA5
LA5-LA7
LB1-LB3
LB3-LB5
LB5-LB7
LC1-LC4
LC4-LC7
1 sec
200 µv

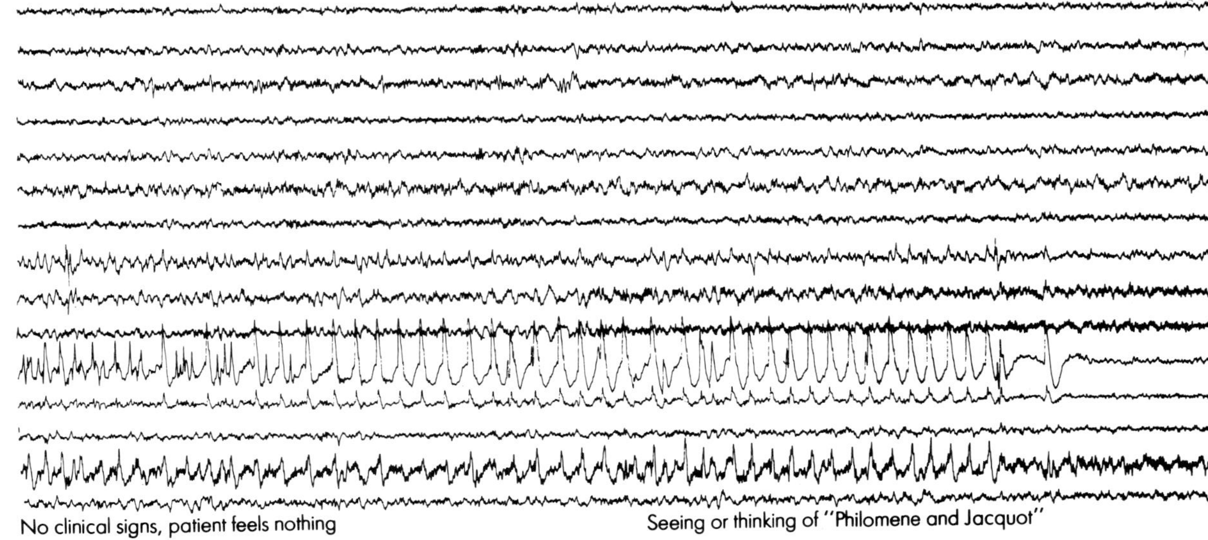

FIG. 2. Patient N.L. Spontaneous minor seizure during which the patient had the experience of seeing or thinking of two comic strip characters. Depth electrode recording. The seizure starts in the left hippocampus (LB1) and spreads to the left parahippocampal gyrus (LC1) and minimally to the left amygdala (LA1). Lower panel is direct continuation of upper one. Abbreviations are the same as in Fig. 1. (From ref. 7, with permission.)

sponse on his part, telling us that he suddenly had experienced something which he could not easily put into words. He likened it to a feeling of falling into water, a feeling as if something had covered his eyes, nose, and mouth. There was no electrical afterdischarge. When stimulation of the same area was repeated without the patient being warned, he exclaimed "Now!" and then asked that the stimulation be repeated, because he had on the tip of his tongue what the experience was all about; however, he could not really describe it when the short stimulation was over. There was again no afterdischarge. Stimulation without warning was repeated once more: As soon as the current was turned on, the patient immediately sat up, opened his mouth with an astonished look on his face, and said that now he knew what it was. The feeling was that of re-experiencing a frightening incident that had taken place when he was 8 years old during the summer holidays when he had gone to Brewer Park in Ottawa, where a boy stronger than he had pushed his head under water. When he described this experience to us, we were first under the impression that he had had a visual hallucination of the scene. However, when he was questioned more closely, this appeared uncertain: He did not really see the boy, but there was no doubt in his mind that it felt "as if he had been there" when the incident happened. There was again no afterdischarge.

It is obvious from this and other instances that what often constitutes the foremost (and to the patient the most compelling) feature of such experiences is this feeling of "being there"—that is, of being personally involved in the hallucinated (or remembered) event rather than remembering the perceptual details, which may remain very vague (7). The substrate for the evocation of these perceptual phenomena is the temporal lobe (2,3,5–10). Both isocortical and limbic stimulation can elicit them. In our experience this occurs, however, most consistently with limbic, particularly amygdaloid, stimulation (7,11).

MEMORY

Epileptic discharge can elicit three different kinds of mnemonic phenomena: (i) an illusion of memory, (ii) a memory flashback, and (iii) interference with memory recording or anterograde memory for the time of the seizure, later experienced as retrograde memory for the attack. Illusion of memory is exemplified by the illusion of familiarity—the "déjà vu" phenomenon. To qualify for being labeled "déjà vu," the experience must be a true illusion; that is, it must obviously clash with what the patient is momentarily experiencing in the real world (4,7). When strictly defined in these terms, the déjà vu phenomenon is the illusion that the present is like the past; that is, a locale which in fact may be totally unfamiliar to the patient (or meeting a person he has never previously met) may incongruously appear to him as if he had been to that particular place (or had seen that particular person) before. There is, however, no memory flashback. I submit that this illusion is in fact an illusion of memory. Encountering suddenly and unexpectedly a familiar locale or person has an affective impact upon us similar to that of sudden fear or of exhilarating astonishment. The main feature of this phenomenon is thus affective, or at least affective-like. Under conditions of everyday life, it is usually associated with an appropriate cognitive content of actually having encountered this situation before. In the case of the déjà vu illusion, the affective component of this experience occurs in isolation without being linked to a specific cognitive content, and the context in which the subject finds himself at the time becomes incongruously linked to the feeling. The patient is very much aware that the feeling is not really in tune with what he is experiencing at the moment, even though a part of his brain seems to tell him otherwise—that what he is experiencing is in fact something out of his personal past. It is important to stick to a strict definition of the déjù vu phenomenon. To extend the meaning of the term to the sense of familiarity that accompanies a memory flashback, where such a feeling is to be expected and therefore does not represent a true illusion, is inappropriate. This distinction is not always clearly made [e.g., by Wieser (5) and by Bancaud (6)]. Failure to make this distinction is of more than semantic interest, because it robs the true déjà vu phenomenon of its lateralizing significance. Indeed, Mullan and Penfield (4) have shown that in the overwhelming majority of instances the illusion of familiarity is elicited by right (or nondominant), but not by left (or dominant), temporal lobe stimulation. In my personal experience (*unpublished observations*) I have found that, with very few exceptions, a true déjà vu illusion was caused either by right temporal lobe seizure discharge or by right temporal lobe stimulation. If strictly defined, this symptom will provide relatively reliable lateralizing information.

The déjà vu illusion in some patients can be so strong that they have the impression that they can predict what is going to happen next. One of our patients (R.H.) suffered from such seizures, which were ushered in by an overwhelming illusion of déjà vu that led to such an illusion of prescience. One night in the course of one of his seizures recorded on telemetry, a nurse carrying a flashlight happened to enter the room just as the attack started. To the nurse's question regarding whether the seizure was like the preceding one, he replied: "Yes, and you are coming in right now, it is all part of it; I mean as soon as I pressed it [i.e., the seizure button], I almost did not, because I knew you were going to come in. It is as if I were reliving all that is happening now. I just knew that you were going to come in with the flashlight on. In a minute there will be more people as if it all happened before, just reliving all this. The more I know what is going to happen the farther it goes and the dizzier I feel . . . it makes me feel strange and weird." The seizure discharge had started in the right hippocampus 15 sec before he pressed the button; it spread to involve the right amygdala, hippocampus, and parahippocampal gyrus, with only modest spread to the temporal isocortex (Fig. 3).

The second type of mnemonic phenomena elicited by ictal discharge is the memory flashback—that is, the sudden emergence of a past event in the patient's mind. The feeling of recall can be so strong that the patient "relives" the experience, as in the example of patient A.M. given above. The vividness of the recall, as in that example, is often more related to the affective impact of the memory than to the detail of what the patient actually is able to visualize or recall. This phenomenon is elicited by temporal lobe discharge and can be reproduced by electrical stimulation of

limbic or isocortical structures, the former being probably more consistently implicated (2,3,5–10).

The third type of involvement of memory mechanisms in seizure discharge is interference with memory recording, leading to anterograde amnesia for the events that occurred during a seizure. This aspect will be discussed later under the rubrics of "loss of consciousness" and automatism.

AFFECT

The choice of the word "affect" instead of "emotion" is deliberate, because the latter term tends to connote a meaning that would restrict affective states to those of high intensity such as fear, anger, or elation. In many instances this is, however, not the case, especially when an affective coloring is associated with a flashback or a hallucination. Among experiential phenomena, affective responses, more often than hallucinations or mnemonic phenomena, occur in isolation or in association with autonomic and viscerosensory manifestations. When occurring in the course of epileptic seizures, they are almost exclusively restricted to those of temporal lobe origin and usually indicate that the ictal discharge involves limbic structures, particularly the amygdala (2–7,9–11).

The most common of these affective responses is fear (7,10), which may range from mild anxiety to outright terror. An example is an observation on patient P.H., who had a consistent aura of fear with her seizures. It often escalated into outright terror with the full enactment of terrified behavior for which she was partly amnestic. The seizure discharge started in the right temporal lobe and involved predominantly the right amygdala and hippocampus (Fig. 4). The feeling of fear was reproduced by amygdaloid stimulation without evoking an afterdischarge.

Much less common are other affective states such as guilt, embarrassment, sadness, anger, exhilaration, mirth, sexual excitement, or a feeling of blissful happiness. An example of a feeling of anxiety mixed with guilt was evoked in patient A.M. upon stimulation of the right hippocampus. He had no hesitation in saying that he had felt something, but at

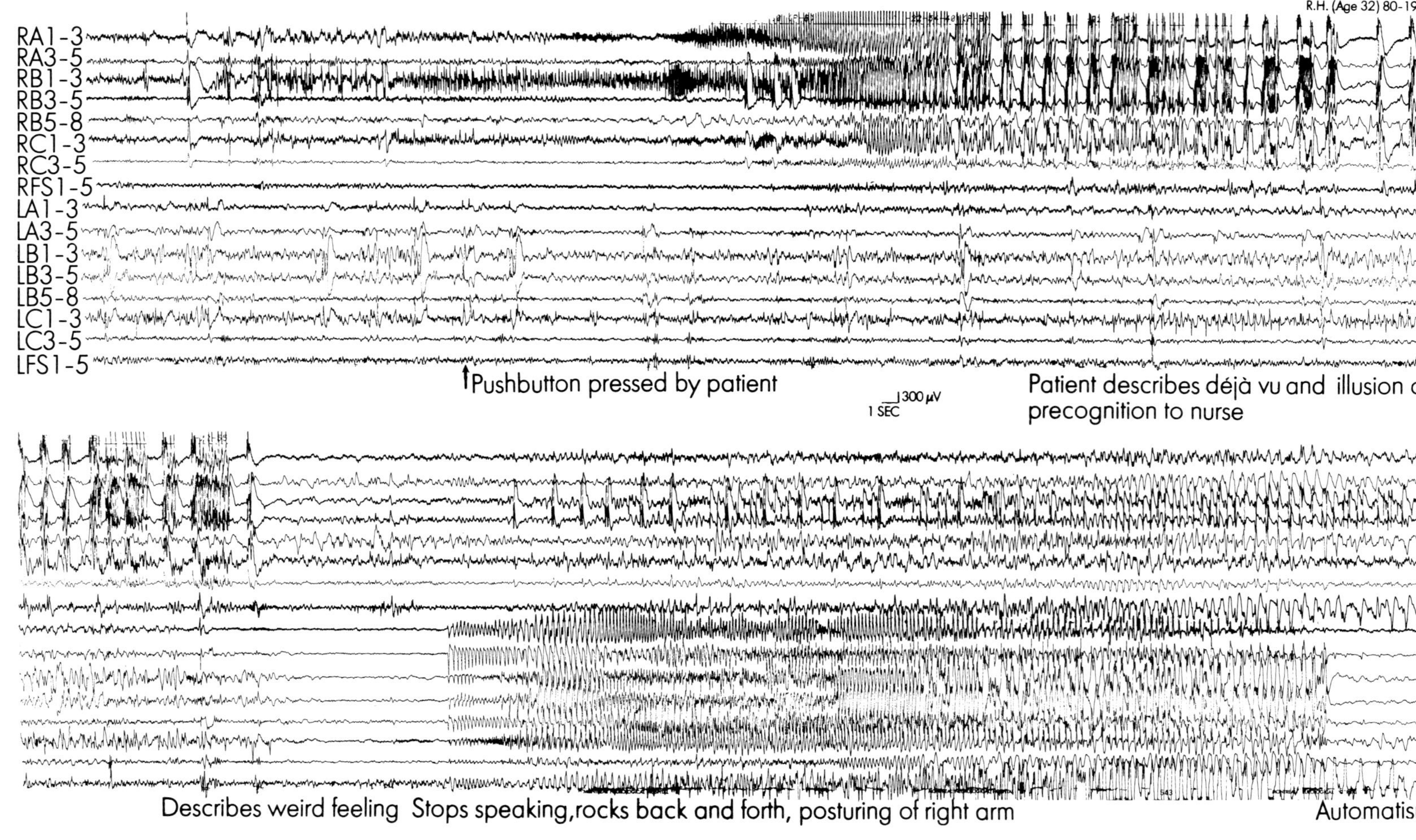
R.H. (Age 32) 80-1989
RA1-3
RA3-5
RB1-3
RB3-5
RB5-8
RC1-3
RC3-5
RFS1-5
LA1-3
LA3-5
LB1-3
LB3-5
LB5-8
LC1-3
LC3-5
LFS1-5
Pushbutton pressed by patient
300 μV
1 SEC
Patient describes déjà vu and illusion of
precognition to nurse
Describes weird feeling Stops speaking,rocks back and forth, posturing of right arm
Automatism

first he had some difficulty in putting the feeling into words. He then likened it to fear and anxiety: ". . . like you are demanding I hand in a report that was due two weeks ago . . . as if I were guilty of some form of tardiness." There was a brief afterdischarge in the stimulated area.

Aggression and Violence

When discussing ictal affective responses, a brief comment concerning ictal aggression or violence is in order. To my knowledge, no well-documented case of well-coordinated and well-directed ictal aggression during a spontaneous seizure has been reported. The often-cited example of violent and destructive behavior observed by Mark et al. (12) occurred in response to electrical stimulation of the amygdala, which induced electrical seizure activity. Whether the spontaneous violent outbursts the same patient displayed on other occasions were seizures remains undetermined. Rather aimless destructive behavior, angry verbal outbursts, or an angry mood has been reported to occur during the course of temporal lobe seizures in only a few patients (13–15). The notion that patients with epilepsy are prone to violence during seizures is probably based on the common observation that in the postictal confusional state a patient may react violently to attempts by well-intentioned witnesses of the attack to restrain him. In his state of confusion he probably misinterprets these attempts as aggressive acts, gets frightened, and reacts in a violent, defensive way (16,17). Such postictal violence is never well directed and usually immediately subsides when the patient is no longer restrained. An excellent review of the subject containing an extensive list of references has been written by Treiman (17). In this review the out-come of the deliberation of a panel of experts on ictal aggression is reported. Epileptologists from four countries, after having reviewed seizures recorded by video monitoring and electroencephalography (EEG), identified 19 patients out of a total of 5400 in whom possibly ictal aggression could be suspected. A group of highly experienced epileptologists reviewed the case histories as well as the video and EEG recordings of the 19 patients and retained 13 for whom a clinical diagnosis of epilepsy could be entertained. Only seven of these patients either displayed destructive behavior directed at objects, threatened other persons, or committed mild violent acts against persons. None committed moderately or severely violent attacks against persons. It is thus quite clear that angry behavior leading to significant violent and aggressive attacks against persons does not usually occur during epileptic seizures (see Chapter 23).

Laughter

A particular affective response occurring during certain seizures is laughter (18–22). It may or may not be associated with a subjectively experienced emotion of mirth. In many cases it is unremembered. It may occur as part of either temporal or frontal lobe seizures. In these cases it often faithfully mimics natural laughter (20,21), although not consistently so. However, pathological laughter may also occur in other conditions such as deep midline lesions without seizures (23,24) or in diffuse encephalopathies associated with epilepsy (19,25). A characteristic of the laughter in the latter two pathological conditions is that it sounds unnatural. Although it may impress observers as being a convincing mimicry of laughter, these patients do not experience mirth; in addition, relatives usually have

---

FIG. 3. Patient R.H. Spontaneous seizure with déjà vu illusion and illusion of prescience. Depth electrode recording. The seizure discharge starts in the right hippocampus (RB1) and spreads to the right parahippocampal gyrus (RC1) and right amygdala (RA1). Spread to the right temporal isocortex (RA3–5, RB3–5, and RC3–5) is modest. The patient describes his illusion to the nurse while right temporal discharge is in progress. The discharge later spreads to the left temporal lobe, at which time the patient stops speaking (lower panel). Abbreviations are the same as in Fig. 1. LFS and RFS: Left and right mesial superior frontal electrodes with contacts 1 in left and right supplementary motor area. (From ref. 7, with permission.)

P.H. (Age 19) 79-0224-1
RA 1-3
RA 3-4
RA 4-6
RB 1-3
RB 3-6
RFS 1-4
RFO 1-4
RFO 4-7
LA 1-3
LA 3-4
LA 4-6
LB 1-3
LB 3-6
LFS 1-4
LFO 1-4
LFO 4-7
Ch 12 | 200 µv
Ch 1-11 and 13-16   1 SEC | 100 µv
Pt. says she feels fear. →

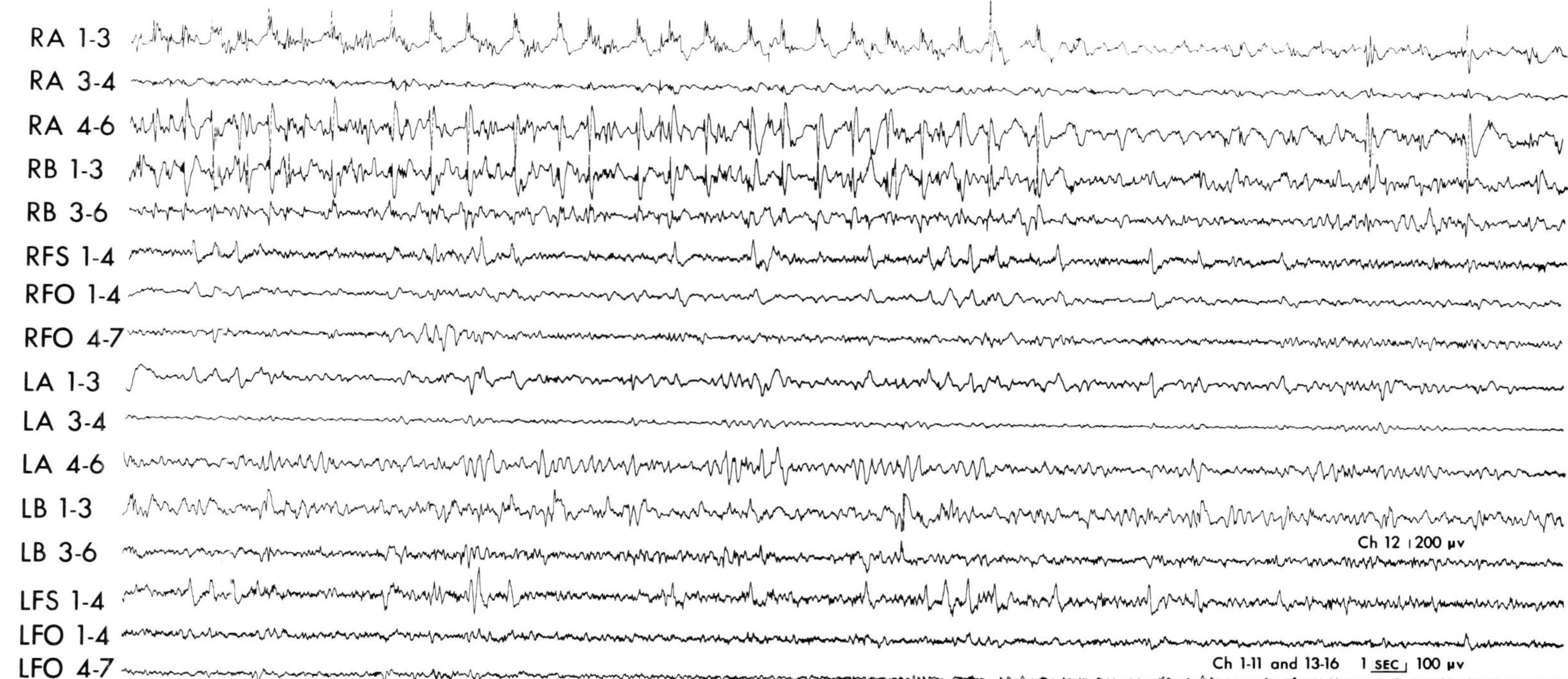

FIG. 4. Patient P.H. Minor seizure with experience of fear. Depth electrode recording. The seizure starts with desynchronization in the right temporal lobe (**upper panel**), followed by build-up of rhythmic seizure activity which predominates in the anterior portion of the temporal lobe, particularly in the amygdala (RA1) and hippocampus (RB1) and anterior temporal isocortex (RA4–6) (**lower panel**). Abbreviations are the same as in Figs. 1 and 3. LFO and RFO: Left and right orbitofrontal cortex with contacts 1 located most medially.

A.T. 83-0762
Stim. RA1-RA2 350 µa
LA1-2
LA2-3
LA3-4
LA4-5
LA5-6
LA6-7
LA7-8
LA8-9
RA1-2
RA2-3
RA3-4
RA4-5
RA5-6
RA6-7
RA7-8
RA8-9

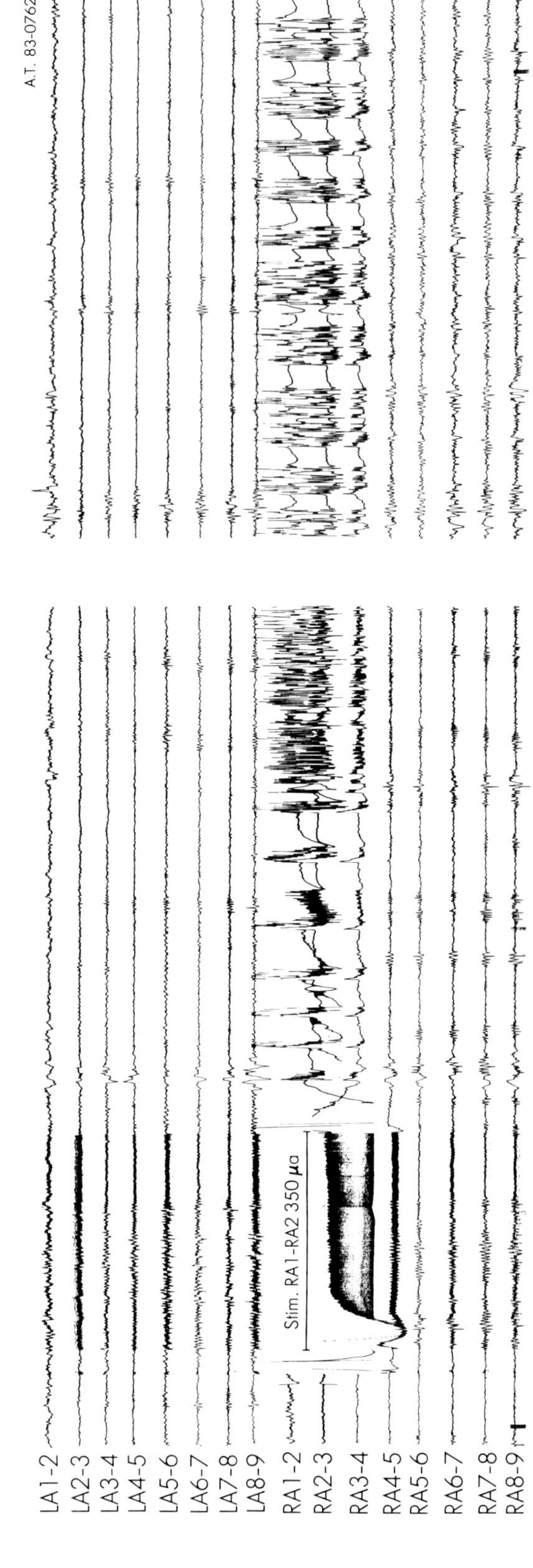

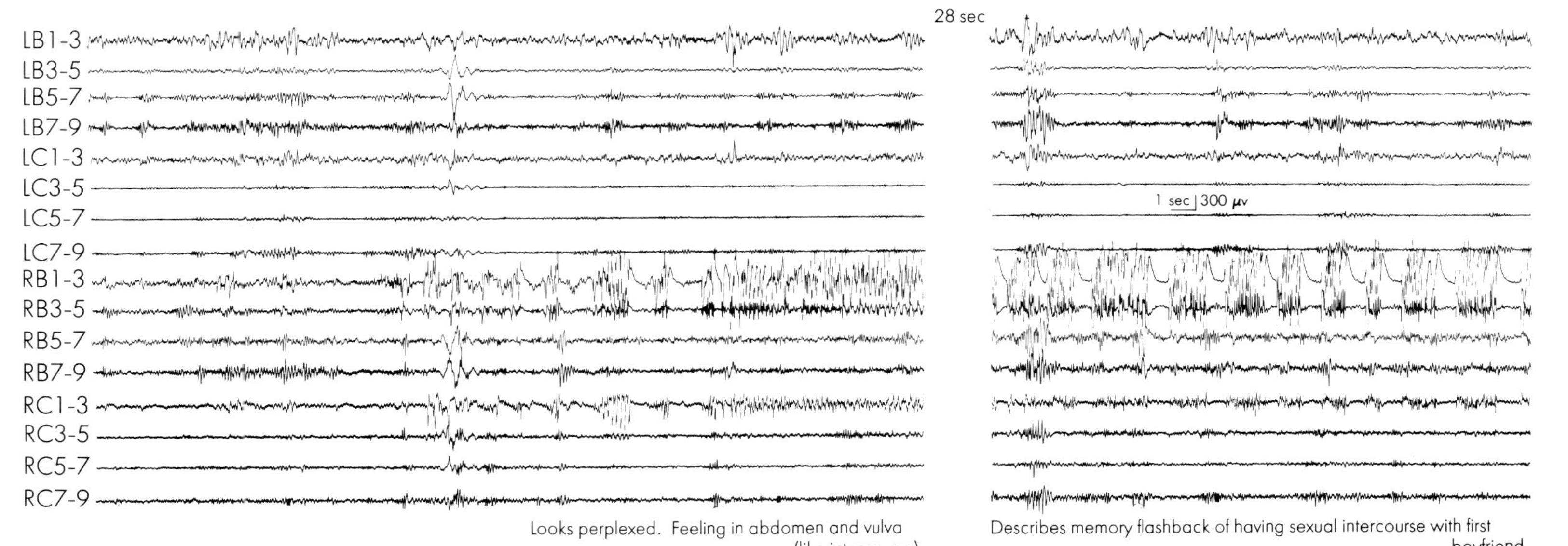

FIG. 5. Patient A.T. Sexual experiential response elicited by right amygdaloid stimulation. Depth electrode recording. The afterdischarge was confined to the right amygdaloid and hippocampal region. Recordings in upper and lower panel are simultaneous (32 channel recording). Abbreviations are the same as in Fig. 1.

no hesitation in stating that the ictal laughter sounds different from the patient's habitual one occurring under appropriate conditions. In a personal observation of a patient with a diffuse encephalopathy associated with a hypothalamic hamartoma, the laughter impressed me as being probably caused by a rapid diaphragmatic clonus, with air being expelled through a nearly closed glottis. It sounded extremely unnatural, yet laughter was the first word that came to one's mind when hearing it. This individual was one of a recently studied group of patients (22) presenting with a curious syndrome (found in some infants and children) characterized by laughing fits and a hypothalamic hamartoma. The EEG of these children usually shows a pattern which is characteristic of a diffuse epileptogenic encephalopathy of the slow spike-and-wave type, which is, in turn, characteristic of secondary generalized epilepsy. This, together with the common presence of mental retardation and severe behavior disorders, suggests that the hypothalamic hamartoma alone, although a characteristic structural feature of the syndrome, cannot fully account for its symptomatology, including the epileptic seizures associated with laughter, and that the underlying pathology, although presently unknown, must be diffuse. The syndrome has been described by several other investigators, many of whom also commented on the high incidence of precocious puberty in these children (for an extensive list of references, see ref. 22). The relation between the laughter and the ictal discharge remains unclear. Is it a positive expression of ictal discharge, or is it a release phenomenon? We do not know.

Sexual Behavior

Ictal sexual manifestations are rare (2, 26,27). Cases of exhibitionism or masturbation either during an ictus or postictally are highly uncommon. Jacome and Risko (28) describe a case of petit mal status with compulsive masturbation in a 41-year-old man. Masturbation or seemingly masturbatory manipulation of the genitalia is, however, rare in this condition as well as in ictal or postictal automatism, a fact that is particularly surprising since much of the automatic movements performed by patients ictally or postictally are directed at their own body or clothing such as rubbing one's nose, scratching, picking on one's clothes or skin, etc. Manipulation of sexual organs may occur in some frontal lobe attacks (29,30), but in my personal opinion there is little evidence that this is truly sexual or masturbatory. It more likely represents a variety of self-manipulation which in most automatisms is directed more commonly at the face or head or at some piece of clothing rather than at the genital region.

Psychosexual phenomena such as a feeling of libido, subjective experience of an erotic sensation in the sex organs (even orgasm), or a memory flashback to an instance of sexual intercourse do occur in some temporal lobe seizures and probably indicate that seizure discharge involves the amygdala (27,31; for more references see ref. 27). Such ictal psychosexual manifestations are virtually confined to women, for reasons that we do not understand (27). I could find only one convincing case of a male in the literature in whom libidinous sexual feelings (as distinguished from mere genital somatosensory or autonomic manifestations) occurred during epileptic seizures (32). Female patients with libidinous psychosexual manifestations only rarely give overt behavioral expression to these feelings. More commonly, they conceal them even from their own physicians, because they are highly embarrassed by them.

One of our patients (A.T.) explored with depth electrodes had seizures of temporal lobe origin which started with a libidinous feeling, a fact she had concealed from her physicians out of embarrassment. It was only when the experience was reproduced by right amygdaloid stimulation during depth electrode exploration that she admitted that it was her habitual aura. She described the experience as a pleasant feeling in her vulva and the inner surface of her thighs, as if she were having sexual intercourse with "X," the boyfriend with whom she had had intercourse for the first time in her life at age 16. There was no visual hallucination and she did not see her partner, and yet she was positive that the experience was that of having intercourse with her old boyfriend. She said that the experience was the evocation of an old memory. There was afterdischarge in the mesial temporal structures on the stimulated side (Fig. 5).

Hunger and Thirst

Among behavioral mechanisms related to affect, one must mention hunger and thirst. Although some patients may have seizures precipitated by eating, I have never, so far, encountered one who reported a feeling of hunger as an aura, nor have I seen a patient who ate or asked for food in the course of a seizure. Gastaut (33), however, described a few observations of ictal hunger occurring as the initial symptom in complex partial seizures, but he stressed that this is only rarely encountered.

The situation is different for drinking. Drinking water is relatively common as an early ictal manifestation of temporal lobe seizures (34), yet patients usually do not report a feeling of thirst; some rationalize their drinking as an attempt to ward off a seizure (33,34). Although this may be a correct explanation in some instances, we have seen examples where drinking seemed to be an integral part of ictal behavior. I first became aware of "ictal drinking" when I encountered a particularly clear example of this in patient A.B., who had frequent, very localized seizure discharges involving the left amygdala and hippocampus while being explored with depth electrodes (16,34). With each of these localized discharges, but only when they involved the amygdala, he would pour himself a glass of water and drink it; when his pitcher was empty he asked for more water (Fig. 6). He did this more than 20 times in a prolonged daytime recording session and did not drink between discharges. He never said he was thirsty, however, and could not give a convincing reason for his frequent drinking. In all cases of drinking associated with seizures, the evidence pointed to a temporal lobe focus; in two patients explored with depth electrodes, the seizure discharge involved the limbic structures of one temporal lobe (34).

EXPERIENTIAL PHENOMENA

Many of the just-discussed perceptual, mnemonic, and affective phenonena occurring during seizures are described by patients in a way suggesting that their subjective quality of immediacy resembles that of everyday-life personal experiences (2,4,7,8,35,36). This stands in contrast to responses elicited by seizure discharge or electrical stimulation of the sensory areas or of the motor cortex. In the latter instances, a patient never reports that what he feels is something embedded in his personal life experience or that it reminds him of some experience in his past. As Penfield (37) put it, "These responses are on a plane quite distinct from his [the patient's] conscious thinking." They are thus somehow unrelated to his personal identity, in contrast to experiential phenomena. These are relatively common (but not universal) manifestations of temporal lobe seizures (3,7,8,11). They always occur at the onset or in the very early stages of the seizure and are therefore usually short-lived. They usually do not outlast the end of an attack—with the rare exception of a strong emotion such as fear, which may occasionally linger on postictally. This is in sharp contrast to another common behavioral manifestation of temporal lobe epilepsy—namely, automatism associated with amnesia, which is sometimes present right from the start of a temporal lobe attack but which more commonly develops only at some point along its course and often continues well into the postictal period without a perceptible break (2,7). Usually only a concomitant EEG recording can tell at which point ictal merges into postictal automatism. Automatism may even be purely postictal, a fact that can unequivocally be demonstrated only by a concurrent EEG recording. We may therefore assume that automatism and amnesia represent evidence for ictal and postictal "paralysis" of normal physiological mechanisms of the temporal lobe. We may also tentatively conclude that, by contrast, experiential phenomena may in fact reflect true positive consequences of ictal discharge. That is, they may result from an activation and not from an abolition of normal physiological processes taking place in the temporal lobe (7); otherwise, like automatism and amnesia, they would also continue into, or could also arise in, the postictal state. The view that experiential phenomena are positive consequences of ictal discharge affecting brain areas implicated in the elaboration of similar experiences occurring under normal conditions is not shared by everyone. Halgren et al. (3) proposed that experiential phenomena represent release phenomena in response to ictal paralysis of tem-

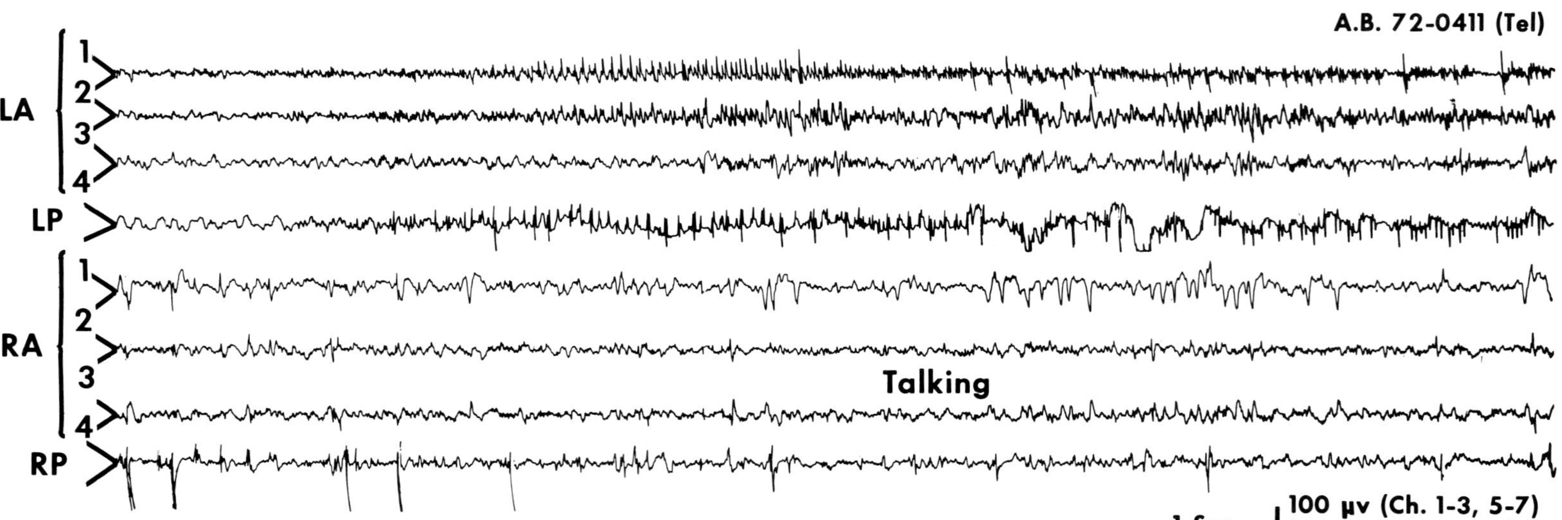

A.B. 72-0411 (Tel)
LA
1
2
3
4
LP
RA
1
2
3
4
RP
Talking
1 Sec.
100 µv (Ch. 1-3, 5-7)
200 µv (Ch. 4 & 8)

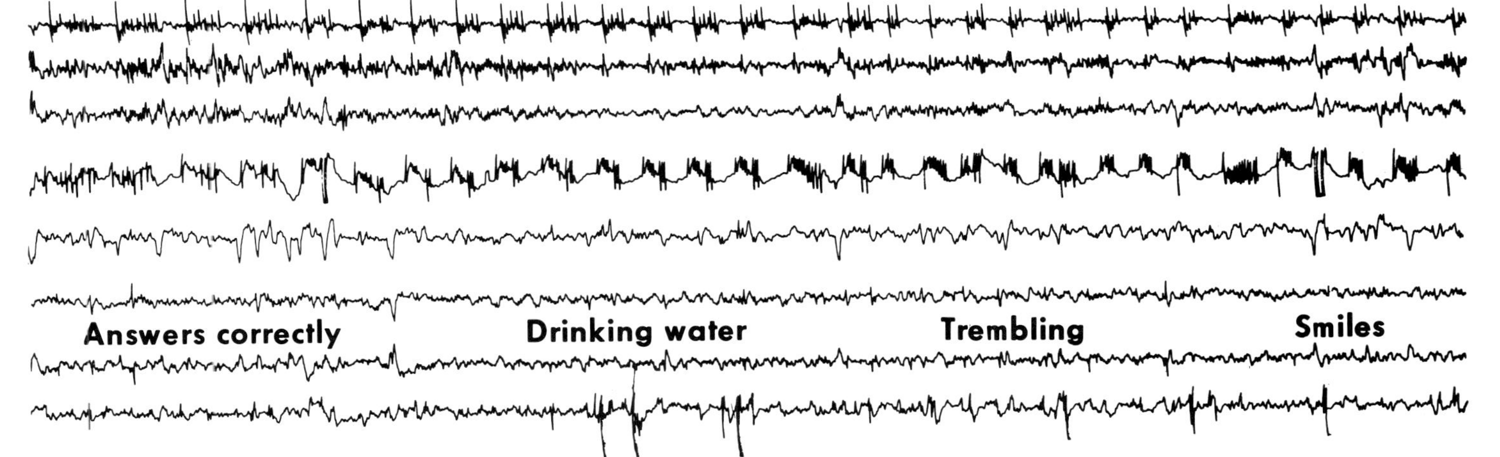

FIG. 6. Patient A.B. Localized seizure discharge in left amygdala and hippocampus eliciting water-drinking. Depth electrode recording. LA and RA: left and right anterior temporal depth electrode strands with deepest contacts (1) in amygdala and contacts 2–4 located increasingly more superficially, 1 cm apart, recording from deep and superficial temporal structures. LP and RP: Recording from contacts 1 and 2 of a more posterior temporal depth electrode strand with contacts 1 and 2 in the left and the right hippocampus. Lower panel is direct continuation of upper one. (From ref. 16, with permission.)

poral lobe mechanisms. Our contrary view that experiential phenomena are positive consequences of temporal lobe ictal discharge (7) is supported by the fact that there is now solid evidence that temporal isocortex, in concert with the limbic structures (i.e., the amygdala and the hippocampus) to which it is mutually and reciprocally interconnected, mediates behavioral mechanisms that link perception, particularly in the visual and auditory modalities with memory and affect (38–51). These circuits are also involved in the reactivation of past memories, in terms of both their purely cognitive and affective dimensions and the recording, consolidation, and recall of memory items (36,51–55). It thus appears likely that perceptual, mnemonic, and affective phenomena concomitant with discharge involving these circuits must be a reflection of an activation of these temporalimbic mechanisms in a manner which, to some extent, must be similar to that which occurs under normal conditions. It would indeed be paradoxical if ictal inactivation of these temporolimbic structures would bring out phenomena known to be dependent upon the normal functioning of these areas.

It may nevertheless on a priori grounds appear improbable that a crude form of neuronal activity of the kind occurring during ictal discharge or artificial electrical stimulation could mimic the normal neuronal activity that underlies such highly differentiated behavioral responses. It is indeed highly unlikely that these responses would occur if all or the majority of neurons normally involved in these complex functions were subject to such crude discharge. The initial and short-lived character of experiential responses, along with their replacement by automatism and amnesia (which so often follow them and which presumably signal a paralysis of the very system involved in evoking them), is in line with the interpretation that these responses represent positive effects of ictal discharge. It is likely that, under normal everyday living conditions, evocation of an experience depends on the formation of a specifically patterned matrix of excitation (and, most likely, of inhibition as well) within widely distributed neuronal populations in large areas of isocortex and of the limbic system. It is now well known that the hippocampal formation and amygdala not only receive, but also emit, projections to vast areas of temporal, frontal, parietal, and occipital isocortex (48,49) which include all the main sensory association areas. These widespread regions could be the substrate within which the postulated widespread matrix of neuronal excitation representing an experience is constructed. In a seizure, but usually only at its onset, localized discharge in a circumscribed part of this widespread system may temporarily be capable of "reproducing" the configuration of such a specific matrix of distributed excitation linked to a specific subjective experience. Perhaps the specific synaptic connectivities in the neuronal structures that form the substrate of these phenomena have been facilitated by repeated ictal activation through a mechanism related to kindling which may thus have served to consolidate them within this cerebral neuronal network (56). This concept of a widely distributed neuronal substrate of experiential phenomena makes it easier to understand why such responses can be elicited by stimulation of isocortical association areas of the temporal lobe

TABLE 1. *Perceptual hallucinations and illusions elicited by electrical stimulation: visual 23, auditory, olfactory 2[a]*

	No afterdischarge, or afterdischarge confined to stimulated structure	Afterdischarge		
Stimulated structure		Limbic spread only	Limbic + neocortical spread	Neocortical spread only
Amygdala	14	2	4	—
Hippocampus	1	—	4	—
Parahippocampal gyrus	—	—	3	—
Neocortex	—	—	—	—

[a]Tables 1 to 3 incorporate the findings reported in refs. 7 and 10.

TABLE 2. *Illusions of memory elicited by electrical stimulation: déjà vu 18, memory recall 16*

Stimulated structure	No afterdischarge, or afterdischarge confined to stimulated structure	Afterdischarge		
		Limbic spread only	Limbic + neocortical spread	Neocortical spread only
Amygdala	14	—	6	—
Hippocampus	2	—	11	—
Parahippocampal gyrus	—	—	—	—
Neocortex	1[a]	—	—	—

[a]Deep temporal stimulation near limbic structures.

(2,4,8), as well as by stimulation of limbic structures (3,7,10). Among the latter, we found the amygdala to be the hottest spot for the reproduction of the whole gamut of experiential phenomena, be they perceptual, mnemonic, or affective (Tables 1–3) (7,10). The distributed matrix of neuronal activation which "represents" the experience may be more crucially related to the specific pattern of its synaptic connectedness on a highly differentiated microanatomical and microphysiological scale than to the precise temporal pattern of neuronal discharge within this system. Specific neurochemical changes at specific synaptic and other neuronal sites within it may also play a role. In light of recent concepts of brain function which invoke parallel distributed processing of perceptual attributes and distributed memories (57–62), the kind of model proposed here appears more acceptable than the view that a specific experience must depend upon precisely timed electrical signals emitted by single neurons in the form of action potentials involving a discretely localized area of brain.

"LOSS" OR "IMPAIRMENT OF CONSCIOUSNESS"

According to the International Classification of Seizures (63), loss or impairment of consciousness is the cardinal sign by which complex partial seizures are to be distinguished from simple partial seizures. One difficulty with assigning so much weight to loss or impairment of consciousness as a criterion of classification is that consciousness cannot be defined in objective terms, and therefore its loss or impairment also escapes strict definition (64,65). Furthermore, from a heuristic point of view, using the concept of "consciousness" as a feature in studies in which one attempts to understand what is going on in the brain during the course of a seizure leads nowhere (65). These difficulties are inherent not only in the study of the mechanism of complex partial seizures, but also in that of absence attacks. It is more fruitful to dispense with the term "loss" or "impairment of consciousness" and to attempt to define in objective behavioral terms the deficit from which

TABLE 3. *Emotions elicited by electrical stimulation: fear 42, anger 1, emotional distress 2*

Stimulated structure	No afterdischarge, or afterdischarge confined to stimulated structure	Afterdischarge		
		Limbic spread only	Limbic + neocortical spread	Neocortical spread only
Amygdala	17	3	3	—
Hippocampus	9	5	1	—
Parahippocampal gyrus	1	1	3	—
Neocortex	2[a]	—	—	—

[a]Probably limbic responses: Stimulation was deep, applied near limbic structures from which identical, but stronger, emotional response (fear) was evoked on stimulation.

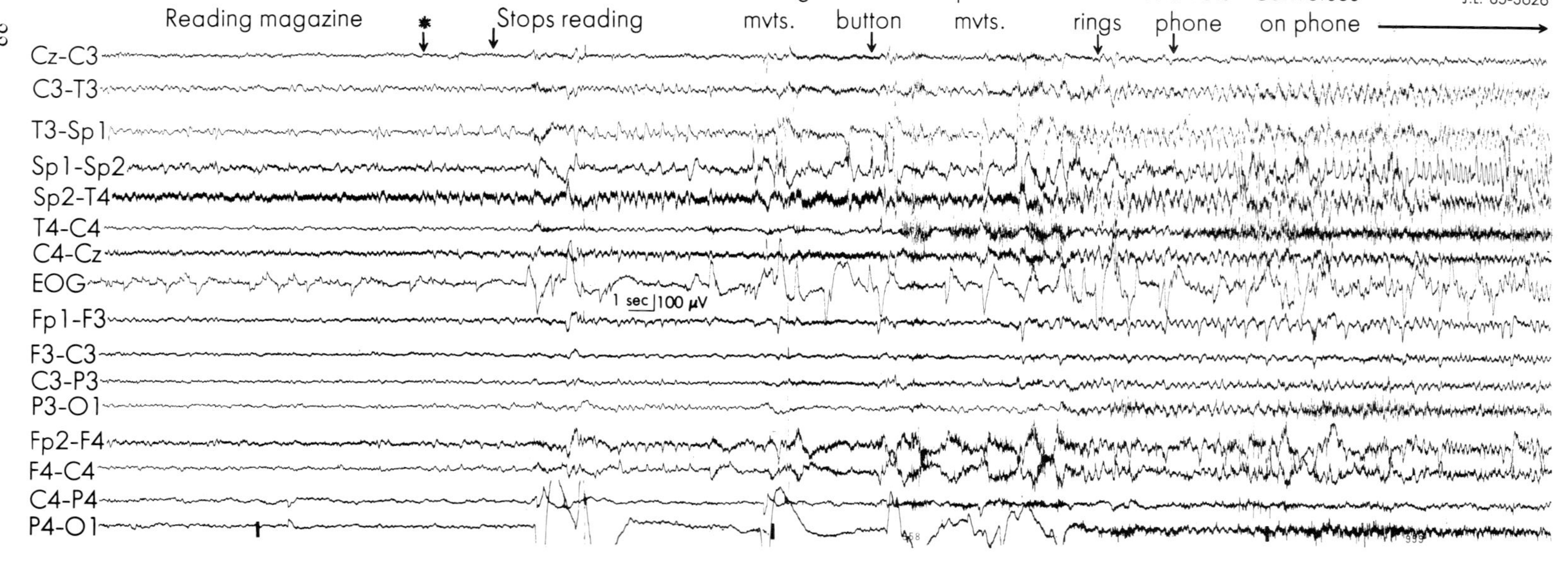

J.L. 85-3626
Reading magazine
Stops reading
Rubbing mvts.
Push button
Purposeless mvts.
Phone rings
Answers phone
Converses on phone
Cz-C3
C3-T3
T3-Sp1
Sp1-Sp2
Sp2-T4
T4-C4
C4-Cz
EOG
Fp1-F3
F3-C3
C3-P3
P3-O1
Fp2-F4
F4-C4
C4-P4
P4-O1
1 sec 100 µV

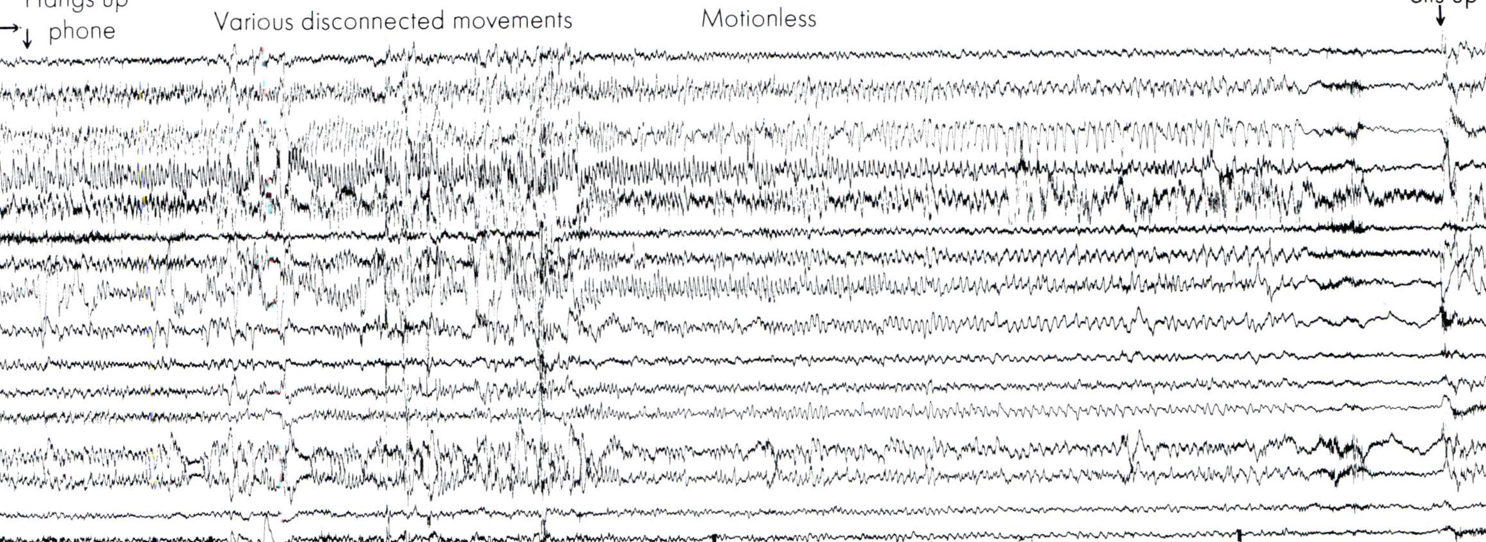

FIG. 7. Patient L.J. Temporal lobe seizure with automatism and amnesia during which the patient's ability to carry on a normal telephone conversation was preserved. Surface EEG recording with scalp and sphenoidal electrodes. Discharge starts in the left temporal region and later spreads to the left parasagittal region and ultimately also to the right hemisphere. Electrode positions labeled according to the 10–20 system. Sp, sphenoidal electrodes; EOG, electro-oculogram; asterisk denotes seizure onset in EEG. Lower panel is direct continuation of upper one.

the patient suffers and which causes him to behave in a manner that suggests to an observer or to himself that he has lost consciousness. It must be admitted that in many instances it is impossible to define exactly which function is impaired during an episode in which consciousness seems to have been lost, but this difficulty should encourage us to try harder to obtain more definitive answers whenever we can. The best method to achieve this end is to not only observe the behavior of a patient during a seizure, but to interact with him in order to test his speech function, his memory, his perceptual and praxic skills, etc. (65). Obviously, this is not possible during a generalized convulsion, where one is forced to fall back on the unhelpful term of loss of consciousness, but even here it may be better to say that the patient was unresponsive and subsequently amnestic of the event rather than to speak of loss of consciousness.

Most often when an observer of a seizure uses the term "loss of consciousness," he in fact observed a state of unresponsiveness. The latter term is much more useful than the former, because it relies on an objective observation and makes no further a priori inferences that cannot be proved to be true. Unresponsiveness is nevertheless not a deficit with a single underlying cause. It may be due to aphasia, as in some temporal or frontal lobe seizures involving speech cortex (65), or it may reflect an inability to perform voluntary movements, as is often the case in absence seizures (65–70), or it may be due to the patient's profound inattentiveness to his surroundings (65,69). There may be other as yet poorly understood causes. It must be admitted that in many cases the precise cause of unresponsiveness cannot be elucidated, even when the patient is tested.

Inattention to interlocutors or to other stimuli in the environment may occur during highly absorbing experiential hallucinations, but it is very rare that one can clearly document this (65). In this case it is, of course, evidence for temporal lobe epileptic discharge. A more global and less specific attentional deficit implicating a number of brain areas—including isocortical association areas, hippocampus, corpus striatum, midline thalamus, and the brainstem reticular formation—may

be the cause of unresponsiveness and other behavioral deficits in absence attacks (69).

An example of unresponsiveness which could have easily been mistaken for loss of consciousness is that of patient F.O., who, in the early part of a spontaneous seizure with widespread left temporal and frontal involvement (as recorded with depth electrodes), was shown a pencil but failed to name it or to respond in any other way. The next day, without any leading questions being asked, the patient accurately remembered most of the circumstances prevailing during the early part of the seizure, particularly that she had been shown a pencil. She said that at that time she had not known what it was, but she now remembered that it had been a pencil. Memory was thus retained, and her failure to respond during the seizure was most likely due to aphasia.

Another deficit which masquerades as loss of consciousness is anterograde amnesia setting in during a seizure and reflecting the patient's inability to record ongoing events in memory. This is most often the hallmark of those seizures in which the patient himself claims to have lost consciousness. That in such cases both responsiveness and cognitive functions may be retained in spite of ongoing ictal discharge can be exemplified by many observations. Such responsiveness can be far from being merely elementary and reflexive and may involve complex behavioral mechanisms which one usually assumes can only be carried out by a conscious individual. A particularly striking example is that of a left-handed patient (L.J.), said to have suffered from temporal lobe seizures with automatism. A spontaneous seizure was recorded on telemetry. It started in the left temporal region and later spread to involve the left parasagittal region and the right hemisphere (Fig. 7). Shortly after seizure onset, she made fumbling movements with her right hand, pushed the seizure button, and continued making fumbling movements, now with both hands. Then the telephone by her bedside rang. She sat up, took the receiver with her left hand and put it to her ear. She then had the following telephone conversation: "Hello" . . . "How are you?" . . . "I only want to know whether you have arrived. Ah, O.K." . . . "Nothing, I shall lie down, and then go to sleep." . . . "Yes, no, no, it's all right, bye-bye." She then hung up. During the early part of the conversation, which lasted for only 17 sec, she continued with her seemingly automatic fumbling movements. After the telephone call, she performed a series of well-coordinated, but somewhat disconnected, movements such as picking up the magazine she had been reading, putting it down again, pressing the push button once more, switching on a light, and covering herself with the bed sheets. She then remained motionless until the seizure discharge came to an end, whereupon she immediately sat up and took the bedpan. The next morning the patient had no recollection of the phone call, and she had no idea with whom she had talked. When shown the video, she was very surprised that she could not remember anything about this phone call. We then contacted her cousin who had called. He had not noticed that anything had been amiss with her. Their conversation had struck him as being entirely normal. This is an example of a temporal lobe seizure with automatism during which the only true deficit was the patient's inability to record in memory an event and her appropriate behavioral response to it, which, under normal circumstances, she would certainly have remembered the next day.

Anterograde amnesia for events taking place during the seizure is most likely caused by bilateral ictal inactivation of the hippocampal formation. Perhaps unilateral hippocampal discharge in an individual in whom the contralateral hippocampus is nonfunctional may also result in anterograde amnesia. It is conceivable that bilateral frontal lobe discharge could also be responsible for an amnestic seizure. Amnesia can also occur in petit mal attacks (71). It is of interest that anterograde amnesia during a seizure can occur while retrograde mnemonic functions remain preserved during the attack, perhaps determining the patient's behavior during the seizure (65).

CONFUSIONAL STATES AND AUTOMATISM

Seizure discharges may be accompanied by behavioral states in which the patient interacts inappropriately with his environment. The most common forms of ictal states expressing themselves in this manner are (a) temporal or frontal lobe automatism (2,5,6,72) and (b) nonconvulsive status. The latter may present either in the form of petit mal status, or complex partial status of temporal or frontal lobe origin (72–83).

Both temporal lobe and frontal lobe automatisms probably reflect interference with the higher functions of these lobes, which prevent the patient from utilizing neuronal mechanisms that are normally involved in elaborating appropriate responses to environmental stimuli. A distinction between temporal and frontal lobe automatism is not easy on clinical grounds alone; however, temporal lobe automatism is usually associated with chewing, lip smacking, and swallowing, whereas gestural and ambulatory automatisms tend to appear late in the seizure or not at all. In frontal lobe automatism, gesturing and deambulation tend to occur early and automatic behavior may be bizarre (5,6,30). These differences are, however, not absolute. Seemingly positive effects of seizure discharge seen in automatism, such as fumbling, face rubbing, picking at one's body or clothes, and purposelessly manipulating objects (and perhaps also chewing and swallowing movements), are probably release phenomena which are normally kept under control by structures in the temporal and/or frontal lobes. Other forms of automatism are more elaborate. They may consist of the performance of overlearned motor behaviors such as undressing, going to bed, uttering expletives, and others which may lead to socially highly embarrassing situations. They are also best interpreted as the consequence of a release phenomenon caused by functional paralysis of mechanisms that normally prevent these behaviors in situations in which they are inappropriate. However, even behaviors that have only recently been learned may be carried out in the course of what is commonly called automatism. Thus the patient F.O., who remembered being shown a pencil she could not name during a seizure (see above), later in the course of the same seizure became amnestic. She could not recall that she had frantically tried to push the seizure button mounted on the side of her armchair, in spite of the fact that she was only capable of using her hand in a clumsy way, with the seizure discharge apparently having led to some motor incoordination. At the time of the seizure covered by anterograde amnesia, she was nevertheless, as her behavior showed, capable of remembering that she had been instructed to press the seizure button when she had an attack. She was evidently determined to follow this instruction in spite of being partially impaired by an ictally determined motor deficit. The seizure discharge in this case involved widespread regions of the left temporal and frontal lobes.

This and many other observations show that during automatism the patient may react in a partially appropriate way (and, at times, even fully appropriately) to stimuli emanating from his environment at the time of the seizure. Thus, his perceptual faculties and motor skills are often intact, at least at a relatively elementary level. This is shown by the observation that how a patient reacts to what he perceives during the automatism may be appropriate in the sense that, for instance, he knows how to avoid danger and how to properly manipulate objects within his reach; yet, in a larger context his behavior may be totally inappropriate, since he cannot utilize the fund of memories and critical knowledge that normally allows us to respond to situations in terms of longer-range goals (i.e., beyond the confines of the momentary situation) and of social appropriateness. Patients are commonly amnestic for behaviors occurring during automatisms no matter how complex they may be and how much they depend upon some fund of memory that must have been available to them at the time of the attack. This is evidence suggesting that memory consolidation is paralyzed even though no retrograde amnesia may be present at the same time (65). The most likely cause is that seizure discharge has interfered with normal hippocampal function. Many of these automatic behaviors extend into the postictal period, an observation which is in accord with the notion that they are to be considered as resulting from a paralysis of function, most likely of the hippocampal system. As the automatic state fades, the patient usually goes through a period of confusion in which he is slow in re-

sponding and disoriented with regard to space and time.

The nature of the confusional state deserves some brief comment. It obviously reflects the fact that the seizure discharge or its postictal aftermath has interfered with the function of structures that normally sustain higher-level cognitive activities. It is likely that there is some interference with perception but not at an elementary level, since patients usually seem to recognize the main perceptual attributes of their surroundings. However, they are not able to relate them to more elaborate cognitive constructs, which require full access to the fund of memories a person utilizes under normal circumstances when scrutinizing the incoming flow of perceptions to which one is continually exposed in daily living. Neuronal dysfunctions are probably widespread and likely involve extensively isocortical association areas and their limbic interconnections, but nothing precise is known about this.

Similar, but more enduring, states of confusion and behavioral slowness can be seen in the three varieties of nonconvulsive status: petit mal status, complex partial status of temporal lobe origin, and complex partial status of frontal lobe origin. Their symptomatologies show many similarities. On clinical grounds, a distinction between the three forms and also their differentiation from other nonepileptic confusional states is difficult to make without a concomitant EEG recording (83).

In petit mal status as in the much shorter absence attacks, a diffuse interference with cortical function takes place. During spike-and-wave discharge, cortical and thalamic neurons are synchronously subject to a regular oscillation between (a) brief periods of excitation corresponding to the spike and (b) much longer periods of inhibition corresponding to the slow-wave components of the spike-and-wave complex (84–86). This neuronal firing pattern is highly abnormal and must severely interefere with normal thalamocortical function. Since it involves all areas of cortex, it is not surprising that higher neuronal functions are severely compromised. In fact, one should instead be surprised at how much patients subject to generalized spike-and-wave discharge are still capable of doing. It is likely that the fundamental deficits seen in petit mal status and in a brief absence seizure are very similar, but because the latter lasts typically only for a few seconds, it is difficult to carry out all the behavioral tests that can be applied to a patient in long-lasting petit mal status. The deficit, although not uniformly the same in all patients, is more akin to dementia (87) than to "loss" or "impairment of consciousness" (85,88). There is often interference with motor performance (slowness in the case of petit mal status), which may be related to the aforementioned apparent inability to initiate voluntary movements seen in absence attacks and attentional deficits (65,69, 70).

In most cases the symptomatology of petit mal status is rather characteristic. There is slowness of mentation, a confusional state associated with continuous eye blinking and occasional myoclonic jerks, signs which are highly suggestive of petit mal status. However, atypical cases are not too uncommon and sometimes may suggest a psychiatric diagnosis (for a detailed list of references see ref. 83). The proper diagnosis is often only made when an EEG is taken at the time when the patient exhibits what appears to be psychotic behavior.

An example of this is the case of D.G., a 13-year-old boy with a long history of absence seizures, some episodes of aggressive and hostile behavior, and others involving staring blankly, speaking gibberish, and urinating and defecating in the living room. Such episodes lasted for 24–48 hr. The behavioral difficulties, even though episodic, were attributed to a difficult home situation, and the patient was under psychiatric care. An episode of abnormal behavior occurred while he was hospitalized at the Montreal Neurological Institute for evaluation of his problem. The patient, who at admission had been cooperative and friendly, one day became hostile and negativistic. He often broke out in tears, used profane language, and called an invisible person "a dirty rat" while shaking his fist at him. He repeatedly said that all this was because his father had divorced his mother. There were occasional myoclonic jerks and fluttering of the eyelids. The boy was disoriented in space;

however, he was able to read from a book and to count correctly, but he perseverated in doing so when asked to perform another task and also in the course of naming objects. While he was in this abnormal behavioral state, the EEG showed continuous generalized bilaterally synchronous 1- to 3-Hz spike-and-wave discharge typical for petit mal status (Fig. 8A). In the course of the EEG recording, the patient suddenly stopped breathing and became cyanosed. The EEG was now dominated by high-amplitude delta waves (Fig. 8B). After a short while he started breathing again spontaneously, sat up, and laughed. The spike-and-wave discharge had almost totally disappeared (Fig. 8C). His skin color turned rosy immediately. A few seconds later the EEG showed 8- to 10-Hz alpha rhythm, with no spike-and-waves (Fig. 8D). The boy's behavior had become entirely normal, and he was in a rather jovial mood. While the EEG symptomatology of this case of petit mal status was entirely typical, most of the associated behavioral phenomena were highly unusual. Equally unusual was the manner in which the status became arrested in response to anoxia resulting from a spontaneous respiratory arrest which may have been induced by the generalized spike-and-wave discharge.

In the case of complex partial status of temporal or frontal origin, the cause for the confusional state is similar to that seen in temporal or frontal lobe automatism (namely, ictal interference with the normal functioning of neuronal mechanisms represented in these lobes), although a few positive signs such as auditory hallucinations or emotional changes (e.g., fear and autonomic signs) may be present in complex partial status of temporal lobe origin (79,81,83; for additional references see the latter paper). Slovenliness, aggressiveness, and sexual disinhibition (89), as well as facetiousness (83), may be seen in frontal lobe complex partial status. These clinical distinctions are, however, of only relative value. I have, for instance, observed a case of petit mal status in whom facetiousness, which is said to be relatively characteristic for frontal lobe nonconvulsive status, was the predominant clinical sign together with constant eye-blinking.

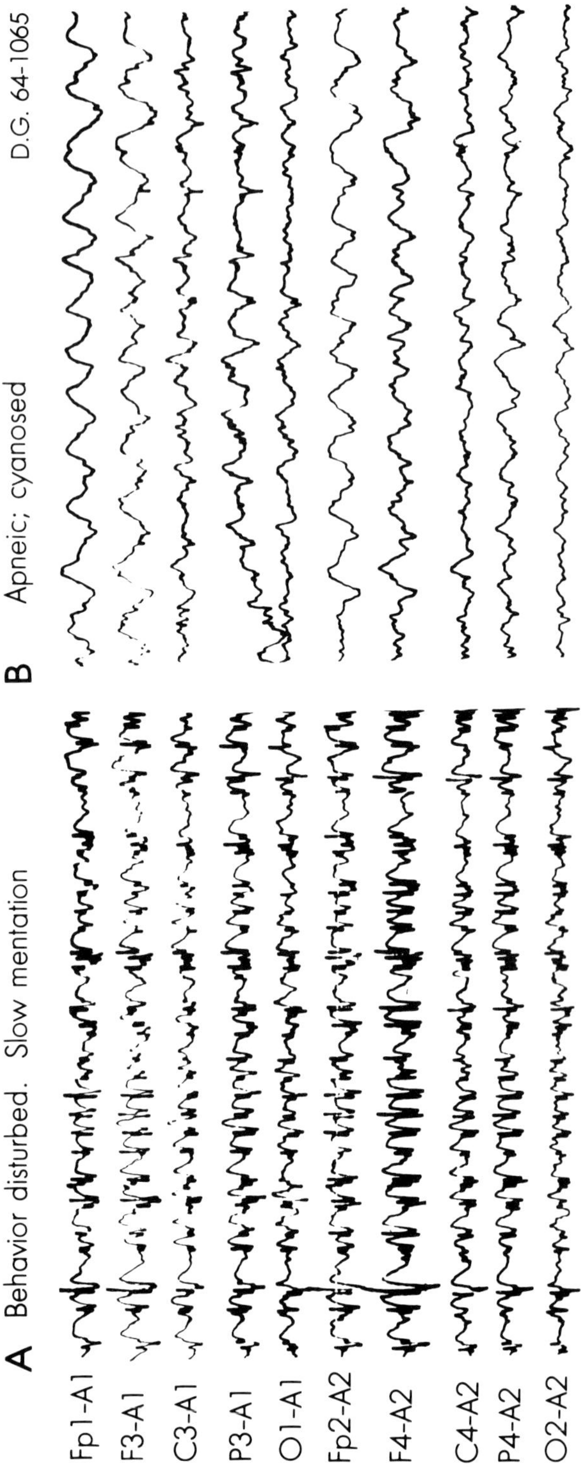

A   Behavior disturbed.   Slow mentation
B   Apneic; cyanosed
D.G. 64-1065
Fp1-A1
F3-A1
C3-A1
P3-A1
O1-A1
Fp2-A2
F4-A2
C4-A2
P4-A2
O2-A2

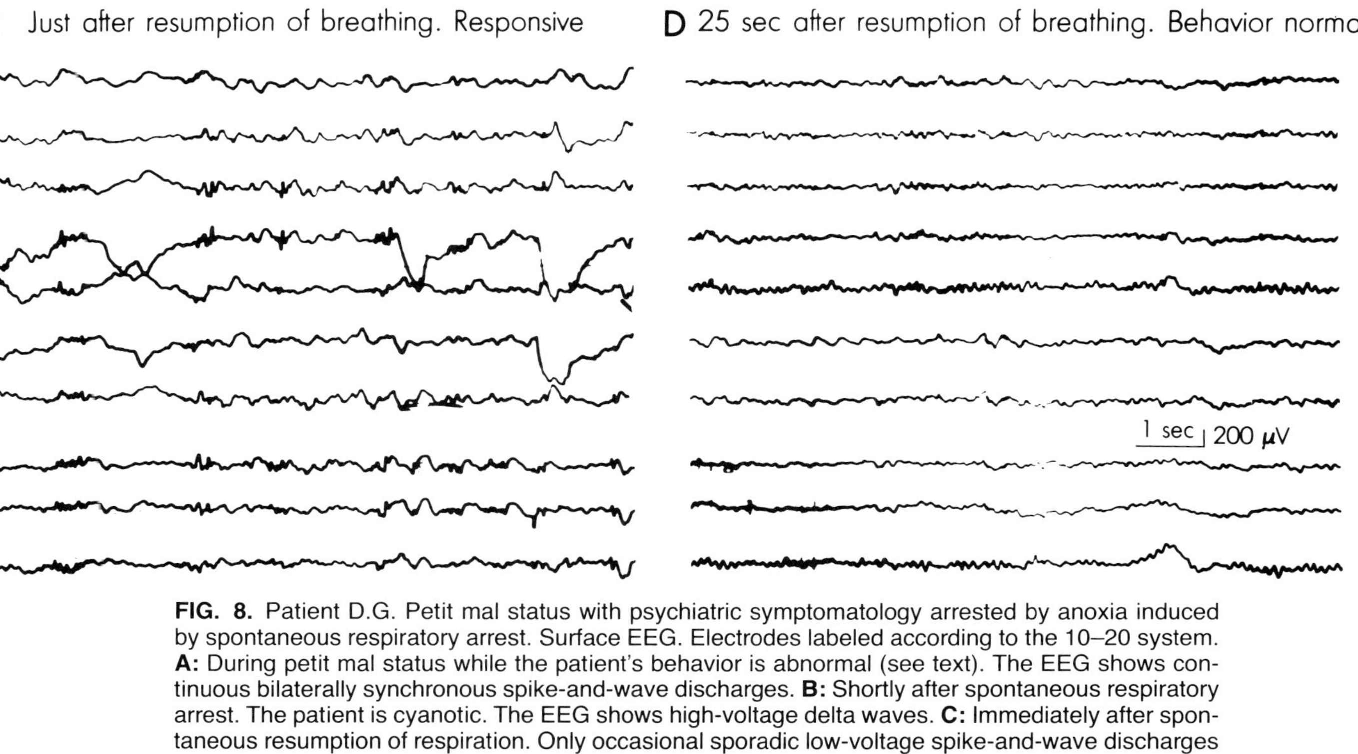

FIG. 8. Patient D.G. Petit mal status with psychiatric symptomatology arrested by anoxia induced by spontaneous respiratory arrest. Surface EEG. Electrodes labeled according to the 10–20 system. **A:** During petit mal status while the patient's behavior is abnormal (see text). The EEG shows continuous bilaterally synchronous spike-and-wave discharges. **B:** Shortly after spontaneous respiratory arrest. The patient is cyanotic. The EEG shows high-voltage delta waves. **C:** Immediately after spontaneous resumption of respiration. Only occasional sporadic low-voltage spike-and-wave discharges are present. **D:** Approximately 25 sec later. The skin color and the patient's behavior have returned to normal. No spike-and-wave discharges. Normal alpha rhythm has returned.

SPEECH

By now it is well known that ictal discharge involving speech cortex never induces speech or the hallicinatory experience of hearing spoken or of reading written words that can be understood by the patient (2,90,91). The effect in the case of ictal involvement of speech cortex is always purely negative, but it reveals itself only when the patient is attempting to use speech in either the expressive or receptive mode. Otherwise he is unaware of his deficit. Sometimes in the case of frontal lobe seizures the speech disturbance is nonfluent. In temporal lobe seizures, speech may be fluent but unintelligible. However, instances like these are rare, and most often there is no way to clinically distinguish with certainty between ictal aphasia of frontal (Broca's area) or temporoparietal (Wernicke's area) origin. One often overlooked aspect is that ictal aphasia may present as mutism and, as has already been mentioned, may then be mistaken for loss of consciousness.

Temporal lobe status, when not involving the limbic structures, may be dominated by dysphasia when involving the speech-dominant temporal lobe. In such a case of temporal lobe status in patient G.L., repeated long stretches of seizure discharge occurred which involved the lateral convexity of the temporal lobe, but not the mesial structures (Fig. 9). The patient had great difficulty in counting forward from 1 to 10 and made a few errors whenever such seizure discharge was present in the EEG. His counting was very slow, and he had difficulty in understanding and answering questions. Whenever the discharge stopped, he performed the above language tasks without any difficulty. This case is interesting because he did not fully satisfy the clinical criteria for complex partial status, since his difficulty seemed to be limited to one involving speech. This correlated very well with epileptiform discharge which involved the convexity of the temporal lobe but which apparently spared the mesial structures.

Uttering of complex speech during a seizure is said to lateralize the origin of complex partial seizures to the speech non-dominant hemisphere (92). It is of interest that patient L.J., who carried on a phone conversation during a temporal lobe seizure with predominant left-sided involvement (see above), was left-handed and on intracarotid amytal testing was found to have bilateral speech representation with right-sided predominance.

CONCLUSION

It is apparent from this review that seizure discharge can directly modify the patient's behavior for the duration of the seizure and for the ensuing period of postictal depression. All facets of higher nervous function can become affected: perception, memory, affect, voluntary movements, and attention, as well as more complex functions such as those involved in selecting behaviors appropriate for the prevailing circumstances—that is, functions that are vital for protecting an individual from physical danger or social opprobrium. Ictal discharge can bring about these changes in two ways: It may exert a positive effect by activating the neuronal substrate of a behavioral mechanism, or it may exert a negative effect by interfering with the proper functioning of such a substrate. Positive effects of ictal discharge usually occur only fleetingly at the beginning of a seizure, when ictal discharge is still confined to relatively circumscribed neuronal cell groups. The effects produced in this positive way are those which the patient experiences subjectively. It appears probable that localized discharge in certain areas can organize in widespread brain regions a matrix of neural activation resembling that underlying similar experiences occurring normally in the course of everyday life. Invasion of these circuits by ictal discharge leads to negative effects (most commonly automatism and amnesia) through interference with neural substrates implicated in higher behavioral mechanisms. Negative effects resulting from ictal discharge can exert their influence in two ways. The first way is direct ictal paralysis of some behavioral functions dependent upon the structure inactivated by the discharge. Thus a neurological deficit may be induced, such as anterograde amnesia, aphasia (both receptive and expressive), lack of initiation of voluntary movements, and confusional states. The latter may be caused by an inability to relate perceptions (which may be somewhat impaired ictally or postictally) to the full

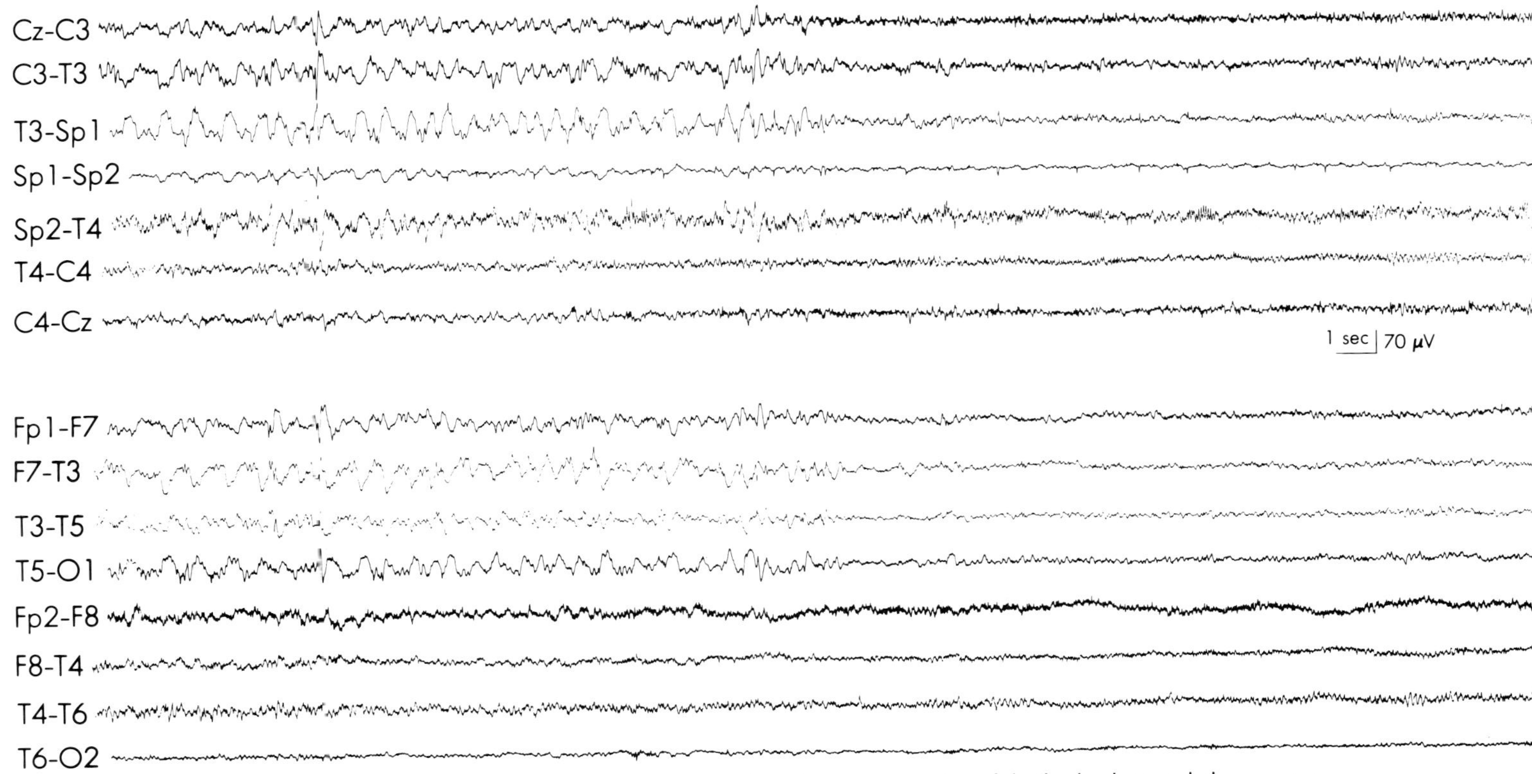

FIG. 9. Patient G.L. Temporal lobe status with prolonged episodes of rhythmic slow and sharp wave discharges involving the convexity of the left temporal lobe during which the patient is dysphasic. Surface EEG recording with scalp and sphenoidal electrodes are labeled as in Fig. 7. In the left half of the EEG sample, the end of an episode of ictal activity is shown during which the patient was markedly dysphasic. The right half shows arrest of epileptic discharge; speech returned to normal. Recordings in upper and lower panel are simultaneous.

range of memories which are available under normal conditions but which are only partially or not at all accessible in the ictal and postictal states. A second, indirect way in which ictal paralysis of a mechanism can produce a behavioral effect is by putting out of action a mechanism which normally restrains some behavioral expressions under circumstances in which they are inappropriate. Ictal paralysis of such controlling mechanisms may then release behaviors from restraint which may manifest themselves as automatisms and confusional states and which may include various forms of inappropriate or even psychotic-like behaviors.

REFERENCES

1. Jackson JH. In: Taylor J, ed. *Selected Writings of John Hughlings Jackson, vol 1: On epilepsy and epileptiform convulsions.* New York: Basic Books, 1958.
2. Penfield W, Jasper H. *Epilepsy and the functional anatomy of the human brain.* Boston: Little, Brown & Company, 1954.
3. Halgren E, Walter RD, Cherlow DG, Crandall PH. Mental phenomena evoked by electrical stimulation of the human hippocampal formation and amygdala. *Brain* 1978;101:83–117.
4. Mullan S, Penfield W. Illusions of comparative interpretation and emotion. *Arch Neurol Psychiatry* 1959;81:269–284.
5. Wieser HG. *Electroclinical features of the psychomotor seizure.* London: Butterworths (Stuttgart: Gustav Fischer), 1983.
6. Bancaud J. Sémiologie clinique des crises épileptiques d'origine temporale. *Rev Neurol* 1987;143:392–400.
7. Gloor P, Olivier A, Quesney LF, Andermann F, Horowitz S. The role of the limbic system in experiential phenomena of temporal lobe epilepsy. *Ann Neurol* 1982;12:129–144.
8. Penfield W, Perot P. The brain's record of auditory and visual experience—a final summary and discussion. *Brain* 1963;86:595–696.
9. Spiers PA, Schomer DL, Blume HW, Mesulam MM. In: Mesulam MM, ed. Temporolimbic epilepsy and behavior. *Principles of behavioral neurology.* Philadelphia: FA Davis, 1985;289–326.
10. Gloor P, Olivier A, Quesney LF. The role of the amygdala in the expression of psychic phenomena in temporal lobe seizures. In: Ben-Ari Y, ed. *The amygdaloid complex.* Amsterdam: Elsevier/North-Holland Biomedical Press, 1981;489–498.
11. Taylor DC, Lochery M. Temporal lobe epilepsy: origin and significance of simple and complex auras. *J Neurol Neurosurg Psychiatry* 1987;50:673–681.
12. Mark VH, Ervin FR, Sweet WH, Delgado J. Remote telemeter stimulation and recording from implanted temporal lobe electrodes. *Confin Neurol* 1969;31:86–93.
13. Ashford JW, Schultz SC, Walsh GO. Violent automatism in a partial complex seizure. *Arch Neurol* 1980;37:120–122.
14. Saint-Hilaire JM, Gilbert M, Bouvier G, Barbeau A. Epilepsy and aggression: two cases with depth electrode studies. In: Robb P, ed. *Epilepsy updated: causes and treatment.* Miami: Symposium Specialists, 1980;145–176.
15. Treiman DM, Delgado-Escueta AV. Aggression during fear and flight in complex partial seizures: a CCTV–EEG analysis. *Epilepsia* 1981;22:246.
16. Gloor P. Electrophysiological studies of the amygdala (stimulation and recording), their possible contribution to the understanding of neural mechanisms of aggression. In: Fields WS, Sweet WH, eds. *Neural bases of violence and aggression.* St. Louis: Warren H Green, 1975;5–40.
17. Treiman DM. Epilepsy and violence: medical and legal issues. *Epilepsia* 1986;27:S77–S104.
18. Daly DD, Mulder DW. Gelastic epilepsy. *Neurology* 1957;7:189–192.
19. Druckmann R, Chao D. Laughter in epilepsy. *Neurology* 1957;7:26–36.
20. Gascon GC, Lombroso CT. Epileptic (gelastic) laughter. *Epilepsia* 1971;12:63–76.
21. Loiseau P, Cohadon F, Cohadon S. Gelastic epilepsy. A review and report of 5 cases. *Epilepsia* 1971;12:313–323.
22. Berkovic SF, Andermann F, Melanson D, Ethier RE, Feindel W, Gloor P. Hypothalamic hamartomas and ictal laughter: evolution of a characteristic epileptic syndrome and diagnostic value of magnetic resonance imaging. *Ann Neurol* 1988;23:429–439.
23. Martin JP. Fits of laughter (sham mirth) in organic cerebral disease. *Brain* 1950;73:453–464.
24. Ironside R. Disorders of laughter due to brain lesions. *Brain* 1956;79:589–609.
25. Chen RC, Forster FM. Cursive epilepsy and gelastic epilepsy. *Neurology* 1973;23:1019–1029.
26. Gastaut H, Collomb H. Etude du comportement sexuel chez les épileptiques psychomoteurs. *Ann Med Psychol (Paris)* 1954;112:657–696.
27. Rémillard G, Andermann F, Testa GF, Gloor P, Aubé M, Martin JB, Feindel W, et al. Sexual ictal manifestations in women with temporal lobe epilepsy: a finding suggesting sexual dimorphism in the human brain. *Neurology* 1983;33:323–330.
28. Jacome DE, Risko MS. Absence status manifested by compulsive masturbation. *Arch Neurol* 1983;40:523–524.
29. Spencer SS, Spencer DD, Williamson PD, Mattson RH. Sexual automatisms in complex partial seizures. *Neurology* 1983;33:527–533.
30. Williamson PD, Spencer DD, Spencer SS, Novelly RA, Mattson RH. Complex partial seizures of frontal lobe origin. *Ann Neurol* 1985;18:497–504.
31. Bancaud J, Favel P, Bonis A, Bordas-Ferrer M, Miravet J, Talairach J. Manifestations sexuelles

paroxystiques et épilepsie temporale. Etude clinique, EEG et SEEG d'une épilepsie d'origine temporale. *Rev Neurol* 1970;123:217–230.

32. Jacome DE, McLain LW, Fitzgerald R. Postural reflex gelastic seizures. *Arch Neurol* 1980;37:249–251.

33. Gastaut H. Les troubles du comportement alimentaire chez les épileptiques psychomoteurs. *Rev Neurol* 1955;92:55–62.

34. Rémillard GM, Andermann F, Gloor P, Olivier A, Martin JB. Water-drinking as ictal behavior in complex partial seizures. *Neurology* 1981;31:117–124.

35. Penfield W. The permanent record of the stream of consciousness. Proceedings of the 14th International Congress of Psychology, Montreal. *Acta Psychol* 1954;47–69.

36. Gloor P. The role of the human limbic system in perception, memory and affect: lessons from temporal lobe epilepsy. In: Doane BK, Livingston KE, eds. *The limbic system: fundamental organization and clinical disorders*. New York: Raven Press, 1986;159–169.

37. Penfield W. The cerebral cortex in man. I. The cerebral cortex and consciousness. *Arch Neurol Psychiatry* 1938;40:417–442.

38. Milner B. Psychological defects produced by temporal lobe excision. *Res Publ Assoc Res New Ment Dis* 1958;36:244–257.

39. Milner B. Visual recognition and recall after right temporal lobe excision in man. *Neuropsychologia* 1968;6:191–209.

40. Milner B. Psychological aspects of focal epilepsy and its neurosurgical management. In: Purpura D, Penry J, Walter R, eds. *Neurosurgical management of the epilepsies. Advances in neurology*, vol 8. New York: Raven Press, 1975;299–332.

41. Kimura D. Right temporal lobe damage. *Arch Neurol* 1963;8:264–271.

42. Mishkin M. Visual mechanisms beyond the striate cortex. In: Russell R, ed. *Frontiers in Physiological Psychology*. New York: Academic Press, 1966;93–119.

43. Mishkin M. Cortical visual areas and their interactions. In: Karczmar AG, Eccles JC, eds. *Symposium on the brain and human behavior*. New York: Springer-Verlag, 1972;187–208.

44. Gloor P. Temporal lobe epilepsy: its possible contribution to the understanding of the functional significance of the amygdala and of its interaction with neocortical–temporal mechanisms. In: Eleftherion BE, ed. *The neurobiology of the amygdala*. New York: Plenum Press, 1972;423–457.

45. Gloor P. Inputs and outputs of the amygdala: what the amygdala is trying to tell the rest of the brain. In: Livingston KE, Hornykiewicz O, eds. *Limbic mechanisms. The continuing evolution of the limbic system concept*. New York: Plenum Press, 1978;189–209.

46. Turner BH, Mishkin M, Knapp M. Organization of amygdalopetal projections from modality-specific cortical association areas in the monkey. *J Comp Neurol* 1980;191:515–543.

47. Ungerleider LG, Mishkin M. Two cortical visual systems. In: Ingle DJ, Goodale MA, Mansfield RJW, eds. *The analysis of visual behavior*. Cambridge, MA: MIT Press, 1982;549–586.

48. van Hoesen GW. The parahippocampal gyrus. *Trends Neurosci* 1982;5:345–350.

49. Amaral DG, Price JL. Amygdalo-cortical projections in the monkey (*Macaca fascicularis*). *J Comp Neurol* 1984;230:465–496.

50. Pandya DN, Yeterian EH. Architecture and connections of cortical association areas. In: Peters A, Jones EG, eds. *Cerebral cortex, vol 4: Association and auditory cortices*. New York: Plenum Press, 1985;3–61.

51. Amaral DG. Memory: anatomical organization of candidate brain regions. In: Plum F, Mountcastle V, eds. *Higher functions of the brain. Handbook of physiology*, Part 1. Washington, DC: American Physiological Society, 1987;211–294.

52. Penfield W, Milner B. Memory deficit produced by bilateral lesions in the hippocampal zone. *Arch Neurol Psychiatry* 1958;79:475–497.

53. Milner B. Amnesia following operation on the temporal lobe. In: Whitty CWM, Zangewill OO, eds. *Amnesia*. London: Butterworths, 1966;109–133.

54. Squire LR. The neuropsychology of memory. *Annu Rev Neurosci* 1982;5:241–273.

55. Squire LR. *Memory and brain*. New York: Oxford University Press, 1987.

56. Gloor P. Epilepsy: relationships between electrophysiology and intracellular mechanisms involving second messengers and gene expression. *Can J Neurol Sci* 1989;16:8–21.

57. Goldman-Rakic. Circuitry of primate prefrontal cortex and regulation of behavior by representational knowledge. In: Plum F, Mountcastle V, eds. *Higher cortical functions. Handbook of Physiology*, Part 1, Ch. 9. Washington, DC: American Physiol Soc, 1987;5:373–417.

58. Goldman-Rakic PS. Topography of cognition: parallel distributed networks in primate association cortex. *Annu Rev Neurosci* 1988;11:137–156.

59. Lynch G. *Synapses, circuits and the beginnings of memory*. Cambridge, MA: The MIT Press, 1987.

60. De Yoe EA, van Essen DC. Concurrent processing streams in monkey visual cortex. *Trends Neurosci* 1988;11:219–276.

61. Livingstone M, Hubel D. Segregation of form, color, movement and depth: anatomy, physiology and perception. *Science* 1988;240:740–749.

62. Rumelhart DE, McClelland JL, and the PDP Research Group. *Parallel distributed processing. Explorations in the microstructure of cognition*, vols 1 and 2. Cambridge, MA: MIT Press, 1988.

63. Bancaud J, Henriksen O, Rubio-Donnadieu F, Seino M, Dreifuss FE, Penry JK. Proposal for revised clinical and electroencephalographic classification of epileptic seizures. *Epilepsia* 1981;22:489–501.

64. Frederiks JAM. Consciousness. In: Vinken PJ, Bruyn GW, eds. *Handbook of clinical neurol-*

ogy, vol 3: Disorders of higher nervous activity. Amsterdam: North-Holland, 1969;49–61.

65. Gloor P. Consciousness as a neurological concept in epileptology: a critical review. *Epilepsia* 1986;27(Suppl 2):S14–S26.

66. Courtois GA, Ingvar DH, Jasper HH. Nervous and mental defects during petit mal attacks. *Electroencephalogr Clin Neurophysiol [Suppl]* 1953;3:87.

67. Shimazono Y, Hirai T, Okuma T, Fukuda T, Yamasu E. Disturbance of consciousness in petit mal epilepsy. *Epilepsia* 1953;2:49–55.

68. Yaeger C, Guerrant JS. Subclinical epileptic seizures, impairment of motor performance and derivative difficulties. *Calif Med* 1957;86:242–247.

69. Mirsky AF. Behavioral and psychophysiological effects of petit mal epilepsy in the light of neuropsychologically based theory of attention. In: Myslobodsky MS, Mirsky AF, eds. *Elements of petit mal.* New York: Peter Lang, 1988;311–340.

70. Myslobodsky MS. Petit mal status as a paradigm of the functional anatomy of awareness. In: Myslobodsky MS, Mirsky AF, eds. *Elements of petit mal epilepsy.* New York: Peter Lang, 1988;71–104.

71. Jus A, Jus J. Retrograde amnesia in petit mal. *Arch Gen Psychiatry* 1962;6:163–167.

72. Williamson PD, Spencer DD, Spencer SS, Novelly RA, Mattson RH. Complex partial status epilepticus: a depth-electrode study. *Ann Neurol* 1985;18:647–654.

73. Lennox W. Petit mal epilepsies, their treatment with tridione. *JAMA* 1945;129:1069–1073.

74. Niedermeyer E, Khalifeh X. Petit mal status ("spike-wave-stupor"). *Epilepsia* 1965;6:250–262.

75. Lob H, Roger J, Soulayrol R, Régis H, Gastaut H. Les états de mal généralisés à expression confusionnelle. In: Gastaut H, Roger J, Lob H, eds. *Les Etats de Mal épileptiques.* Paris: Masson, 1967;91–109.

76. Passouant P, Cadilhac J, Ribstein M, Delange M, Castan P. Les états de mal partiels. In: Gastaut H, Roger J, Lob H, eds. *Les Etats de Mal épileptiques.* Paris: Masson, 1967;152–181.

77. Lugaresi E, Pazzaglia P, Tassinari CA. Differentiation of "absence status" and "temporal lobe status". *Epilepsia* 1971;12:77–87.

78. Andermann F, Robb JP. Absence status. *Epilepsia* 1972;13:177–187.

79. Wieser HG. Temporal lobe or psychomotor status epilepticus. A case report. *Electroencephalogr Clin Neurophysiol* 1980;48:558–572.

80. Treiman DM, Delgado-Escueta AV. Complex partial status epilepticus. In: Delgado-Escueta AV, Wasterlain CG, Treiman DM, Porter RJ, eds. *Status Epilepticus. Advances in neurology,* vol 34. New York: Raven Press, 1983;69–81.

81. Wieser HG, Hailemariam S, Regard M, Landis T. Unilateral limbic epileptic status activity: stereo EEG, behavioral and cognitive data. *Epilepsia* 1985;26:19–29.

82. Guberman A, Cantu-Reyna G, Stuss D, Broughton R. Nonconvulsive generalized status epilepticus: clinical features, neuropsychological testing, and long-term follow-up. *Neurology* 1986;36:1284–1291.

83. Rohr-le-Floch J, Gauthier G, Beaumanoir A. Etats confusionnels d'origine épileptique. Intérêt de l-EEG fait en urgence. *Rev Neurol (Paris)* 1988;6–7:425–436.

84. Avoli M, Gloor P, Kostopoulos G, Gotman J. An analysis of penicillin-induced generalized spike and wave discharges using simultaneous recordings of cortical and thalamic single neurons. *J Neurophysiol* 1983;50:819–837.

85. Gloor P. Neurophysiological mechanism of generalized spike-and-wave discharge and its implication for understanding absence seizures. In: Myslobodsky MS, Mirsky AF, eds. *Elements of petit mal epilepsy.* New York: Peter Lang, 1988;159–209.

86. Gloor P, Fariello RG. Generalized epilepsy: some of its cellular mechanisms differ from those of focal epilepsy. *Trends Neurosci* 1988;11:63–68.

87. Nightingale S, Welch JL. Psychometric assessment in absence status. *Arch Neurol* 1982;39:516–519.

88. Gloor P. Generalized epilepsy with spike and wave discharge: a reinterpretation of its electrographic and clinical manifestations. *Epilepsia* 1979;20:571–588.

89. Boone KB, Miller BL, Rosenberg L, Durazo A, McIntyre H, Weil M. Neuropsychological and behavioral abnormalities in an adolescent with frontal lobe seizures. *Neurology* 1988;38:583–586.

90. Penfield W, Roberts L. *Speech and brain mechanism.* Princeton, NJ: Princeton University Press, 1959.

91. Ojemann GA. Brain organization for language from the perspective of electrical stimulation mapping. *Behav Brain Sci* 1983;6:189–206.

92. Koerner M, Laxer KD. Ictal speech, postictal language dysfunction, and seizure lateralization. *Neurology* 1988;38:634–636.

Advances in Neurology, Vol. 55, edited by
D. Smith, D. Treiman, and M. Trimble,
Raven Press, Ltd., New York © 1991.

2

Neurochemical Substrates of Ictal Behavior

Brian S. Meldrum

Department of Neurology, Institute of Psychiatry, London SE5 8AF, England

Seizure activity is associated with a wide range of biochemical changes in the brain, most of which correlate directly with enhanced neuronal activity in the excitatory and inhibitory pathways directly involved in epileptic discharges. These include changes in energy consumption (CMR_{O_2}, CMR_{glu}), changes in concentration of metabolites concerned in glucose metabolism, changes in ionic distribution, and changes in the concentration and turnover of various neurotransmitters (inhibitory and excitatory amino acids, monoamines, peptides, etc). There are also changes in various second messenger systems, in gene expression, and in pathophysiological processes that may contribute to long-term changes in neuronal behavior or to processes leading to neuronal cell death. All these processes will vary in severity according to the intensity and duration of local seizure activity, and they will require variable periods for their restitution postictally. Correlating biochemical changes with behavior requires an integration of our knowledge of neurochemistry as it relates to neuronal activity, and of the anatomy of seizure activity and the relation between behavior and the integrated activity of the brain. This chapter summarizes some of the evidence currently available.

CHANGES IN ENERGY METABOLISM

An increase in cerebral metabolic rate for oxygen and glucose (CMR_{O_2} and CMR_{glu}, respectively) has frequently been reported to accompany seizures in man and in experimental animals (1–3). The severity and time course of such changes show some variation,

but in general they are remarkably consistent even when comparing seizures that are clinically and electrographically diverse. In rats with sustained seizure activity induced by bicuculline, the CMR_{O_2} is increased 2.7 times during the first 20 min (4) whereas the CMR_{glu} is initially increased fourfold (5). This is associated with a marked increase in cerebral blood flow (CBF) which commonly exceeds the increase in CMR_{O_2}, leading to an increase in P_{O_2} in the sagittal sinus blood. The increased blood flow is a consequence of local vasodilation (under both neuronal and metabolic control). Thus regional CBF measurements indicate the brain areas involved in the seizure activity.

There is a rapid increase in cerebral lactate concentration (doubling in 10 sec in bicuculline seizures in the rat), accompanied by an increase in the lactate/pyruvate ratio. Study of the intermediates of glycolysis confirms the early enhancement of the glycolytic rate, with marked activation of phosphofructokinase (1). Brain glucose and glycogen content both fall within the first few minutes of seizure activity. Glucose flux into the brain is also enhanced.

Brain creatine concentration rises and phosphocreatine content falls. This appears to be mainly a consequence of a reduction in intracellular pH (Fig. 1). Brain ATP and ADP levels and the calculated energy charge show little change, provided that the seizures are not associated with impaired respiratory or cardiovascular function (1).

In the presence of hypoglycemia (spontaneous or induced by insulin), the increase in CMR_{O_2} is less well maintained and the seizure

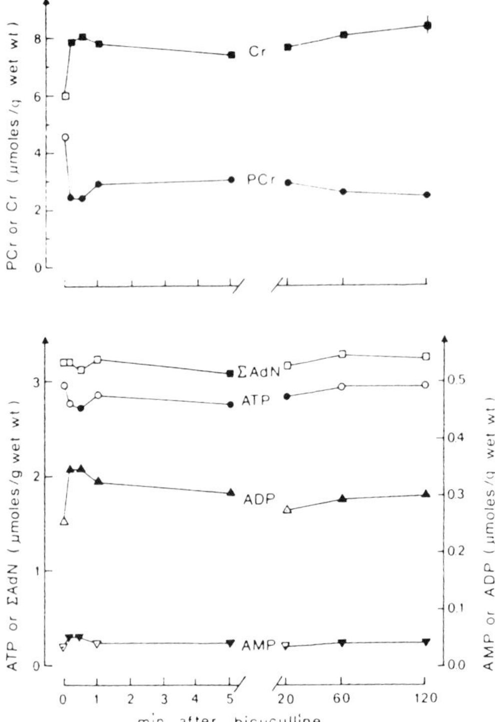

FIG. 1. Changes in the concentrations of PCr, creatine, ATP, ADP, and AMP, as well as in the sum of adenine nucleotides (ΣAdN), in rat brain during seizures induced by an intravenous injection of bicuculline. Filled symbols indicate statistically significant changes ($p < 0.05$). Control values (in μmol g^{-1} wet wt; $n = 10$) are: PCr, 4.59 $\pm$ 0.06; creatine, 6.01 $\pm$ 0.06; ATP, 2.95 $\pm$ 0.03; ADP, 0.257 $\pm$ 0.002; AMP, 0.030 $\pm$ 0.001. (From ref. 1, with permission.)

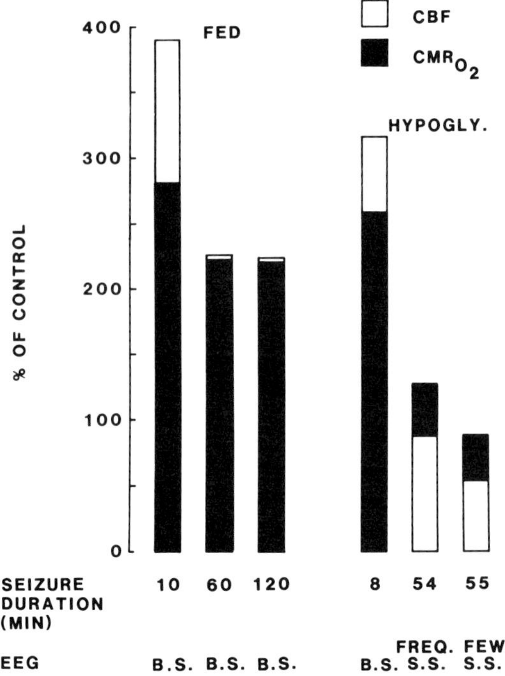

FIG. 2. Overall cerebral blood flow (CBF) and oxygen consumption (CMR$_{O_2}$; % of control) during the progression of bicuculline seizures in fed rats and insulin-induced hypoglycemic rats. B.S., burst suppression seizure discharge on the electroencephalogram (EEG); S.S., single spikes. (From ref. 3, with permission.)

activity itself becomes reduced [as assessed by the severity of the paroxysmal activity on the electroencephalogram (EEG); see fig. 2]. Prolonged seizures induced by bicuculline in the rat lead to cytopathological changes in hippocampal pyramidal neurons. These changes are less severe if arterial hypotension or hypoglycemia lead to a reduction in seizure activity (6).

Studies of regional CBF or glucose metabolism provide an indication of the focal origin and spread of seizure activity. Changes in CBF or in CMR$_{glu}$ have been widely used in animal models of epilepsy to chart the spatial extent of seizure activity. Similar studies can now be made in humans by means of PET (positron emission tomography) or SPECT (single-photon emission computerized tomography) (7,8). There are, however, limitations in spatial resolution (which are most marked for SPECT) and in temporal resolution (which are most marked for PET).

The 2-Deoxyglucose Method in Experimental Seizures

This method involves (a) the administration of ^{14}C- or ^{3}H-labeled 2-deoxyglucose (2DG) during the seizure period, (b) sacrifice 45 min later, and (c) autoradiography of frozen brain sections (9). Phosphorylated 2DG accumulates at a rate proportional to glucose phosphorylation; measurements of arterial 2DG and glucose content allow calculation of the regional CMR$_{glu}$. This method shows a clear pattern of regional enhancement of glucose metabolism that is widely assumed to give a picture of the brain regions directly involved in the seizure activity. It has been used in generalized and focal seizures in rodents (10,11) and in focal motor seizures in monkeys (12). These studies show a marked metabolic activation in the amygdala and hippocampus in the initial stages of limbic seizures induced by electrical or chemical (kainic acid) stimulation. With the development of more generalized motor activity, activation occurs also in basal ganglia and thalamic limbic structures (e.g., mediodorsal nucleus). Focal seizures induced by application of penicillin to the motor cortex of pubescent monkeys are associated with metabolic activation in the ipsilateral putamen, the globus pallidus, the substantia nigra, and the contralateral cerebellar cortex (12). Metabolic activation is also prominent in the substantia nigra (pars reticulata) in generalized seizures induced electrically or by bicuculline.

Fluorodeoxyglucose Studies in Humans

PET using [18F]fluorodeoxyglucose permits imaging of the regional glucose utilization in the human brain. The application of the technique to the study of functional cerebral anatomy in epilepsy is reviewed by Henry et al. (7). In a typical procedure, cerebral metabolism is averaged over a period of 30–45 min to produce a single image, the quantitative interpretation of which requires a steady state throughout the period. Many of the values in Table 1 are presumably lower than the true metabolic rate associated with seizure activity because the seizure activity was not sustained throughout but was instead replaced by a period of postictal metabolic depression. Apart from this effect, the results for regional and generalized seizures are comparable to those obtained with 2-DG in experimental seizures in animals. It is noteworthy that the bilaterally synchronous three-per-second spike-and-wave discharges induced by hyperventilation in patients with petit mal seizures are associated with a 2.5- to 3.5-fold increase in CMR_{glu} (13). This is in spite of the fact that the abnormal synchronized cortical activity may be predominantly inhibitory in nature.

Ionic Changes

Studies with ion-selective microelectrodes have produced a very consistent picture of the

TABLE 1. *Regional metabolic rates during partial and generalized seizures in man[a]*

			Ictal $rCMR_{glu}$ or $rCMR_{O2}$			
Seizure	n	Ictal EEG (%)[b]	Measurement	Focal (% change)[c]	Surround	Reference
Partial	3	—	$rCMR_{glu}$	↑ (30–60%)	⅓ ↑ General	14
Partial	2	—	$rCMR_{glu}$	↑ (82–130%)	½ ↑ General ½ Distal	15
Partial	1	4%	$rCMR_{glu}$	↓ (−12%)	↓ (−8%)	16
Partial (recurrent)	4	34–50%	$rCMR_{glu}$	↑ (206–487%)	²⁄₄ ↓ (−42 to −15%) ²⁄₄ ↑ (43–111%)	
Partial (continuous)	1	100%	$rCMR_{glu}$	↑ (116%)	↑ (60%)	
Partial (continuous)	1	100%	$rCMR_{glu}$	↑ (100 500%)	↑	17
Generalized (absence)	4	—	$rCMR_{glu}$	—	Global ↑ (100–200%)	13
Generalized (ECT)	1	—	$rCMR_{glu}$	—	↑ Global	17
Partial	2	—	$rCMR_{O2}$	↑ (150%)	½ ↑ General	18
Partial and generalized	6	—	$rCMR_{O2}$	↑ Focal + multifocal	½ ↑ Distal ⁴⁄₆ ↑ Distal	19

[a]$rCMR_{glu}$, regional cerebral metabolic rate for glucose; $rCMR_{O2}$, regional cerebral metabolic rate for oxygen; EEG, electroencephalogram; ECT, electroconvulsive therapy.
[b]Percentage of ictal events in EEG recording during the 30 min of $rCMR_{glu}$ determination.
[c]Percent increase above interictal value.
Reproduced from ref. 3, with permission.

nature of changes in extracellular ion concentration that accompany seizure activity (20). There is a rapid increase in extracellular $[K^+]$ that soon stabilizes at a plateau of 9–13 mM. Extracellular $[Ca^{2+}]$ falls from a normal level of 1.3 to 0.7–1.1 mM (21). Exceptionally, $[Ca^{2+}]_o$ can fall to 0.25 mM in the frontal cortex of the baboon *Papio papio* during photically induced seizure activity (22). At such a low level of $[Ca^{2+}]_o$, synaptic activity will be suppressed. Extracellular $[Mg^{2+}]$ also falls during seizures. Studies with brain slices have shown that a reduced $[Ca^{2+}]$ and $[Mg^{2+}]$ and an enhanced $[K^+]$ concentration comparable to that seen *in vivo* during seizures favors the occurrence of epileptiform activity. It is likely that the changes in extracellular cation concentration occurring in gray matter with onset of epileptic discharges make a significant contribution to the maintenance of local seizure activity.

NEUROTRANSMITTER METABOLISM

Changes have been reported relating to the major fast inhibitory and excitatory systems [mediated by the amino acids (gamma-aminobutyric acid) (GABA) and glycine (inhibitory) and glutamate and aspartate (excitatory)] and to the modulatory systems (mediated by the monoamines and peptides).

Inhibitory Amino Acid Neurotransmitters

Changes in the concentration of the inhibitory transmitters GABA and glycine vary considerably according to the seizure model studied (23). An increase in GABA content occurs in sustained seizures induced by pentylenetetrazol or bicuculline (1,24,25) (Fig. 3). Experiments employing a GABA-transaminase inhibitor have established that there is a threefold increase in the metabolic turnover of GABA during bicuculline-induced seizures (26).

Excitatory Amino Acid Neurotransmitters

The cerebral concentrations of glutamate and aspartate decrease during prolonged seizure activity induced by pentylenetetrazol or

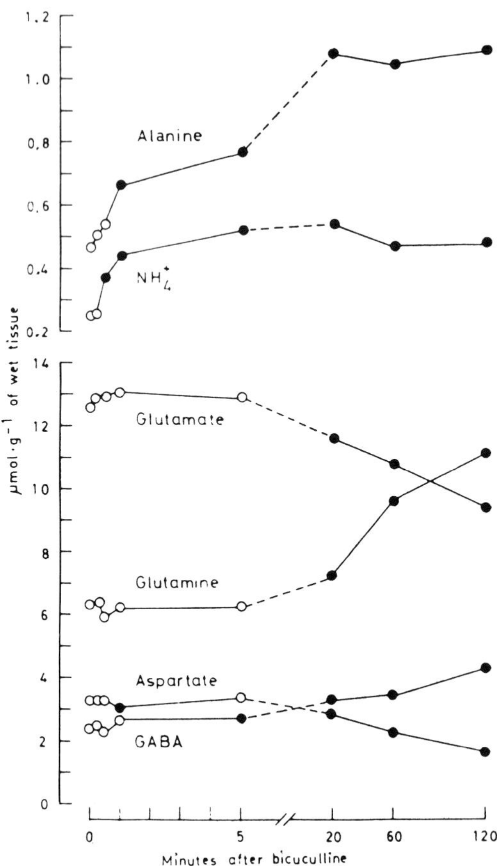

FIG. 3. Changes in cerebral cortex concentrations of ammonia and amino acids during bicuculline-induced seizures. Control values (in μmol g^{-1} wet wt; $n = 10$) are: alanine, 0.518 ± 0.019; aspartate, 3.34 ± 0.04; glutamine, 6.16 ± 0.09; glutamate, 12.73 ± 0.14; NH$_4^+$ 0.234 ± 0.013. Filled symbols indicate values significantly different from control ($p < 0.05$). (From ref. 1, with permission.)

bicuculline (1,24,25). At the same time, glutamine concentration increases. An increased ammonia concentration probably contributes to enhanced conversion of glutamate to glutamine. An increased synaptic release of glutamate and aspartate is almost certainly a consequence, as well as a cause, of sustained burst firing. Studies of extracellular concentration of amino acids during status epilepticus have shown increases in taurine, alanine, and phosphoethanolamine but tend to show little or no change in glutamate concentration

(27), apparently because of very efficient reuptake.

Monoamines

Studies of the regional levels of the various monoamine neurotransmitters (and their metabolites) in the brain during seizures have yielded an extraordinary diversity of results. The use of enzyme inhibitors to block the synthesis or further metabolism of the neurotransmitter (with measurement of the precursor, monoamine, or metabolites) can help in the interpretation of changes in monoamine concentration (28). The effects of electroshock seizures on neurotransmitter metabolism and receptor function have been reviewed by Green and Nutt (29). There appear to be little or no changes in dopamine metabolism during electrically or chemically induced seizures. Enhanced noradrenaline turnover has been reported in chemically induced seizures (28) but is not a consistent finding. An extraordinary variety of changes in tryptophan, L-5-hydroxytryptamine, and 5-hydroxyindoleacetic acid have been described during electrically or chemically induced seizures (29,30).

Peptides

There is an enormous diversity of peptides found in the brain. Their role in neuronal function is not well understood. Some have a direct excitatory action, whereas others appear to modulate fast excitation and inhibition. Several peptides vary in concentration in association with epileptic activity (e.g., dynorphin, enkephalins, somatostatin, substance P, neurotensin) (31–33). Three hours after the induction of seizures in the rat by systemic kainic acid, somatostatin, neurotensin and substance P appear to be markedly reduced in frontal cortex and hippocampus (by immunocytochemistry). We have found a transient decrease in neuropeptide Y during bicuculline-induced seizures (see Fig. 4).

The enkephalins modify seizure threshold, and both anticonvulsant and proconvulsant effects have been described (34,35). One possibility that has aroused discussion is that a release of enkephalins contributes to postictal behavioral changes (36). Motor deficits and raised seizure threshold postictally appear to be related to activation of mu and kappa opioid receptors; morphine facilitates the motor effects, whereas naloxone blocks them.

Seizure activity can also induce relatively

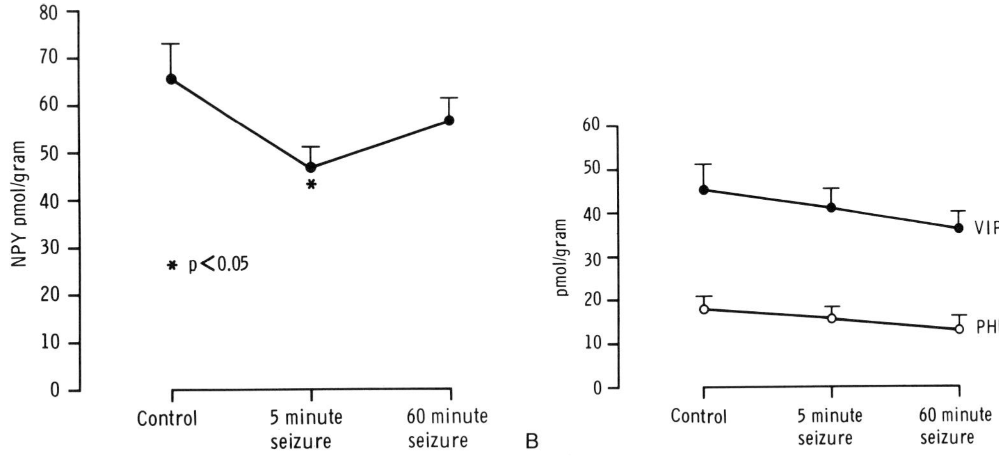

FIG. 4. Changes in peptide content in the hippocampus during sustained seizures induced by bicuculline in the rat. Peptide content was determined by radioimmunoassay on hippocampal homogenates from rat brain prior to or 5 or 60 min after onset of seizures. Graphs show (**A**) an early fall in neuropeptide Y (NPY) content and (**B**) no statistically significant change in vasoactive intestinal peptide (VIP) and PHI. Measurements of somatostatin, cholecystokinin, substance P, bombesin, and neurotensin also showed no change. (Data from M. Evans, J. Allen, S. R. Bloom, G. Roberts, and B. S. Meldrum, *unpublished observations.*)

long-lasting changes in brain peptides. In an immunocytochemical study of the rat hippocampus, Gall (37) showed that prolonged focal seizure activity (induced by electrolytic lesions or intracerebroventricular kainic acid) was followed by a marked increase in enkephalin immunoreactivity in the mossy fiber system whereas dynorphin and cholecystokinin immunoreactivities were markedly reduced. The increase in enkephalin is attributable to enhanced synthesis. This may be a consequence of the activation of ornithine decarboxylase activity during seizure activity (see section entitled "Protein Synthesis," below). The reduction in somatostatin in amygdala/pyriform cortex seen after kainic acid seizures can also be very prolonged (30 days) (32).

Adenosine

There are marked increases in brain adenosine content early in experimentally induced seizures. A three- to fivefold increase in adenosine content is reported during the first minute of bicuculline-induced seizures (38,39), and a 30-fold increase occurs following electroshock in rats (40). These increases are partly the result of breakdown of nucleotides as indicated by parallel increases in AMP and in inosine and hypoxanthine. An increase in extracellular adenosine has considerable functional significance. Through an action on presynaptic receptors the synaptic release of glutamate is reduced. This reduction of excitatory transmission has an antiepileptic effect but may also modify normal function.

Second Messenger Systems

There are dramatic changes in most second messenger systems early in seizure activity, and these entrain multiple secondary events. There are, for example, marked increases in cAMP and cGMP, which will modify activity in the cAMP- and cGMP-dependent protein kinases and thus modify activity in many receptor and enzyme systems (see Table 2).

The increase in cAMP levels follows seizure onset and is thought to be a consequence of formation and release of adenosine and perhaps enhanced adrenergic activity. Adenosine antagonists can decrease the cAMP increase in mouse brain (41).

cGMP is present in forebrain in lower concentration than is cAMP, but it is relatively higher in cerebellum. Increases in cGMP content induced by convulsant drugs can precede electrographic seizure onset. In cerebellar slices and cell cultures, application of excitatory amino acids can induce marked increases in cGMP content. It has recently been shown (55) that glutamate acts on N-methyl-D-aspartate (NMDA) receptors on cerebellar cells, thereby causing the release of a diffusible factor (thought to be endothelium-derived relaxing factor, nitric oxide) which provokes the increase in cGMP, apparently through activation of guanylate cyclase in glia and nerve terminals. A similar sequence of events with enhanced glutamate release and activation of NMDA receptors probably occurs during the initiation of seizure activity.

There is a remarkable breakdown of phospholipids associated with seizure activity (see Table 3 and ref. 65). There are dramatic in-

TABLE 2. *Increases in cyclic nucleotide levels at the onset of experimental seizures*

Seizure model	Cortex		Cerebellum		References
	cAMP	cGMP	cAMP	cGMP	
Electroshock	5×		3–4×	4–5×	41–43
Bicuculline	2–4×	3.5×			44, 45
Pentylenetetrazol	2.5–7×	2–3×	2–9×	2.5–15×	46–50
Homocysteine	2.5×				51
Isoniazid	2.5×	2–5×	3×	5×	52
3-Mercaptopropionate	3×	1.7×			53
Penicillin	NC[a]	13[b]×			54

[a]NC, no change.
[b]Ictal change in focus versus contralateral cortex.
Reproduced from ref. 3, with permission.

TABLE 3. *Increases in cortical free fatty acid and prostaglandin levels at the onset of experimental seizures[a]*

Seizure model	FFA	AA	PGF_{2a}	PGE_2	References
Bicuculline	2–4×	13–17×	—	—	56–58
Electroshock	2.5×				59
		5–14×	18×		60
					61
Picrotoxin	—	—	32×	—	62
Isoniazid	—	—	19×	—	62
Carbachol	1.5×	3×	70×	—	63
Pentylenetetrazol	2×	3–5×	—	—	50, 59, 63
			4–150×	4–40×	46, 61–64

[a]FFA, total free fatty acids; AA, arachidonic acid; $PGF_{2\alpha}$, prostaglandin $F_{2\alpha}$; PGE_2, prostaglandin E_2. Reproduced from ref. 3, with permission.

creases in the concentration of diacyglycerol and of free fatty acids—especially arachidonic acid, which then serves as precursor for a wide range of physiologically active metabolites such as prostaglandins, hydroxyeicosatetraenoic acids (HETEs), and leukotrienes. The initiating events for these cascades appear to be of two kinds. Neurotransmitters act on receptors linked via G proteins to phospholipase C, which hydrolyzes phosphoinositides to yield diacylglycerol and inositol 1,4,5-tris-phosphate. Glutamate can produce this effect by acting on the so-called quisqualate metabotropic receptor (66). Diacylglycerol is a modulator of protein kinase C.

The other major initiating step is activation of phospholipase A2, apparently via an increase in intracellular $[Ca^{2+}]$. The intracellular $[Ca^{2+}]$ is raised through Ca^{2+} entry via agonist-operated Ca^{2+} channels (such as the NMDA-receptor complex) and via voltage-dependent Ca^{2+} channels, as well as through Ca^{2+} release from intracellular stores.

PROTEIN SYNTHESIS

Regional protein synthesis can be estimated by the *in vivo* incorporation of labeled amino acid precursors ($[^3H]$tyrosine or $[^{14}C]$leucine) into protein and its visualization by autoradiography. Studies of this kind have shown impairment of protein synthesis during or subsequent to seizure activity in the rat and marmoset (67,68). The regional distribution of decreased or absent protein synthesis tends to correspond to the regions of greatest metabolic activation as shown by the deoxyglucose method, but with some unexplained variation and patchiness. The rate of protein synthesis depends on the cellular GDP/GTP ratio, with GDP increases being inhibitory (69). Any decrease in ATP level alters the GDP/GTP ratio (through the NDP kinase reaction), so that decreases in energy charge decrease protein synthesis.

Synthesis of some proteins is, however, increased following seizures. It has long been known that ornithine decarboxylase activity increases markedly in the brain 2–12 hr after electroshock or other seizures (70,71). This increase results from induction of enzyme synthesis; it leads to enhanced synthesis of polyamines such as spermidine, and it may be the mechanism that controls the increased synthesis of enkephalin following seizures (37,71). There is also evidence from immunocytochemical studies of the c-fos protein that the synthesis of this regulatory protein can be activated by seizure activity (72); c-fos messenger RNA is elevated in mouse brain 60 min after convulsions are initiated with pentylenetetrazol, apparently through increases in cytosolic and nuclear $[Ca^{2+}]$, thereby activating gene expression. The increases in c-fos are most marked in the nuclei of neurons in the cortex and limbic system.

Endocrine Changes Associated with Seizures

Seizures are associated with changes in the plasma concentration of several hormones. These arise from spread of seizure activity to the amygdala and to hypothalamic nuclei or other regions directly controlling the release from the pituitary of hormones or releasing factors. This is clearly the mechanism leading to the increase in plasma prolactin that occurs after electroconvulsive therapy (ECT) or spontaneous generalized seizures (73,74). The increases in prolactin and in vasopressin (75) are still seen after fully modified ECT, indicating that they arise from the electrical seizure activity and are not secondary to the peripheral events of a generalized seizure. In contrast, increases seen in plasma growth hormone, in adrenocorticotropic hormone (ACTH), and in cortisol following unmodified ECT are reduced if modified ECT is used, thus indicating a contribution from systemic events (76).

Generalized seizures are associated with marked activation of the autonomic nervous system (77). This has important effects on glucose metabolism. Increases in plasma epinephrine and norepinephrine can occur very early after seizure onset (within 1–5 min) (78). Blood glucose concentration commonly rises during prolonged seizures (79). This is a consequence of increased plasma epinephrine, sympathetic activation of hepatic glycolysis, and a rise in plasma glucagon. This hyperglycemia can, in turn, promote insulin release and be followed by a secondary hypoglycemia (80).

Behavioral Significance of Metabolic Changes

The majority of the biochemical changes described above are a reflection of enhanced neuronal and synaptic activity. It will be appreciated that there is enhanced activity in both excitatory and inhibitory pathways during seizure activity. In particular, during the spread of seizure activity, excitation either within gray matter (cortex) or in a network of deep nuclei may be surrounded by enhanced inhibition. Examples include (a) enhanced inhibition in the contralateral cortex and (b) activation of the inhibitory outputs of the substantia nigra pars reticulata.

Indeed, the marked increase in glucose utilization in the substantia nigra is likely to reflect primarily enhanced activity in GABAergic neurons. Thus behavioral manifestations of seizures are determined by enhanced excitation and synchronicity in certain

excitatory systems and also by enhanced inhibition affecting other pathways or structures. These two phenomena are manifest clinically when seizure activity directly involves the motor system. Thus tonic motor activity or rhythmic myoclonus involves particular motor groups (reflecting excitatory activity), or there is a sudden arrest of movement or loss of muscle tone (reflecting inhibitory activity). For focal motor seizures there is of course a good correlation between the regions of the motor cortex involved and the motor manifestations. There are also other motor syndromes indicative of particular patterns of seizure spread, such as the raised contralateral arm and contraversive head turning associated with frontal seizures involving the supplementary motor cortex. Precise anatomical correlations are harder to specify for seizures associated with more complex cognitive or behavioral manifestations. Thus the impairment of memory associated with complex partial seizures (81) could be caused by excessive excitation or excessive inhibition, or by the loss of normal function in limbic structures necessary to memory.

A further complicating factor is the variable time course of events in different brain areas: Some areas or nuclei may show continuing epileptic activity, other areas may show postictal depression of function, and others may show partial recovery. The behavioral concomitants of such complex interactive events may be unpredictable and not consistent between different ictal episodes.

SUMMARY

Ictal activity is associated with (a) very marked changes in energy metabolism and neurotransmitter turnover and (b) complex secondary effects on second messenger systems and the control of protein synthesis. These events both reflect the abnormal patterns of excitatory and inhibitory activity and entail further modifications of neuronal function. More refined *in vivo* measurements of neurochemical changes and their anatomy will be required if we are to correlate the more subtle ictal behavioral abnormalities with their underlying events.

ACKNOWLEDGMENT

The author's research has been supported by the Wellcome Trust, the Medical Research Council, and the British Epilepsy Association.

REFERENCES

1. Chapman AG, Meldrum BS, Seisjö BK. Cerebral metabolic changes during prolonged epileptic seizures. *J Neurochem* 1977;28:1025–1035.
2. Meldrum BS. Metabolic effects of prolonged epileptic seizures and the causation of epileptic brain damage. In: Rose FC, ed. *Metabolic disorders of the nervous system*. London: Pitman Medical, 1981;175–187.
3. Chapman AG. Cerebral energy metabolism and seizures. In: Pedley TA, Meldrum BS, eds. *Recent advances in epilepsy 2*. Churchill Livingstone: Edinburgh, 1985;19–63.
4. Meldrum BS, Nilsson B. Cerebral blood flow and metabolic rate early and late in prolonged epileptic seizures induced in rats by bicuculline. *Brain* 1976;99:523–542.
5. Borgström L, Chapman AG, Siesjö BK. Glucose consumption in the cerebral cortex of rat during bicuculline-induced status epilepticus. *J Neurochem* 1976;27:971–973.
6. Blennow G, Brierley JB, Meldrum BS, Siesjö BK. Epileptic brain damage. The role of systemic factors that modify cerebral energy metabolism. *Brain* 1978;101:68/–/00.
7. Henry TR, Engel J, Mazziotta JC. PET studies of functional cerebral anatomy in human epilepsy. In: Meldrum BS, Ferrendelli JA, Wieser HG, eds. *Anatomy of epileptogenesis*. London: John Libbey, 1988;155–178.
8. Lee BI, Markand ON, Wellman HN, Siddiqui AR, et al. HIPDM–SPECT in patients with medically intractable complex partial seizures: ictal study. *Arch Neurol* 1988;45:397–402.
9. Sokoloff L, Reivich M, Kennedy C, Des Rosiers MH, Patlak CS, Pettigrew KD, Sakurada O, Shinohara M. The [^{14}C]deoxyglucose method for the measurement of local cerebral glucose utilization: theory, procedure, and normal values in the conscious and anesthetized albino rat. *J Neurochem* 1977;28:897–916.
10. Engel J, Wolfson L, Brown L. Anatomical correlates of electrical and behavioral events related to amygdaloid kindling. *Ann Neurol* 1978;3:538–544.
11. Handforth A, Ackermann RF. Electrically induced limbic status and kindled seizures. In: Mcldrum BS, Ferrendelli JA, Wieser HG, eds. *Anatomy of epileptogenesis*. London: John Libbey, 1988;71–87.
12. Caveness WF, Kato M, Malamut BL, Hosokawa S, Wakisaka S, Raymond R, O'Neill BS. Propagation of focal motor seizures in the pubescent monkey. *Ann Neurol* 1980;7:213–221.
13. Engel J, Lubens P, Kuhl DE, Phelps ME. Local cerebral metabolic rate for glucose during petit mal absences. *Ann Neurol* 1985;17:121–128.
14. Theodore WH, Newark ME, Sato S, Brooks R, Patronas N, De La Paz R, DiChiro G, Kessler R.M., Margolin R, Manning RG, Channing M, Porter RJ. [^{18}F]Flurodeoxyglucose positron emission tomography in refractory complex partial seizures. *Ann Neurol* 1983;14:429–437.
15. Kuhl DE, Engel J, Phelps ME, Selin C. Epileptic patterns of local cerebral metabolism and perfusion in humans determined by emission computed tomography of ^{18}FDG and ^{13}NH$_3$. *Ann Neurol* 1980;8:348–360.
16. Engel J Jr, Kuhl DE, Phelps ME, Rausch R, Nuwer M. Local cerebral metabolism during partial seizures. *Neurology* 1983;33:400–413.
17. Engel J Jr, Kuhl DE, Phelps ME. Patterns of human local cerebral glucose metabolism during epileptic seizures. *Science* 1982;218:64–66.
18. Depresseux JC, Franck G, Sadzot B. Regional cerebral blood flow and oxygen uptake rate in human focal epilepsy. In: Baldy-Moulinier M, Ingvar DH, Meldrum BS, eds. *Current problems in epilepsy. I. Cerebral blood flow, metabolism and epilepsy*. London: John Libbey, 1984;76–81.
19. Franck G, Sadzot B, Depresseux JC, et al. Regional cerebral blood flow and oxygen uptake rate in human focal epilepsy and status epilepticus. In: Delgado-Escueta AV, et al., eds. *Basic mechanism of the epilepsies. Advances in neurology, Vol. 44*. New York: Raven Press, 1986;935–948.
20. Heinemann U, Konnerth A, Pumain R, Wadman WJ. Extracellular calcium and potassium concentration changes in chronic epileptic brain tissue. In: Delgado-Escueta AV, Ward AA, Woodbury DM, Porter RJ, eds. *Basic mechanisms of the epilepsies. Advances in neurology, vol 44*. New York: Raven Press, 1986;641–661.
21. Heinemann U, Hamon B. Calcium and epileptogenesis. *Exp Brain Res* 1986;65:1–10.
22. Pumain R, Menini C, Heinemann U, Louvel J, Silva-Barrat C. Chemical synaptic transmission is not necessary for epileptic seizures to persist in the baboon, *Papio papio. Exp Neurol* 1985;89:250–258.
23. Meldrum BS, Swan JH, Ottersen OP, Storm-Mathisen J. Redistribution of transmitter amino acids in rat hippocampus and cerebellum during seizures induced by L-allylglycine and bicuculline: an immunocytochemical study with antisera against conjugated GABA, glutamate and aspartate. *Neuroscience* 1987;22:17–27.
24. Chapman AG, Westerberg E, Premachandra M, Meldrum BS. Changes in regional neurotransmitter amino acid levels in rat brain during seizures induced by L-allylglycine, bicuculline, and kainic acid. *J Neurochem* 1984;43:62–70.
25. Whisler KE, Tews JK, Stone WE. Cerebral amino acids and lipids in drug-induced status epilepticus. *J Neurochem* 1968;15:215–220.
26. Chapman AG, Evans MC. Cortical GABA turnover during bicuculline seizures in rats. *J Neurochem* 1983;41:886–889.

27. Lehmann A, Hagberg H, Jacobson I, Hamberger A. Effects of status epilepticus on extracellular amino acids in the hippocampus. *Brain Res* 1985;147–151.
28. Calderini G, Carlsson A, Nordström C-H. Monoamine metabolism during bicuculline-induced epileptic seizures in the rat. *Brain Res* 1978; 157:295–302.
29. Green AR, Nutt DJ. Psychopharmacology of repeated seizures: possible relevance to the mechanism of action of electroconvulsive therapy. In: Iversen LL, Iversen SD, Snyder SH, eds. *Handbook of psychopharmacology*, vol 19. New York: Plenum Press, 1987;375–419.
30. Essman WB. *Neurochemistry of cerebral electroshock*. New York: John Wiley & Sons, 1973.
31. Hong JS, Yoshikawa K, Kanamatsu T, McGinty JF, Mitchell CL, Sabol SL. Repeated electroconvulsive shocks alter the biosynthesis of enkephalin and concentration of dynorphin in the rat brain. *Neuropeptides* 1985;5:557–560.
32. Sperk G, Wieser R, Widmann R, Singer EA. Kainic acid induced seizures: changes in somatostatin, substance P and neurotensin. *Neuroscience* 1986;17:1117–1126.
33. Wolf-Dieter R, Heuschneider G, Sperk G, Riederer P. Biochemical events in spontaneous seizures in the Mongolian gerbil. *Metab Brain Dis* 1989;4:3–7.
34. Meldrum B, Menini C. Effect of morphine, enkephalins, β-endorphin, and related compounds on seizure thresholds. In: Morselli PL, Lloyd KG, Löscher W, Meldrum M, Reynolds EH, eds. *Neurotransmitters, seizures and epilepsy*. New York: Raven Press, 1981;23–35.
35. Meldrum BS, Menini C, Naquet R, Riche D, Silva-Comte C. Absence of seizure activity following focal cerebral injection of enkephalins in a primate. *Regul Pept* 1981;2:383–390.
36. Caldecott-Hazard S, Engel J. Limbic post-ictal events: anatomical substrates and opioid receptor involvement. *Prog Neuropsychopharmacol Biol Psychiatry* 1987;11:389–418.
37. Gall C. Seizures induce dramatic and distinctly different changes in enkephalin, dynorphin, and CCK immunoreactivities in mouse hippocampal mossy fibers. *J Neurosci* 1988;8:1852–1862.
38. Chapman AG. Free fatty acid release and metabolism of adenosine and cyclic nucleotides during prolonged seizures. In: Morselli PL, Lloyd KG, Löscher W, Meldrum BS, Reynolds EH, eds. *Neurotransmitters, seizures & epilepsy*. New York: Raven Press, 1981;165–173.
39. Winn HR, Welsh EJ, Rubio R, Berne RM. Changes in brain adenosine during bicuculline-induced seizures in rats. Effects of hypoxia and altered systemic blood pressure. *Circ Res* 1980; 47:568–577.
40. Schultz V, Lowenstein JM. The purine nucleotide cycle. Studies of ammonia production and interconversions of adenine and hypoxanthine nucleotides and nucleosides by rat brain *in situ*. *J Biol Chem* 1978;253:1938–1943.
41. Sattin A. Increase in the content of adenosine 3',5'-monophosphate in mouse forebrain during seizures and prevention of the increase by methylxanthines. *J Neurochem* 1971;18:1087–1096.
42. Lust WD, Goldberg ND, Passonneau JV. Cyclic nucleotides in murine brain: the temporal relationship of changes induced in adenosine 3',5'-monophosphate and guanosine 3',5'-monophosphate following maximal electroshock or decapitation. *J Neurochem* 1976;26:5–10.
43. McCandless DW, Feussner GK, Lust WD, Passonneau JV. Metabolite levels in the brain following experimental seizures: the effects of isoniazid and sodium valproate in cerebellar and cerebral cortical layers. *J Neurochem* 1979;32: 755–760.
44. Rehncrona S, Siesjö BK, Westerberg E. Adenosine and cyclic AMP in cerebral cortex of rats in hypoxia, status epilepticus and hypercapnia. *Acta Physiol Scand* 1978;104:453–463.
45. Siesjö BK, Ingvar M, Folbergrová J, Chapman AG. Local cerebral circulation and metabolism in bicuculline-induced status epilepticus: relevance for development of cell damage. In: Delgado-Escueta AV, Wasterlain CG, Treiman DM, Porter RJ, eds. *Status epilepticus. Mechanisms of brain damage and treatment. Advances in neurology*, vol 34. New York: Raven Press, 1983;217–230.
46. Folco GC, Longiave D, Bosisio E. Relations between prostglandin E_2, F_{2a} and cyclic nucleotides levels in rat brain and induction of convulsions. *Prostaglandins* 1977;13:893–900.
47. Ferrendelli JA, Kinscherf DA. Cyclic nucleotides in epileptic brain: effects of pentylenetetrazol on regional cyclic AMP and cyclic GMP levels *in vivo*. *Epilepsia* 1977;18:525–531.
48. Gross RA, Ferrendelli JA. Effects of reserpine, propranolol, and aminophylline on seizure activity and CNS cyclic nucleotides. *Ann Neurol* 1979;6:296–301.
49. Palmer GC, Jones DJ, Medina MA, Stavinoha WB. Anticonvulsant drug actions on *in vitro* and *in vivo* levels of cyclic AMP in the mouse brain. *Epilepsia* 1979;20:95–104.
50. Ingvar M, Söderfeldt B, Kalimo H, Olsson Y, Seisjö BK. Metabolic, circulatory, and structural alterations in the rat brain induced by sustained pentylenetetrazol seizures. *Epilepsia* 1984;25:191–204.
51. Folbergrová J. Cyclic 3',5'-adenosine monophosphate in mouse cerebral cortex during homocysteine convulsions and their prevention by sodium phenobarbital. *Brain Res* 1975;92:165–169.
52. McCandless DW, Feussner GK, Lust WD, Passonneau JV. Metabolic levels in brain following experimental seizures: the effect of maximal electroshock and phenytoin in cerebellar layers. *J Neurochem* 1979;32:743–753.
53. Folbergrová J. Cyclic GMP and cyclic AMP in the cerebral cortex of mice during seizures induced by 3-mercaptopropionic acid: effects of anticonvulsants agents. *Neurosci Lett* 1980; 16:291–296.

54. Raabe W, Nicol S, Gumnit RJ, Goldberg ND. Focal penicillin epilepsy increases cyclic GMP in cerebral cortex. *Brain Res* 1978;144:185–188.

55. Garthwaite J, Charles SL, Chess-Williams R. Endothelium-derived relaxing factor release on activation of NMDA receptors suggests role as intercellular messenger in the brain. *Nature* 1988;336:385–388.

56. Chapman AG, Ingvar M, Siesjö BK. Free fatty acids in the brain in bicuculline-induced status epilepticus. *Acta Physiol Scand* 1980;110:335–336.

57. Siesjö BK, Ingvar M, Westerberg E. The influence of bicuculline-induced seizures on free fatty acid concentrations in cerebral cortex, hippocampus, and cerebellum. *J Neurochem* 1982;39:796–802.

58. Bazan NG, Morelli de Liberti SA, Rodriguez de Turco EB. Arachidonic acid and arachidonyl-diglycerols increase in rat cerebrum during bicuculline-induced status epilepticus. *Neurochem Res* 1982;7:839–843.

59. Bazan NG Jr. Changes in free fatty acids of brain by drug induced convulsions, electroshock and anaesthesia. *J Neurochem* 1971;18:1379–1385.

60. Zatz M, Roth RH. Electroconvulsive shock raises prostaglandins F in rat cerebral cortex. *Biochem Pharmacol* 1975;24:2101–2103.

61. Berchtold-Kanz E, Anhut H, Heldt R, Neufang B, Hertting G. Regional distribution of arachidonic acid metabolites in rat brain following convulsive stimuli. *Prostaglandins* 1981;22:65–79.

62. Spagnuolo C, Terzi C, Galli C. Differential response of brain $PGF_{2\alpha}$ synthesis to methionine sulfoximine in respect of other convulsant drugs. *Pharmacol Res Commun* 1978;10:541–544.

63. Marion J, Wolfe LS. Increase *in vivo* of unesterified fatty acids, prostaglandin $F_{2\alpha}$ but not thromoboxane B_2 in rat brain during drug induced convulsions. *Prostaglandins* 1978;16:99–110.

64. Steinhauer HB, Hertting G. Lowering of the convulsive threshold by non-steroidal anti-inflammatory drugs. *Eur J Pharmacol* 1981;69:199–203.

65. Bazan NG, Birkle DL, Tang W, Reddy TS. The accumulation of free arachidonic acid, diacylglycerols, prostaglandins, and lipoxygenase reaction products in the brain during experimental epilepsy. In: Delgado-Escueta AV, Ward AA, Woodbury DM, Porter RJ, eds. *Basic mechanisms of epilepsies. Advances in neurology, vol 44.* New York: Raven Press, 1986;879–902.

66. Sugiyama H, Ito I, Hirono C. A new type of glutamate receptor linked to inositol phospholipid metabolism. *Nature* 1987;325:531–533.

67. Kiessling M, Kleihues P. Regional protein synthesis in the rat brain during bicuculline-induced epileptic seizures. *Acta Neuropathol (Berl)* 1981;55:157–162.

68. Wasterlain CG, Dwyer BE, Fujikawa D. Metabolic studies of neonatal seizures in newborn marmoset monkeys: a possible role in the pathogenesis of brain damage for mismatch between flow and metabolism. In: Baldy-Moulinier M, Ingvar DH, Meldrum BS, eds. *Cerebral blood flow metabolism & epilepsy.* London: John Libbey, 1984;121–129.

69. Dwyer BE, Wasterlain CG. Regulation of brain protein synthesis during status epilepticus. In: Delgado-Escueta AV, Wasterlain CG, Treiman DM, Porter RJ, eds. *Status epilepticus. Mechanisms of brain damage and treatment. Advances in neurology, vol 34.* New York: Raven Press, 1983;297–304.

70. Pajunen AEI, Hietala OA, Viiansalo EL, Piha RS. Ornithine decarboxylase and S-adenosyl-L-methionine decarboxylase in mouse brain: effect of electrical stimulation. *J Neurochem* 1978;30:281–283.

71. Baudry M, Lynch G, Gall C. Induction of ornithine decarboxylase as a possible mediator of seizure-elicited changes in genomic expression in rat hippocampus. *J Neurosci* 1986;6:3430–3435.

72. Morgan JI, Cohen DR, Hempstead JL, Curran T. Mapping patterns of c-fos expression in the central nervous system after seizure. *Science* 1987;237:192–197.

73. Abbott RJ, Browning MCK, Davidson DLW. Serum prolactin and cortisol concentrations after grand mal seizures. *J Neurol Neurosurg Psychiatry* 1980;43:163–167.

74. Öhman R, Walinder J, Balldin J, Wallin L, Abrahamsson L. Prolactin response to electroconvulsive therapy. *Lancet* 1976;2:936–937.

75. Raskind M, Orenstein H, Weitzman RE. Vasopressin in depression. *Lancet* 1979;i:164.

76. Meldrum BS. Endocrine consequences of status epilepticus. In: Delgado-Escueta AV, Wasterlain CG, Treiman DM, Porter RJ, eds. *Status epilepticus. Advances in neurology, vol 34.* New York: Raven Press, 1983;399–403.

77. Meldrum BS. Pathophysiology. In: Laidlaw J, Richens A, eds. *A textbook of epilepsy,* 2nd ed. Edinburgh: Churchill Livingstone, 1982;456–487.

78. Weil-Malherbe H. The effect of convulsive therapy on plasma adrenaline and noradrenaline. *J Ment Sci* 1955;101:156–162.

79. Meldrum BS, Horton RW. Physiology of status epilepticus in primates. *Arch Neurol* 1973;28:1–9.

80. Meldrum BS, Horton RW, Bloom SR, Butler J, Keenan J. Endocrine factors and glucose metabolism during prolonged seizures in baboon. *Epilepsia* 1979;20:527–534.

81. Gallassi R, Morreale A, Lorusso S, Pazzaglia P, Lugaresi E. Epilepsy presenting as memory disturbances. *Epilepsia* 1988;29:624–629.

Advances in Neurology, Vol. 55, edited by
D. Smith, D. Treiman, and M. Trimble,
Raven Press, Ltd., New York © 1991.

3

Interictal Psychiatric Disorders

Neurochemical Aspects

E.H. Reynolds

Department of Neurology, Maudsley and King's College Hospitals, London SE5 8AZ, England

The metabolic basis of the interictal behavioral and psychiatric disorders of epilepsy must ultimately be confirmed by the study of patients. Here one immediately comes up against a seemingly formidable obstacle—a drug problem! Almost any metabolic disturbance which is detected in patients with epilepsy must be suspected to be, and usually is, due to antiepileptic drug therapy. Of course, it is possible to study untreated seizure patients, but for the most part they do not suffer from the behavioral and psychiatric disorders in question.

However, as discussed in detail in other chapters of this book (Chapters 13–15), evidence has accumulated in the last two decades that most antiepileptic drugs do contribute significantly to some of the interictal mental disorders (1–4). Studies in normal volunteers, as well as in newly diagnosed and chronic patients with epilepsy, have revealed subtle effects of the drugs on mood, cognition, and behavior in some patients, precipitating frank psychiatric disorder. Furthermore, amongst the many metabolic consequences of chronic antiepileptic drug therapy (5,6), it has been possible to relate some to the mental effects of the drugs (2,7). Some of the metabolic changes due to antiepileptic drug therapy (e.g., folate deficiency) are also relevant to the study of psychiatric disorders outside the field of epilepsy, as I will illustrate. Thus there can be, and is, a fruitful interchange of information and ideas from the study of both epilepsy and non-epilepsy populations. The fact that seizures (electroconvulsive therapy) are used as a form of treatment for some psychiatric disorders remains a key issue in this interchange (8).

In this review I will discuss some of the metabolic consequences of antiepileptic drug therapy that may be relevant to the behavioral and mental effects of the drugs, and, where appropriate, I will also relate them to studies of similar biochemical changes in non-epileptic psychiatric disorders. One area which could be relevant but which will not be covered in this discussion is the influence of the drugs on hormonal metabolism, the behavioral consequences of which have received very little attention.

MONOAMINES

It is appropriate to begin by examining the possible role of the serotonergic, dopaminergic, and other monoamine systems which have dominated metabolic thinking in relation to psychiatry for over 25 years. The evidence is rather sparse and, in some respects, controversial.

Cerebrospinal Fluid (CSF) Monoamine Metabolites

Chadwick and Crawford (9) have reviewed several studies of the concentrations of homovanillic acid (HVA) and 5-hydroxyindolacetic acid (5HIAA), as well as one study of 4-hydroxy-3-methoxyphenylethyleneglycol (MHPG), in the CSF of epilepsy patients. The concentrations of these metabolites are thought to reflect, to some degree, the turnover of catacholamines and serotonin in brain and spinal cord. No definite abnormalities have been detected for HVA or MHPG in treated or untreated patients with epilepsy. Some studies have suggested a lowering of 5HIAA in drug-treated patients, but Chadwick et al. (10) reported a trend in the opposite direction which became significant in patients exhibiting signs of drug toxicity. I am not aware of any systematic attempt to relate changes in CSF amine metabolites to mental changes in epilepsy. Furthermore, there would be difficulty in knowing whether any putative abnormalities are due to altered turnover of monoamines or to changes in the egress of the metabolites from the CSF.

Monoamine Precursors

An alternative approach to exloring monoamine metabolism in patients is to measure precursors such as plasma free tryptophan, which is known to influence serotonin turnover. Pratt et al. (11) have reported that carbamazepine significantly elevates plasma free tryptophan levels compared to those in untreated epilepsy patients or in normal controls, whereas phenytoin and phenobarbitone have the opposite effect (Table 1). Further-more, the rise in free tryptophan is correlated to blood levels of carbamazepine (Fig. 1). These investigators have suggested that the opposite effects of these drugs on tryptophan metabolism may be related to the different effects of the drugs on mood and mental function [i.e., the psychotropic effect of carbamazepine (Chapter 16) and the depressant effects of phenobarbitone and phenytoin (Chapters 13, 14)].

BIOLOGICAL ANTAGONISM

It is appropriate to consider Meduna's concept of biological antagonism here, because this is an area where monoamines as well as several other metabolic factors may play a role (8,12,13). The clinical aspects of the psychoses of epilepsy and of biological antagonism are discussed in Chapters 8 and 9. I will restrict myself to a discussion of the physiological, pharmacological, and metabolic evidence in support of Meduna's hypothesis, which I first attempted in 1968 (8).

We are presented with a curious paradox in the study of epilepsy. Although there is an increased prevalence of mental disorders in subjects with epilepsy, electroconvulsive therapy (ECT) is widely regarded as a useful treatment for some psychiatric disorders, especially depression, and its effectiveness is thought to depend on the production of generalized seizure activity. Indeed, amongst other reasons, it was the improvement in the mental state of

TABLE 1. *Plasma tryptophan concentrations in drug-treated and untreated epilepsy patients and normal volunteers[a]*

Subjects	Number of subjects	Bound tryptophan (μg/ml)	Free tryptophan (μg/ml)	Bound/free ratio
Normal volunteers	33	8.76	1.33	6.59
Epilepsy patients				
Untreated	15	7.67‡	1.32	5.83
On PB	7	7.82	1.01†	7.76
On DPH	38	7.41§	1.15†	6.44
On CBZ	20	9.86*	2.70*	3.65*

[a]Data are expressed as the antilog mean. PB, phenobarbitone; DPH, phenytoin; CBZ, carbamazepine. *All comparisons with CBZ are significant ($p < 0.001$) except with bound plasma tryptophan for PB group ($p < 0.005$) and normal volunteers ($p < 0.025$). Other comparisons with normal volunteers: †$p < 0.05$, ‡$p < 0.025$, §$p < 0.001$. (From ref. 11, with permission.)

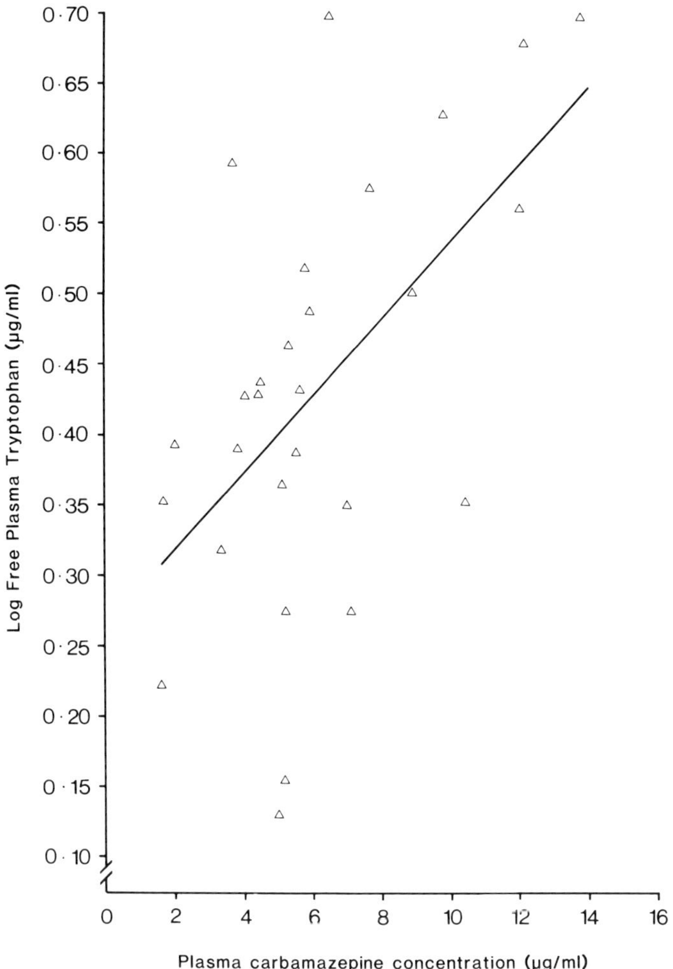

FIG. 1. Relationship between plasma carbamazepine and plasma free tryptophan in patients with epilepsy. (From ref. 11, with permission.)

some patients with catatonic schizophrenia following spontaneous seizures that led Meduna (14) to introduce convulsive therapy. Hill (15), in his study of the electroencephalogram (EEG) in episodic behavior disorders, comments that besides catatonic schizophrenics, in whom paroxysmal EEG activity may be found in up to 25%, other occasional patients with behavior or psychopathic disorders with paroxysmal EEG findings may benefit psychologically from the occurrence of epileptic seizures. He proposed that the paroxysmal spike or spike-and-wave activity in the catatonic schizophrenic may represent a "homeostatic" response on the part of the organism, with the EEG changes disappearing with psychological recovery. Stevens (16,17) has also commented that all that spikes are not necessarily epilepsy, and that such spike activity might have "restitutive" functions. In seizure patients, special interest has centered on a subgroup in whom psychotic episodes seem to alternate with seizures—as, for example, reviewed by Landolt (18), who also described the "forced normalization" of the EEG in which epileptic activity may disappear as seizures cease and the patient becomes psychotic. I have pointed out (8) that

TABLE 2. *Evidence of biological antagonism between epilepsy and schizophrenia*[a]

	Epilepsy	Schizophrenia
Neurophysiology		
EEG	Forced normalization (Landolt)	Homeostatic (Hill)
Neuropharmacology		
Antiepileptic drugs		
Barbiturates	Therapeutic	Aggravation
Phenothiazines	Aggravation (convulsant)	Therapeutic
Neurochemistry		
Dopamine agonists	Therapeutic	Aggravate
Dopamine antagonists	Aggravation	Therapeutic
Methionine	?Therapeutic	Aggravation
Methionine-sulfoximine	Convulsant	?Therapeutic
Folic acid	Aggravation (convulsant)	Therapeutic

[a]Modified from ref. 8, with permission.

Landolt's "forced normalization" observations are the inverse of Hill's "homeostatic" proposals (Table 2).

Some pharmacological considerations also support the concept of an inverse relationship between epilepsy and schizophrenia. For example, it is well known that phenothiazines, the main pharmacological weapon in the treatment of schizophrenia, have convulsant properties and may precipitate seizures in some patients (19). Furthermore, antiepileptic drugs and barbiturates exert a consistently unfavorable effect in schizophrenic psychoses, and they may occasionally play a role in precipitating schizophrenia-like psychoses in epilepsy patients (20).

There is also a surprising amount of biochemical data which support the concept of biological antagonism (Table 2). One of the most consistent metabolic findings in schizophrenia is that the administration of methionine aggravates some 40% of patients (21). It is well known that the methionine antagonist methionine-sulfoximine is a potent convulsant which has been used in experimental studies of seizure mechanisms (22). Less well substantiated is a possible therapeutic effect of methionine in epilepsy (23) and of methionine-sulfoximine in schizophrenia (24). There is now abundant experimental evidence that folic acid and its derivatives have potent excitatory properties which are used for the experimental study of epilepsy (25–27). There is also evidence (*vide infra*) that folic acid deficiency can aggravate schizophrenia and other psychiatric disorders and that this can be rectified by folate replacement (28). Finally, as Trimble and Meldrum (13,29) point out, dopamine antagonists (including phenothiazines) are therapeutic in schizophrenia and reduce seizure threshold, whereas dopamine agonists (such as L-dopa or amphetamines) have the reverse effect, elevating seizure threshold but aggravating or precipitating psychoses (Fig. 2).

GAMMA-AMINOBUTYRIC ACID (GABA)

The role of the inhibitory neurotransmitter, GABA, in seizure mechanisms has been of widespread theoretical, experimental, and practical interest for many years. This has culminated in the development of vigabatrin, a GABA-transaminase inhibitor, as a promising new antiepileptic drug for the treatment of chronic epilepsy (30). But what of the role of GABA in interictal psychological disorders? Clinical studies with vigabatrin suggest that it may be implicated at least with respect to mood disorders. In a review of 1147 patients treated with vigabatrin, "nervousness" was reported in 3.5% and depression in 2.7% (P. J. Lewis, *personal communication*, 1989). In 127 children treated with the drug, excitement or agitation was reported in 8.8% (31). In an open and double-blind study of the effect of vigabatrin on seizures (32) and mood (33) in

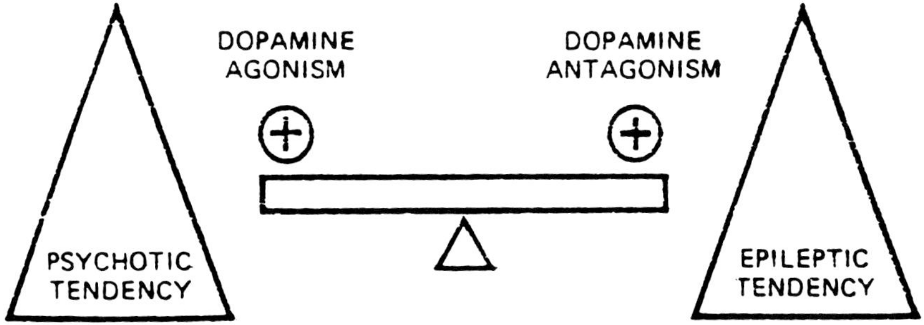

FIG. 2. Relationship between epilepsy, psychosis, and dopamine. (From ref. 13, with permission.)

chronic epilepsy, standard psychometric assessments included the Beck Inventory for Depression, the Mood Adjective Check List (MACL), and the Spielberger State Anxiety Inventory (STAI). In the open phase, 4 out of 24 (17%) patients were withdrawn from the study because of depression. Overall, there was a significant increase in anxiety on the STAI, as well as a trend toward increases in depression scores on the Beck and MACL, despite the improvement in seizure control that occurred in two-thirds of the patients. In 14 patients out of the original 24 who then proceeded to a double-blind phase (i.e., 7 ran-

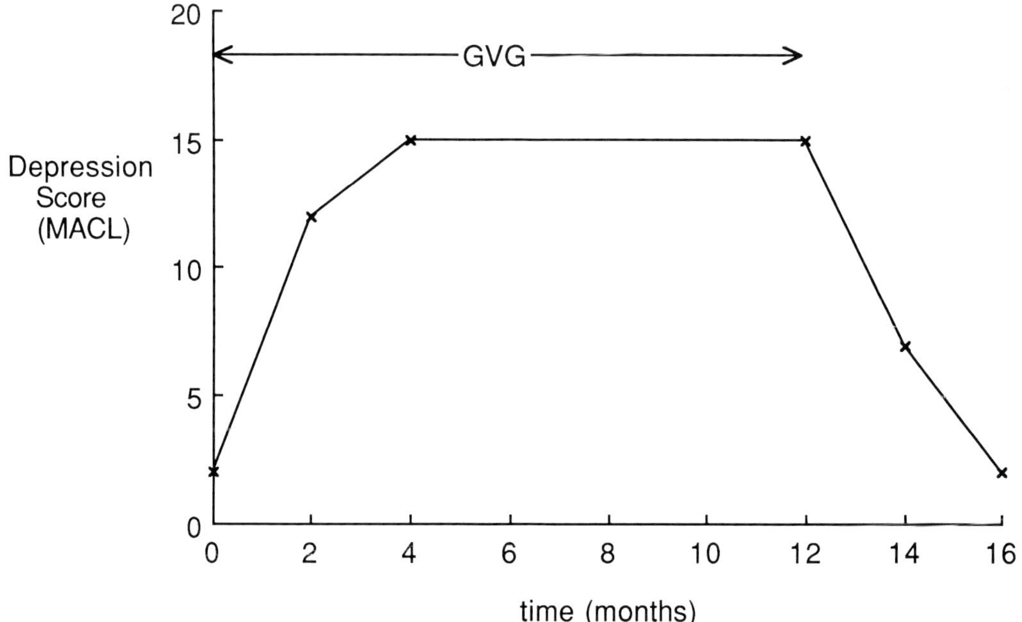

FIG. 3. Relationship between depression and vigabatrin administration in a 22-year-old female patient with temporal lobe epilepsy.

domized to stay on vigabatrin and 7 to switch to placebo), no significant differences in mood scores between the drug and placebo were seen, but the numbers in the two groups were small and the depressive reactors had been screened out. It should also be stressed that the majority of patients receiving vigabatrin experience no change in mood, or an improvement in mood or well-being, associated with better seizure control. It is possible that patients who experience a depressive reaction, an example of which is illustrated in Fig. 3, are more vulnerable for constitutional or psychosocial reasons. Nevertheless, the role of GABA is reinforced by the study of Nurnberger et al. (34), who administered one to four doses of GABA (0.1 to 1.0 mg/kg) or placebo intravenously to normal subjects and to euthymic bipolar affective disorder patients. Mood was assessed on the Profile of Mood States, and all subjects reported dysphoria with GABA—especially an increase in Tension score and decrease in Elation score, which was not seen with placebo. This anxiogenic effect of GABA, as well as the anxiety depressive reactions with vigabatrin, is of interest in view of the antianxiety effects of benzodiazepines, some of whose actions are linked to the GABA receptor (35).

FOLIC ACID

It is well established that antiepileptic drug therapy, mainly with phenytoin and barbiturates, leads to a fall in serum, red blood cell, and CSF folate in a high proportion of patients (36,37). This subject drew me into the field of epilepsy 25 years ago, and from our earliest studies it seemed plausible that drug-induced folate deficiency had implications for the mental state of some epilepsy patients (7,38). The association between the fall in folate levels and various mental disorders—especially depression and dementia, but also some psychoses—seemed remarkable; and the rare, drug-induced megaloblastic anemia was invariably accompanied by neuropsychiatric complications which also usually responded to folic acid therapy (7,36). An open study of folic acid therapy for 6 months in 26 epilepsy outpatients with low serum folate levels (with-

out hematological complications) suggested that the main effect of the vitamin was on drive, initiative, motivation, mood alertness, and sociability (7,39).

Although the neurological and psychiatric complications of folate deficiency from all its causes are now more widely accepted (40–42), the subject has remained more uncertain within the field of epilepsy. The main reason for this is that several placebo-controlled trials of folate in epilepsy subjects with low serum folate levels proved negative, including one in which I participated (36,37). Several possible factors may have contributed to the difficulties and controversies within this field:

1. It is now apparent that even in the presence of folate deficiency or vitamin B_{12} deficiency, from all their causes severe enough to produce megaloblastic anemia, as many as one-third have no neurological complications (43).

2. A serum folate level is a less reliable guide to folate status than is a red blood cell folate level, and thus a low serum folate level may be of no immediate neuropsychiatric significance in more than one-third of patients.

3. Changes in mental state induced by the vitamin are often slow to occur over many months, and clinical trials should therefore probably be undertaken for at least 6 months (28). This is also true of mental changes induced by alterations (especially reduction) of antiepileptic drug therapy, as Thompson and Trimble (44) have described.

4. The type of mental change most frequently seen with the vitamin (i.e., changes in drive, mood, etc.) will not be detected by the standard I.Q.-type psychometric techniques which were employed in the earlier folate trials. This type of mental change is also seen with alterations in antiepileptic drug therapy (e.g., reducing polytherapy or switching from phenytoin to carbamazepine), for which new psychometric techniques have since been developed (4).

5. In seizure subjects, perhaps even more so than in non-seizure subjects, many biological and psychosocial factors contribute to mental illness, making it difficult to establish the precise role of any individual factor (12).

In the last decade, four further studies—one in children (45), two in adults (46,47), and one in the community (48)—have all again emphasized the close association between (a) folate deficiency in epilepsy subjects and (b) that in patients with mental disorder, mainly depression. The latter study is of particular interest, because it overcame the criticism of selection bias in hospital- or institution-based investigations and also employed precise standardized assessments of mental function—in particular the Goldberg Clinical Interview Schedule. The investigators showed, for example, that low serum folate in patients with epilepsy is correlated with depression but not anxiety.

Outside the studies of epilepsy there has been growing literature relating folate deficiency to various neuropsychiatric disorders in patients with megaloblastic anemia, as well as in the fields of psychiatry, neurology, and geriatrics (37,40,43,49,50). Although depression is the most frequently reported complication, the range of disorders is similar to that seen with vitamin B_{12} deficiency and includes dementia, organic psychoses, peripheral neuropathy, and even, rarely, subacute combined degeneration of the spinal cord. Recently, Carney et al. (51) have examined red blood cell folate levels in a series of 243 consecutive admissions to an acute psychiatric unit in a district general hospital. Definite folate defi-

ciency (red blood cell folate level >150 ng/ml) was seen in 12%. A borderline deficiency state (red blood cell folate level >200 ng/ml) was found in as many as 31%. As in the earlier studies of serum folate, low red blood cell folate was again mainly associated with depression, although low values were sometimes seen in any diagnostic category. As always, the question arises as to why so many psychiatric patients have definite or borderline folate deficiency (52). The most plausible explanation is that the deficiency is due to a poor diet secondary to the psychological disorder. Although this may be true of many patients (perhaps even the majority), it is probably an oversimplification of the complete explanation. Attempts to show that the deficiency is dietary in origin have not been very successful (53–55). In this connection the association of depression and folate deficiency in patients with epilepsy is of special interest because the deficiency is, to a very large extent, *drug*-induced. Drugs, barbiturates, and alcohol may possibly contribute to the deficiency in non-epilepsy psychiatric subjects, but it was notable in the red blood cell folate study that the levels in depressed patients, who were not obviously malnourished, were similar to those in an alcoholic group who were more apparently malnourished. Clearly,

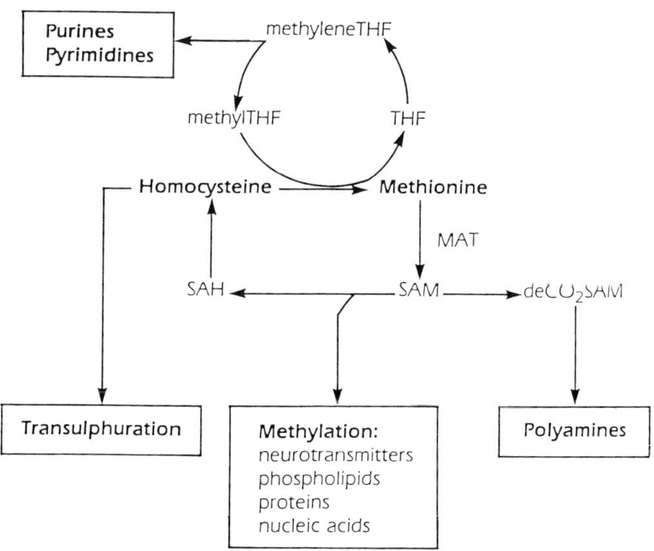

FIG. 4. Relationship between folate cycle, *S*-adenosylmethionine, and methylation.

there is much to learn about the causes of folate deficiency in psychiatric patients, and the possible role of malabsorption has not been examined.

Whatever the causes of the folate deficiency, the significance of the deficiency in relation to the underlying psychological disorder is another issue of considerable interest. Even when the deficiency state is secondary to the psychiatric illness, it is possible that it will eventually aggravate the mental state. I have emphasized the close links between folate deficiency and mood disorder. Recent evidence suggesting that *S*-adenosylmethionine (SAM) has antidepressant properties (*vide infra*) lends credence to the view that folate deficiency, through its links with SAM and methylation in the nervous system (Fig. 4), as well as via other mechanisms, can play an etiological role (39,49,56,57). Support for this view comes from a double-blind placebo-controlled trial of folate replacement (28). Forty-one patients (24 with depressive illness and 17 with schizophrenia) with red blood cell folate levels >200 mg/ml were randomly and blindly allocated to methylfolate (15 mg daily) or placebo for 6 months in addition to standard psychiatric treatment, including psychopharmacological measures. In both the depressed and schizophrenic subgroups, the addition of methylfolate was associated with significantly better clinical and social recovery. The main effect of the vitamin again was on mood, and there was evidence that the longer the treatment the more apparent were the differences with the placebo group. Methylfolate is the form of folate that is transported into the nervous system, and it would clearly be of interest to undertake studies with this folate derivative in epilepsy subjects.

FOLIC ACID SAM

The folate cycle is a mechanism for synthesizing methyl groups which eventually find their way via the synthesis of methionine to SAM, which is the methyl donor in innumerable methylation reactions in the nervous system, involving monoamines, polyamines, neurotransmitters, membrane phospholipids, proteins, and nucleoproteins (56) (Fig. 4). With my interest in folate, I was therefore intrigued 10 years ago to learn of the Italian studies suggesting that SAM had antidepressant properties (56,58). This observation, together with my own and other studies linking folate deficiency to depression, strongly suggests that methylation in the nervous system is implicated in mood and affective disorders (56,57). The Italian claims for SAM have since been supported by studies in the United Kingdom (59,60) as well as by recent trials in the United States (61).

Until 3 years ago, SAM had only been available for parenteral administration; my colleagues and I (62) have undertaken some pilot observations in epilepsy subjects. We gave SAM openly (200 mg per day, intravenously) to three chronic epilepsy patients, and the observations are summarized in Table 3. All three had long-standing chronic partial seizures resistant to currently available antiepileptic drugs. The first patient, a 45-year-old woman on phenytoin and carbamazepine, was also depressed. Between the fourth and eighth injection, her mood and activity improved considerably; at this point she decided to visit some relatives in another part of the country, thus terminating the study. The second patient, a young woman who was mentally retarded, had already had an unsuccessful right

TABLE 3. *Chronic epilepsy patients: open SAM (200 mg per day, intravenously)*

Case	Sex	Age	Seizures	Drugs[a]	Mental state	Injections	Response
1	F	45	Chronic partial	CBZ DPH	Depressed	8	Mood elevation
2	F	22	Chronic partial (right hemispherectomy)	CBZ	Low I.Q.; drowsy and withdrawn	14	Arousal
3	M	24	Chronic partial (Sturge-Weber)	CBZ DPH	I.Q. 50; mute, withdrawn	3	Activation

[a]CBZ, carbamazepine; DPH, phenytoin.

TABLE 4. *Chronic epilepsy patients: SAM versus placebo (8–14 days), single-blind*

Case	Sex	Age	Seizures	Drugs[a]	Mental state	Response
1	F	18	Chronic partial	CBZ	Withdrawn	+
2	M	22	Drop attacks	CBZ	Normal	−
3	F	25	Chronic partial	—	Normal	−
4	M	19	Drop attacks, chronic partial	PB, SV	Retarded	+ (Overactive)

[a]CBZ, carbamazepine; PB, phenobarbitone; SV, sodium valproate. Response: −, activation; +, elevated mood.

hemispherectomy for drug-resistant partial seizures. She now presented an unusual problem of drowsiness which had persisted despite reduction of her antiepileptic medication to carbamazepine alone. Within 24 hr of the first injection of SAM, she was much more alert and remained so throughout the course of daily injections, although the effect was beginning to fade by the end of the 2 weeks. The third patient had drug-resistant seizures associated with Sturge-Weber syndrome and was transferred from an institution for the mentally retarded, where he had been mute and withdrawn for several months. After the third injection he spoke his first words, which were that he did not want any more injections. He was subsequently treated with methylfolate orally for his drug-induced folate deficiency, and he continued to show considerably more interest, activity, and communication. Between them, these three patients exhibited three of the central features of SAM—namely, its effects on arousal (case 2), on activation (case 3), and on mood (case 1).

We then undertook a single-blind study comparing SAM (200 mg per day, intravenously) against placebo (intravenous saline) for 8–14 days in four additional chronic epilepsy patients (Table 4). Two of the four showed an effect of SAM on mental function. An 18-year-old girl who was previously quiet and withdrawn displayed much improved interest, improved motor and social activity, and elevated mood during the second week on SAM. A 19-year-old retarded young man became very overactive and elated between the fourth and seventh injections of SAM, and we were concerned that he was becoming hypomanic. During the second week the hypomanic features subsided, but the overall improvement in mood and activity continued.

We observed carefully the effect of SAM on seizure frequency in our patients, because there is evidence that folic acid can aggravate seizure control in some epilepsy patients (39,63) and in experimental models (25,26,27,64). However, we did not observe any adverse effect of SAM on seizure control in these patients. Nor did we observe any striking beneficial effects on seizures, although there was a suspicion of a late rebound deterioration of seizure control during the placebo phase. No effect of SAM on phenytoin or carbamazepine blood levels was observed.

These preliminary observations on the effect of SAM in subjects with epilepsy are in keeping with the reports of an influence of SAM on mood and arousal and suggest that more extensive and longer-term studies with the newly available *oral* SAM (65) would be of interest in epilepsy subjects with and without mood disturbances, and also with and without drug-induced folate deficiency.

FOLIC ACID, GABA, SEIZURES, AND DEPRESSION

I have discussed the role of folate and of GABA in interictal mental disorders, but both are also implicated in seizure mechanisms. The possible role of GABA in seizure mechanisms is well known and is discussed in detail in Chapter 2. Although the convulsant effect of folic acid in patients with epilepsy has been a somewhat contentious subject (37,39), there is now abundant evidence that folates have potent excitatory properties in several species and can be utilized as experimental models of epilepsy (25–27). Folic acid enhances the electrical kindling of seizures in the rat (66) and can even be used on its own to kindle seizures (67).

The mechanism of the excitatory properties

of folates is uncertain, but there is growing evidence that they may do so by blocking or reversing GABA-mediated inhibition. Utilizing a microelectrophoretic technique on single neurons of the cat cerebral cortex, Davies and Watkins (68) showed that the vitamin, especially the formyl derivative, could reverse the inhibitory effects of GABA by up to 80%. Hill and Miller (69) then reported that folic acid antagonized presynaptic inhibition in the rat cuneate nucleus. Clifford and Ferrendelli (70) suggested that the excitatory actions of folates were more likely to be the result of disinhibition than of direct excitation. Otis et al. (71) confirmed that the application of folic acid to neurons results in a reduction of the GABA-mediated inhibitory postsynaptic potentials, as well as resulting in a reduction of the response to iontophoretically applied GABA. In a series of experiments in the rat employing intra-neocortical administration, Van Rijn and co-workers (72,73) showed that the epileptic phenomena induced by folates resemble those induced by disinhibitory compounds (i.e., bicuculline, strychnine, penicillin, and picrotoxin) but differ in many respects from those induced by direct excitatory drugs (i.e., kainic acid, carbachol, and neostigmine). The same investigators also reported that folates reverse the inhibiting effect of GABA on the binding of the cage-convulsant ^{3}H-*t*-butylbicycloorthobenzoate (^{3}H-TBOB) to the GABAa-receptor complex. Furthermore, the rank order of this *in vitro* effect by the different folate derivatives correlated with the rank order of epileptogenicity determined by their *in vivo* studies.

In view of the opposing effects of folates and GABA at the synaptic level, it is tempting to suggest that this relationship is relevant not only to their respective excitatory and inhibitory role in seizure mechanisms, but also to their opposing influence on mood—namely, the mood elevating effects of folates and the mood depressing and anxiogenic effects of GABA and vigabatrin.

REFERENCES

1. Reynolds EH. Iatrogenic disorders in epilepsy. In: Williams D, ed. *Modern trends in neurology,* vol 5. London: Butterworths, 1970;271–286.

2. Reynolds EH. Mental effects of antiepileptic medication. *Epilepsia* 1983;24(Suppl 2):S85–S95.

3. Trimble MR, Reynolds EH. Anticonvulsant drugs and mental symptoms. *Psychol Med* 1976;6:169–178.

4. Trimble MR, Reynolds EH. Neuropsychiatric toxicity and anticonvulsant drugs. In: Matthews WB, Glaser GH, eds. *Recent advances in clinical neurology,* vol 4. Edinburgh: Churchill Livingstone, 1984;261–280.

5. Reynolds EH. Chronic antiepileptic toxicity. *Epilepsia* 1975;16:319–352.

6. Schmidt D. *Adverse effects of antiepileptic drugs.* New York: Raven Press, 1982.

7. Reynolds EH. Mental effects of anticonvulsants, and folic acid metabolism. *Brain* 1968;91:197–214.

8. Reynolds EH. Epilepsy and schizophrenia. Relationship and biochemistry. *Lancet* 1968;1:398–401.

9. Chadwick D, Crawford P. Clinical, biochemical and pharmacological factors in seizures. In: Trimble MR, Reynolds EH, eds. *What is epilepsy? The clinical and scientific basis of epilepsy.* Edinburgh: Churchill Livingstone, 1986; 53–66.

10. Chadwick D, Jenner P, Reynolds EH. Serotonin metabolism in human epilepsy: the influence of anticonvulsant drugs. *Ann Neurol* 1977;1:218–224.

11. Pratt JA, Jenner P, Johnson AL, et al. Anticonvulsant drugs alter plasma tryptophan concentrations in epileptic patients: implications for antiepileptic action and mental function. *J Neurol Neurosurg Psychiatry* 1984;47:1131–1133.

12. Reynolds EH. Biological factors in psychological disorders associated with epilepsy. In: Reynolds EH, Trimble MR, eds. *Epilepsy and psychiatry.* Edinburgh: Churchill Livingstone, 1981;264–290.

13. Trimble MR, Meldrum BS. Monoamines, epilepsy and schizophrenia. In: Obiols J, Ballus E, Gonzales M, Pujol J, eds. *Biological psychiatry today.* Amsterdam: Elsevier, 1979;470–475.

14. Meduna L. *Die Konvulsionstherapie der Schizophrenie.* Halle: Carl Marhold, 1937.

15. Hill D. EEG in episodic, psychotic and psychopathetic behaviour. *Electroencephalogr Neurophysiol* 1952;4:419–442.

16. Stevens JR. All that spikes is not fits. In: Shagass C, Gershon S, Friedhoff AJ, eds. *Psychopathology and brain dysfunction.* New York: Raven Press, 1975;183–198.

17. Stevens JR. All that spikes is not fits. In: Trimble MR, Reynolds EH, eds. *What is epilepsy. The clinical and scientific basis of epilepsy.* Edinburgh: Churchill Livingstone, 1986;97–115.

18. Landolt II. Serial electroencephalographic investigations during psychotic episodes in epileptic patients and during schizophrenic attacks. In: Lorentz de Haas, ed. *Lectures on epilepsy.* Amsterdam: Elsevier, 1958;91–133.

19. Toone BK, Fenton GW. Epileptic seizures induced by psychotropic drugs. *Psychol Med* 1977;7:265–270.

20. Stevens JR. Risk factors for psychopathology in

individuals with epilepsy. In: Koella WP, Trimble MR, eds. *Temporal lobe epilepsy, mania, and schizophrenia and the limbic system. Advances in biological psychiatry,* vol 8. Basel: Karger, 1982;56–80.

21. Cohen SM, Nichols A, Wyatt R, Pollin W. The administration of methionine to chronic schizophrenic patients: a review of 10 studies. *Biol Psychiatry* 1974;8:209–225.

22. Tower DB. *Neurochemistry of epilepsy.* Springfield, IL: Charles C Thomas, 1960.

23. Kalousek J, Kohout J, Pinta Z, Boska F. *Cesk Neurol* 1963;26:21.

24. Heath RG, Nesselhof W, Timmons E. *Arch Gen Psychiatry* 1966;14:213.

25. Hommes OR, Hollinger JL, Jansen NJT, et al. In: Convulsant properties in folate compounds: some considerations and speculations. In: Botez MI, Reynolds EH, eds. *Folic acid in neurology, psychiatry and internal medicine.* New York: Raven Press, 1979;285–316.

26. Arends J, Hommes O, Doesburg W, et al. Folate activated partial epilepsy: a model for drug study. In: Dam MM, Gram L, Penry JK, eds. *Advances in epileptology: XIIth Epilepsy International Symposium.* New York: Raven Press, 1981;653–669.

27. Kaijima M, Riche D, Rousseva S, et al. Electroencephalographic, behavioural and histopathologic features of seizures induced by intra-amygdala application of folic acid in cats. *Exp Neurol* 1984;86:313–321.

28. Godfrey P, Toone BK, Flynn T, Carney MWP, Laundy M, Bottiglieri T, Chanarin I, Reynolds EH. Methyl folate enhances recovery from psychiatric illness. *Lancet* 1990;336:392–395.

29. Trimble MR. The relationship between epilepsy and schizophrenia: a biochemical hypothesis. *Biol Psychiatry* 1977;12:299–304.

30. Richens A. Vigabatrin. In: Levi RH, Mattson RH, Meldrum BS, Penry JK, Dreifuss FE, eds. *Antiepileptic drugs,* 3rd ed. 1989;in press.

31. Livingston JH, Beaumont D, Arzimanoglou A, Aicardi J. Vigabatrin in the treatment of epilepsy in children. *Br J Clin Pharmacol* 1989;27(Suppl 1):113S–118S.

32. Ring H, Heller A, Farr I, Reynolds EH. Vigabatrin: rational treatment for chronic epilepsy. *J Neurol Neurosurg Psychiatry* 1990;In press.

33. Birbeck KA, Ossetin J, Ring H, et al. Vigabatrin and mood. Paper presented to 18th Epilepsy International Congress, New Delhi, 1989.

34. Nurnberger JI, Berrettini WH, Simmons-Alling S, et al. Intravenous GABA administration is anxiogenic in man. *Psychiatry Res* 1986;19:113–117.

35. Enna SJ, Karbon EW. GABA receptors: an overview. In: Olsen RW, Venter JC, eds. *Benzodiazepine–GABA receptors and chloride channels: structural and functional properties.* New York: Alan R Liss, 1986;41–56.

36. Reynolds EH. Diphenylhydantoin: haematologic toxicity. In: Woodbury DM, Penry JK, Schmidt P, eds. *Antiepileptic drugs,* 1st ed. New York: Raven Press, 1972;247–262.

37. Reynolds EH. Neurological aspects of folate and vitamin B12 metabolism. In: Hoffbrand AV ed. *Clinics in haematology,* vol 5. London: WB Saunders, 1976;661–696.

38. Reynolds EH. Anticonvulsant therapy, folic acid metabolism and mental symptoms. Proceedings of IVth World Congress of Psychiatry. *Excerpta Med Int Cong Ser* 1966;150:1733–1735.

39. Reynolds EH. Effects of folic acid on the mental state and fit frequency of drug treated epileptic patients. *Lancet* 1967;1:1186–1188.

40. Botez MI, Reynolds EH, eds. *Folic acid in neurology, psychiatry and internal medicine.* New York: Raven Press, 1979.

41. Lishman WA. *Organic psychiatry,* 2nd ed. Oxford: Blackwell, 1988.

42. Trimble MR. *Biological psychiatry.* Chichester: Wiley, 1988.

43. Shorvon SD, Carney MWP, Chanarin I, Reynolds EH. The neuropsychiatry of megaloblastic anaemia. *Br Med J* 1980;281:1036–1042.

44. Thompson EJ, Trimble MR. Anticonvulsant drugs and cognitive functions. *Epilepsia* 1982;23:531–544.

45. Trimble MR, Corbett J, Donaldson D. Folic acid and mental symptoms in children with epilepsy. *J Neurol Neurosurg Psychiatry* 1980;43:1030–1034.

46. Rodin E, Schmaltz S. Folate levels in epileptic patients. In: Parsonage M, Grant RHE, Craig AG, Ward AA, eds. *Advances in epileptology: XIVth Epilepsy International Symposium.* New York: Raven Press, 1983;143–153.

47. Robertson MM, Trimble MR. Depressive illness in patients with epilepsy: a review. *Epilepsia* 1983;24(Suppl):S109–S116.

48. Edeh J, Toone BK. Antiepileptic therapy, folate deficiency and psychiatric morbidity: results of a survey in general practice. *Epilepsia* 1985;26:434–440.

49. Carney MWP. Serum folate values in 423 psychiatric patients. *Br Med J* 1967;IV:512–516.

50. Reynolds EH. Folic acid and neuropsychiatry. *Farm Terapia* 1985;2:163–168.

51. Carney MWP, et al. Red cell folate concentrations in psychiatric patients. *J Affective Disorders* 1990;19:207–213.

52. Carney MWP, Sheffield BF. Associations of subnormal serum folate and vitamin B12 and effects of replacement therapy. *J Nerv Ment Dis* 1970;150:404–412.

53. Reynolds EH, Preece JM, Bailey J, Coppen A. Folate deficiency in depressive illness. *Br J Psychiatry* 1970;117:287–292.

54. Thornton WE, Thornton BP. Folic acid, mental function and dietary habits. *J Clin Psychiatry* 1978;39:315–322.

55. Ghadirian AM, Ananth J, Engelsmann F. Folic acid deficiency and depression. *Psychosomatics* 1980;21:926–929.

56. Reynolds EH, Stramentinoli G. Folic acid, S-adenosylmethionine and affective disorder. *Psychol Med* 1983;13:705–710.

57. Reynolds EH, Carney MWP, Toone BK. Methylation and mood. *Lancet* 1984;2:196–198.

58. Agnoli A, Andreoli V, Casacchia M, Serbo R.

Effect of *S*-adenosyl-L-methionine (SAMe) upon depressive symptoms. *J Psychiatr Res* 1976;13: 43–54.

59. Carney MWP, Martin R, Bottiglieri T, et al. The switch mechanism in affective illness and SAM. *Lancet* 1983;1:820–821.

60. Carney MWP, Edeh J, Bottiglieri T, et al. Affective illness and *S*-adenosylmethionine: a preliminary report. *Clin Neuropharmacol* 1986;9:379–385.

61. Bell KM, Plom L, Bunney WE, et al. *S*-Adenosylmethionine treatment of depression; a controlled clinical trial. *Am J Psychiatry* 1988; 145:1110–1114.

62. Reynolds EH, Carney WMP, Toone BK, et al. Transmethylation and neuropsychiatry. In: Mato JM, ed. *Biochemical, pharmacological and clinical aspects of transmethylation. Cell biology reviews*, vol 2. 1987;93–102.

63. Reynolds EH. Anticonvulsants, folic acid and epilepsy. *Lancet* 1973;1:1376–1378.

64. Smith DB, Carl GF. Anticonvulsant–folate interactions. In: Dam M, Gram L, Penry JK, eds. *Advances in epileptology: XIIth Epilepsy International Symposium*. New York: Raven Press, 1981;671–678.

65. Carney MWP, Chary TKN, Bottiglieri T, et al. Switch mechanism in affective illness and oral *S*-adenosylmethionine. *Br J Psychiatry* 1987; 150:724–725.

66. Miller AA, Goff D, Webster RA. Predisposition of laboratory animals to epileptogenic activity of folic acid. In: Botez MI, Reynolds EH, eds. *Folic acid in neurology, psychiatry and internal medicine*. New York: Raven Press, 1979;331–334.

67. O'Donnell RA, Leach MJ, Miller AA. Folic acid induced kindling in rats: changes in brain amino acids. In: Blair JA, ed. *Chemistry and biology of pteridines*. Berlin: Walter de Gruyter, 1983;801–805.

68. Davies J, Watkins JC. Facilitatory and direct excitatory effects of folate and folinate on single neurons of cat cerebral cortex. *Biochem Pharmacol* 1973;22:1667–1668.

69. Hill RG, Miller AA. Antagonism by folic acid of presynaptic inhibition in the rat cuneate nucleus. *R J Pharmacol* 1974;50:425–427.

70. Clifford BD, Ferrendelli JA. Neurophysiologic effects of folate compounds in hippocampus *in vitro*. *Brain Res* 1983;266:209–216.

71. Otis LC, Madison DV, Nicoll RA. Folic acid has a disinhibitory action in the rat, hippocampal slice preparation. *Brain Res* 1985;346:281–286.

72. Van Rijn CM, Van der Velden TJAM, Rodrigues de Miranda JF, et al. The influence of folic acid on the picrotixin-sensitive site of the GABAa–receptor complex. *Epilepsy Res* 1988;2:215–218.

73. Van Rijn CM. Folic acid, epilepsy and the GABAa-receptor complex. *PhD thesis*, Catholic University of Nijmegen, 1989.

Advances in Neurology, Vol. 55, edited by
D. Smith, D. Treiman, and M. Trimble,
Raven Press, Ltd., New York © 1991.

4

Are Complex Partial Seizures a Sequela of Temporal Lobe Dysgenesis?

Arnold B. Scheibel

*Departments of Anatomy and Cell Biology, Psychiatry and Biobehavioral Sciences, and Brain
Research Institute, UCLA Center for the Health Sciences, Los Angeles, California 90024*

*The present contains nothing more than the
past, and what is found in the effect was already in the cause.*
Henri Bergson, *L'Evolution Créatrice*, 1907

The purpose of this chapter is to reexamine
the still puzzling problem of temporal lobe seizures and to try to develop a conceptual
framework within which their etiology and
pathogenesis may better be understood. The
task is formidable, especially when viewed in
terms of the broad spectrum of neurologists,
neurosurgeons, and pathologists who have already confronted the challenge over the past
century. It is probably fair to say that some
degree of consensus has begun to emerge regarding those pathological entities bearing a
putative substrate relationship to complex
partial seizures. In addition, a body of data
has developed which is beginning to shed
some light on the physiological bases for the
seizure equivalent states. Beyond these, however, a unifying hypothesis which might more
closely relate the nature of the structural
changes to their causes, on the one hand, and
to their functional expression at the behavioral level, on the other hand, has remained
out of reach.

In what follows, I will argue that one or
more developmental faults arising during embryogenesis may set the stage for the development of many, if not all, cases of temporal
lobe epilepsy, both as a physiological brain
disorder and as a cause of unusual psycholog-

ical phenomena. These will be contrasted
with a group of structural alterations which
appear to develop during the course of the
syndrome and which are undoubtedly a consequence of it.

HISTORICAL OVERVIEW

A number of useful reviews of the neuropathological changes found in brain tissue
from patients with complex partial seizures
have appeared in the past decades, including
those of Spielmeyer (1), Stauder (2), Margerison and Corsellis (3), Gastaut (4), Penfield
and co-workers (5–9), Falconer et al. (10),
Brown (11), and Babb and Brown (12). Much
of this information is familiar and will only be
summarized here. Added to it are data from
our own research (13–15), thereby preparing
the way for a synthesis which may highlight
some interrelationships among disorders of
embryological development which appear to
have received insufficient attention.

As early as 1825, the presence of structural
alterations in the hippocampi of patients with
epilepsy had been noted by Bouchet and Cazauvieilh (16). The sclerotic changes which
they described, however, were not considered
by them to be specifically related to the seizures and psychotic behavior shown by their
14 autopsied patients. More careful anatomic
descriptions by Meynert (17), Pfleger (18),
and Sommer (19) contributed to knowledge of
the finer structure of these areas, especially in
the epilepsy patient. Sommer identified the

pyramidal neurons of that area now considered to include prosubiculum and at least part of CA1 (20) as being particularly subject to loss (Sommer's sector). Sommer's original descriptions also included cell loss in the rest of Ammon's horn, but he appeared uncertain about the extent and significance of changes in the end folium structure (CA4) and dentate gyrus. Most significantly, he emphasized the potential vulnerability of hippocampal structures to pathological alterations and linked such changes, at least conceptually, to temporal lobe seizures.

Nineteen years later, Bratz (21) published a careful histological analysis of brain tissue specimens from 50 epilepsy patients. Among these, 50% showed hippocampal atrophy and cell loss; of this group of 25 patients, only about 50% had bilateral changes. Bratz emphasized the extensive loss of hippocampal pyramidal cells throughout the cornu Ammonis, but he described some degree of cell sparing in CA2 (Bratz' sector) and in CA4. Since fully half of his series showed other patterns of pathology (syphilitic gummae, parasitic cysts, etc.) without obvious hippocampal cell loss or sclerosis, he argued that hippocampal atrophy could not be the inevitable consequence of temporal lobe seizures and might better be considered as one of its causes. This basically "modern" position was not widely accepted at the time and has only

achieved some degree of acceptance in the last 30 years.

Among those championing the idea that seizures caused hippocampal cell loss and sclerosis was Spielmeyer. In two rather short but influential papers (1,22), he argued that the sclerotic changes were secondary to severe vascular alterations and hypoxia brought on by seizuring activity. Using a patient who died after suffering 2 days of status epilepticus as his model, he demonstrated degenerating hippocampal pyramidal cells and phagocytosis as evidence of an actively destructive process. He further suggested that the unusual vulnerability of Sommer's sector to this hypoxic insult could be attributed to an idiosyncratic pattern of vascularization in this area. These ideas, attractive as they seemed, could not stand the test of time, and there is now fairly general agreement that prolonged hypoxia is not a regular concomitant of temporal lobe seizures. Similarly, it has not been possible to provide convincing anatomical or physiological evidence to support the notion of a uniquely deficient vascular supply to hippocampus, despite both (a) the high packing density of both pyramidal cells and dentate granules and (b) the geometrically complex embryogenesis of the hippocampal plate (23–26) (Fig. 1). Of particular importance in this regard have been the observations of the Penfield group (8), who were among the first to

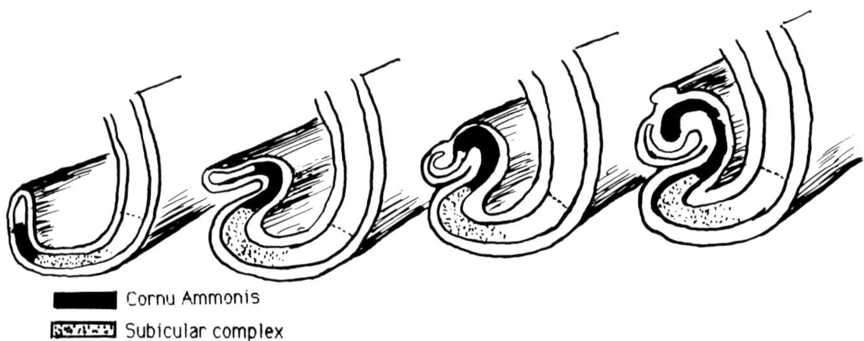

FIG. 1. Diagrammatic drawings tracing the development of the hippocampus and related structures as seen in coronal sections. The extent of cornu Ammonis and of subicular complex are indicated. Note that the dentate gyrus (unmarked), which is originally the most medial portion of the hippocampal plate, becomes detached during the secondary curvature (4th diagram) and wraps around the end of the developing hippocampal cell lamina as the external surfaces of dentate gyrus and subiculum come into close contact, thereby forming the hippocampal fissure. (Modified from ref. 71, with permission.)

document the occurrence of rapidly developing vasodilatation and hyperemia during temporal lobe ictus, rather than vascular spasm and oxygen starvation.

Increasingly convincing correlations between temporal lobe pathology (particularly hippocampal sclerosis) and complex partial seizures were provided by the reports of Stauder (2) and Margerison and Corsellis (3). The former demonstrated a 100% correlation between hippocampal sclerosis and proven temporal lobe seizures in 29 patients, but in only 3 of 18 patients without psychomotor epilepsy. On the basis of these findings, he concluded that the auras and dreamy states which characterized the syndrome were directly related to hippocampal pathology. Thirty years later, the clinical and pathological study of Margerison and Corsellis (3) reached similar conclusions. Again, a striking majority of patients with complex partial seizures had sclerotic hippocampi (85% of 22 patients), and further support was thereby provided for hippocampectomy as a rational mode of therapeutic intervention.

An attractive hypothesis bearing on the challenging question of the origin of hippocampal sclerosis had been advanced somewhat earlier by the Penfield group (7,27). They suggested that compression of the fetal head and formation of an intracranial pressure cone during the birthing process might temporarily compromise blood supply to the temporal lobe, thereby resulting in the development of incisural sclerosis. This notion has not been supported by further investigation (10,12) but did serve to reemphasize the significance of the ventromedial surface of the temporal lobe in partial seizures.

Detailed quantitative clinicopathological studies by Babb, Brown, Crandall, and their associates (see, e.g., refs. 12, 28, and 29) have introduced some degree of rigor into this field. By combining results from chronic multiple superficial and depth recording electrode stations, from batteries of psychological tests, and from neuropathological analysis of surgically removed tissue with both light and electron microscopy, they have demonstrated a tight correspondence between seizure behavior and specific pathology. For example, in three cases with 100% focal onset of electrophysiologically documented seizures limited to the anterior hippocampus, significant degrees of sclerosis and cell loss (i.e., a loss of at least 50% of the neurons) were found in, and only in, this region. Conversely, the presence of obvious sclerosis and cell loss at the posterior resection line (four cases) implied the presence of further pathology in the unresected tissue. In such patients, electrographic studies had shown seizure activity developing simultaneously in anterior and posterior hippocampi, and the results of surgery were less successful. From studies such as these, Babb and Brown (29) concluded that ". . . seizure-generating tissue is linked to hippocampal sclerosis, and as the site of the damage varies, the site of the seizure focus varies. No doubt that explains surgical failures, if damage is widespread in temporal lobe or bilaterally."

The presence and distribution of multiple pathological foci have constituted one of the major treatment challenges in this syndrome. Several lines of evidence argue for the presence of some degree of bilateral hippocampal damage in all drug-refractory human temporal lobe seizure patients. Three major neuropathological studies of autopsy material from confirmed temporal lobe epilepsy patients provide information about bilateral involvement, including those of (a) Sano and Malamud (30), who reported 86%, (b) Mouritzen-Dam (31), reporting 88%, and (c) Margerison and Corsellis (3), reporting 47%. Hippocampal pathology may therefore be considered significantly bilateral although seldom symmetric (28,31).

Over the last three decades, eight major studies have been in essential agreement over the presence of at least one significant neuropathological substrate for temporal lobe seizures. Approximately two-thirds of all patients examined in these reports (range of 58–75%, with an average of 65%) show hippocampal cell loss and sclerosis. However, it has become equally clear that other significantly seizure-related pathological entities may be present, particularly in the extrahippocampal portions of the temporal lobes. Such lesions include gliomas, hamartomas, and heterotopias.

In a series of 129 specimens examined by Babb and Brown (29), 30% included lesions such as hamartomas (12.5%), gliomas (12%), or hetertopias (5%). Two hundred and two discrete lesions were found among a total of 878 cases collected over an almost 50-year period at the Montreal Neurological Institute and reported by Mathieson (32). Excluding the 50 which represented sequelae of trauma or infection, almost 18% represented focal disturbances such as vascular malformations, gliomas and gangliogliomas, heterotopias, tuberous sclerosis lesions, and other small masses. The possible pathogenic significance of discrete focal lesions such as hamartomas has been emphasized by Falconer and Cavanagh (33).

Stepping back somewhat from the minutiae of the various reports, one is struck by the regularity with which a group of developmental malformations appears to constitute the only apparent neuropathological correlate of the temporal lobe ictal state in fully one-third of the cases examined. It seems appropriate, therefore, to raise the following question. Is there a possibility that at least some of the remaining two-thirds of cases of complex partial seizures, those whose only obvious pathological changes consist of hippocampal cell loss and mesial temporal sclerosis, might also represent embryogenetic faults? Before addressing this possibility in detail, we will outline several structural changes which are seen with more variable frequency in these cases, one of which may again suggest developmental defect, albeit of a different type, and the other of which appears to reflect the long-term effects of repeated ictal events.

MICROVASCULAR CHANGES

In approximately one-third of the specimens from two series of cases of temporal lobe epilepsy which we have had the opportunity to examine, we have noted a group of changes in the capillary bed of cerebral cortex (15). The most obvious and dramatic changes were initially noticed in Golgi-stained tissue specimens. The findings were then confirmed and extended in studies with the scanning electron microscope and are epitomized by Fig. 2.

The changes appear as sac-like outpouch-

ings from the small vessels, particularly those whose diameter ranges from 5 to 20 μm. The structures may be single and isolated, or continuous like a string of beads. The isolated enlargements are found most frequently at vessel bifurcations and usually in the crook or angle formed by the branching. Those found along the course of a single unbranched vessel may appear as symmetrical swellings or in some cases as extended sacs or pouches, sometimes with a neck-like narrowing. When we first described them, it was difficult to differentiate them from swollen perivascular cells such as pericytes. Subsequent studies with more sensitive staining techniques showed that they were as translucent as the vessel wall from which they formed the protruding extensions. Scanning electron microscopy confirmed our impressions and showed, in addition, that the fine perivascular neural plexus which characterizes the abluminal wall of such vessels was often continuous over these structures. We were surprised to see that in many cases there were small concentrations of dark pigment or masses of erythrocytes in the brain parenchyma, immediately adjacent to the vascular enlargement.

Although these structures are still under investigation as appropriate tissue specimens are obtained, it is hard to avoid the conclusion that they represent microaneurysmal faults in the vessel walls. The mural structure of such vessels differs, of course, from larger arteries such as those which make up the circle of Willis. Aneurysms at various branch points of this circle are well known and are usually attributed to congenital or genetic faults in the intramural smooth muscle sheets, faults most likely to occur at these points of bifurcation. However, it is not unreasonable to hypothesize that the capillary wall defects which we have noted may also represent some type of developmental structural anomaly (perhaps in the capillary basement membrane) which allows progressive herniation of the vascular endothelium, with consequent leakage and occasional "blow out."

These findings may have special significance in light of the fact that iron salts and hemosiderin appear to be epileptogenic agents that are almost as effective as alumina cream (34,35). It has also been shown that in-

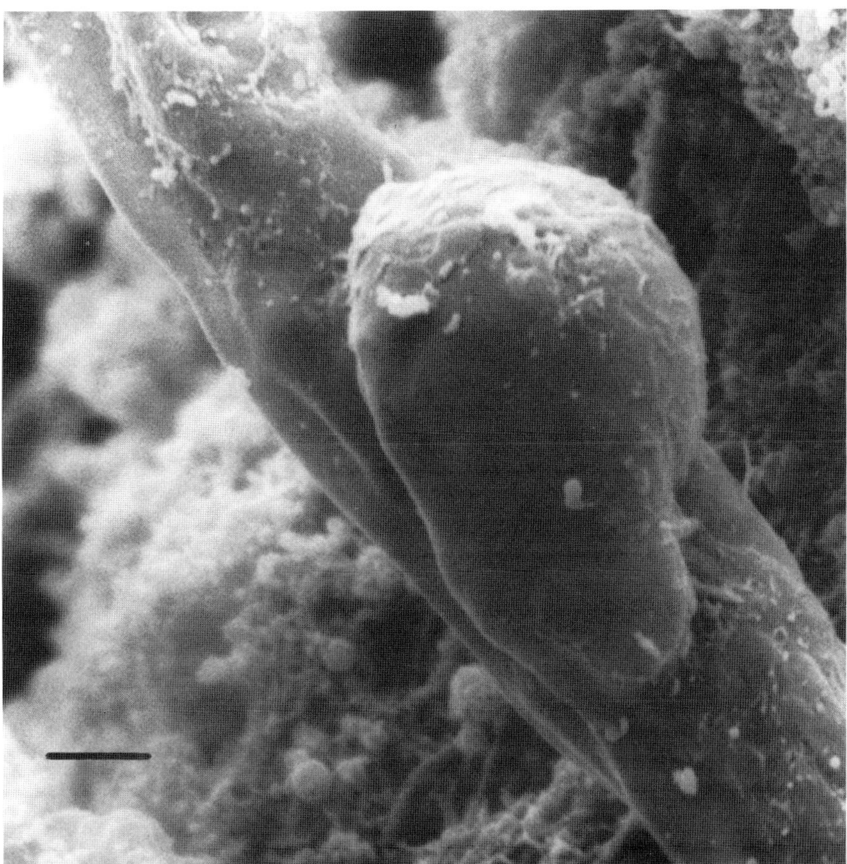

FIG. 2. Scanning electron microscopic view of aneurysm-like outpouching from a small vessel in block of medial temporal lobe tissue removed from a patient with complex partial seizures. Scale bar represents 2.5 mm. Rapid Golgi variant. × 8000. (Slightly modified from ref. 15, with permission.)

troduction of small amounts of blood into cortical tissue has a profound effect on the electrocorticogram (36,37). It is therefore conceivable that chronic, episodic escape of erythrocytes through developmental defects in small cortical vessels, into the surrounding parenchyma, may constitute another possible pathogenic factor in epileptogenesis.

PROGRESSIVE DENDRITIC CHANGES

Dendritic changes have been seen in approximately one-half of a group of 12 cases of complex partial seizures from which we have been able to study tissue specimens. The alterations have been noted characteristically in hippocampus and dentate gyrus, but not in adjacent parahippocampal tissue. Golgi-impregnated preparations have been particularly useful in this study, since neuronal cell body changes and glial alterations only seem to occur very late in the process (14).

The earliest changes are characterized by irregular zones of dendrite spine loss along sections of the dendrite tree of hippocampal pyramids and dentate granules. The sectors of spine loss are at first isolated, and sometimes only one or two dendrite stems of a neuronal dendrite ensemble are affected. In more advanced situations, the entire dendrite spine complement may be lost and dendrites begin to appear irregular or nodulated in outline (Fig. 3). At what we assume to be a further stage of development, there is active fragmentation or loss of dendrite shafts, sometimes with the appearance of projecting leaf-like excrescences. Cell bodies may begin to appear irregular and swollen, losing their characteristic triangular appearance; in addition, the dendrite ensemble appears shrunken and distorted (Fig. 4). Although we have no quanti-

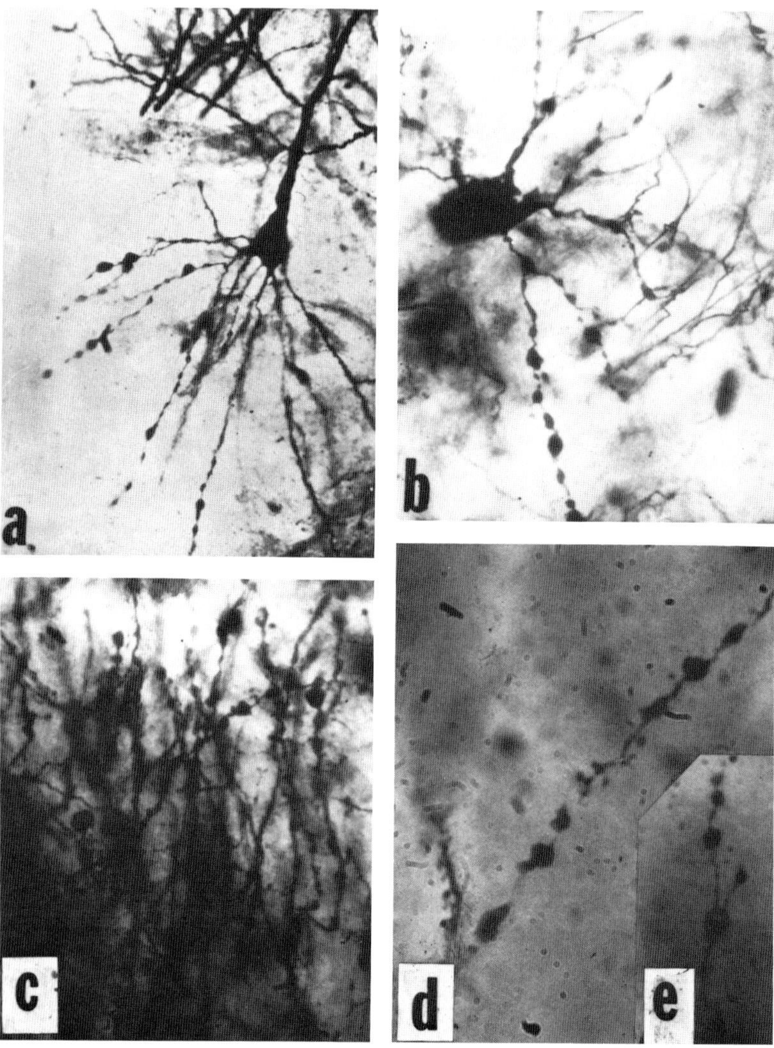

FIG. 3. Structural alterations in dendrites of the hippocampus of adult patients with temporal lobe epilepsy. (**a**) Spine loss and nodulation in the basilar dendrites of a hippocampal pyramidal cell. ×250. (**b**) Nodular string-of-bead changes in the dendrite system of a nonpyramidal hippocampal neuron. ×400. (**c**) Nodular changes along the apical shafts of several hippocampal (CA1) pyramidal neurons. ×400. (**d**) Advanced nodular string-of-beads changes along the apical dendrite of a single pyramidal neuron in CA1. ×600. (**e**) Advanced nodulation at the bifurcating apical tip of a CA1 pyramid. Rapid Golgi variant. ×600. (From ref. 14, with permission.)

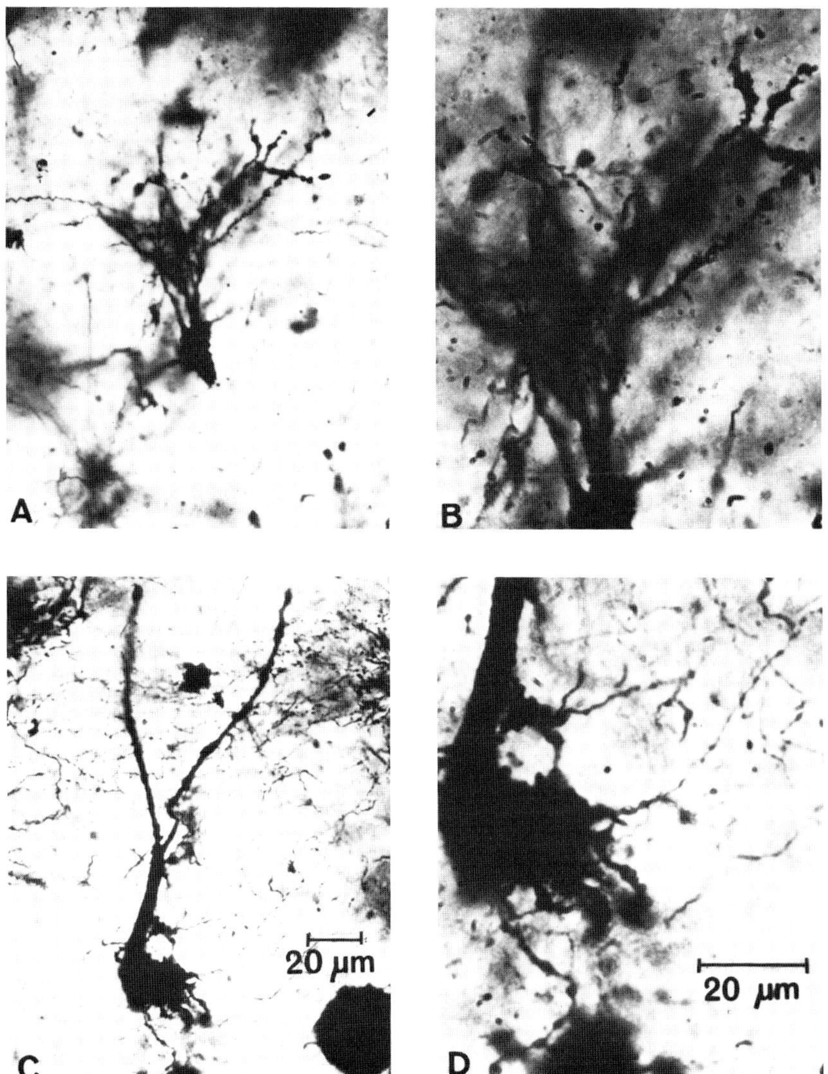

FIG. 4. Advanced deteriorative changes in two neurons from the adult hippocampus in a patient with temporal lobe epilepsy. (**A** and **B**) Small pyramidal cell in CA2 showing marked shrinkage of apical dendrite system with spine loss and terminal nodulation. (**C** and **D**) Pyramidal cell from CA1 showing advanced degree of loss of apical dendrites and virtually complete loss of basilar dendrite ensemble. Rapid Golgi variant. Magnifications: **A** and **C**, ×200; **B** and **D**, ×450. (From ref. 14, with permisson.)

tative data, we have the strong impression that during these latter phases of the process, gliosis becomes a prominent feature of the surrounding parenchyma. In addition, we have observed that the extent and intensity of dendritic and neuronal changes seem to vary as a positive function of the length of time during which the patient has had epilepsy. It is clear that these alterations do not occur in every patient with complex partial seizures; it is equally obvious that the changes are not idiosyncratic for ictus, since similar dendritic changes have been noted in a wide range of problems, including alcoholism and nutritional insufficiency (38). Nonetheless, they may well be indices of periods of disturbed metabolism which accompany chronic repetitive ictal phenomena in the limbic system.

THE CLASH OF DATA

Several factors stand out in most of the literature surveyed. Above all, temporal lobe epilepsy seems to be a syndrome which characteristically develops in early life. A number of recent reviews agree that at least 50% of patients develop seizures in the first decade. In the series studied by Margerison and Corsellis (3), the mean age of onset was 6 years. Of these, 65% showed mesial temporal sclerosis and 20–25% had localized hamartomatous lesions. Falconer et al. (10) emphasized the importance of at least one premonitory infantile convulsion usually attributed to teething, fever, colic, etc., as a frequent part of the history (13 out of 47 cases). However, only 10% of children who suffer infantile convulsions go on to develop an established epileptic syndrome.

A positive family seizure history is also frequent, although the incidence varies somewhat among the reports. The Falconer group (10) noted that 6 out of 47 cases (~13%) had a family history, whereas Margerison and Corsellis (3) reported 44%. Average values drawn from case series reported in a number of studies suggests that reasonable values for familial incidence range from 12% to 20%.

Falconer et al. (10) found a confirmed history of birthing injuries and perinatal head trauma relatively unimpressive (7 out of 47 cases) and suggested that this figure was similar to that reported in nonictal groups.

The relevant literature suggests that of all patients with complex partial seizures who have been subject to temporal lobe resection approximately two-thirds (58–75%) have shown mesiotemporal sclerosis. In a second group representing 20–25% of resected patients, focal lesions such as hamartomas, heterotopias, focal vascular anomalies, and nodules of tuberous sclerosis have been demonstrated. Thus, the majority of patients with temporal lobe epilepsy (80–90%) appear to harbor one (and sometimes more than one) of these pathological entities. It seems very likely that the focal lesions of the second group represent genetic or congenital faults which develop during embryogenesis. The central unsolved question as to etiology and pathogenesis of temporal ictus must then devolve upon the origin and nature of mesiotemporal sclerotic lesions.

As already indicated, there remains a notable divergence of opinion on this subject. The possibility of vascular spasm secondary to the ictus with prolonged hypoxia and progressive cell damage, a theory advanced by Spielmeyer (1,22) and Scholz (35,39,40) almost 60 years ago, remains thinkable but not convincing. The demonstration [by Penfield's group (8) and subsequently by a number of others] that local cortical hyperemia rather than vasoconstriction accompanies ictus makes the notion of hypoxic damage less likely. Cavanagh and Meyer (41) were impressed by the high incidence of mesiotemporal sclerosis in those patients whose ictal episodes started before the age of 4 years, particularly in those whose earliest episodes might have involved status epilepticus. It seemed not unreasonable to postulate that very severe convulsions at an early age might cause neuronal loss and gliosis, especially if the rapidly developing hippocampal neurons are particularly sensitive to hypoxia at this stage of life.

Spielmeyer (22) had described the presence of phagocytes and degenerating neurons in a patient who came to postmortem examination following 2 days of continuous status epilepticus. He compared the widespread destruction caused by this long-continuing electrical storm to that following other conditions resulting in massive hippocampal damage such as carbon monoxide poisoning and endophlebitis. He concluded that the pathology was the direct result of an inadequate vascular supply to Ammon's horn, marked by (a) idiosyncratic twisting of the septal artery which presumably occurred during embryogenesis and (b) a pattern of inadequately collateralized end arteries which rendered the hippocampus uniquely susceptible to ischemia. These assumptions were largely refuted by Scharrer (23) using the carbon monoxide-poisoned oppossum brain as a model of the massive hypoxic event. He demonstrated that the vascular supply pattern to the hippocampus was not unique, since end arteries were found widely throughout the cortex. Furthermore, the resulting pattern of hippocampal damage developed in the experimental model was bilaterally symmetric, in contradistinction to the characteristic asymmetry of lesions in the human epileptic hippocampus. Here it should be reemphasized that patterns of mesiotemporal sclerosis are frequently bilateral but rarely symmetric (i.e., >10%) (29) and that the cell loss, where it does exist, is sufficiently small to allow unilateral resection to produce essentially complete freedom from seizures in 75% or more of cases depending on the series reported.

With regard to the hypothesized inadequacy of the capillary tree, the vascular bed supplying hippocampus is no less rich than that supplying other cerebral areas in rats (24) and humans (25). In an early quantitative study, Cobb (26) demonstrated that the capillary plexus among the hippocampal pyramidal cells is greater than that supplying the adjacent dentate granule layer. This is of considerable interest because in temporal lobe epilepsy patients the hippocampal pyramidal cells characteristically undergo greater loss than do the dentate cells. Note also that studies by Massarweh et al. (42) indicate that periods of hypoxia produced by carotid ligation in postnatal mice result in ischemic necrosis of the internal layer of dentate granule cells but spare the hippocampal pyramidal cells in CA1 and CA3. Thus available data do not appear to support the assumption of a hippocampus that is uniquely vulnerable to seizure-induced ischemia. And when the induced insult is sufficiently massive to produce cell destruction, the resulting patterns of cell loss differ significantly, both within the individual hippocampus and in their bilateral pattern, when compared with the pattern found in patients with complex partial seizures.

Studies by Chugani and Phelps (43) and by Kennedy and Sokoloff (44) document an increase in cerebral glucose demand and oxygen consumption during infancy. However, in a well-controlled study of 362 Danish children with definitive diagnoses of febrile convulsions, Lee et al. (45) found that only 15 (4%) of these children subsequently developed epilepsy; of these 15, only three (20%) showed partial seizures. Since this incidence did not differ from that of a random population of epilepsy patients, the investigators concluded that there was no causal relationship between infantile febrile convulsions and temporal lobe epilepsy.

We are faced with a spectrum of observations which argue both for and against the possibility of temporal lobe epilepsy as an acquired syndrome. The thoughtful paper of Falconer et al. (10) is particularly useful insofar as it highlights the ambivalent quality of the data. These investigators emphasize the marked tendency for patients with mesial temporal sclerosis to have had seizure episodes in infancy or early childhood (13 out of 47 cases) and for this pathology to be characteristically unilateral or at least highly asymmetric. They also stress the idiosyncratic distribution of the pathology. In its least robust form, neuronal loss and gliosis are limited to Sommer's sector, with some degree of gliosis in the amygdala. More advanced sclerotic pictures include patchy cell loss in uncus, in amygdala, in more extensive portions of the cornu Ammonis (but with relative sparing of CA2), in the fusiform gyrus, and even in the more lateral gyri of the temporal lobe. In the second and third cortical layers, neocortical thickness may be reduced and cell loss can be found. As already noted, the seizuring cortex does not ordinarily appear to become anoxic (8,46); however, experimental evidence indicates that if the ictus were sufficiently severe and long-lasting to result in hypoxia and diminished brain glucose levels, the pattern of resulting cortical damage would be very different (23).

Falconer et al. (10) also emphasize the rather small incidence of difficult birthing histories in their patients (7 out of 47), a frequency similar to that found in a non-epileptic control series. In addition, they find little evidence to support either (a) the concept of mechanical compression of anterior choroidal and posterior cerebral arteries during the process of parturition, as suggested by Earle et al. (27), or (b) the idea of birth-induced tentorial herniation secondary to increased intracranial pressure, advanced by Scholz (40) and others.

DEFECTIVE NEUROEMBRYOGENESIS

The possibility that temporal lobe epilepsy may result from defective embryogenesis was suggested as early as the first decade of the 20th century by Alzheimer (47) and by Rancke (48). Veith and Wricke (49) have called attention to the high incidence of cortical microdysgenesis (37%) in patients with temporal lobe epilepsy compared to a 4% incidence in a non-epileptic population. They noted a significant increase (up to 10,000/mm³) in the density of neurons in the molecular layer of all three frontal gyri—a highly abnormal state resembling that of the immediately prenatal cortex. Equally impressive was the even greater density of residual neurons in frontal white matter. They interpreted the existence of these dystopic cell rests as strong evidence for disordered neurogenesis. In addition, 20–25% of the lesions which they identified were hamartomas, an equally persuasive index of defective cortical development. Approximately two-thirds (65%) of this patient group showed mesiotemporal sclerosis, and 44% of these patients had a positive family history. Particularly impressive is the significant degree of overlap between patients showing frontal lobe dysgenesis and those exhibiting specific mesiotemporal lobe pathology.

The lesion termed "mesial temporal sclerosis" is characterized by extensive neuronal loss (>50%) (29) with a rather specific distribution, along with varying amounts of glial proliferation. However, it should be noted that recent quantitative studies indicate that hippocampal cell loss is also found in conjunction with focal, usually extrahippocampal, lesions which are considered to be developmental in origin. Babb and Brown (29) reported a 22–30% diminution in hippocampal neurons, along with a similar neuronal deficit (20–36%), in the prosubiculum of ictal patients with identified glioma or hamartoma. Such levels of reduced cell number are seldom recognizable by qualitative estimation and require the type of rigorous quantification introduced by Mouritzen-Dam (31) and Babb and Brown (29). In the presence of heterotopias, however, cell loss in both hippocampus and prosubiculum may reach or exceed 50%. In a group of unpublished studies based on air encephalograms, Udvenhelyi, Falconer, and Serafetinides noted that the hemisphere containing the focal lesion was usually smaller than that of the opposite side, suggesting a defect in growth and development. These data are cited primarily to emphasize the frequency with which hippocampal cell loss appears coincidentally with lesions which are almost certainly the result of developmental anomalies. It might be added that mesial temporal sclerosis may also be found in young "non-epileptic mental defectives" (49), thereby emphasizing the fact that seizures are not a necessary antecedent of this pathological pattern.

Our own interest in the possibility that complex partial seizures may represent one of the more florid aspects of temporal lobe dysgenesis is based not only on consideration of this body of conflicting data, but also on our investigation of structural changes in the hippocampus of schizophrenic patients.

SCHIZOPHRENIA AS A DISORDER OF EMBRYOGENESIS

Approximately a decade ago, we had the opportunity to examine a number of specimens of temporal lobe tissue from a group of chronically hospitalized schizophrenic patients and to compare them with a control group of nonschizophrenics from the same setting (50). Each member of the former group (10 patients) showed an idiosyncratic type of neurohistological pattern characterized by significant degrees of disarray in the hippocampal pyramidal cells. This was initially observed in Golgi stains of hippocampus but was also readily recognizable in routine Nissl-stained sections (Fig. 5). Quantitative studies revealed that the alteration in neuronal organization was especially robust in the anterior third of the pes hippocampus and was most obvious at interface zones, particularly those between prosubiculum and CA1 and between CA1 and CA2, although islands of disarray could be found almost anywhere within the cornu Ammonis (51). Subsequent analysis indicated that the changes were bilateral (52). The characteristically anterior location of this structural alteration was reminiscent of the earlier findings of Heath (53) and Sem-Jacob-

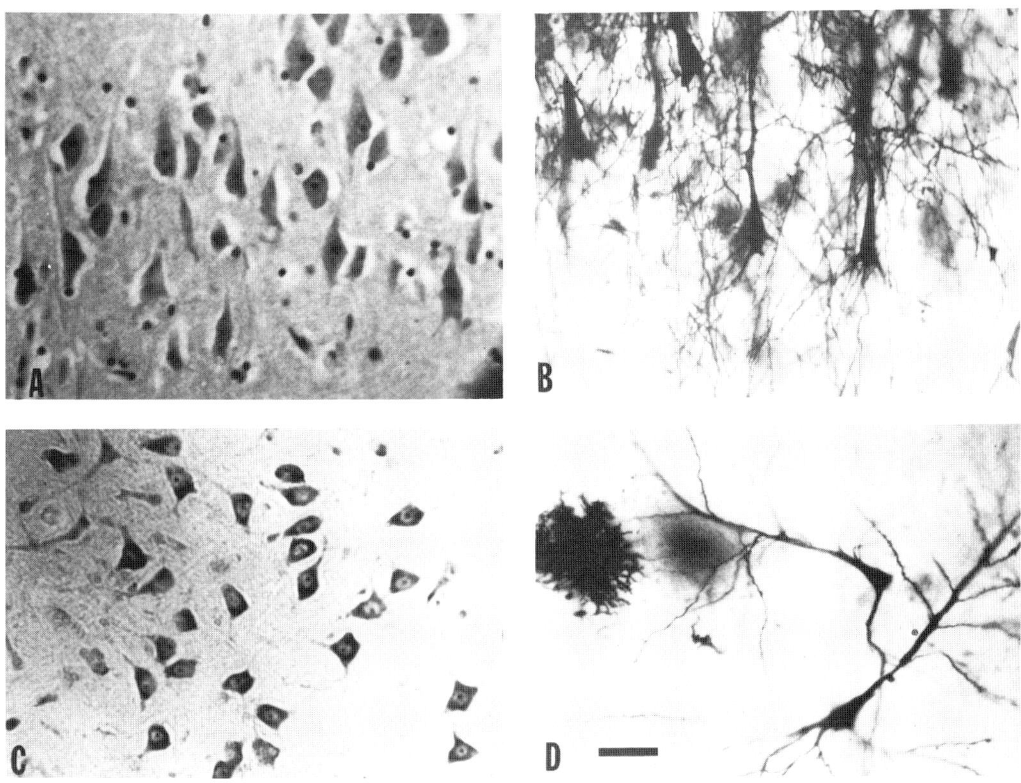

FIG. 5. Comparison of hippocampal specimens from nonschizophrenic (**A** and **B**) and schizophrenic (**C** and **D**) patients. Thionine stain is used in **A** and **C**; Golgi stain is used in **B** and **D**. Note the cell body and dendritic disarray in **C** and **D**. Scale bar represents 25 mm.

sen et al. (54,55), who had reported the presence of deep paroxysmal spiking activity in anterior temporal lobe and posterior frontal lobe stations during florid psychotic manifestations.

Several considerations made it seem likely that the hippocampal disarray reflected problems in neuroembryogenesis and more specifically in the migration of primitive neurons (neuroepithelial cells) into the presumptive hippocampal plate, a process significantly dependent on the integrity of neuronal cell adhesion molecules or NCAM (56). Faults in the utilization or maturation of NCAMs during embryogenesis have recently been demonstrated in two genetic mutant mice, reeler and staggerer, both of whom show disorganized structure in cerebral and/or cerebellar cor-

tices (57,58). We hypothesized that maternal and/or fetal exposure to a toxic or destructive agent during the period of cell migration might account for this effect, probably in the presence of some type of genetic vulnerability (59).

Careful long-term epidemiological studies reported from Scandinavia by Mednick et al. (60) indicated that in a large cohort of pregnant women exposed to a flu-like virus, those who suffered their infection during the second trimester of pregnancy were >300% more likely to have an offspring who eventually became schizophrenic than were those infected during the first or third trimesters. We were intrigued by the fact that influenza virus is one of a small number of viruses characteristically producing the enzyme capsular neuraminidase, which has the almost unique capability of significantly affecting the binding properties of NCAM. Because migration of primitive neurons into the hippocampal plate occurs during the second trimester of pregnancy (61), the apparently greater morbidity of fetuses who shared maternal exposure to the flu at this time could be related, at least on a putative basis, to this infectious event. Thus, the reeler and staggerer mice served as a conceptual model, or caricature, for our conception for the development of a histological substrate in which schizophrenia might later develop.

We are presently pursuing this hypothesis in several ways; that is, we are (a) looking for minute copy numbers of viral genome in schizophrenic patients and (b) trying to create an animal model more directly by infecting pregnant female mice with influenza virus at various times during pregnancy. If our notion has validity, we would expect to see some degree of cortical (including hippocampal) cell disarray develop when infection occurred during the time period critical to cell migration.

Schizophrenia and temporal lobe epilepsy are, in many ways, substantially dissimilar afflictions, and this brief presentation of our schizophrenia hypothesis (59) is meant more to serve as an exemplar to an approach than to serve as a substantive disease model. Nonetheless, there are basic parallels between the two which can prove instructive and which may, in the long run, point toward more profound similarities than are at first apparent.

Above all, both diseases appear to be associated with dysfunction of the medial margin or limbic component of the temporal lobe. Changes in hippocampal structure are obvious in the majority of cases of both syndromes that have been examined and may eventually turn out to be present in all. Alterations may also exist in parahippocampus, in amygdala, and, to an extent that is still far from clear, in association areas of the prefrontal and temporal neocortex. This remarkable centering of histologic anomalies in limbic structures seems almost certainly dependent upon disordered neuroembryogenesis in the schizophrenias and, we believe, highly likely to be so in at least the majority of temporal lobe epilepsies. What factors operating during embryological development might be responsible for this situation?

Although the ultimate organization of the hippocampus is generally considered to be simpler than that of neocortex, its embryogenesis presents certain unique features which may be relevant to our enquiry. The presumptive hippocampal plate, developing on the medial wall of the telencephalic vesicle, undergoes a process of folding during which the original external surfaces of the dentate gyrus and the juxtahippocampal sector (i.e., the subicular complex) become closely applied to each other along the banks of the rapidly obliterating hippocampal sulcus (Fig. 1). Cellular proliferation in the ventricular zone or ependymal layer is initially similar to that in other portions of the developing telencephalon, but several idiosyncratic patterns soon develop. Coincident with the buckling of the hippocampal plate, the anlage of dentate cells become separate from the remainder of the original hippocampal primordia and then follow their own developmental pattern. Although the original dentate granule cells are generated at approximately the same time as are those of the hippocampus (62–64), proliferation of dentate cells continues well into postnatal life.

It is now well established that the time windows for migration of primitive neurons into the primordial hippocampal plate and the neighboring subiculum show considerable variation. In their overview of hippocampal development in the rodent, Stanfield and Cowan (65) indicated that the major migrational events in CA1 and CA3 seem to occur over a fairly broad period of time (i.e., from embryonic day 10 to day 18). However, in the small intervening zone of CA2, migration appears to be essentially completed within a single 24-hr period on embryonic day 15 (Fig. 6). Rakic and Nowakowski (64) reported that in the developing Rhesus macaque, migration of primitive neurons into CA1 (the regio superior) is spread over a reasonably long time period (i.e., from embryonic day 38 through day 70). The same process in adjoining areas CA2, CA3, and CA4 (the regio inferior) occurs more rapidly between embryonic days 38 and 56.

Although migration along radial glial stalks

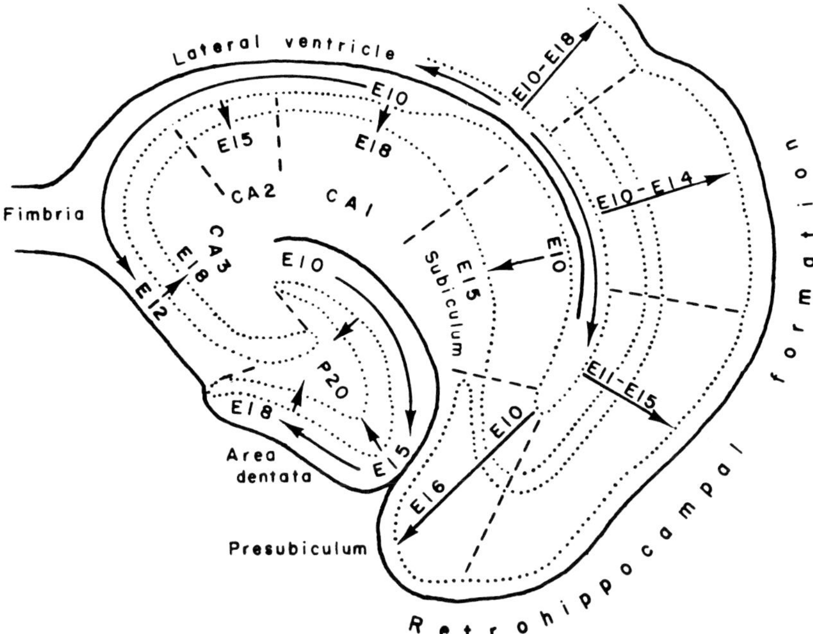

FIG. 6. Drawing of the hippocampal–dentate complex and retrohippocampal formation showing approximate times of migration of primitive neurons for each of the sectors in the mouse. Note the variation in time windows for each of the sectors involved. "E" denotes embryonic day; "CA1," "CA2," and "CA3" denote cornu Ammonis 1, 2, and 3. (From ref. 63, with permission.)

occurs in the hippocampal–subicular complex as it does in neocortex, the mechanics of the process may be somewhat different. In the Rhesus monkey, Nowakowski and Rakic (66) estimated that migration occurs at a rate of about 15 μm/day as compared to the considerably faster 115 μm/day found in the nearby neocortex. Furthermore, migrating hippocampal neurons appear to relinquish their contact with the radial glial fibers before they reach the end of their migration into the bottom of the Ammonic plate, at least in the CA1 sector (65). This appears to contrast markedly with neocortical cells which maintain their contact with radial glial fibers until they come to the end of their migration at the top of the cortical plate (58). Additionally, there is some evidence that hippocampal neurons may undergo a second phase of migration which reverses the position of considerable numbers of neurons during a terminal phase of hippocampal plate development (67). Finally, a number of observations on development and maturation of cells in the regio inferior (CA2,

CA3, CA4) can be interpreted as indicating a different mechanism of cell assembly in this part of the hippocampus. To such patterns of developmental variation must be added the well-known persistence of dentate neurogenesis well into the postnatal period. All of these considerations demonstrate the complex orchestration of biological processes which are involved in development of limbic structures.

SOME APPARENT SIMILARITIES BETWEEN TEMPORAL LOBE EPILEPSY AND SCHIZOPHRENIA

For more than two decades, investigators have concerned themselves with the question as to whether temporal lobe epilepsy and schizophrenic psychoses were related, either in terms of a basic personality configuration or through interictal manifestations (see Chapter 9). We do not plan to comment directly on this still controversial area. However, in going over the data, it appears to us that a number of parallels exist in the phenomena which characterize the two syndromes. Their enumeration may be useful at this time.

1. There appears to be evidence of familial or genetic components in each syndrome. In the case of temporal lobe disease, a very broad range of figures has been quoted, ranging from about 4% to 25% in parents or other first-degree relatives. What is inherited is not clear. Some have suggested either (a) a lower general threshold to cortical ictal response or (b) seizure susceptibility (68). Lindsay (69) favors a somewhat more discrete explanation in the sense that what is inherited may be a genetic susceptibility to convulsions in the presence of fever.

An equally broad range of incidence values has been quoted in the schizophrenias, where from 12% to 25% of first-degree relatives show either an overt psychotic history or other evidence of character or personality disturbance. In monozygotic twins, up to 50% concordance has been reported. There is no agreement as to whether the syndrome reflects a single genetic fault (possibly an autosomal dominant with variable penetrance) or a polygenic problem. In either case, it is totally conjectural as to whether the trait which is passed on can actually be considered a "schizophrenic gene or gene cluster," or whether it may have a broader range of phenotypic expressions (e.g., human leukocyte antigen (HLA)-related immunocompetence problems). At this point, our own preference is for gene traits which may influence the manner in which the fetus responds to maternal viral exposure. The heritable factor would thereby influence the possible development of later psychotic disease, through changes produced in the developing hippocampus by viral exposure during the period of hippocampal cell migration.

2. In each syndrome the hippocampus is a prominent site of structural anomalies, although it is not the only focus of pathological change. In temporal lobe disease the most prominent changes appear to include massive neuronal drop-out (or nonappearance) in the prosubiculum, CA1, and CA3, with some degree of cell sparing in CA2 and a variable picture in CA4 (the endblade) (Fig. 7). These alterations are often bilateral but are seldom, if ever, symmetrical; usually, only one lobe shows quantitatively significant degrees of

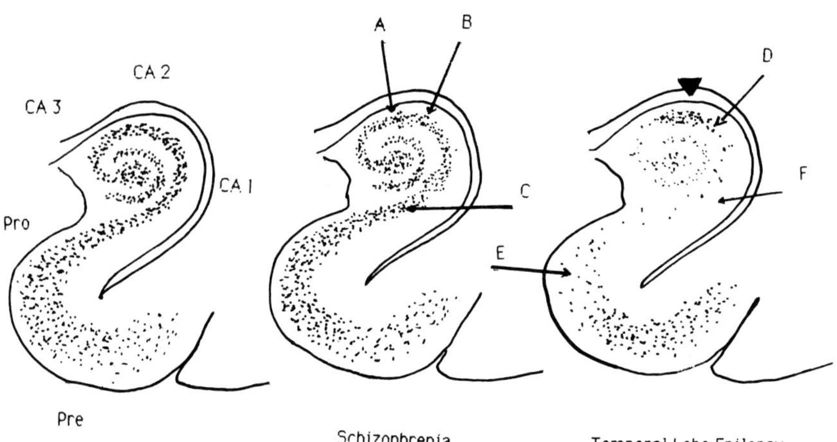

FIG. 7. Drawings comparing cellular alterations in the hippocampus of patients with schizophrenia and temporal lobe epilepsy. In the former, areas of neuronal disarray are maximal at the interfaces between prosubiculum and CA1 (C), between CA1 and CA2 (B), and between CA2 and CA3 (A). In the latter, neuronal loss is usually maximal in the prosubiculum lying between E and F (*arrows*) and in CA1 lying between F and D (*arrows*). Cell sparing is usually found in CA2 (*arrowhead*). Cell loss is variable in CA3 and in the filum (endblade). "Pre" denotes presubiculum; "Pro" denotes prosubiculum; "CA1," "CA2," and "CA3" denote cornu Ammonis 1, 2, and 3.

cell fall-out or nonappearance. Additionally, there may be (a) focal cell rests in adjacent temporal neocortex, (b) alterations in structure of the cortical gray and white matter in amygdala, prefrontal lobe, etc., and (c) small but measurable differences in the size of the principally affected temporal lobe as compared to that on the other side.

The schizophrenic hippocampus is also anomalous, although the alterations are different. The most prominent change seems to consist in the bilateral disarray of hippocampal pyramidal cells, seen particularly at the interface zones between prosubiculum and CA1, CA1 and CA2, and CA2 and CA3 (Fig. 5). These are also frequently accompanied by gross changes in relative size relationships between temporal lobe and ventricle (ventricular–brain ratio) and by possible (although not yet quantitatively verified) alterations in prefrontal cytoarchitectonics.

3. Both syndromes characteristically manifest themselves in the young. A very sizable proportion (30–50%) of patients with complex partial seizures have developed their ictus before the age of 10 years. Schizophrenia is also a disease of youth, although it is more likely to become obvious at or after the onset of puberty, or in the late teens and early twenties.

4. Both syndromes are characterized by electrical storms in the anterior temporal cortex. An enormous body of data documents the temporal and spatial patterns of complex partial seizures, both during the seizure phase and during interictal periods. Documentation is very much more scarce in the case of schizophrenia, but three different laboratories have reported the presence of abnormal spike discharges in anterior temporal lobes and in orbitofrontal cortex during periods of psychotic behavior (53,54,70).

5. Both syndromes may be accompanied by a rather wide variety of behavioral and psychological signs and symptoms. It is difficult to decide how these should be compared, since the range is so great. Patients with complex partial seizures may have auras such as olfactory hallucinations, ill-defined visceral sensations, dreamy states, automatisms, transient thinking deficits and confusional states, amnesias, and short periods of bizarre or aggressive behavior. But for the most part, the psychological and related motor phenomena are temporary and seldom outlast the electrical storm by more than a brief interval. Schizophrenic patients may have any or all of these; however, the hallucinations are usually auditory, and the splitting of affect from thought content is idiosyncratic. So also is the blocking of speech and flow of thought trains, as well as the delusional systems which characterize the inner life of so many patients. Added to these "positive symptoms" may be those of even more malignant import, the so-called "negative symptoms" characterized by withdrawal and inaccessibility, lack of affect, and progressive deterioration. But most of all, the individual schizophrenic episode or "break" extends through considerable time periods—often weeks or months. Even with the periods of remission, which may be seen with or without neuroleptic therapy, recurrence of florid psychotic states may be expected in most patients. Considering the robust differences in the underlying histological, physiological, and neurochemical substrates, the relative incongruence of the clinical picture is not surprising.

As suggested above, the schizophrenic syndrome is considered not necessarily as a closely related disease process but rather as an example of another long-term, incapacitating syndrome apparently related to limbic lobe dysfunction. The most tempting parallels are those which suggest defective embryogenesis developing in response to some untoward intrauterine event and resulting in relatively early developing syndromes characterized by structural–functional abnormalities and behavioral and psychological dysfunction.

CONCLUSIONS

Complex partial seizures have become a topic of remarkably durable interest in the neurological and neurosurgical fields. Particularly intriguing are the glimpses which this syndrome seems to provide of relationships between definable brain lesions and aberrant electrical and behavioral activity. The relatively low degree of responsiveness to pharmacotherapy shown by patients with the syndrome, and the often spectacular response to surgical intervention, have conspired to provide almost unique opportunities for simultaneous research and therapeusis. Nonetheless, the problems of etiology and pathogenesis remain thorny ones. At present, the literature probably contains several thousand reported cases, but these are always post hoc and frozen frame in nature. We still have not been privileged to follow the course of development of the process, nor is it entirely clear where and when we would set up our camera tripod, if we could. Conventional wisdom looks to the birthing process or to the very first years of life as the time frame when the initial insult occurs. Yet no robust statistic supports any special prevalence of birth-related injury, and none of the pathophysiologic mechanisms proposed as crucial to the development of brain pathology has stood the test of subsequent investigation. Some studies have provided data suggesting persuasive correlations between temporal lobe epilepsy and infantile febrile seizures. But again, equally well-founded studies find no such correlation and point to the enormous numbers of infants who experience infantile seizure episodes but who do not go on to develop complex partial seizures. In their thoughtful review, Babb and Brown (29) conclude that, despite the conflicting evidence, some hippocampal damage must occur early in life, and this undoubtedly leads to synaptic reorganization with the formation of "epileptic circuits."

One of the most impressive features of brain tissue from temporal lobe epilepsy patients, examined either *in situ* or under the microscope, is the frequency with which evidence of defective neuroembryogenesis appears. Whether limited to modest degrees of atrophy in temporal lobe, to changes in the ventricular–brain ratio, to alterations in neuronal arrangement and packing density in temporal and frontal cortices, or to the presence of aberrant cell and tissue rests (hamartomas, heterotopias, etc.) in white or gray matter, a significant proportion of brain tissue specimens from patients with complex partial seizures reveals evidence of neuronal dysgenesis. It has already been noted that hippocampal embryogenesis shows a number of features which are idiosyncratic and that neuronal migration, perhaps the most critical step in cortical development, follows an especially complex spatial and temporal scenario during hippocampal development. On

this basis it seems reasonable to propose that mesiotemporal sclerosis might also represent a problem in hippocampal embryogenesis and that the infantile seizures, reported by some to be a remarkably frequent harbinger of the later temporal lobe epileptic state, may actually represent the earliest manifestation of a structural–functional defect already present in the limbic cortex.

Here, for purposes of argument at least, let us borrow conceptually from our recent work with schizophrenias (50,51,59). Perhaps the rather stereotypic pattern of mesiotemporal sclerosis with its maximum involvement of the H1 field (prosubiculum and CA1) and CA3, with less intensive involvement of CA2 and the endblade (CA4), reflects a specific configuration of temporal lobe dysgenesis. The cause remains conjectural, but the remarkable sensitivity of the developing nervous system to toxic or infective agents, especially in the absence of a competent blood–brain barrier, may provide the necessary clue. In the case of the schizophrenias, careful epidemiological studies from Scandinavia established a putative link between maternal infection with a flu-like virus during the second trimester of pregnancy and a 300% increase in the incidence of schizophrenia in the offspring (60). We suggest that some similar process occurring during fetal development may produce a somewhat different pathoanatomic and pathophysiologic pattern than that which provides the substrate for development of complex partial seizures. As we have hypothesized in the case of the schizophrenias, the small yet significant genetic component may again represent not so much a gene or gene cluster coding for "seizurability," but rather one affecting immunocompetence in the fetus which may help determine neuronal response to foreign antigens during neuroembryogenesis. The pathological picture is one of apparent limbic neuronal loss (or nonappearance) combined with some degree of gliosis and varying degrees of aberrant cell rests and focal accumulations throughout the temporal and frontal lobes. Genetic or congenital faults in development of the cerebrovascular walls may also be involved. Most of these changes can be conceived of as secondary to defective migration of primitive neurons into the cortical plate during the second trimester of pregnancy. Detailed epidemiological studies, both retrospective and prospective, might go far toward showing whether the hypothesized events have actually occurred during the intrauterine life of individuals who later develop temporal lobe epilepsy.

SUMMARY

1. Complex partial seizures are closely associated with a group of discrete neuropathological entities which include focal lesions (such as hamartomas and heterotopias) and small vascular lesions, all of which are generally considered to have been present at birth.

2. The pathological change most frequently found in patients with temporal lobe epilepsy is mesiotemporal sclerosis. Although this pathological alteration in subicular and hippocampal structures has been attributed to any one of a number of perinatal or postnatal insults, we suggest that it also may represent a sequela of disturbed neuroembryogenesis.

3. We suggest that many, perhaps most, cases of temporal lobe epilepsy may resemble other major disorders of cognition and behavior (such as schizophrenia) in representing the sequelae of temporal lobe dysgenesis.

REFERENCES

1. Spielmeyer W. The anatomic substratum of the convulsive state. *Arch Neurol Psychiatry* 1930; 23:869–875.
2. Stauder KH. Epilepsie und Schlafenlappen. *Arch Psychiatr Nervenkr* 1936;104:181–211.
3. Margerison JH, Corsellis JAN. Epilepsy and the temporal lobes. *Brain* 1966;89:499–530.
4. Gastaut H. So-called "psychomotor" and "temporal" epilepsy. *Epilepsia* 1953;5:59–99.
5. Penfield W, Ward A. Epileptogenic lesions. *Arch Neurol Psychiatry* 1948;60:20–36.
6. Penfield W, Flanigin H. Surgical therapy of temporal lobe seizures. *Arch Neurol Psychiatry* 1950;64:492–500.
7. Penfield W, Baldwin M. Temporal lobe seizures and the technic of subtotal temporal lobectomy. *Ann Surg* 1952;136:625–634.
8. Penfield W, Jasper H. *Epilepsy and the functional anatomy of the human brain.* Boston, MA: Little, Brown & Company, 1954.
9. Penfield W, Paine K. Results of surgical therapy for focal epileptic seizures. *Can Med Assoc J* 1955;73:515–531.
10. Falconer MA, Serafetinides EA, Corsellis JAN. Etiology and pathogenesis of temporal lobe epilepsy. *Arch Neurol* 1964;10:233–248.
11. Brown WJ. Structural substrates of seizure focus in the human temporal lobe. In: Brazier MAB, ed. *Epilepsy: its phenomena in man.* New York: Academic Press, 1973;339–374.
12. Babb TL, Brown WJ. Neuronal, dendritic, and vascular profiles of human temporal lobe epilepsy correlated with cellular physiology *in vivo.* In: Delgado-Escueta AV, et al., eds. *Advances in neurology, vol 44: Basic mechanisms of the epilepsies—Molecular and cellular approaches.* New York: Raven Press, 1986;949–966.
13. Scheibel M, Scheibel AB. Hippocampal pathology in temporal lobe epilepsy. A Golgi study. In: Brazier MAB, ed. *Epilepsy: its phenomena in man.* New York: Raven Press, 1973;311–337.
14. Scheibel M, Crandall P, Scheibel AB. The hippocampal–dentate complex in temporal lobe epilepsy. *Epilepsia* 1974;15:55–80.
15. Scheibel AB, Paul L, Fried I. Some structural substrates of the epileptic state. In: Jasper HH, van Gelder NM, eds. *Basic mechanisms of neuronal hyperexcitability.* New York: Alan R Liss, 1983;109–130.
16. Bouchet, Cazauvieilh. De l'epilepsie considerée dans ses rapports avec l'alienation mentale. Récherche sur le nature et le siège de les deux maladies. memoire qui a emporte le prix au concours établi par M. Esquirol. *Arch Gen Med* 1825;9:510–542.
17. Meynert T. Studien über das Pathologisch-Anatomische Material der Wiener Irren-Anstalt. *Vierteljahrsschr Psychiatr* 3:381–402.
18. Pfleger L. Beobachtungen über Schrumpfung und Sklerose des Ammonshorns bei Epilepsie. *Allg Z Psychiatr* 1880;36:359–365.
19. Sommer W. Erkrankung des Ammonshorns als Aetiologisches Moment der Epilepsie. *Arch Psychiatr Nervenkr* 1880;10:631–675.
20. Lorente de Nó R. Studies on the structure of the cerebral cortex. II. Continuation of the study of the ammonic systems. *J Psychol Neurol (Leipz)* 1934;46:113–177.
21. Bratz E. Ammonshornbefunde der Epileptischen. *Arch Psychiatr Nervenkr* 1899;31:820–836.
22. Spielmeyer W. Die Pathogenese des Epileptischen Krampfes. *Z Gesamte Neurol Psychiatr* 1927;109:501–520.
23. Scharrer E. Vascularization and vulnerability of the cornu Ammonis in the opossum. *Arch Neurol Psychiatry* 44·483–506.
24. Craigie EH. The vascular supply of the archicortex of the rat. I. The albino rat (*Mus norgevicus albinus*). *J Comp Neurol* 1930;51:1–11.
25. Hiller F. Über die Krankhaften Veränderungen im Zentralnervensystem nach Kohlenoxydvergiftung. *Z Gesamte Neurol Psychiatr* 1928;117:698–727.
26. Cobb S. The cerebral circulation. VII. A quantitative study of the capillaries in the hippocampus. *Arch Surg* 1929;18:1200–1209.
27. Earle KM, Baldwin M, Penfield W. Incisural

sclerosis and temporal lobe seizures produced by hippocampal herniation at birth. *Arch Neurol Psychiatry* 1953;69:27–42.

28. Babb TL, Lieb JP, Brown WJ, Pretorius J, Crandall PH. Distribution of pyramidal cell density and hyperexcitability in the epileptic human hippocampal formation. *Epilepsia* 1984;25:721–728.

29. Babb TL, Brown WJ. Pathological findings in epilepsy. In: Engel J Jr, ed. *Surgical treatment of the epilepsies.* New York: Raven Press, 1987;511–540.

30. Sano K, Malamud N. Clinical significance of sclerosis of the cornu Ammonis. *Arch Neurol Psychiatry* 1953;70:40–53.

31. Mouritzen-Dam A. Hippocampal neuron loss in epilepsy and after experimental seizures. *Acta Neurol Scand* 1982;66:601–642.

32. Mathieson G. Pathology of temporal lobe foci. In: Penry JK, Daly DP, eds. *Advances in neurology, vol 11: Complex partial seizures and their treatment.* New York: Raven Press, 1975; 163–181.

33. Falconer MA, Cavanagh JB. Clinicopathological considerations of temporal lobe epilepsy due to small focal lesions. *Brain* 1959;82:483–504.

34. Reid SA, Sypert GW, Boggs WM, Willmore LJ. Histopathology of the ferric-induced chronic epileptic focus in cat: a Golgi study. *Exp Neurol* 1979;66:205–219.

35. Scholz W. Über die Entstehung des Hirn-Befundes bei der Epilepsie. *Z Gesamte Neurol Psychiatr* 1933;145:471.

36. Fifkova E, Van Harreveld A. Long-lasting morphological changes in dendritic spines of dentate granular cells following stimulation of entorhinal area. *J Neurocytol* 1977;6:211–230.

37. Hammond E, Ramsey R, Villareal H, Wilder B. Effects of intracortical injection of blood and blood components on the electrocorticogram. *Epilepsia* 1980;21:3–14.

38. Monti A. Sur les altérations du systeme nerveux dans l'inanition. *Arch Ital Biol* 1895;24:347–360.

39. Scholz W. Selective neuronal necrosis and its topistic patterns in hypoxemia and oligemia. *J Neuropathol Exp Neurol* 1953;12:249–261.

40. Scholz W. Contributions of patho-anatomical research to the problem of epilepsy. *Epilepsia* 1959;1:36–61.

41. Cavanagh JB, Meyer A. Aetiological aspects of Ammon's horn sclerosis associated with temporal lobe epilepsy. *Br Med J* 1956;2:1403–1407.

42. Massarweh W, Schwartz P, Vinters H, Dwyer B, Fujikawa D, Wasterlain C. Selective vulnerability of the dentate gyrus in a neonatal rat model of hypoxia-ischemia. 1990;submitted for publication.

43. Chugani HT, Phelps ME. Maturational changes in cerebral function in infants determined by 18 FDG position emission tomography. *Science* 1986;231:840–843.

44. Kennedy C, Sokoloff L. An adaptation of the nitrous oxide method to the study of the cerebral circulation in children. Normal values for cerebral blood flow and cerebral metabolic rate in childhood. *J Clin Invest* 1957;36:1130–1137.

45. Lee K, Diaz M, Melchior JC. Temporal lobe epilepsy—not a consequence of childhood febrile convulsions in Denmark. *Acta Neurol Scand* 1981;63:231–236.

46. Dymond AM, Crandall PH. Oxygen availability and blood flow in the temporal lobes during spontaneous epileptic seizures in man. *Brain Res* 1976;102:191–196.

47. Alzheimer A. Die Gruppierung der Epilepsie. *Allg Z Psychiatr* 1907;53:418.

48. Rancke O. Beiträge zur Kenntnis der Normalen und Pathologischen Hirnrindenbildung. *Beitr Pathol Anat* 1910;47:51–60.

49. Veith G, Wricke R. Cerebrale Differenzierungsstörungen bei Epilepsie. In: *Jahrbuch 1968.* Köln-Opladen: Westdeutschr. Verlag, 1968;515–534.

50. Scheibel AB, Kovelman JA. Disorientation of the hippocampal pyramidal cell and its processes in the schizophrenic patient. *Biol Psychiatry* 1981;16:101–102.

51. Kovelman JA, Scheibel AB. A neurohistological correlate of schizophrenia. *Biol Psychiatry* 1984; 19:1601–1621.

52. Conrad A., et al. Hippocampal pyramital cell disarray in schizophrenia as a bilateral phenomenon. *Arch Gen Psych*;in press.

53. Heath RG. Correlation of electrical recordings from cortical and subcortical regions of the brain with abnormal behavior in human subjects. *Confin Neurol* 1958;18:305–313.

54. Sem-Jacobsen CW, Peterson MC, Lazarte JA, Dodge HW Jr, Holman CB. Intracerebral electrographic recordings from psychotic patients during hallucinations and agitation. *Am J Psychiatry* 1955;112:278–288.

55. Sem-Jacobsen CW, Peterson MC, Lazarte JA, Dodge HW Jr, Holman CB. Electroencephalographic rhythms from the depths of the parietal, occipital and temporal lobes in man. *Electroencephalogr Clin Neurophysiol* 1956;8:263–278.

56. Rutishauser U, Thierry JP, Braekenbury R, Edelman GM. Surface molecules mediating interactions among embryonic neural cells. In: Schmitt FO, ed. *The neurosciences: Fourth study program.* New York: Rockefeller University Press, 1979;735–746.

57. Edelman GM, Chuong CM. Embryonic to adult conversion of neural cell adhesion molecules in normal and staggerer mice. *Proc Natl Acad Sci USA* 1982;79:7036–7040.

58. Pinto-Lord MC, Eurard P, Caviness US Jr. Obstructed neuronal migration along radial glial fibers in the neocortex of the reeler mouse. A Golgi–EM analysis. *Dev Brain Res* 1982;4:379–393.

59. Conrad A, Scheibel AB. Schizophrenia and the hippocampus, the embryological hypothesis extended. *Schizophr Bull* 1987;13:577–587.

60. Mednick SA, Machon RA, Huttenen M, Bonnet D. The 1957 Helsinki type A-2 influenza epi-

demic and adult schizophrenia. *Arch Gen Psychiatry* 1988;45:189–292.

61. Sidman RL. Cell–cell recognition in the developing central nervous system. In: Schmitt FO, Worden FG, eds. *The neurosciences: Third study program*. Cambridge, MA: M.I.T. Press, 1974;743–758.

62. Angevine JB Jr. Time of neuron origin in the hippocampal region: an autoradiographic study in the mouse. *Exp Neurol (Suppl)* 1965;2:1–70.

63. Angevine JB Jr. Critical cellular events in the shaping of neural centers. In: Schmitt FO, ed. *The neurosciences: Second study program*. New York: Rockefeller University Press, 1970;62–72.

64. Rakic P, Nowakowski RS. The time of origin of neurons in the hippocampal region of the Rhesus monkey. *J Comp Neurol* 1981;196:99–128.

65. Stanfield BB, Cowan WM. The development of the hippocampal region. In: Peters A, Jones EG, eds. *Cerebral cortex*, vol 7. New York: Plenum Press, 1988;91–131.

66. Nowakowski RS, Rakic P. The site of origin and route and rate of migration of neurons in the hippocampal region of the Rhesus monkey. *J Comp Neurol* 1981;196:129–154.

67. Smart IHM. Radial unit analysis of hippocampal histogenesis in the mouse. *J Anat* 1982;135:763–793.

68. Doose H, Gerken H, Horstmann T, Volzke E. Genetic factors in spike-wave absences. *Epilepsia* 1973;14:57–75.

69. Lindsay JMM. Genetics and epilepsy. A model from critical path analysis. *Epilepsia* 1971;12:47–54.

70. Hanley J, Berkhout J, Crandall P, Rickles WR, Walter RD. Spectral characteristics of EEG activity accompanying deep spiking in a patient with schizophrenia. *Electroencephalogr Clin Neurophysiol* 1970;28:90.

Advances in Neurology, Vol. 55, edited by
D. Smith, D. Treiman, and M. Trimble,
Raven Press, Ltd., New York 1991.

5

Psychosis and the Temporal Lobe

Janice R. Stevens

*Neuropsychiatry Branch, NIMH Neurosciences Center at St. Elizabeth's,
Washington, D.C. 20032*

Psychosis, like epilepsy, is a symptom of disordered brain function. Psychosis, also like epilepsy, is of particular interest to investigators of brain activity because it gives the observer access to functions of normally suppressed ("forbidden") circuits of the brain. Let us begin with some definitions.

Psychosis is defined by Webster as "mental disease, any serious mental derangement" (1). For purposes of this discussion, psychosis will be more sharply defined to include disorders characterized by impaired reality testing, hallucinations, delusions, or bizarre behavior. The many known causes of psychosis include all of the etiologic categories reviewed in the differential diagnosis of other medical disorders—genetic, developmental metabolic, infectious, traumatic, neoplastic, vascular, toxic, deficiency, hematologic, immunogenic, psychological, and "idiopathic."

Defining the temporal lobe should be less difficult than defining psychosis. Readily identified by inspection of the brain, the smooth contours of the temporal cortex enclose, as is well known, two of the major structures of the limbic system: amygdala and hippocampus. These two structures, in turn, project to hypothalamus, mammillary bodies, cingulate gyrus, striatum (including nucleus accumbens, olfactory tubercle, and bed nucleus of the stria terminalis), septum, orbital cortex, temporal neocortex, frontal lobe, and thalamus. Any discussion of psychosis and the temporal lobe must include these and other projections and reciprocal relationships

of the limbic system concealed within its depths.

PSYCHOSIS

For this discussion, the psychoses may be conveniently divided as follows: (a) schizophrenia; (b) mania and depression; (c) paranoid hallucinatory; and (d) confusional. Schizophrenia and manic–depressive psychoses are distinguished by their occurrence in clear consciousness, generally without definite precipitating factors and with a history positive for similar illness in 5–25% of first- and second-degree relatives. Known organic precipitants or "coarse brain disease" are considered exclusion factors for these "functional" psychoses. In contrast, the paranoid hallucinatory disorders, which are distinguished from the schizophrenias by a relative preservation of affect, attention, and cognitive abilities, may occur during or following a very wide variety of brain insults and of toxic, environmental, and endogenous precipitants (including seizures). My task in this chapter will be to try to establish some psychological and anatomic correlations between psychoses and the sites of the brain that may constitute their substrates. In this endeavor we begin by examining the relationships between certain psychoses and known focal lesions of the brain, traumatic brain injury, neoplasms, infections, and neurologic syndromes.

Brain Injury

Summarizing the data from 3552 young men who were brain injured in the Russian–Finnish War, Achte et al. (2) reported occurrence of postinjury psychosis in 8.9% of the total, with schizophrenia and paranoid psychosis each accounting for 2% and 40%, respectively, of the total psychotic group. This is a prevalence two to four times that expected for men in this age group. In contrast, affective (mood) psychoses occurred in only 1% of the total head-injured group (12% of the psychotics). In comparison with a nonpsychotic group of brain-injured men from the same population sample, temporal lobe lesions were only slightly increased in the psychotic group (20.4 versus 17.6%). Dementia was more frequently associated with frontal lobe injuries. Basal injuries showed a significant correlation with Korsakoff-type psychosis. The distribution of other anatomical localizations for various psychotic subgroups did not differ from that in the brain-injured nonpsychotic series.

Achte et al. (2) emphasized that the subsequent occurrence of schizophrenia did not appear to be related to localization of the brain injury, length of post-traumatic coma, or occurrence of seizures. In 42.3% of the cases the psychosis did not appear until 10 or more years after the injury. Hillbom (3), analyzing the same material, noted that patients with psychiatric disturbances of all kinds more often had left-sided injuries than did the entire group (46.7 versus 29.7%). Frontal lesions were slightly underrepresented in association with psychosis, and temporal localization was significantly more frequent among those with psychosis (43.5 versus 17.6% in patients with open head injuries). In contrast, fewer injuries of sensorimotor areas and cerebellum appeared in the psychiatrically disturbed group than in the total population of head injuries without psychosis. Neither Achte et al. (2) nor Hillbom (3) could relate the occurrence of psychosis to the presence of a seizure disorder even though some 40% of the 3552 men in this series suffered at some time from seizures. In summary, left hemisphere, temporal lobe, and basal lesions were overrepresented in patients with diverse psychoses compared with the nonpsychotic brain-injured group,

but no specific localization of lesions for schizophrenia or for paranoid or affective (mood) psychosis could be discerned in this large, well-studied group.

Tumor

In the days before noninvasive imaging or even skull films were routinely obtained in the general run of hospitalized mental patients, brain tumors were discovered at autopsy in as many as 13% of patients as compared with 1–1.5% in the general population (4). Patients with brain tumors may have a variety of organic as well as phenomenologically typical "functional" psychoses. Schizophrenia-like illnesses were diagnosed in 70 patients with cerebral tumors in the archival review by Davison and Bagley (4), who compared the tumor localization in the schizophrenia-like cases with that in an unselected series of 6000 cases of cerebral tumor. As compared to all other cerebral tumor types, only pituitary adenomas were significantly associated with schizophrenia. As for localization, catatonic states were associated with third ventricle tumors, whereas hallucinations were associated with temporal lobe and suprasellar tumors. Epilepsy was not a significant factor. In their discussion, Davison and Bagley (4) remark:

> It should be noted that the apparent irrelevance of epilepsy in the etiology of psychoses associated with cerebral trauma and tumor is further evidence in support of the thesis that epileptic psychoses are etiologically related to the underlying cerebral lesion rather than to the occurrence of fits.

Rather, the tumor data suggest, as do the trauma data, that it is the location of the cerebral lesion (temporal lobe, hypothalamus) that contributes importantly to the development of the psychosis.

In Malamud's series of 245 brain tumors, mental symptoms occurred in 75–80% with temporal and frontal lesions and in 90% of those with third ventricle tumors (5). Schizophrenia-like psychoses were associated with tumors in hippocampus, amygdala, and cingulate gyrus, whereas depression was associated with masses in temporal, hippocampal, or orbital gyrus. Malamud noted no relationship between symptoms and laterality of the lesion. There was a high incidence of seizures in the temporal lobe cases.

Infection

Psychoses occur with a variety of infections affecting the brain (4). Specifically, schizophrenia-like psychoses have also been reported to accompany a very wide variety of cerebral infections. Historically, encephalitis lethargica, which occurred in pandemic form worldwide following the influenza epidemic after World War I, was most often associated with psychiatric problems in children. These included hyperactivity and conduct disorders that often responded to amphetamines. Catatonic motor behavior and schizophrenia-like states were described in older patients and were often followed by Parkinsonism. Narcolepsy was also a frequent sequel and was accompanied by schizophrenia in some cases. The pathological findings in acute encephalitis lethargica were those of a typical gray matter encephalitis principally affecting midbrain (including tegmentum, substantia nigra, and ocular cranial nerve nuclei) but also affecting basal ganglia and cortex in some cases (6). Following the acute inflammatory lesions, intense gliosis appeared in both tegmentum and nigral region of the midbrain and posterior hypothalamus. The most common neurological sequelae were Parkinsonism in adults and behavior disorders in children. Seizures were not a common symptom or sequel.

Both paranoid–hallucinatory and hebephrenic subtypes of schizophrenia were described, and, contrary to expectations of the current dopamine hypotheses of schizophrenia, Parkinsonism was not uncommonly associated with the psychosis (7).

Menninger (8) noted an increased incidence of schizophrenia following the influenza pandemic that followed World War I. Another encephalitis that often imitated schizophrenia was the parenchymatous encephalitis of syphilis, termed "general paresis"; this disorder could present with every form of psychiatric disorder, including mania, depression, and schizophrenic syndromes. Because general paresis, like many of the viral encephalitides, causes a diffuse inflammatory reaction, nerve cell loss, and proliferation of microglia and astrocytes in many brain areas, it is not very helpful in aiding localization for any specific psychosis. Single and multiple case reports of psychosis in association with other specific brain infections have appeared—notably herpes simplex encephalitis, an inflammation that attacks principally the temporal lobe. Depressive disorders, but rarely depressive psychoses, have been reported following both systemic and meningitic infections with Epstein–Barr virus (9).

Heredodegenerative Disorders Associated with Psychosis

Typical schizophrenia-like disorders have been reported in numbers considerably exceeding chance in Huntington's chorea and Wilson's disease, both of which are disorders whose principal anatomic target is the basal ganglia (and neither of which is associated with seizures). In contrast, psychoses in patients with multiple sclerosis, principally a disorder of the cerebral and spinal white matter, are not increased beyond chance expectation (4).

EPILEPSY

My own interest in the relationship between epilepsy and mental disorders began with the paper by Gibbs et al. (10) that reported a dramatically increased incidence of a variety of psychiatric problems in what was then called *psychomotor epilepsy* [subsequently renamed *temporal lobe epilepsy* (TLE)] and which has since been subsumed under the general category of *complex partial seizures* (CPS). Gibbs et al.'s findings were based on electroencephalograms (EEGs) in more than 11,000 patients, all referred to the EEG Laboratory of the Northwestern University Neuropsychiatric Department. Gibbs and Gibbs (11) reported a vastly increased frequency of significant neuropsychiatric disorders (especially personality disturbances and unclassified psychosis) occurring in 40–50% of their patients with psychomotor epilepsy as compared with only 1–2% of patients with other types of epilepsy (Fig. 1). Although the frequency of schizophrenia among patients with psychomotor epilepsy was four times that of patients

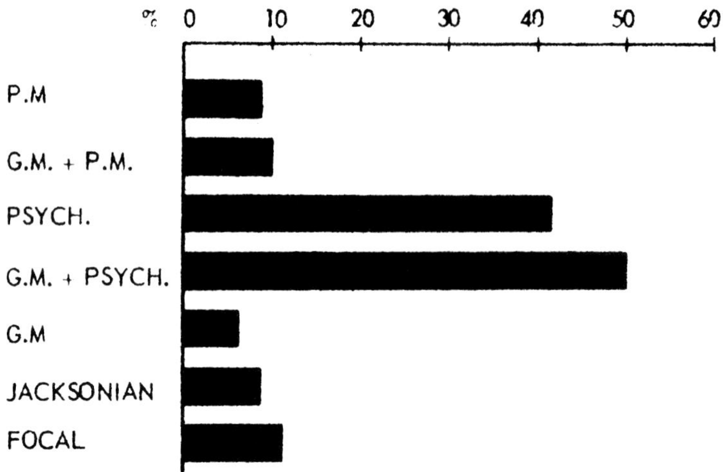

FIG. 1. Incidence of psychiatric symptoms (personality disturbances and psychoses) in various types of epilepsy. *N* = 11,612. P.M., petit mal; G.M., grand mal; PSYCH., psychomotor. (From ref. 11, with permission.)

with grand mal epilepsy, it was still only 1% in their combined psychomotor plus psychomotor–grand-mal patients, or essentially the same as the prevalence of schizophrenia in the general U.S. population (Table 1).

I was a resident in neurology at Yale in those early days when the Gibbs' first reports appeared. I immediately set out to explore the significance of their startling statistics on the marked increase in psychopathology among patients with the psychomotor–temporal-lobe epilepsies. This, I thought, must be a clue to the pathophysiology of disturbed behavior. Apparently I was not the only one to be so stimulated. Following the Gibbses' publications, many case reports appeared supporting their observation of a special relationship between psychomotor epilepsy and psychopathology. However, when we embarked on studies to analyze the elements that might determine this special relationship, we were surprised to discover that using age- and socio-economic-matched patients with psychomotor and grand mal epilepsy we could not demonstrate the overrepresentation of psychopathology they had shown in the psychomotor patients (12,13). Although there were exceptions (14), other controlled studies generally agreed (Table 2) (15–18). Looking back now on that discrepancy, there appear to be a number of

reasons why the Gibbses' data have been difficult to replicate in controlled studies.

1. As I only very recently learned, 75% of the total number of patients with epilepsy studied by the Gibbses were under 20 years of age and were therefore not likely to have yet developed psychoses or other major psychopathology (Frederick Gibbs, *personal communication*, February 1989). But only about 5% of this young age group were diagnosed with psychomotor epilepsy, which the Gibbses considered to be overwhelmingly a disorder of adults. Thus, by the nature of their population, nearly all of the psychomotor patients, but only 25% of all other seizure patients, fell into the age groups (20+ years) where adult psychopathologic syndromes were likely to be diagnosed. Therefore, although the 40–50% incidence of significant psychopathology in the psychomotor patients may be reasonably accurate for their sample, the very low rates of psychopathology in grand mal and other epilepsies (Table 3) may reflect a low rate of reported psychiatric diagnoses in the children who were referred for EEG testing for epilepsy. Assuredly, it reflects the fact that more than 75% of generalized epilepsy patients were children and were thus very unlikely to be diagnosed as psychotic.

TABLE 1. *Psychiatric findings in psychomotor epilepsy*[a]

Psychiatric findings	Psychomotor		Psychomotor and grand mal		Anterior temporal focus	
	Number of cases	Percentage	Number of cases	Percentage	Number of cases	Percentage
Unclassified psychosis	49	7.2	170	9.4	169	10.0
Manic–depressive psychosis (manic)	8	1.2	17	0.9	15	0.9
Manic–depressive psychosis (depressed)	6	0.9	15	0.8	15	0.9
Depression	14	2.1	37	2.0	60	3.6
Suicidal tendencies	19	2.8	42	2.3	46	2.7
Schizophrenia	2	0.2	14	0.8	5	0.3
Schizoid tendencies	3	0.3	4	0.2	7	0.4
Paranoid tendencies	17	2.5	46	2.5	40	2.4
Delusions	0	0.0	5	0.2	5	0.3
Unclassified neurosis	36	5.3	66	3.7	78	4.7
Anxiety neurosis	3	0.3	6	0.3	5	0.3
Obsessive neurosis	0	0.0	2	0.1	2	0.1
Compulsive neurosis	2	0.2	3	0.1	2	0.1
Alcoholism	1	0.1	20	1.1	16	0.9
Hysteria	4	0.6	7	0.4	8	0.4
Behavior problems	51	7.5	68	3.8	63	3.8
Personality disturbance	83	12.2	293	16.2	203	12.1
Passive–dependent attitude	4	0.6	33	1.8	22	1.3
Fearfulness	4	0.6	14	0.8	11	0.6
Tearfulness	1	0.1	4	0.2	6	0.3
Nervousness	15	2.2	58	3.2	36	2.1
Emotional instability	5	0.7	12	0.7	10	0.5
Enuresis	0	0.0	8	0.4	5	0.3
Hyperactivity	3	0.4	6	0.3	12	0.7
Irritability	7	1.0	110	6.1	90	5.4
Temper tantrums	9	1.3	33	1.8	27	1.6
Rage attacks	1	0.1	27	1.5	14	0.9
Assaultive tendencies	6	0.8	14	0.8	17	1.1
Homicidal tendencies	5	0.7	8	0.4	10	0.5
Psychopathy	2	0.3	8	0.4	6	0.3
Abnormal sexual behavior	0	0.0	2	0.1	2	0.1
Nightmares	0	0.0	4	0.2	3	0.2
Hallucinations	18	2.7	39	2.1	44	2.6
Déjà vu	1	0.1	6	0.3	4	0.2
Confusion	7	1.0	29	1.6	15	0.9
Lethargy	3	0.4	8	0.4	6	0.3
Memory defect	3	0.4	47	2.5	44	2.6
Mental deficiency	29	4.3	216	12.0	179	10.7
Hypersomnia (not due to drugs)	19	2.8	23	1.2	19	1.1
Electroshock therapy for psychosis	10	1.5	19	1.1	24	1.4
No significant psychiatric findings (exclusive of mental deficiency)	377	55.6	906	50 0	707	42.2

[a]Incidence of various psychiatric findings in a group of patients with clinical seizures of the psychomotor type and no other type of clinical seizure (678 cases), in a group with clinical seizures of the psychomotor and grand mal type (1806 cases), and in a group with a focus of spike seizures activity in the anterior temporal area (psychomotor type of focus) and no other type of seizure discharge (1675 cases). The first two groups are mutually exclusive, but the third (i.e., the electroencephalographically selected group) includes the majority of the cases in the two clinically selected groups. (From ref. 11, with permission.)

TABLE 2. *Generalized epilepsy, temporal lobe epilepsy, and psychosis: controlled studies*[a]

Study	N	Comparison	Results
Small et al. (13)	50	Psychiatric and psychometric evaluation; psychomotor and GE	No differences in psychotic incidence
Stevens (12)	100	History of admission to a psychiatric hospital	Psychosis: TLE 31%, GE 29% Focal nontemporal: 8%; more schizophrenia in TLE; more apathy in GE
Bruens (15)	19	TLE, GE, TLE–GE; diagnosis at psychiatric hospital	Psychoses 6% in TLE and in GE; 33% in TLE–GE
Standage and Fenton (16)	37	Present State Examination (PSE) TLE versus non-TLE	No differences
Kristensen and Sindrup (35)	192	TLE with psychosis; TLE without psychosis	More visceral seizures; organic; deep limbic pathology in TLE with psychosis
Shukla et al. (14)	132	TLE and GE clinical diagnosis from epilepsy clinic in India	Schizophrenia diagnosed in 17% of TLE; 4% of GE
Toone et al. (18)	69	Psychosis with epilepsy; psychosis without epilepsy	No difference in family history; less catatonia, less premorbid abnormality in psychosis with epilepsy
Perez et al. (42)	24	Psychiatric profile (PSE): 17 TLE and 7 GE, all with psychosis	Diagnosis of nuclear (Schneiderian) schizophrenia in 11 of 17 TLE and in 0 of 7 GE (more affective blunting and regression in GE)

[a]GE, generalized epilepsy; TLE, temporal lobe epilepsy.

2. The Gibbses' EEG Laboratory was located in a neuropsychiatric hospital whose surgeons had a special interest in the treatment of TLE associated with psychiatric disorders and who were among the first to perform temporal lobectomies on these patients (19,20).

3. The psychiatric diagnoses on these patients were made by their referring physicians. Many symptoms and behaviors during psychomotor seizures are so similar to those of neurosis, psychosis, and personality and conduct disorders that these ictal manifestations are likely to have been misdiagnosed as interictal psychiatric problems in many cases (Table 1). The extremely low incidence of behavioral and other psychiatric diagnoses reported for patients with generalized epilepsy is more difficult to understand and may, as already mentioned, reflect the diagnostic habits of physicians who referred children for EEG, principally for epilepsy (Table 3).

4. Patients with typical temporal lobe auras (e.g., olfactory, gustatory, déjà vu) preced-ing generalized ("grand mal") seizures were nevertheless classified as having grand mal (generalized) epilepsy in the Gibbs' series, thus placing a number of patients in the grand mal category when they might otherwise have been classified as having TLE. Because the incidence of grand mal epilepsy in patients with psychiatric disorders was reportedly very low compared to that in patients with psychomotor–TLE disorders, these individuals with temporal lobe auras, if included in psychomotor–temporal-lobe epilepsy category, might have considerably decreased the incidence of psychopathology in the latter.

5. The Gibbses themselves were not blind to the psychiatric diagnosis when they interpreted the EEGs.

These comments are in no way meant to detract from the monumental and pioneering contributions of the Gibbs' and their collaborators to the early development of the EEG and to clinical EEG correlations. They may, however, provide some explanation as to why

TABLE 3. *Psychiatric symptoms in grand mal epilepsy*[a]

Psychiatric symptoms	Number of cases	Percentage
Unclassified psychosis	39	0.7
Manic–depressive (manic)	1	—
Manic–depressive (depressive)	1	—
Depression	7	—
Suicidal tendencies	2	—
Unclassified neurosis	93	1.6
Anxiety neurosis	21	0.4
Alcoholism	17	0.3
Behavior problems	126	2.2
Personality disturbance	16	0.3
Passive–dependent attitude	1	—
Fearfulness	27	0.4
Tearfulness	3	—
Nervousness	5	—
Enuresis	3	—
Hyperactivity	9	—
Irritability	14	0.3
Temper tantrums	40	0.7
Breath-holding	14	—
Rage attacks	6	—
Assaultive tendencies	1	—
Psychopathy	7	—
Nightmares	7	—
Hallucinations	5	—
Confusion	7	—
Memory defect	13	0.3
Lethargy	2	—
Mental deficiency	331	5.7
No significant psychiatric findings	5280	94.3

[a]Incidence of psychiatric symptoms in patients with generalized tonic–clonic convulsions and no other type of clinical seizure (5598 cases). (From ref. 11, with permission.)

subsequent controlled studies of TLE, generalized epilepsy (GE), and behavior have generally not supported the striking preponderance of psychiatric disturbances they reported with psychomotor–temporal-lobe epilepsy as compared to those reported with GE.

This brief analysis of the important material of the Gibbs' points out one of the most serious problems in attempting a study of relationships between epilepsy and psychopathology. The wide variation in incidence of clinically significant psychiatric disorders in individuals with epilepsy depends almost entirely on the source of the patient sample. The lowest incidence is found in community surveys of epilepsy. In one such survey it was found that 25–30% of the persons with seizures had never sought medical attention even though it was both available and free of charge (21). These patients worked and lived relatively normal lives. Yet, according to Zielinski (21) the majority of these individuals had partial seizures, generally of temporal origin. The highest frequency of psychiatric disorders is found in surveys of epilepsy made in mental hospitals, in institutions for persons with epilepsy or for retarded persons, and in clinics specializing in the treatment of intractable seizure disorders. Between these two extremes are the individuals with epilepsy who seek medical care in general medical and neurologic hospitals and clinics and whose rate of admission to mental hospitals is 10 times that of individuals with epilepsy from the community field studies (21).

Surveys made in general practices in Great Britain or Scandinavia (where National Health Insurance prevents the automatic segregation of the indigent, who are generally the most disabled) yield a prevalence of around 2% psychosis and 9% clinically significant nonpsychotic psychiatric problems among adults with epilepsy. This figure is similar to that found in the general population (22). In a survey of psychiatric morbidity in 14 general practices in Great Britain, Pond et al. (23) found that 29% of 245 children and adults with epilepsy had psychiatric problems. These were principally conduct disorders in children and neuroses in adults. Seven percent had been hospitalized for psychiatric illness (half of whom were diagnosed as having TLE). Because many studies assert that it is not epilepsy, but TLE, that is significantly associated with psychopathology, it is important to recognize that the prevalence of TLE in each study population varies enormously and thus must be considered before comparing results between investigators. Thus, Gudmundsson's (24) field study of all epilepsy patients (including children and adults) in Iceland yielded 987 cases; only 6.3% were diagnosed as having psychomotor or temporal-lobe epilepsy, whereas 55% were diagnosed as having GE. In contrast, Smith et al. (25) reported that only 5% of patients in the Veterans Administration (VA) multicenter study of 622 newly diagnosed adults with epilepsy had GE! The psychopathology found in 50% of the sample studied by Gudmundsson would be expected to include very few patients with TLE, whereas a majority of those with psychopathology in the VA study must have TLE unless TLE offered some protection against such psychopathology. In other words, the significance of both the psychopathology and the TLE rate must be judged against an appropriate age/socioeconomic-matched field or hospital sample examined in the same way by the same investigators and using the same definitions of both epilepsy and psychopathology subtypes.

Among 72 patients with epilepsy admitted to a British mental hospital, Betts (26) reported that the main psychiatric diagnoses were depression (n = 22), organic brain syndrome (n = 22), and personality disorder (n = 15). Three were diagnosed as having paranoid psychosis, and none were diagnosed as having schizophrenia. In a study of a chronic mental hospital population of 13,000, there were 78 with epilepsy and psychosis: 28 with paranoid psychosis; 20 with "furors"; and 15 with paranoid schizophrenia, half of whom had the onset of their schizophrenia prior to the onset of the epilepsy. Most of these patients had TLE, and right-sided lesions were more common than left-sided ones (27).

Twelve years later, almost all of these patients who survived were mentally well.

Psychopathology in Children with Epilepsy

Some surveys of children with epilepsy have disclosed an elevated incidence of associated psychiatric disturbances (principally conduct disturbances) and mental retardation (28). Although Rutter et al. (28) reported a higher incidence of psychiatric disturbances in children with TLE, Whitman et al. (29), using a standardized questionnaire and interview, found that patients with TLE and primary GE were subject to similar incidence and types of psychiatric problems. Lindsay et al. (30) reported a high incidence of hyperactivity and rage attacks among 100 children with TLE (a majority of whom also had generalized seizures, mental retardation, or neurologic problems). There were 12 children in their sample with only TLE, and these were reportedly psychologically healthy. Although 70% of the original group of children no longer had clinically significant psychiatric disturbances in adult life, nine had developed schizophrenia (31). Four of those later diagnosed as schizophrenic had childhood I.Q. scores ranging between 50 and 70; also, all had originally had severe GE or frequent temporal lobe seizures as children, with attacks continuing into adult life (two died with status epilepticus). Eight of these nine patients were males, and seven of the nine had left temporal EEG foci; the other two had bilateral foci. Further analysis of the very high incidence of future schizophrenia in these children, like that of the postlobectomy psychoses discussed later in this chapter, may give important clues to the pathophysiology of schizophrenia-like psychoses.

EPILEPSY AND SCHIZOPHRENIA

The observation that schizophrenia and epilepsy rarely occurred in the same individual— or that if they did, the psychosis was less severe—gave rise to the use of convulsive therapies in psychiatry (32). In 1963, Slater and Beard (33) challenged this belief in the mutual antagonism of schizophrenia and epilepsy. They reported that schizophrenia-like psychoses appeared in an unexpectedly large number of patients with epilepsy referred to the National and Maudsley Hospitals in London. They reported that these psychoses tended to appear around 14 years after onset of the epilepsy and affected a greater number of patients with TLE than with other epilepsies.

This landmark study promoted and continues to generate great interest in the relationship between schizophrenia and TLE. There are however, a number of problems that cast doubt on the special relationship between TLE and schizophrenia alleged by Slater and Beard (33). First, the coincidence of 69 cases of epilepsy and schizophrenia-like psychosis in the greater London area, while perhaps unlikely if it had been a random population survey (where approximately 250 such persons would be expected among a population of 10 million), is not so remarkable when it is recognized that Slater and Beard's (33) patients were found among patients already referred for epilepsy. Moreover, many were referred for intractable and complicated epilepsy to two major London hospitals that were specialized centers for nervous and mental disease, and where, during this period, patients with epilepsy and psychiatric disturbances were of special interest to the neurosurgical staff. Moreover, one-third of the 69 patients

in this study were diagnosed as having GE, not TLE—a proportion not much different from the 60–65% TLE we found in a university referral clinic for adult epilepsy (12). The interval of 14 years between the onset of epilepsy and the beginning of psychosis, cited by Slater and Beard (33) as evidence for the special relationship between the two disorders, corresponds closely to the peak ages of onset of both epilepsy and schizophrenia (34); other studies have reported a range of 2–50 years, with a mean (which is thus rather meaningless) of 14–16 years. Finally, some 70% of the 69 patients had evidence of focal or diffuse structural changes, manifest principally by dilated cerebral ventricles or sulci. Similar findings were reported by Kristensen et al. (35), who noted that evidence for subcortical atrophy was one of the factors distinguishing patients with TLE plus psychosis from patients with TLE without psychosis.

A number of controlled studies have been published in which the relationship of TLE and GE to schizophrenia has been examined. A majority of these studies fail to demonstrate either an increase or decrease in the incidence of schizophrenia in patients with epilepsy (26,36), and several large studies have shown a decreased incidence of epilepsy among schizophrenics (Table 4).

TABLE 4. *Epilepsy, schizophrenia, and psychosis*

Prevalence of psychosis in general population:	4.5%	(2.2–9.5%; ref. 36)
Prevalence of psychosis in epileptic individuals:	1.1%	(N = 1073; ref. 36)
	7%	(N = 987; ref. 24)
Prevalence of schizophrenia in general population:	0.1–0.8%	(N = >2500[b]; ref. 39)
Prevalence of schizophrenia in epileptics:	0.75%	(N = 1073; ref. 36)
Prevalence of schizophrenia in patients with TLE[a]:	1.8%	(N = 666; ref. 58)
	1%	(N = 2500; ref. 11)
Prevalence of epilepsy in general population:	0.5%	(N = >1000; ref. 21)
Prevalence of epilepsy in schizophrenia:	0.33%	(N = 50,000; ref. 37)
Prevalence of TLE among clinic adults (>15 years) with epilepsy:	60–76%	(N = 2978; ref. 38)
Prevalence of TLE among hospitalized epileptic psychiatric patients:	50–84%	(N = 136; ref. 41) (N = 57; ref. 57) (N = 100; ref. 12)
Prevalence of TLE in Schizophrenia-like psychosis + epilepsy:	75%	(N = 69; ref. 33)

[a]TLE, temporal lobe epilepsy.
[b]Based on rate/1000.

One of the most interesting of these reports is from London, where Perez et al. (42) studied 24 adult patients with psychosis and epilepsy, consecutively referred to the Neuropsychiatry Department of the National Hospital, Queen Square. Seventeen of these patients had complex partial seizures and EEG diagnosis of TLE, and seven had GE. Diagnosed by the Present State Examination (PSE) and classified by the Catego program (43), the patients with TLE, especially those with left-sided EEG foci, were much more likely to receive a diagnosis of "nuclear" schizophrenia than were those with GE. The investigators noted that affect was generally preserved in most of these patients and that they were able to live and work in the community without psychotropic medication. In contrast, the GE patients with psychoses had more evidence of social and cognitive deterioration, but none were judged as having "nuclear" schizophrenia. Affective disorders were equally common in both groups and were not associated with laterality of focus.

In interpreting this study, it is important to recognize how the definition of "nuclear schizophrenia" differs from the more classical definitions of schizophrenia. The diagnosis of PSE "nuclear schizophrenia" depends on the presence of at least one of Schneider's seven First-Rank Symptoms (FRS) for diagnosis (thought intrusion, thought broadcast, thought commentary, thought withdrawal, voices talking about the patient, primary delusions, and delusions of control or of alien penetration). Since five of these seven symptoms are concerned with verbal phenomena, it is perhaps not surprising that patients with left temporal lobe disturbance are overrepresented in this cohort. Use of the FRS diagnosis of schizophrenia has been criticized by a number of investigators—notably Carpenter and Strauss (44), who noted that many patients with other psychiatric disorders met the FRS criteria whereas almost half of the patients diagnosed as having schizophrenia by more traditional criteria did not. Given the nonspecificity of the FRS, the Perez et al. (42) correlation of left-sided TLE with some of these symptoms favors an association of these symptoms with dysfunction of the left temporal lobe and its projections as they suggest,

but it does not prove a correlation with schizophrenia.

ELECTROENCEPHALOGRAPHIC STUDIES

Although Hans Berger, discoverer of the human EEG, was a psychiatrist who hoped the secret of psychosis might emerge from the study of electrical activity of the brain, conventional EEG has not contributed greatly to our understanding of psychoses in general and schizophrenia in particular. Not unexpectedly, most of the organic toxic and confusional psychoses are associated with diffuse, moderate slowing in the EEG. Concerning schizophrenia, early reports stress decreased alpha, increased theta, slowing, and occasional spike-and-wave activity over one or both temporal lobes. More than half of the EEGs from patients with schizophrenia are, however, within normal limits. Computerized EEG spectra now emphasize these findings in technicolor maps, showing evidence of lateralized asymmetry. Isolated frontal slowing seen on the computerized maps of schizophrenic patients is almost surely a product of eye movement artifact. As in TLE, however, the real action may lie beneath the surface and rarely reach scalp or cortical electrodes. Thus Kendrick and Gibbs (19), Heath (45), and Sem-Jacobsen (46) reported abnormal spike activity in deep brain nuclei during psychotic episodes. During a prolonged telemetered EEG from a severely psychotic young schizophrenic with no history of seizures, we recorded at least one clear-cut episode of paroxysmal rhythmic left, followed by right temporal hypersynchronous activity consistent with deep temporal spiking or hypersynchrony (47). Dr. Joseph Faber of Prague recently sent me photographs of a young schizophrenic with depth electrodes in the hippocampus showing spike activity similar to that reported by Heath. The scalp EEG evidence, although sparse (because most schizophrenics have normal or only mildly abnormal surface EEGs), is consistent with the anatomic and clinical data that point to abnormality in deep limbic structures and their projection sites as the substrate of schizophrenia-like psychoses (19,45,46).

Ramani and Gumnit (48) had the opportunity to study the scalp EEG of 10 epilepsy patients who developed psychoses while being treated in hospital for seizures. In nine patients the interictal psychosis was indistinguishable from schizophrenia: Five of these patients had complex partial seizures, and the other four showed evidence of GE. One patient showed the normalization of the EEG described by Landolt (49). Four patients showed bilateral temporal spike-and-wave activity, one showed right temporal activity, one showed left temporal activity, and the remaining patients showed bilateral synchronous frontal and central complexes. Of the 38 patients admitted with a history of psychoses to Ramani and Gumnit's large epileptic unit, 63% were diagnosed as having complex partial seizures (CPS). This was almost exactly the same proportion of CPS as in their general clinic population of patients with epilepsy without psychoses.

A predominance of left-sided foci in TLE patients developing schizophrenia or schizophrenia-like psychoses has been reported by Flor-Henry (50), Ounsted and Lindsay (31), Sherwin (51), and Toone and Driver (52) but not by Kristensen et al. (35), Jensen and Larsen (53), Serafetinides and Falconer (54), Parnas and co-workers (34,55), or Betts (27). The explanation of this discrepancy may lie with the differences in diagnostic criteria employed by the different investigators. The English generally use FRS, whereas the Scandinavians do not. Thus Parnas et al. (34) found that left-sided foci were underrepresented in their five TLE patients with classical schizophrenia but overrepresented in patients diagnosed as having paranoid-hallucinatory psychosis (a psychosis distinguished from schizophrenia by absence of thought disorder, affective flattening, and deterioration).

DEPRESSION

Depression is widely reported in patients with epilepsy, both by interview and by psychological tests such as the Minnesota Multi-phasic Personality Inventory (MMPI). Manic–depressive behavior (both manic and depressed types) was diagnosed in nearly 4% of patients with psychomotor and psychomotor–grand-mal epilepsy by Gibbs et al. (10), a figure four times higher than that found in the general population. Among more than 4000 GE patients, no depression or bipolar disorder was reported by Gibbs and Gibbs (11). However, this discrepancy may be explained, as noted above, by the preponderance of children in the entire sample and by the failure of referring physicians to note psychiatric diagnoses in patients referred for epilepsy.

Although the percentage who were psychotic was not specified, depression was the most common psychiatric diagnosis in Betts' (27) 72 cases of adults with epilepsy admitted to a mental hospital. In their review of suicide and epilepsy, Mathews and Barabas (56) estimated the frequency of death by suicide among individuals with epilepsy to be 5%—approximately three to four times the U.S. general population average (1.4%). Although the review by Barraclough (57) reported that patients with TLE were at 25 times the risk for suicide as compared to that for the general population (and at five times the risk compared to that of individuals with other epilepsies), it is notable that three of the four TLE samples in this study are drawn from nonrepresentative sources of individuals with epilepsy. These include two temporal lobe surgery series and the childhood TLE series of Ounsted and Lindsay (31), which, as already noted, included children with a variety of organic syndromes in addition to TLE. The remaining series of 666 adult TLE (TLE only, with no other organic syndromes) patients studied by Currie et al. (58) from a neurology clinic in London recorded three suicides among 54 deaths. It is not possible to compare this TLE group with other types of epilepsy in the Barraclough review, since the other studies cited did not report their suicides by TLE and other epilepsy types. Thus the definitive study on suicide with respect to TLE and other epilepsies remains to be done.

Robertson and Trimble (59), while reporting a high incidence of depressive neurosis in patients with epilepsy, did not find an excess of manic–depressive psychosis and found no relationship between the depressive neurosis (or psychoses) and the type of epilepsy. Few studies have supported Flor-Henry's (50) interesting proposal that a right temporal focus is associated with depressive disorders.

EXPERIMENTAL STUDIES

If the dramatic increase in psychopathology reported by the Gibbs' among patients with psychomotor seizures was not sufficient to interest the student of brain and abnormal behavior in the temporal lobe, the experimental studies in animals would certainly do so. Several volumes, rather than a single chapter, would be required to review the voluminous literature demonstrating the relationship of the temporal lobes and the subtemporal limbic structures to emotions and behavior. Bard and Mountcastle's (60) observations on the savage states induced in cats following medial temporal ablations, as well as Kluver and Bucy's (61) classic report on the taming, hyperorality, hypersexuality, and hypermetamorphism in primates following bilateral anterior temporal lobectomy, have contributed to the "limbic system" concept of MacLean and Delgado (62). The studies of Egger and Flynn (63) on amygdala "push–pull" control of hypothalamically elicited attack behavior, as well as Kling et al.'s (64) remarkable reports of altered behavior following limbic lesions, have fostered enormous interest in the limbic system as an anatomic substrate for emotional, hierarchical, and self- and species-preserving behaviors.

Depth Electrode Studies in Humans

Studies of the limbic system in humans have nearly all been carried out in individuals with medically intractable TLE. Surface and deep electrodes acutely or chronically implanted in various parts of the system have shown that many, if not all, of the subjective sensations (i.e., hallucinations, delusions, thought-blocking, and stereotypes) observed in schizophrenia and schizophrenia-like psychoses can occur during spontaneous seizures arising in the deep temporal lobe structures or have been elicited by stimulation of these structures. Auditory hallucinations in the third person (a hallmark of schizophrenia) are, however, only rarely elicited by stimulation of deep temporal sites (65). Weiser (66) reported that spontaneous seizures arising from hippocampus and amygdala associated with auditory hallucinations also show abnormal electrical activity in the primary auditory area and basal ganglia.

Electrolytic lesions in medial amygdala or hypothalamus in human subjects prone to episodic pathologic rage were reportedly successful in suppressing rage attacks (67–69), but this type of therapy has been largely discontinued as a result of objections by a segment of the population that would not tolerate this treatment of abnormal human behavior.

With all the evidence we have seen pointing to deep temporal lobe limbic sites for psychoses, it is not surprising that temporal lobe surgery was also undertaken for schizophrenia in the past. These operations were nearly uniformly unsuccessful and were soon given up (19). In contrast, following frontal white matter ablations that isolated the frontal lobe from the dorsal medial thalamus, relief was reported with regard to some of the more severe delusional fears and terrifying derogatory hallucinations. Relief of these disabling symptoms in schizophrenics was also reported following orbital white matter lesions, sometimes mistakenly called *substantia innominotomy,* which severed the connection of the amygdala with the orbital cortex. This operation is still carried out to relieve intractable suffering of certain schizophrenics with severe terrors or agonizing somatic symptoms (70). Surgical treatment for intractable depression, on the other hand, appeared to be most successful following anterior cingulotomy severing connections between the hippocampus, the frontal lobe, the septum, and the hypothalamus (71).

POST-TEMPORAL
LOBECTOMY PSYCHOSIS

Temporal lobectomy for focal epilepsy of temporal lobe origin is now a routine and highly successful treatment for carefully chosen cases in more than two dozen centers in the United States and as many in other countries. Reports from a number of centers indicate that patients with TLE and psychoses do not generally show improvement in the psychoses following temporal lobectomy even though seizures are ameliorated. Certain types of psychopathology, such as irritability and rage attacks (if present) in patients with TLE, are oftentimes greatly improved after temporal lobectomy or by restricted hippocampo-amygdalotomy, especially if the seizures are arrested. The latter procedure has also been reported successful in at least one case of typical schizophrenia-like psychosis in association with epilepsy (H. G. Weiser, *personal communication,* February 1989). Even more interesting and puzzling is the fact that both depression and schizophrenic paranoid–hallucinatory states may occur for the first time following temporal lobe resection for seizures. The postoperative depression usually occurs quite soon after the surgery and may be severe and resistant enough to require convulsive therapy. Paranoid–hallucinatory states which occurred *de novo* in 3 of 14 patients with TLE in our series following temporal lobectomy occurred months to years after the surgery and generally responded well to dopamine-blocking (neuroleptic) therapy.

Postlobectomy psychoses have been reported in up to 12% of cases in other series (53), but their cause and frequency remain as yet unknown (Table 5).

The occurrence of schizophrenia-like psychoses after removal of the damaged temporal lobe focuses attention on what could be happening in the projection sites of that resected lobe after removal. We used to think that there was no regeneration in the central nervous system after injury and that injuries of adult brain are followed by gliosis, not by axonal sprouting. However, sprouting of catecholamine fibers to occupy septal sites following section of the fimbria, as reported by Raisman (72) in the rat, raises new possibilities for both physiologic and pathologic repair in the adult mammalian brain. That such regeneration also takes place in other neurotransmitter systems and in the human brain is evident from recent work of Cotman and co-workers (73,74), who have shown sprouting of the acteylcholine system after septal lesions and in the molecular layer of the hippocampus in Alzheimer's disease in humans.

ANATOMIC STUDIES OF SCHIZOPHRENIA

Although dilated ventricles and cortical sulcal widening were reported in a percentage of patients with schizophrenia and other psychoses on the basis of pneumoencephalogram or autopsy findings more than 50 years ago, it was not until the advent of noninvasive imaging by computerized tomography that structural abnormalities in the brain were widely recognized by the psychiatric community. More than 50 such studies have now been published, and a majority demonstrate mild-to-moderate ventricular dilatation (often demonstrable only by measurement), principally affecting the body of the lateral ventricles and the third ventricle (75). When we turn

TABLE 5. *Mental state of temporal lobe epilepsy (TLE) patients following unilateral temporal lobectomy*

Series	Length of study	N	Abnormal prior to lobectomy	Improved after lobectomy	Psychotic prior to lobectomy	Psychotic after lobectomy	New psychosis
Bailey, 1957 (94)	2–6 years	63	53	14	12	19	7
Jensen and Larsen, 1975 (95)	2–5 years	74	63	15	11	20	9
Polkey, 1983 (96)	2–5 years	40	16	8	0	3	3
Stevens, 1988 (97)	20–30 years	14	8	2	0	4	4
Taylor (Falconer series), 1972 (98)	5 + years	100	87	19	16	19	3

to anatomical studies on autopsy material, measurements can be more exact. Bogerts et al. (76) examined serial sections of the brains of 13 schizophrenic patients and nine matched controls from the Vogt collection in Dusseldorf, Germany. They reported a significant decrease in volume of the parahippocampal gyrus, hippocampus, amygdala, and internal pallidal segment, along with narrowing of the paraventricular nuclei of the thalamus and hypothalamus, in patients with chronic schizophrenia. Notable in their material is the fact that, in contrast to the rather uniform pathology of Huntington's chorea or Parkinson's disease, individual schizophrenic patients have variable pathology affecting only one, two, three, or more of the above areas. Gliosis has also been reported from scattered and variable areas both within and outside the limbic system and its projections (77,78), whereas other reports emphasize pathology in hippocampus and entorhinal cortex (79–82).

Introduction of relatively specific pharmacologic agents useful in the treatment of nearly all types of psychoses reawakened the interest of psychiatrists with regard to brain pathology and chemistry. Discovery of neuroleptics, and that their potency against psychoses is directly proportional to their ability to block dopamine (D2) receptors in the brain, called attention to brain dopamine (DA) pathways and projections as being potentially important substrates of psychosis. As is well known, the major cerebral DA pathways arise in the substantia nigra (A9) and ventral tegmental area (VTA, A10), ascending to innervate the neostriatum and ventral (limbic) striatum, respectively. These basal ganglia nuclei account for more than 85% of the DA projection sites in the brain. Smaller, less well known pathways from VTA innervate amygdala, hippocampus, parts of frontal cortex, entorhinal cortex, hypothalamus, and periventricular regions of the third ventricle and midbrain.

To choose any one or more of these DA terminal sites as the probable anatomic substrate of schizophrenia and schizophrenia-like psychoses would be a random process were it not for the information gained from study of the anatomic lesions associated with psychoses. As we have already seen, tumor, infection, heredodegenerative disease, and epilepsy make relatively very small contributions to the occurrence of schizophrenia. The similarity of auras of temporal lobe seizures to many of the subjective symptoms and experiences of individuals with schizophrenia, as well as the elicitation of symptoms strikingly similar to those of schizophrenic patients by stimulation of deep limbic structures, emphasizes the importance of the temporal lobe and of the subcortical limbic structures and their projections as the substrates of psychotic experience. Putting the DA hypothesis of psychosis together with the clinical parallels between TLE and schizophrenic experience, I proposed a number of years ago that pathology of schizophrenia should be found in the DA-rich projection sites of the limbic system in the ventral (limbic) striatum (83). Although two studies have reported a modest decrease in neurons in the nucleus accumbens in schizophrenia (84,85), it is the elevation in D2 receptors in this region and neostriatum that have been the most consistent pathologic finding in schizophrenic brains (86). Because neuroleptic treatment also increases D2 receptors in these regions, the significance of this finding in schizophrenic brains has remained moot for more than a decade. There is also reportedly increased DA and homovanillic acid in the amygdala, particularly on the left side of schizophrenic brains (87).

The pathologic findings in schizophrenic brains, which include diminished temporal lobe volume, decrease in hippocampal pyramidal cells, and narrowing of the entorhinal cortex, could provoke "downstream" regeneration or degeneration or produce altered receptors in projection sites in dorsal and ventral (limbic) striatum, hypothalamus, etc.

One clue to the etiology of psychoses is the importance of DA-blocking agents, all of which lower convulsive threshold and ameliorate productive psychotic symptoms. The action of DA on cell firing is generally inhibitory. This suggests that while excessive excitatory neuronal discharge causes seizures, excessive inhibition—maintained by increased dopaminergic or other inhibitory transmitters (e.g., norepinephrine, gamma-aminobutyric acid)—contributes to psychosis. There is support for this hypothesis from clinical observation of psychoses appearing in some individuals as clinical seizures decrease

(33,35,49,50,88), as well as from experimental investigations with amygdala kindling that have shown enhanced dopaminergic activity in amygdala projection sites (89,90). Positron emission tomography (PET) demonstrates hypometabolism consistent with inhibition of local neuronal activity in specific areas in schizophrenia and both surrounding and at a distance from the epileptic focus in patients with epilepsy and psychosis (91–93).

Many of these projection sites are in the very areas where Heath and others reported spike activity in the brains of schizophrenic patients and in epilepsy patients with psychoses (45,46).

CONCLUSIONS

This review of the relationships between temporal lobe pathology and psychosis indicates that pathologic changes in the temporal lobe and in its deep and frontal lobe projection sites may contribute to occurrence of psychosis in patients with tumor, trauma, and certain heredodegenerative disorders. Evaluation of the epilepsy literature with respect to TLE (or CPS) and psychoses still leaves us in doubt as to the particular relationship between TLE and psychopathology because there are serious problems of sampling and diagnosis of both epilepsy and psychopathology. Among the few large epidemiologic field (i.e., nonhospital or nonclinical) studies of epilepsy, the diagnosis of TLE or CPS was made in only 30–40% of cases, yet the percentage of adults with TLE or CPS in specialty clinics for epilepsy is around 65–85%. Does this mean that a much larger percentage of patients with TLE report to specialty clinics because they are more severely affected, or does it mean that many GE cases diagnosed outside of the hospital or clinic actually have TLE with secondary generalization?

Among patients with psychoses and epilepsy, patients with TLE outnumber patients with other epilepsies 2 to 1, but this may only reflect the higher percentage of TLE in patients in hospital and clinic samples. If we compare their numbers with the percentage of patients with TLE in community surveys, TLE is greatly overrepresented in psychiatric cohorts. But if we compare the frequency of TLE in patients with psychoses with the frequency of TLE among epilepsy patients reporting to specialty clinics for epilepsy, the incidence is practically the same. These patients in the specialty clinics are also much more often psychiatrically impaired and have more severe intractable epilepsies when compared to those surveyed in the field studies. In contrast, in the latter as many as one-third of all epilepsy patients do not feel the need for medical care, nor do they seek it, because their seizures are not sufficiently troublesome. Moreover, a majority of those who carry on without care have partial epilepsy— usually of the temporal lobe type. Clearly, better epidemiologic studies of large numbers of patients with TLE and other epilepsies diagnosed in the same uniformly acceptable fashion are required to answer the question, "Does TLE predispose to psychosis?"

Davison and Bagley (4), in their archival review of 782 published reports concerned with organic brain disease and schizophrenia, cautioned that the vast majority of patients displaying a schizophrenic syndrome have no detectable brain disease. Modern neuropathologic and imaging studies have somewhat altered this perspective, focusing attention on neurochemical and relatively modest structural changes. Most patients with epilepsy (including TLE) do not have, or will never develop, schizophrenia-like psychoses. The contribution of epilepsy, trauma, and tumor to the occurrence of schizophrenia is very, very small. When psychoses and epilepsy do occur together, it appears that brain damage or dysfunction in critical areas beyond the temporal lobe is a common denominator. Among patients who develop psychoses, it is hypothesized that pathological changes (degeneration, sprouting, excessive excitation or inhibition, or receptor change) in amygdala–hippocampal projection sites in striatum, basal forebrain, hypothalamus, thalamus, or frontal lobe are possible links between temporal lobe pathology and psychoses. A number of factors reviewed in this chapter led to this hypothesis: (a) Psychosis occurs following surgical resection of the temporal lobe, even when seizures are arrested; (b) dilated lateral and third ventricles exist in a significant number of patients with schizophrenia, signifying pathology beyond the temporal lobe; and (c) brain diseases associated with schizophrenia often spare the temporal lobe but involve basal ganglia, midbrain, and hypothalamus, all of which are projection sites of deep temporal structures.

In closing, I should like to express my agreement with those two distinguished Englishmen Kenneth Davison and Christopher Bagley, who concluded their valuable review as follows: "After considering the seemingly incompatible hypotheses of affinity, antagonism and chance association of epilepsy and schizophrenia, we are forced to conclude that all three are correct" (4).

ACKNOWLEDGMENTS

I gratefully acknowledge the technical assistance of Ms. Sheila Johnson, and I am grateful to Drs. Lewellyn Bigelow, Kenneth Rickler, and Daniel Weinberger for reviewing the manuscript.

REFERENCES

1. *Webster's new collegiate dictionary.* Springfield, MA: G & C Merriam, 1960.
2. Achte KA, Hillbom E, Aalberg V. Psychoses following war brain injuries. *Acta Psychiatr Scand* 1969;45:1–18.
3. Hillbom E. After effects of brain injuries. *Acta Psychiatr Scand* 1960;suppl 142:1–195.
4. Davison K, Bagley CR. Schizophrenia-like psychoses associated with organic disorders of the central nervous system: a review of the literature. In: Herrington RN, ed. *British Journal of Psychiatry special publication,* no. 4. Headley Bros Ltd, Ashford, Kent. 1969;113–184.
5. Malamud N. Psychiatric disorder with intracranial tumors of limbic system. *Arch Neurol* 1967;17:113–123.
6. Buzzard EF, Greenfield JG. Lethargic encephalitis: its sequelae and morbid anatomy. *Brain* 1919;42:305–338.
7. Fairweathers DS. Psychiatric aspects of the post encephalitic syndrome. *J Ment Sci* 1947;93:201–254.
8. Menninger K. The schizophrenic syndrome as a product of acute infectious disease. *Arch Neurol Psychiatry* 1928;20:464–481.
9. Hendler N, Leahy W. Psychiatric and neurologic sequelae of infectious mononucleosis. *Am J Psychiatry* 1978;135:842–844.
10. Gibbs FA, Gibbs EL, Furster B. Psychomotor epilepsy. *Arch Neurol* 1948;60:331–339.
11. Gibbs FA, Gibbs EL. *Atlas of electroencephalography,* vol II. Cambridge, MA: Addison-Wesley, 1952.
12. Stevens JR. Psychiatric implications of psychomotor epilepsy. *Arch Gen Psychiatry* 1966;14:461–471.
13. Small JS, Milstein V, Stevens JR. Are psychomotor epileptics different? *Arch Neurol* 1962;7:330–338.
14. Shukla GD, Srivastava ON, Katiyar BC. Sexual disturbances in temporal lobe epilepsy: a controlled study. *Br J Psychiatry* 1979;134:288–292.
15. Bruens JH. Psychoses in epilepsy. *Psychiatr Neurol Neurochir* 1971;74:174–192.
16. Standage KF, Fenton GW. Psychiatric symptom profiles of patients with epilepsy: a controlled investigation. *Psychol Med* 1975;5:152–160.
17. Parnas J, Korsgaard S. Epilepsy and psychosis. *Acta Psychiatr Scand* 1982;66:89–99.
18. Toone BK, Garralda ME, Ron MA. The psychoses of epilepsy and the functional psychoses: a clinical and phenomenological comparison. *Br J Psychiatry* 1982;141:256–261.
19. Kendrick JF, Gibbs FA. Origin, spread and neurosurgical treatment of the psychomotor type of seizure discharge. *J Neurosurg* 1957;14:270–284.
20. Simmel ML, Counts S. Clinical and psychological results of anterior temporal lobectomy in patients with psychomotor epilepsy. In: Baldwin M, Bailey P, eds. *Temporal lobe epilepsy.* Springfield, IL: Charles C Thomas, 1958;530–550.
21. Zielinski JJ. Epidemiologic overview of epilepsy morbidity, mortality and clinical implications. In: Blumer D, ed. *Psychiatric aspects of epilepsy.* Washington, DC: American Psychiatric Press, 1984;67–98.
22. Fenton GW. The EEG, epilepsy and psychiatry. In: Trimble MR, Reynolds EH, eds. *What is epilepsy?* London: Churchill Livingstone, 1986;139–159.
23. Pond DA, Bidwell BH, Stein L. A survey of epilepsy in 14 general practices. I. Demographic and medical data. *Psychiatr Neurol Neurochir* 1960;63:217–236.
24. Gudmundsson G. *Epilepsy in Iceland: a clinical and epidemiological investigation. Acta Neurol Scand.* Copenhagen: Munksgaard, 1966; 43(suppl):1–124.
25. Smith DB, Craft BR, Collins J, Mattson RH, Cramer JA and the VA Epilepsy Cooperative Study Group 118). Behavioral characteristics of epilepsy patients compared with normal controls. *Epilepsia* 1986;27:760–768.
26. Betts TA. A follow-up study of a cohort of patients with epilepsy admitted to psychiatric care in an English city. In: Harris P, Maudsley C, eds. *Epilepsy: Proceedings of the Hans Berger Centenary Symposium.* Edinburgh: Churchill Livingstone, 1974;326–338.
27. Betts TA. Epilepsy and the mental hospital. In: Reynolds EH, Trimble MR, eds. *Epilepsy and psychiatry.* Edinburgh: Churchill Livingstone, 1981;175–184.
28. Rutter M, Graham P, Yule W. *A neuropsychiatric study in childhood.* Philadelphia: JB Lippincott, 1970.

29. Whitman S, Hermann BP, Black RB, Chhabria S. Psychopathology and seizure type in children with epilepsy. *Psychol Med* 1982;12:843–853.

30. Lindsay J, Ounsted C, Richards P. Long-term outcome in children with temporal lobe seizures. II. Marriage, parenthood and sexual indifference. *Dev Med Child Neurol* 1979;21:433–440.

31. Ounsted C, Lindsay J. The long term outcome of temporal lobe epilepsy in childhood. In: Reynolds EH, Trimble MR, eds. *Epilepsy and psychiatry.* Edinburgh: Churchill Livingstone, 1981;185–215.

32. Von Meduna LJ. *Die konvulsionstherapie der schizophrenie.* Halle: Carl Marhold, 1937.

33. Slater E, Beard G. The schizophrenia like psychoses of epilepsy. *Br J Psychiatry* 1963;109:95–150.

34. Parnas J, Korsgaard S, Krautwald O, et al. Chronic psychosis in epilepsy: a clinical investigation of 29 patients. *Acta Psychiatr Scand* 1982;66:282–293.

35. Kristensen O, Hein Sindrup E. Psychomotor epilepsy and psychosis (Parts I and II). *Acta Neurol Scand* 1978;57:361–379.

36. Bartlett JEA. Chronic psychosis following epilepsy. *Am J Psychiatry* 1957;114:338–343.

37. Kat W. Uber den gegensatz epilepsie-schizophrenie und das kombinierte vorkommen diser. *Krankheiten Psychiatr Bl* 1937;41:733–745.

38. Gastaut H, Gastaut JL, Goncalves e Silva GE, Fernandez-Sanchez GE. Relative frequency of different types of epilepsy: a study employing the classification of the International League Against Epilepsy. *Epilepsia* 1975;16:457–461.

39. Eaton WW. Epidemiology of schizophrenia. *Epidemiologic Rev* 1985;7:105–126.

40. Toone BK, Dawson J, Driver MV. Psychoses of epilepsy: a radiological evaluation. *Br J Psychiatry* 1982;140:244–248.

41. Bash KW, Mahnig P. Admissions for epilepsy to a psychiatric clinic over a decade. In: Canger R, Angeleri F, Penry JK, eds. *Advances in epileptology: XIth Epilepsy International Symposium.* New York: Raven Press, 1980;233–236.

42. Perez MM, Trimble MR, Murray NMF, Reider I. Epileptic psychosis: an evaluation of PSE profiles. *Br J Psychiatry* 1985;146:155–163.

43. Wing JK, Cooper JE, Sartorius N. *The description and classification of psychiatric symptoms.* London: Cambridge University Press, 1974.

44. Carpenter WT Jr, Strauss JS. Cross-cultural evaluation of Schneider's first-rank symptoms of schizophrenia: a report from the International Pilot Study of Schizophrenia. *Am J Psychiatry* 1974;131:682–687.

45. Heath RG. *Studies in schizophrenia.* Cambridge, MA: Harvard University Press, 1954.

46. Sem-Jacobsen CW. Depth electrographic observations on psychotic patients. A system related to emotional behavior. *Acta Psychiatr (KBh)* 1959;34:412–416.

47. Stevens JR, Bigelow L, Denney D, Lipkin J, Livermore AH Jr, Rauscher F, Wyatt RJ. Telemetered EEG–EOG during psychotic behaviors of schizophrenia. *Arch Gen Psychiatry* 1979;36:251–262.

48. Ramani VV, Gumnit RJ. Intensive monitoring of epileptic patients with interictal psychosis in epilepsy. *Ann Neurol* 1982;11:613–622.

49. Landolt H. Serial electroencephalographic investigations during psychotic episodes in epileptic patients and during schizophrenic attacks. In: de Haas L, ed. *Lectures on epilepsy.* New York: Elsevier, 1958;91–131.

50. Flor-Henry P. Psychosis and temporal lobe epilepsy. *Epilepsia* 1969;10:363–395.

51. Sherwin I. *Psychosis associated with epilepsy: significance of the laterality of the epileptogenic lesion.* London: British Medical Association, 1981.

52. Toone BK, Driver MV. Psychosis and epilepsy. *Res Clin Forums* 1980;2:121–127.

53. Jensen I, Larsen JK. Mental aspects of temporal lobe epilepsy. Follow-up of 74 patients after resection of a temporal lobe. *J Neurol Neurosurg Psychiatry* 1979;42:256–265.

54. Serafetinides EA, Falconer MA. The effects of temporal lobectomy in epileptic patients with psychosis. *Br J Psychiatry* 1962;108:584–593.

55. Parnas J, Korsgaard S. Epilepsy and psychosis. A review. *Acta Psychiatr Scand* 1982;66:89–99.

56. Mathews WS, Barabas G. Suicide and epilepsy: a review of literature. *Psychosomatics* 1981;22:515–524.

57. Barraclough B. Suicide and epilepsy. In: Trimble MR, Reynolds EH, eds. *Epilepsy and psychiatry.* New York: Churchill Livingstone, 1981;72–76.

58. Currie S, Heathfield KWG, Henson RA, Scott DF. Clinical course and prognosis of temporal lobe epilepsy. A survey of 666 patients. *Brain* 1971;94:173–190.

59. Robertson MM, Trimble MR. Depressive illness in patients with epilepsy: a review. *Epilepsia* 1983;24(Suppl 2):S109–S116.

60. Bard P, Mountcastle VB. Some forebrain mechanisms involved in expression of rage with special reference to suppression of angry behavior. *Res Publ Assoc Nerv Ment Dis* 1948;27:362–404.

61. Kluver H, Bucy PC. An analysis of certain effects of bilateral temporal lobectomy in the rhesus monkey, with special reference to "psychic blindness." *J Psychol* 1938;5:33–54.

62. MacLean PD, Delgado JMR. Electrical and chemical stimulation of frontotemporal portion of limbic system in the waking animal. *Electroencephalogr Clin Neurophysiol* 1953;5:91–100.

63. Egger MD, Flynn JP. Effects of electrical stimulation of the amygdala on hypothalamically elicited attack behavior in cats. *J Neurophysiol* 1963;26:705–720.

64. Kling AJ, Orbach J, Schwarz N, Towne J. Injury to the limbic system and associated structures in cats. *Arch Gen Psychiatry* 1960;3:391–420.

65. Halgren E, Walter RD, Cherlow DG, Crandall PH. Mental phenomena evoked by electrical stimulation of the human hippocampal formation and amygdala. *Brain* 1978;101:83–117.

stimulation of the human hippocampal formation and amygdala. *Brain* 1978;101:83–117.

66. Weiser HG. Depth recorded limbic seizures and psychopathology. *Neurosci Biobehav Rev* 1983; 7:427–440.

67. Narabayashi H, Nagao T, Saito Y, Yoshida M, Nagahata M. Stereotaxic amygdalotomy for behavior disorders. *Arch Neurol* 1963;9:1–16.

68. Balasubramaniam V, Kanaka TS, Ramanujam PB, et al. Sedative neurosurgery. *Neurology (India)* 1970;18(Suppl 1):45–52.

69. Mark VH, Sweet W, Ervin F. Deep temporal lobe stimulation and destructive lesions in episodically violent temporal lobe epileptics. In: Fields WS, Sweet WH, eds. *Neural bases of violence and aggression*. St. Louis: Warren Green, 1975;379–391.

70. Knight G. Stereotactic tractotomy in the surgical treatment of mental illness. *Neurol Neurosurg Psychiatry* 1965;28:304.

71. Ballantine HT Jr, Levy BS, Dagi TF, Giriunas IB. Cingulotomy for psychiatric illness: report of 13 years' experience. In: Sweet WH, Obrador S, Martin-Rodriguez JG, eds. *Neurosurgical treatment in psychiatry, pain, and epilepsy*. Baltimore: University Park Press, 1975;333–353.

72. Raisman G. Neuronal plasticity in the septal nuclei of the adult rat. *Brain Res* 1969;14:25–48.

73. Cotman C, Nieto-Sampedro M, Harris EW. Synapse replacement in the nervous system of adult vertebrates. *Physiol Rev* 1981;61:644–782.

74. Geddes JW, Monaghan DT, Cotman CW, Lott IT, Kim RC. Plasticity of hippocampal circuitry in Alzheimer's disease. *Science* 1985;230:1178–1180.

75. Reveley MA. CT scans in schizophrenia. *Br J Psychiatry* 1985;146:367–371.

76. Bogerts B, Meertz E, Schonfeldt-Bausch R. Basal ganglia and limbic system pathology in schizophrenia. A morphometric study of brain volume and shrinkage. *Arch Gen Psychiatry* 1985;42:784–791.

77. Stevens JR. Neuropathology of schizophrenia. *Arch Gen Psychiatry* 1982;39:1131–1139.

78. Stevens JR. Epilepsy and psychosis: neuropathological studies of six cases. In: Trimble MR, Bolwig TG, eds. *Aspects of epilepsy and psychiatry*. New York: John Wiley & Sons, 1986;117–146.

79. Kovelman JA, Scheibel AB. A neurohistological correlate of schizophrenia. *Biol Psychiatry* 1984; 19:1601–1621.

80. Jakob H, Beckmann H. Prenatal development disturbances in the limbic allocortex in schizophrenics. *J Neural Transm* 1986;65:154–161.

81. Falkai P, Bogerts B. Cell loss in the hippocampus of schizophrenics. *Eur Arch Psychiatr Neurol* 1986;236:154–161.

82. Brown R, Colter N, Corsellis JAN, et al. Postmortem evidence of structural brain changes in schizophrenia: Differences in brain weight, temporal horn area, and parahippocampal gyrus compared with affective disorder. *Arch Gen Psychiatry* 1986;43:36–42.

83. Stevens JR. An anatomy of schizophrenia? *Arch Gen Psychiatry* 1973;29:177–189.

84. Pakkenberg B. Post-mortem study of chronic schizophrenic brains. *Br J Psychiatry* 1987;151: 744–752.

85. Dom R, de Saedeler J, Bogerts B, Hopf A. Quantitative cytometric analysis of basal ganglia in catatonic schizophrenics. In: Perris C, Struwe G, Jansson B, eds. *Biological psychiatry*. New York: Elsevier/North-Holland, 1981; 723–726.

86. Lee T, Seeman P. Elevation of brain neuroleptic/dopamine receptors in schizophrenia. *Am J Psychiatry* 1980;137:191–197.

87. Reynolds GP. Increased concentrations and lateral asymmetry of amygdala dopamine in schizophrenia. *Nature* 1983;305:527–529.

88. Wolf P, Trimble MR. Biological antagonism and epileptic psychosis. *Br J Psychiatry* 1985;146: 272–276.

89. Sato M, Okamoto M. Dopaminergic kindling and electrical kindling. In: Wada JA, ed. *Kindling 2*. New York: Raven Press, 1981;105–122.

90. Csernansky JG, Holman CA, Bonnet KA, Grabowsky K, King R, Hollister LE. Dopaminergic supersensitivity at distant sites following induced epileptic foci. *Life Sci* 1983;32:385–390.

91. Franzen G, Ingvar DH. Absence of activation in frontal structures during psychological testing of chronic schizophrenics. *J Neurol Neurosurg Psychiatry* 1975;38:1027–1032.

92. Weinberger DR, Berman KF, Zec RF. Physiologic dysfunction of dorsolateral prefrontal cortex in schizophrenia. I. Regional cerebral blood flow evidence. *Arch Gen Psychiatry* 1986;43: 114–125.

93. Gallhofer B, Trimble MR, Frackowiak R. A study of cerebral blood flow and metabolism in epileptic psychosis using PET and oxygen. *J Neurol Neurosurg Psychiatry* 1985;48:201–206.

94. Bailey P, Green JR, Amador L, Gibbs FA. Treatment of psychomotor states by anterior temporal lobectomy. A report of progress. *Res Pub Nerv & Ment Dis* 1953;31:341–346.

95. Jensen I, Larsen JK. Mental aspects of temporal lobe epilepsy. *J Neurol, Neurosurg, Psych* 1979; 42:256–265.

96. Polkey CE. Effects of anterior temporal lobectomy apart from the relief of seizures: a study of 40 patients. *J Roy Soc Med* (London) 1983; 76:354–358.

97. Stevens JR. Psychiatric consequences of temporal lobectomy for intractable seizures: a 20–30-year follow-up of 14 cases. *Psychol Med* 1990;20(in press).

98. Taylor DC. Mental state and temporal lobe epilepsy. A correlative account of 100 patients treated surgically. *Epilepsia* 1972;727–765.

Advances in Neurology, Vol. 55, edited by
D. Smith, D. Treiman, and M. Trimble,
Raven Press, Ltd., New York © 1991.

6

Neurobiological Evidence for Epilepsy-Induced Interictal Disturbances

Jerome Engel, Jr.,* Richard Bandler,†
Neil C. Griffith,‡ and Sally Caldecott-Hazard*

*Departments of Neurology and Anatomy, Laboratory of Environmental and Biomedical
Sciences, and the Brain Research Institute, UCLA School of Medicine,
Los Angeles, California, 90024; †Department of Anatomy, University of Sydney,
New South Wales, Australia; and ‡Epilepsy Unit, Westmead Hospital, Westmead,
New South Wales, Australia

There remains considerable resistance to the concept of epilepsy-induced neurobiological substrates of behavioral disturbances. This can be partly attributed to a well-meaning desire on the part of many to avoid assertions that would negatively affect the image of persons with epilepsy. Throughout history, patients with epilepsy have been treated as outcasts because of fear of contagion and also because it was believed that epilepsy was a result of demonic possession and punishment for sins (1,2). More recently, epilepsy was treated as a form of insanity (3). These misconceptions, which persist to some degree in all cultures, result in discriminations against persons with epilepsy, thereby contributing greatly to their handicap. Consequently, observations that imply a causal relationship between epilepsy and unacceptable interictal behavior can reinforce the stigma. On the other hand, to deny that such a relationship might exist would result in failure to search for a preventable or treatable source of considerable disability among persons with epilepsy. Therefore, it is most appropriate to pursue both clinical and experimental investigations that provide an opportunity for identifying ways in which recurrent epileptic seizures could lead to enduring disturbances in interictal behavior. However, there is overriding concern that the results of such studies be interpreted with extreme caution and reported in a responsible manner, with every effort made to avoid conclusions that could be misinterpreted to the detriment of those who suffer from epilepsy.

This chapter is primarily concerned with evidence suggesting that enduring cerebral dysfunction can result from recurrent epileptic seizures, and that this dysfunction might underlie certain interictal behavioral disturbances that have been associated with epilepsy in the literature (4–27). The important contribution of environmental factors to the psychosocial disturbances suffered by persons with epilepsy, well documented by Taylor and Lochery and by Hermann and Whitman (Chapters 10 and 27, *this volume*), will not be repeated here. However, confounding neurobiological factors, such as pharmacodynamic actions of antiepileptic drugs and direct effects of underlying pathological lesions, as well as unrecognized ictal events, will be considered here first, as alternative neurobiological substrates of behavior disturbance in epilepsy that must be differentiated from the consequences of epilepsy per se. Arguments will then be made that epilepsy may be uniquely capable of producing enduring functional disruption of cerebral activity. Although definitive conclusions cannot be reached at this time, suggestive studies have led to testable hypotheses which should stimulate active basic and clinical research in this area.

CONFOUNDING NEUROBIOLOGICAL FACTORS

Pharmacological Effects

Pharmacological agents used to treat epilepsy have adverse effects on behavior which may be dose-related or which may reflect hypersensitivity or idiopathic reactions (28–30). These relationships are discussed in greater detail by several authors elsewhere in this volume. Dose-related side effects such as sedation, cognitive impairment, and depressed mood commonly occur with some classes of drugs such as the barbiturates and benzodiazepines, but this is less commonly seen with carbamazepine and valproate (31,32). Barbiturates, and to a lesser extent benzodiazepines, also produce hyperactivity in children and are associated with irritability, aggressive behavior, and confusion in the elderly. Phenytoin (33) and valproate (29) can produce progressive encephalopathy with reversible impairment of intellectual function unassociated with nystagmus or ataxia. Drug-induced personality changes and psychoses most commonly occur with primidone and ethosuximide, and the depression commonly induced by phenacemide has greatly limited the usefulness of this drug. Specific disturbances in cognitive function, such as aphasia and recent memory deficit, can also occur as reversible dose-related drug effects with all antiepileptic medications, in direct relation to their ability to cause nonspecific sedation and mental impairment. Such unmasking of preexisting subclinical disturbances can be distinguished from progressive neurological deficits related to an underlying lesion when symptoms correspond to serum drug levels and coexist with other more commonly encountered dose-related toxic signs and symptoms. The mechanisms by which such interictal behavioral disturbances are produced by these medications are presumed to reflect direct actions on the brain. However, this may not always be the case.

Antiepileptic drugs have numerous systemic effects that could indirectly influence cerebral function. For instance, interictal behavioral disturbances may accompany drug-induced hypocalcemia, autoimmune disturbances, hyper- and hypoparathyroid disease, and systemic lupus erythematosus. Chronic administration of antiepileptic drugs alters neuroendocrine function (which could have effects on sexual and other behaviors) (34,35) and lowers folic acid and B_{12} levels (29); however, the importance of this effect on the development of behavioral disturbances remains controversial, and replacement of folic acid may reduce the efficacy of pharmacotherapy (36). Behavioral abnormalities also could herald rare side effects of some drugs (e.g., hyperglycemia, pseudolymphoma, and hepatic necrosis). All antiepileptic drugs exacerbate symptoms of porphyria, which gives rise to psychiatric symptoms. The cosmetic side effects of phenytoin (37) should not be overlooked as a cause of poor self-image and lack of confidence.

Considerable literature is accumulating concerning the interaction between epileptic seizures and sleep (38). Although it is generally appreciated that sleep can exacerbate epileptic seizures in many patients (39), demonstrated effects of seizures on sleep are less widely known. Studies on experimental animals have shown that the development of chronic epileptic seizures is associated with a disruption of sleep, characterized specifically by a decrease in the amount of rapid eye movement (REM) sleep. Clinical data suggest that similar sleep disruption occurs in at least some patients with epilepsy (38). REM deficit may, in turn, induce personality disturbances, affective symptoms, and even psychosis (40). Some commonly used antiepileptic medications, particularly the barbiturates and the benzodiazepines, also reduce REM time (41); this effect may be enhanced by the common practice of giving these medications at bedtime. Consequently, behavioral disturbances associated with these medications in epileptic patients could reflect, in part, an exacerbation of sleep disruption. A preexisting REM deficit may be sufficiently worsened in some patients by bedtime hypnotic drugs, producing interictal behavioral manifestations. The contribution of antiepileptic drug and epilepsy-induced disturbances of sleep patterns on interictal behavior of persons with epilepsy deserves more research attention than it has received to date.

When depression occurs following administration of antiepileptic medication, it may be related to consequent relief from seizures. Affective disturbances have been observed following successful surgical treatment of epilepsy, and as many as one-third of patients may experience depression lasting for months and, rarely, even years (12,42). Although this can in some cases be attributed to difficulties adjusting to a life without epileptic seizures, often it is clearly out of proportion to situational factors and has even been successfully treated with electroconvulsive shock therapy (ECT) (12). The same neurobiological mechanisms responsible for the beneficial effect of ECT on endogenous depression may contribute, in reverse, to the appearance of enduring depression in patients whose habitual seizures have suddenly ceased as a result of surgical or pharmacological intervention. Animal investigations elucidating possible substrates of this phenomenon are discussed later in this chapter.

Direct Effects of Underlying Lesions

Neurological, intellectual, and cognitive deficits often reflect the location and severity of the underlying neuropathological lesion. In general, more extensive lesions produce more profound behavioral disturbances; however, it is also true that more extensive lesions are more likely to give rise to epilepsy. For instance, the risk of seizures persisting in clumsy patients, in patients with severe hypertonia, and in patients with cerebral palsy is 2, 5, and 10 times greater, respectively, than in patients without motor handicap (43), and there is an inverse relationship between the incidence and severity of seizures and I.Q. (44). Given this direct correlation between the ablative effects of an underlying lesion and its epileptogenicity, it is often difficult to determine the degree to which any interictal behavioral deficits result from the lesion itself, as opposed to the epileptogenic process which the lesion might induce.

More interesting than the severity of the lesion is the evidence that the appearance, and perhaps even the character, of interictal behavioral disturbances might depend in part on the anatomical location of the underlying neuropathological process. Although the suggestion that certain personality traits may be characteristic of temporal lobe epilepsy (5) is controversial, there is increasing agreement that some of these personality traits are more likely to occur in patients with mesial temporal electroencephalographic (EEG) spike foci (13) and that they may be particularly related to lesions in the limbic system responsible for generating fear responses (10). In one study, the suicide rate among patients with epilepsy was reported to be 5% higher than that in the general population, but 25% higher among patients with temporal lobe epilepsy (4). Implications of a relationship between lesions in the limbic system and the appearance of interictal behavioral disturbances is not surprising, given the importance of the limbic system in the development of social behavior. It is impossible from these clinical studies, however, to differentiate between direct and epileptic effects of epileptogenic lesions on limbic system development, particularly because patients with small lesions of the mesial temporal lobe usually do not come to the attention of physicians unless they have seizures. A study comparing the psychosocial history of individuals with small structural lesions of one mesial temporal lobe discovered at autopsy, with and without epilepsy, might help to resolve this issue. Even then, however, any differences found might also be attributed to genetic or acquired factors that predispose a brain to develop epilepsy if a lesion appears, rather than to the epilepsy itself.

Hemispheric specialization has been considered important in the manifestation of interictal disturbances; left hemisphere lesions have been associated with schizophrenia (7,19), and right hemisphere lesions have been associated with manic–depressive illness (7). These observations are consistent with arguments that disruption of the language-dominant hemisphere should give rise to thought disorders (26) but that disruption of the nondominant hemisphere should give rise to disturbances of emotion (45). Results of other studies, however, have contested this view (14,46). Many such investigations of hemispheric specialization in patients with epilepsy are compromised by difficulties in lateralizing normal, as well as epileptic, function. Not only do interictal EEG spikes, ictal EEG onsets, and even structural lesions occasionally falsely lateralize the epileptogenic region (47), but there is a relatively high incidence of pathological shifting of normal hemisphere functions in patients with partial epilepsy (48). On the other hand, reports that mood and affect are more often disordered among patients with left hemispheric lesions (14) are usually based on instruments that depend on language and that might only identify depression of the language-dominant hemisphere.

An interesting observation is the increased incidence of schizophrenia among patients with epilepsy secondary to hamartomas. One explanation of this relationship derives from controversial karyotype studies which have associated the extra Y chromosome with psychopathology and also with ectodermal dysplasias (49), including hamartomas of the brain. Consequently, the occurrence of both schizophrenia and a cerebral hamartoma in the same patient could be due to a single chromosomal defect and would not necessarily imply that either the hamartoma or resultant seizures caused the schizophrenia. The enormous complexities involved in attempting to evaluate the importance of anatomical factors is further illustrated by the observation by Taylor (26) that schizophrenia is most likely to occur in left-handed women with seizures who have a hamartoma in the left mesial temporal lobe. Either the lesion itself or the epileptogenic process might disrupt function in the left hemisphere, causing pathological left-handedness and also disturbed thought, the latter of which is dependent upon language. Taylor postulated that sexual dimorphism in hippocampal development results in a critical period for functional disruption in women, which is more likely to coincide with the onset of epileptic disturbances. Of course, all of these factors could simultaneously contribute to the appearance of schizophrenia.

ICTAL EVENTS THAT APPEAR TO BE INTERICTAL

Simple partial seizures can give rise to affective, autonomic, and psychic symptoms that can mimic psychiatric disturbances (50). Prolonged unilateral limbic seizures can produce these symptoms in clear consciousness, and without EEG changes recorded from scalp electrodes (51). Sensory or autonomic phenomena reflecting prolonged simple partial seizures generated from extratemporal sites are also commonly unassociated with obvious EEG changes (52) and could be misinterpreted or embellished by patients in a manner that would lead to disturbed behavior. Simple partial status epilepticus without obvious motor components, therefore, might be mistaken for an interictal behavior disorder, particularly if the symptoms did not also occur paroxysmally preceding more obvious ictal events (i.e., auras preceding complex partial or generalized seizures). Correct diagnosis of ictal events that give rise to alterations in behavior without associated EEG changes requires a high degree of suspicion on the part of the physician. When prolonged interictal behavioral disturbances resemble habitual auras in patients with known epilepsy, simple partial status epilepticus should be considered and attempts should be made to reverse the condition with intravenous benzodiazepines. There are no clear guidelines for suspecting or diagnosing simple partial status epilepticus in other situations, since many nonepileptic behaviors may also resolve with intravenous diazepam.

Patients with epilepsy can occasionally exhibit bizarre behaviors such as multiple personality disorders (53,54), possession states (54), and fugue states (poriomania) (55), which have been considered (by some investigators) to occasionally reflect continuous or serial epileptic seizures. Since an ictal state has not been substantiated in most cases, these events are more correctly referred to as "seizure-related." The so-called episodic dyscontrol syndrome (56,57) also occurs in patients with epilepsy, and intermittent outbursts may be controlled by antiepileptic drugs. However, there is no evidence that these paroxysmal behaviors are epileptic events. At times, such behaviors may appear during postictal confusional states and should be classified as "peri-ictal." When postictal dysfunction is prolonged, this could contribute to symptoms considered to be interictal, as discussed in the next section.

SPECIFIC INFLUENCES
OF EPILEPTOGENESIS

Resistance to the concept that epileptic events themselves can give rise to enduring disturbances in behavior relates to similar resistance to the concept that epileptogenesis is a progressive process. Certainly not all epileptic conditions are associated with progressive symptoms. However, there is considerable evidence from both animal and clinical data to indicate that many epileptic phenomena reflect dynamic processes. In acquired epilepsy, a latent period of months to many years between induction of a localized cerebral insult and the appearance of a chronic epileptic condition is well known (58). This period was referred to by Penfield and Jasper (59) as "ripening of the scar"; it presumably reflects injury-induced reorganization of neuronal integration, predisposing to enhanced excitation and synchronization. These pathophysiological alterations occur gradually, usually without clinical manifestation, until spontaneous seizures appear. Since there are clearly progressive changes in this situation that exist from the time of the initial insult to the appearance of an epileptic disorder, it is reasonable to assume that this progressive process then continues. Indeed, it would be unreasonable to assume that the process would stop at the time the first seizure occurred.

Because of the confounding factors introduced by the presence of a structural lesion in most patients, and also because of the inevitable pharmacological intervention, it is extremely difficult to document a progressive nature of epileptic disturbances in humans. Although infantile hemiplegia occurs with epileptic seizures, developmental delay occurs with cryptogenic infantile spasms, and behavioral regression occurs with cryptogenic Lennox–Gastaut syndrome, all in the absence of an apparent underlying structural pathological process, there is no evidence that these functional disturbances result solely from the epilepsy per se. Two extensive studies of the natural history of temporal lobe epilepsy—one of 666 patients from London (60), and the other of 100 patients from Oxford (61–64)—documented worsening of the epileptic condition, accompanied by a deterioration of function,

when seizures continued. However, both series included a subset of patients for whom seizures were reduced or abolished as a result of anterior temporal lobectomy. These patients did not experience deterioration, suggesting that recurrent epileptic seizures determined the poor behavioral outcome.

Recurrent seizures also induce homeostatic mechanisms that act to reduce epileptic hyperexcitability. These are the mechanisms that presumably terminate ictal events, prevent ictal spread, and persist to maintain the interictal state. Some interictal behavioral disturbances appear to develop as side effects of these homeostatic reactions. The most common example of this is postictal dysfunction, which can range from localized neurological deficits (such as focal paresis, or aphasia) to anterograde amnesia, less specific confusion, automatisms, emotional changes, and psychosis. Prolonged postictal psychosis occurs (6), and transient neurological deficits following complex partial status epilepticus can occasionally last for months (65,66). Such reversible, but enduring, postictal alterations in cerebral function might explain the following common observations after successful surgical treatment of complex partial seizures: (a) Apparently persistent memory deficits usually improve (67), (b) I.Q. increases an average of 10 points (67), and (c) other behavioral disturbances such as aggression, hyposexuality, and problems with interpersonal relationships may also disappear (12,25,67, 68). The interpretation is inescapable that the localized epileptogenic brain tissue was not only malfunctioning but was also adversely influencing other cerebral structures at a distance in order to produce the observed behavioral deficits. Once the epileptogenic tissue was removed, the distant brain recovered. Whereas ablative lesions cause specific deficits, plasticity of the central nervous system (particularly in children) can compensate for such destructive effects. However, the intermittent nature of functional disruption caused by epileptic activity could prevent corrective plastic changes and be a much more potent factor in the development of abnormal behavior.

Epileptic seizures might also indirectly induce chronic behavioral disturbances by their effects on the neuroendocrine system (35,69,70) and on sleep (38), as mentioned earlier in this chapter.

The progressive nature of some epileptogenic processes and the detrimental effect of epilepsy-induced homeostatic mechanisms are difficult to document in patients. However, extensive animal research has clearly demonstrated that these phenomena exist. Secondary epileptogenesis, which can occur spontaneously (e.g., as the "mirror focus") (71) or can be brought under experimental control in the form of kindling (72–75), provides opportunities to study the relatively consistent evolution of epileptic mechanisms in the laboratory. Although the clinical relevance of secondary epileptogenesis is still debated (76–78), it would be logical to assume that the potential exists (at least in some patients) for repetitive epileptiform discharges to facilitate subsequent propagation along specific pathways, and that this could serve as a substrate of persistent altered interictal behavior. For instance, kindled excitability of mesial temporal projection fields could conceivably account for those interictal personality traits which have been described as a reversed Klüver–Bucy syndrome (8). Considerable evidence indicating that inhibitory mechanisms are enhanced during the interictal state is now also accumulating from experimental animal models and from patients (79). These apparent homeostatic mechanisms would be expected to exert influences on cerebral function that might be manifested as interictal behavioral disturbances. The disruptive effect of intermittent epileptiform activity on distant brain development has also been demonstrated in the animal laboratory: The appearance of adult lateral geniculate neuron responses to visual stimulation is prevented when epileptic foci are produced in visual cortex of the immature rabbit (80,81).

The contribution of experimental animal studies to understanding possible neurobiological bases of three specific interictal behavioral disturbances commonly addressed in the clinical literature—depression, schizophrenia, and aggression—will now be presented.

Depression

Although depression is known to be a common interictal symptom in patients with epilepsy, its greater representation in this patient group as compared to that in patients with other equally disabling disorders has only recently been recognized (17,82). One study suggested that depressed mood was as high as 75%, and somatic symptoms of depression as high as 60%, in patients with epilepsy (21). Although reaction to illness may contribute greatly to the occurrence of depression among persons with epilepsy (83,84), when patient populations with and without epilepsy were matched for vocational disability, depression was twice as common and suicide more than four times as common in the population with epilepsy (82,85). Depression in epilepsy is discussed elsewhere in this volume (see Chapter 12).

Experimental animal studies that provide insights into mechanisms of the beneficial effects of ECT on endogenous depression may help explain the occurrence of depression in patients with epilepsy between recurrent seizures, as well as after sudden relief from seizures (86). Endogenous opioids are known to be released during seizures (87–89) and may function as natural mood elevators (90,91). It has been postulated that the beneficial effect of ECT on clinical depression is mediated, at least in part, by the resultant elevated levels of endogenous opioids (92,93). Patients with recurrent seizures could conceivably become physiologically dependent on these intermittent, excessively high levels of endogenous opioids and could develop depression as a withdrawal response to reduction of these abnormal levels when seizures do not occur, either during the interictal period or following effective therapeutic intervention (86,94). Indeed, localized enduring disturbances in opioid function have now been demonstrated in patients with temporal lobe epilepsy; positron emission studies, using the mu opioid receptor ligand [^{11}C]carfentanil, have revealed that the interictal hypometabolic zone is associated with enhanced opioid receptor binding (95). Up-regulation of opiate receptors has also been seen in animals following repeated opioid administration (96).

Research utilizing experimental animal models of depression (97,98), in association with experimental epilepsy, may ultimately provide insights into the neuronal mechanisms of this serious clinical complication of epilepsy.

Schizophrenia

The prevalence of psychosis in epilepsy is under continual debate, but it has been estimated to be 10–15% in patients with severe, uncontrolled temporal lobe epilepsy (19) and to be 5–9% for epilepsy in general (99,100). Controversy concerning whether epilepsy is associated with a unique schizophreniform psychosis (15,20) is discussed in detail elsewhere in this volume (see Chapter 9). Nevertheless, resective surgical treatment that succeeds in abolishing habitual complex partial seizures does not usually alter the symptoms of coexisting chronic schizophrenia (25) (although postictal psychosis is abolished). This observation does not refute the possibility that schizophrenia in epileptic patients results from the epileptogenic process; rather, it indicates only that the schizophrenic disturbance is usually permanent at the time of surgery. Schizophrenia can take a considerable period of time to develop following the onset of epileptic seizures, and it is impossible to determine whether successful surgical treatment early in the course of the condition would have prevented the later appearance of schizophrenic symptoms.

Psychosis has been reported to alternate with seizures in some patients, such that psychiatric symptoms are absent while patients are having seizures but are present when seizures stop; however, this is not necessarily a common finding (16). The possibility that schizophrenia and seizures may be mutually exclusive in some patients is consistent with the view that schizophrenic symptoms are, at least in part, dopamine-mediated (101) whereas most seizures are dopamine-inhibited (102). This inverse relationship between schizophrenia and seizures is discussed elsewhere in this volume (see Chapters 3 and 5) and argues for the possibility that seizure-induced homeostatic mechanisms could contribute to the appearance of psychotic symptoms. The forced normalization of Landolt (103) refers to the occasional disappearance of interictal epileptiform transients from the EEG during psychotic episodes, which Wolf (see Chapter 8, *this volume*) has interpreted as evidence that these psychotic symptoms reflect subcortical seizure activity.

Schizophrenic-like symptoms have been produced in cats by repeated electrical stimulation of ventral tegmental dopaminergic projections to the nucleus accumbens of the forebrain septal region (104). Although it is not possible to prove that this represents an animal model of schizophrenia, it does suggest that intermittent stimulation similar to that which might occur during recurrent seizures can produce enduring changes in dopamine-mediated behavior. Amygdaloid kindling in cats, a technique that results in seizures, has been shown to induce prolonged interictal alterations in dopamine receptor sensitivity which was demonstrated by enhanced stereotypy with administration of methamphetamine (105). Since recurrent limbic seizures in these experimental animals, similar to recurrent epileptiform discharges in patients with temporal lobe epilepsy, appear to potentiate dopamine-mediated behaviors (i.e., induce dopamine receptor supersensitivity), the development of chronic schizophrenia in some patients could conceivably be epilepsy-induced.

Aggression

In this volume, Treiman (see Chapter 21) discusses the fact that "aggression" is a term that has been used widely, and imprecisely, in reference to behavioral disturbances that occur in association with epilepsy. Three animal models of epilepsy-related aggressive behaviors can be reasonably well defined: postictal disturbances that represent hyperreactivity rather than directed aggression, and interictal disturbances that are similar to the well-studied phenomena of predatory attack and of defensive rage.

Postictal behavioral disturbances in patients can most often be ascribed to a Todd's phenomenon, appearing as transient paralysis of function and focal neurological deficits (106). These symptoms presumably reflect postictal inactivation of cortical regions involved in the ictal event, which usually include bilateral structures with complex partial seizures. Postictal automatisms, therefore, most likely reflect diencephalic-mediated behaviors released from higher cortical control. During the period of disorientation after a complex partial seizure, patients can react violently to perceived threats such as attempts, at restraint. This has been interpreted as aggressive behavior, although it is nondirected. Such reactivity is less likely to occur following a generalized convulsion, since postictal dysfunction in this situation also involves the motor system.

Postictal aggression characterized by reactive biting has been reported following amygdaloid-kindled seizures in rats (107). As in the human postical state, this is not a directed attack but is, instead, a hyperreactive phenomenon which can include explosive jumping, rarely occurring spontaneously but easily provoked during the postictal phase by touching or rough handling (108,109). Postictal explosive motor behavior can be exacerbated by pretreatment with naloxone and can be suppressed by pretreatment with morphine (108,109). Significant enhancement of this postictal phenomenon occurs with morphine withdrawal precipitated by pretreatment with naloxone in morphine-addicted rats (108,109). Although this indicates that endogenous opioids are involved in mediating postictal explosive motor behavior, their actual role is complicated.

Another postictal change that may be mediated more directly by endogenous opioids is the so-called multiple-squeak response of rats to painful stimulation. In contrast to the tail-flick and other spinal cord reflex withdrawal reactions to pain, the multiple-squeak response is believed to require some degree of cerebral processing and is used as a measure of affective function (110). The multiple-squeak response is transiently suppressed following amygdaloid-kindled seizures, and the duration of this suppression is shortened by pretreatment with naloxone (109,111). These findings suggest that some postictal disturbances in affective display are mediated by endogenous opioid mechanisms.

The anatomical substrates of predatory attack and defensive rage have been extensively studied in the cat (112–114). Predatory attack is the directed and stereotyped quiet biting behavior that cats use to kill rats. Defensive rage is the equally stereotyped response of cats to perceived threat. The typical defense reaction starts with an initial threat display (the "Halloween" cat) which consists of pupillary dilatation, piloerection, retraction of the ears,

arching of the back, drawing in of the neck, and vocalization (hissing, howling, growling), but without attack or flight. If the threatening stimulus comes closer or becomes potentially more harmful, the behavior of the cat may change from a threat display to an actual attack or flight. Both predatory attack and the different categories of defensive behavior can be elicited by electrical stimulation of specific sites either in the hypothalamus or in the midbrain. Predatory attack is elicited by stimulation of the lateral hypothalamus or of the ventral midbrain tegmentum, whereas defensive behaviors are elicited by stimulation of the medial hypothalamus or the midbrain periaqueductal gray region (PAG) and adjacent tegmentum.

With electrical stimulation, one cannot distinguish effects due to stimulation of fibers of passage from those due to stimulation of neuronal cell bodies. Recently, however, it has been found that the integrated patterns of somatic and autonomic changes characteristic of two subcategories of defense—namely, threat display and escape/flight—can be evoked by microinjections of excitatory amino acids into distinct, restricted parts of the midbrain PAG (115–118). Because it is well established that excitatory amino acids excite cell bodies and their dendritic processes, but not axons of passage (119), these results indicate that different defensive reactions are mediated by neuronal cell bodies found within different and distinct parts of the midbrain PAG.

These findings are of particular interest with respect to the postictal endogenous opioid-mediated behaviors discussed in the previous paragraphs, since the restricted PAG regions mediating the different categories of defense are each major sites of endogenous opioid receptors and endogenous opioid-containing cell bodies (120–122). Indeed, opioid peptides have been reported to suppress defensive rage in cats when microinjected into PAG (123) or into the bed nuclei of the stria terminalis (124). Consequently, an opioid mechanism for defensive rage behavior in cats would appear to be similar to that of postictal hyperreactivity in rats (108,109).

Stimulation-induced predatory attack and defensive rage can also be modulated by stimulation of specific sites in the limbic system, particularly the amygdala and hippocampus

(125). Furthermore, amygdaloid kindling in the cat can postictally increase or decrease the threshold for hypothalamic-induced defensive rage, depending on the site of kindling stimulation (126), and can produce an enduring reduction in predatory attack behavior accompanied also by an increased defensive reactivity (127).

Based on these observations, an experimental model has been developed for limbic-epilepsy-induced enduring disturbances in interictal defensive reactivity (94,128–130). Epilepsy was produced by microinjection of kainic acid (KA) into the dorsal hippocampus of cats. An acute phase lasting 3–8 days (average duration of 6 days) was characterized by recurrent partial seizures which usually began in the left hippocampus and amygdala. The partial seizures consisted of behavioral arrest, pupillary dilatation, contralateral circling, ipsilateral twitching of facial muscles, and salivation. For many of the cats, the clinical signs of partial seizure activity also included components of defensive behavior— that is, piloerection, ear retraction, hissing, and growling, as well as directed striking or biting if the cat was handled. Oftentimes, partial seizures were followed by generalized convulsions. The number of seizures that occurred varied from day to day, and individual cats were unpredictable as to the frequency and severity of their seizure activity.

Following the acute period, the cat entered a more stable chronic period during which time they had fewer recurrent partial seizures. The seizures, however, manifested the same behavioral patterns seen during the acute phase and were associated with ictal EEG discharges recorded directly from electrodes in the hippocampus and the amygdala. The chronic period could be further subdivided into the *epileptic phase* (i.e., the period when partial seizures recurred at regular intervals) and the *latent phase* [i.e., the period when no spontaneous seizures were observed for several days (minimum of 3 days) to weeks]. Significantly, during the epileptic phase the cats showed a clear emotional lability during the periods between seizures. That is, although they appeared behaviorally normal if handled in an affectionate manner, any trivial provocation, such as sudden movement or pinch of the skin, elicited an explosive defensive rage

reaction. This heightened emotional reactivity was not associated with epileptiform EEG changes in the amygdala or hippocampus, and it appeared to be interictal. Furthermore, this interictal defensiveness exhibited a degree of laterality, being particularly marked when the cat was approached from the side that was contralateral to the epileptogenic lesion (Fig. 1). This argues against a nonspecific cause of the behavior, such as general debilitation or discomfort. As well, the thresholds for hypothalamic or PAG electrical-stimulation-induced defense reactions were lowered interictally.

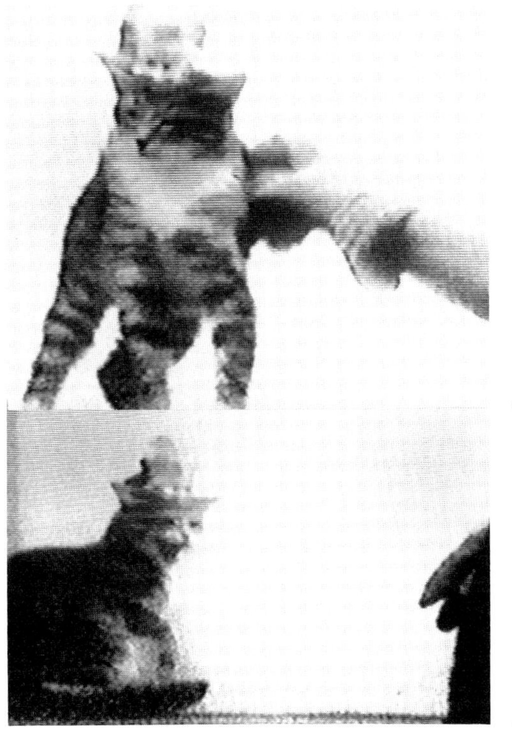

FIG. 1. Demonstration of lateralized hyperreactivity. Photographs were taken from a videotape recording of a cat with a chronic, kainic acid-induced epileptogenic lesion in the left hippocampus. **A:** When the cat was approached on the left (ipsilateral) side, it responded by rubbing up against the offered hand and purring. **B:** When an attempt was made to touch the cat on the right (contralateral) side, it assumed a defensive posture (ears back, piloerection, and pupillary dilatation), hissed, and struck at the offered hand with the right paw.

In contrast, during the latent phase the emotional reactivity of the cats returned to normal, and the thresholds for electrical brain stimulation-induced defensive reactions also returned toward baseline. This indicates that the interictal emotional lability seen during the epileptic phase was not simply the result of a structural lesion in the hippocampus or elsewhere. The interictal emotionality changes were also not caused by the occurrence of seizures per se, since generalized convulsions induced by single or repeated electrical stimulation of the hippocampus or amygdala did not consistently alter emotional reactivity (128). Presumably, the limbic excitability changes that characterize the epileptic phase also predispose the cat to the enduring alterations in interictal emotionality.

Recently, using high-performance liquid chromatography, changes in several putative neurotransmitter amino acids have been measured in cisternal cerebrospinal fluid (CSF) of cats that were made epileptic, as above, by intrahippocampal injections of KA (129). It was found that during the chronic epileptic phase, CSF gamma-aminobutyric acid (GABA) levels were significantly decreased as compared with pre-KA levels. In contrast, CSF levels of other amino acids—taurine, aspartic acid, and glutamic acid—were not significantly changed. The decrease in CSF GABA was clearly not due to occurrence of seizures per se, since CSF GABA levels were found to be significantly elevated during the time of the most intense acute seizure activity—namely, the first 6 days post-KA. Insofar as CSF GABA concentration can be considered to reflect brain GABA concentration (131,132), these data suggest that a decrease in brain GABA may contribute to the interictal emotional lability of cats which have been made epileptic by intrahippocampal injections of KA. Interestingly, the increase in interictal defensiveness in the cats with epilepsy is similar to the increased defensiveness which can be evoked by intraventricular, midbrain PAG, or medial hypothalamic microinjections of GABA antagonists in the rat (112,133–135). Furthermore, defensive rage behavior in cats can be suppressed by microinjections of the GABA agonist muscimol into PAG (136).

It would be inappropriate to suggest that the altered interictal defensiveness of these epileptic cats represents a model of aggressive behavior in patients with epilepsy. The latter is clearly a less specific social response, influenced by multiple factors such as gender, I.Q., and environmental circumstances (24). In contrast, the heightened interictal defensiveness in cats reflects engagement of a species-specific "hard-wired" behavior. This may be due to epilepsy-induced alteration in emotional tone, which could be manifested in various ways in humans (e.g., irritability, insecurity, impulsivity, depression, sexual dysfunction), depending on determinant physiological, psychological, and social conditions. Whether the pathophysiology of this experimentally induced phenomenon is in fact related to the basic mechanisms of disturbances in affect which are reported to occur interictally in patients with limbic epilepsy (5,6) remains speculative at best.

SUMMARY

It is not in the best interest of persons with epilepsy to deny the possibility that seizures could cause enduring behavioral disturbances. Rather, it is essential to pursue clinical and animal investigations in order to identify any such changes that might occur and to elucidate their mechanisms. Many testable hypotheses can be developed from existing evidence.

Antiepileptic medication may produce interictal behavioral disturbances in patients with epilepsy by indirect mechanisms. Some aberrant behaviors could be due to medication-induced systemic disorders, neuroendocrine dysfunction, or REM deficit, whereas depression following successful treatment with drugs, as well as with surgery, may be related more specifically to cessation of seizures.

The underlying neuropathological process also induces neurological and mental deficits, but it is not always possible to differentiate those behavioral disturbances due to destructive effects of the lesion from those due to recurrent epileptic seizures. Behavioral disturbances are associated more frequently with epileptogenic lesions in limbic structures than with those elsewhere in the brain, but a relationship between hemispheric lateralization of the epileptogenic lesion and specific interictal behavioral symptoms remains controversial.

When considering the effects of seizures per se on interictal behavior, it is important to realize that some "interictal" behavioral disturbances may actually be ictal events. Prolonged affective, autonomic, and psychic disturbances can occur in clear consciousness with unilateral limbic seizures that are not associated with scalp EEG changes.

When epilepsy is acquired as a result of cerebral damage, the epileptogenic process takes time to develop before spontaneous seizures appear. It is more reasonable to assume that this progressive process continues than to postulate that it stops completely at the time the first seizure occurs. Epilepsy-induced protective homeostatic mechanisms that act to terminate ictal events, prevent ictal spread, and maintain the interictal state may also disrupt interictal function. Furthermore, seizures could indirectly influence interictal behavior as a result of their effects on neuroendocrine function and sleep.

Because of confounding biological factors, it is difficult to document the association of any epilepsy disorder, by itself, with progressive behavioral disturbances in humans. Secondary epileptogenesis, protective homeostatic mechanisms, and epilepsy-induced disturbances in development can be readily demonstrated, however, in experimental animal models.

In experimental animals, endogenous opioids are released during seizures and mediate some postictal behaviors. A physiological dependency on high levels of endogenous opioids released during seizures could produce depression as a withdrawal symptom interictally or when seizures no longer occur as a result of successful therapy. Experimental animal models of depression exist to test hypotheses concerning pro- and antidepressant effects of epileptogenesis.

Experimental models of epilepsy have demonstrated that recurrent seizures can lead to enduring changes in dopamine receptor sensitivity which suggest a possible mechanism for the development of schizophrenia in patients with epilepsy.

Postictal hyperreactivity has been studied in kindled rats and may reflect endogenous opioid withdrawal phenomena. The neurobiological bases of predatory attack and defensive rage behaviors in cats have been well defined, involve limbic, hypothalamic, and midbrain structures, and can can be modified by endogenous opioids and GABA. Interictal defensive rage appears to be exacerbated in cats with epileptogenic hippocampal lesions, indicating that such limbic hyperexcitability can modulate affective tone. Such emotional changes in humans would come under cortical control and might be manifested as more subtle and variable disturbances in behavior.

ACKNOWLEDGMENTS

This work was supported by grants NS-02808, NS-15654, and NS-20867 from the National Institutes of Health, grant MH-37916 from the National Institute of Mental Health, contract DE-AC03-76-SF00012 from the Department of Energy, and a grant from the Australian National Health and Medical Research Council. Dr. Engel was a recipient of a Guggenheim fellowship.

REFERENCES

1. Jelik WG. The epileptic's outcast role and its background: a contribution to the social psychiatry of seizure disorders. *J Operat Psychol* 1979;10:127–133.
2. Temkin O. *The falling sickness.* Baltimore: Johns Hopkins University Press, 1945.
3. Berrios GE. Epilepsy and insanity during the early 19th century. *Arch Neurol* 1984;41:978–981.
4. Barraclough B. Suicide and epilepsy. In: Reynolds EH, Trimble MR, eds. *Epilepsy and psychiatry.* London: Churchill Livingstone, 1981;72–76.
5. Bear DM, Fedio P. Quantitative analysis of interictal behavior in temporal lobe epilepsy. *Arch Neurol* 1977;34·454–467.
6. Blumer D, Benson DF. Psychiatric manifestations of epilepsy. In: Benson DF, Blumer D, eds. *Psychiatric aspects of neurologic disease,* vol II. New York: Grune & Stratton, 1982;25–48.
7. Flor-Henry P. Epilepsy and psychopathology. In: Granville-Grossman K, ed. *Recent advances in clinical psychiatry—2.* London: Churchill Livingstone, 1976;262–294.
8. Gastaut H, Morin G, Leserre N. Etude du

comportement des epileptiques psychomoteurs dans l'intervalle de leurs crises: les troubles de l'activitie globale et de la socialite. *Ann Med Psychol* 1955;113:1–27.

9. Gibbs FA. Ictal and nonictal psychiatric disorders in temporal lobe epilepsy. *J Nerv Ment Dis* 1951;113:522–528.

10. Hermann BP, Dikman S, Schwartz MS, Karnes WE. Interictal psychopathology in patients with ictal fear: a quantitative investigation. *Neurology* 1982;32:7–11.

11. Hermann BP, Reil P. Interictal personality and behavioral traits in temporal lobe and generalized epilepsy. *Cortex* 1981;17:125–128.

12. Hill D, Pond DA, Mitchell W, Falconer MA. Personality changes following temporal lobectomy for epilepsy. *J Ment Sci* 1957;103:18–27.

13. Nielsen H, Kristensen O. Personality correlates of sphenoidal EEG-foci in temporal lobe epilepsy. *Acta Neurol Scand* 1981;64:289–300.

14. Perini GI, Mendius R. Depression and anxiety in complex partial seizures. *J Nerv Ment Dis* 1984;172:287–290.

15. Perez MM, Trimble MR. Epileptic psychosis-diagnostic comparison with process schizophrenia. *Br J Psychiatry* 1980;137:245–249.

16. Ramani SV, Gumnit RJ. Intensive monitoring of interictal psychosis in epilepsy. *Ann Neurol* 1982;11:613–622.

17. Robertson MM, Trimble MR. Depressive illness in patients with epilepsy: a review. *Epilepsia* 1983;24(Suppl 2):S109–S116.

18. Rodin E, Schmaltz S. The Bear–Fedio personality inventory and temporal lobe epilepsy. *Neurology* 1984;34:591–596.

19. Sherwin I, Peron-Magnan P, Bancaud J, Bonis A, Talairach J. Prevalence of psychosis in epilepsy as a function of laterality of the epileptogenic lesion. *Arch Neurol* 1982;39:621–625.

20. Slater E, Beard AW. The schizophrenia-like psychoses of epilepsy. *Br J Psychiatry* 1963;109:95–150.

21. Standage KF, Fenton GW. Psychiatric symptom profiles of patients with epilepsy: a controlled investigation. *Psychol Med* 1975;5:152–160.

22. Stevens JR. Psychiatric implications of psychomotor epilepsy. *Arch Gen Psychiatry* 1966;14:461–471.

23. Stevens JR, Hermann BP. Temporal lobe epilepsy psychopathology and violence: the state of the evidence. *Neurology* 1981;31:1127–1132.

24. Taylor DC. Aggression and epilepsy. *J Psychosom Res* 1969;13:229–236.

25. Taylor DC. Mental state and temporal lobe epilepsy: a correlative account of 100 patients treated surgically. *Epilepsia* 1972;13:727–765.

26. Taylor DC. Factors influencing the occurrence of schizophrenia-like psychosis in patients with temporal lobe epilepsy. *Psychol Med* 1975;5:249–254.

27. Trimble MR. Personality disturbance in epilepsy. *Neurology* 1983;33:1332–1334.

28. Hirtz DG, Nelson KB. Cognitive effects of an-

tiepileptic drugs. In: Pedley TA, Meldrum BS, eds. *Recent advances in epilepsy 2*. London: Churchill Livingstone, 1985;161–182.

29. Reynolds EH. Mental effects of antiepileptic medication: a review. *Epilepsia* 1983;24(Suppl 2):S85–S96.

30. Rivinius TM. Psychiatric effects of the anticonvulsant regimens. *J Clin Psychopharmacol* 1982;2:165–192.

31. Mattson RH, Cramer JA, Collins JF, et al. Comparison of carbamazepine phenobarbital phenytoin and primidone in partial and secondarily generalized tonic–clonic seizures. *N Eng J Med* 1985;313:145–151.

32. Trimble MR, Thompson PJ. Anticonvulsant drugs, cognitive function, and behavior. *Epilepsia* 1983;24(Suppl 1):S55–S63.

33. Trimble MR, Reynolds EH. Anticonvulsant drugs and mental symptoms. *Psychol Med* 1976;6:69–178.

34. Franceschi M, Perego L, Cavagnini F, Cattaneo AG, Invitti C, Caviezel F, Strambi LF, Smirne S. Effects of long-term antiepileptic therapy on the hypothalamic–pituitary axis in man. *Epilepsia* 1984;25:46–52.

35. Toone B. Sexual disorders in epilepsy. In: Pedley TA, Meldrum BS, eds. *Recent advances in epilepsy 3*. New York: Churchill Livingstone, 1987;233–259.

36. Carl GF, Smith DB. Interaction of phenytoin and folate in the rat. *Epilepsia* 1983;24:494–501.

37. Falconer MA, Davidson S. Coarse features in epilepsy as a consequence of anticonvulsant therapy. *Lancet* 1973;2:1112–1114.

38. Sterman MB, Shouse MN, Passouant P, eds. *Sleep and epilepsy*. New York: Academic Press, 1981.

39. Janz D. Epilepsy and the sleeping–waking cycle. In: Magnus O, de Lorentz AM, eds. *The epilepsies. Handbook of clinical neurology 15*. Amsterdam: North-Holland, 1974;457–490.

40. Dement W, Henry P, Cohen H, Ferguson J. Studies on the effect of REM deprivation in humans and in animals. In: Kety S, Evarts E, Williams H, eds. *Sleep and altered states of consciousness, ARNMD, vol XLV*. Baltimore: Williams & Wilkins, 1967;456–468.

41. Johnson LC. Effects of anticonvulsant medication in sleep pattens. In: Sterman MB, Shouse MN, Passouant P, eds. *Sleep and epilepsy*. New York: Academic Press, 1982;381–394.

42. Horowitz MJ, Cohen FM. Temporal lobe epilepsy: effect of lobectomy on psychosocial functioning. *Epilepsia* 1968;9:23–41.

43. Sillanpaa M. The significance of motor handicap in the prognosis of childhood epilepsy. *Dev Med Child Neurol* 1975;17:52–57.

44. Corbett J. Epilepsy and mental retardation. In: Reynolds EH, Trimble MR, eds. *Epilepsy and psychiatry*. London: Churchill Livingstone, 1981;138–146.

45. Ross ED. Functional–anatomic organization of

the affective components of language in the right hemisphere. *Arch Neurol* 1981;38:561–569.

46. Mendius JR, Engel J Jr. Studies of hemispheric lateralization in patients with partial epilepsy. In: Benson DF, Zaidel E, eds. *The dual brain.* New York: The Guilford Press, 1985;263–276.

47. Engel J Jr. Approaches to localization of the epileptogenic lesion. In: Engel J Jr, ed. *Surgical treatment of the epilepsies.* New York: Raven Press, 1987;75–95.

48. Rausch R, Walsh GO. Right hemisphere language in right-handed patients. *Arch Neurol* 1984;41:1077–1080.

49. Razavi L. Cytogenic and somatic variation in the neurobiology of violence: epidemiological, clinical and morphogenic considerations. In: Fields WS, Sweet WH, eds. *Neural bases of violence and aggression.* St. Louis: WH Green, 1975;205–272.

50. Commission on Classification and Terminology of the International League Against Epilepsy. Proposal for revised clinical and electroencephalographic classification of epileptic seizures. *Epilepsia* 1981;22:489–501.

51. Wieser HG, Hailemariam S, Regard M, Landis T. Unilateral limbic epileptic status activity: stereo EEG behavioral and cognitive data. *Epilepsia* 1985;26:19–29.

52. Devinsky O, Kelly K, Porter RJ, Theodore WH. Clinical and electroencephalographic features of simple partial seizures. *Neurology* 1988;38:1347–1352.

53. Benson DF, Miller BL, Signer SF. Dual personality associated with epilepsy. *Arch Neurol* 1986;43:471–474.

54. Mesulam MM. Dissociative states with abnormal temporal lobe EEG. Multiple personality and the illusion of posession. *Arch Neurol* 1981;38:176–181.

55. Mayeux R, Alexander MD, Benson DF, Brandt J, Rosen J. Poriomania. *Neurology* 1979;29:1616–1619.

56. Monroe RR. *Episodic behavioral disorders: a psychodynamic and neurophysiologic analysis.* Cambridge, MA: Harvard University Press, 1970.

57. Rickler KC. Episodic dyscontrol. In: Benson DF, Blumer D, eds. *Psychiatric aspects of neurological disease, vol II.* New York: Grune & Stratton, 1982;49–73.

58. Jennett B. *Epilepsy after non-missile head injuries, 2nd ed.* Chicago: William Heinemann, 1975.

59. Penfield W, Jasper H. *Epilepsy and the functional anatomy of the human brain.* Boston: Little, Brown & Company, 1954.

60. Currie S, Heathfield WG, Henson RA, Scott DF. Clinical course and prognosis of temporal lobe epilepsy—a survey of 666 patients. *Brain* 1971;94:173–190.

61. Lindsay J, Ounsted C, Richards P. Long-term outcome in children with temporal lobe sei-

zures. I. Social outcome and childhood factors. *Dev Med Child Neurol* 1979;21:285–298.

62. Lindsay J, Ounsted C, Richards P. Long-term outcome in children with temporal lobe seizures. II. Marriage, parenthood and sexual indifference. *Dev Med Child Neurol* 1979;21:433–440.

63. Lindsay J, Ounsted C, Richards P. Long-term outcome in children with temporal lobe seizures. III. Psychiatric aspects in childhood and adult life. *Dev Med Child Neurol* 1979;21:630–636.

64. Ounsted C, Lindsay L, Norman R. *Biological factors in temporal lobe epilepsy. Clinics in developmental medicine,* no. 22. London: Spastics Society of Medical Education and Information Unit in association with William Heinemann Medical Books, 1966.

65. Engel J Jr, Kuhl DE, Phelps ME, Rausch R, Nuwer M. Local cerebral metabolism during partial seizures. *Neurology* 1983;33:400–413.

66. Engel J Jr, Ludwig BI, Fetell M. Prolonged partial complex status epilepticus: EEG and behavioral observations. *Neurology* 1978;28:863–869.

67. Rausch R, Crandall PH. Psychological status related to surgical control of temporal lobe seizures. *Epilepsia* 1982;23:191–202.

68. Walker AE, Blumer D. Long-term behavioral effects of temporal lobectomy for temporal lobe epilepsy. *McLean Hosp J (Special Issue)* 1977;85–103.

69. Herzog AG, Russell V, Vaitukaitis JL, Geschwind N. Neuroendocrine dysfunction in temporal lobe epilepsy. *Arch Neurol* 1982;39:133–135.

70. Sperling MR, Pritchard PB III, Engel J Jr, Daniel C, Sagel J. Prolactin in partial epilepsy: an indicator of limbic seizures. *Ann Neurol* 1986;20:716–722.

71. Morrell F. Secondary epileptogenic lesions. *Epilepsia* 1959/1960;1:538–560.

72. Goddard GV, McIntrye DC, Leech CK. A permanent change in brain function resulting from daily electrical stimulation. *Exp Neurol* 1969;25:295–330.

73. Wada JA, ed. *Kindling.* New York: Raven Press, 1976.

74. Wada JA, ed. *Kindling 2.* New York: Raven Press, 1981.

75. Wada JA, ed. *Kindling 3.* New York: Raven Press, 1986.

76. Engel J Jr, Cahan L. Potential relevance of kindling to human partial epilepsy. In: Wada JA, ed. *Kindling 3.* New York: Raven Press, 1986;37–54.

77. Goldensohn ES. The relevance of secondary epileptogenesis to the treatment of epilepsy: kindling and the mirror focus. *Epilepsia* 1984;25(Suppl 2):S156–S173.

78. Morrell F. Secondary epileptogenesis in man. *Arch Neurol* 1985;42:318–335.

79. Engel J Jr, Wilson CL. Evidence for enhanced synaptic inhibition in human epilepsy. In: Nis-

ticó G, Morselli PL, Lloyd KG, Fariello RG, Engel J Jr, eds. *Neurotransmitters, seizures, and epilepsy. III.* New York: Raven Press, 1986;1–10.

80. Baumbach HD, Chow KL. Visuocortical epileptiform discharges in rabbits: differential effects on neuronal development in the lateral geniculate nucleus and superior colliculus. *Brain Res* 1981;209:61.

81. Chow KL, Baumbach HD, Glanzman DL. Abnormal development of the lateral geniculate neurons in rabbit subjected to either eyelid closure or corticofugal paroxysmal discharges. *Brain Res* 1978;146:489.

82. Benson DF, Mendez MF, Engel J Jr, Signer SF, Zimmermann B. Affective symptomatology in epilepsy. *Int J Neurol* 1985/1986;19/20:30–39.

83. Dodrill CB, Batzel LW. Interictal behavioral features of patients with epilepsy. *Epilepsia* 1986;27(Suppl 2):S64–S76.

84. Schiffer RB, Babigian HM. Behavioral disorders in multiple sclerosis, temporal lobe epilepsy, and amyotrophic lateral sclerosis. *Arch Neurol* 1984;41:1067–1069.

85. Mendez MF, Cummings J, Benson F. Depression in epilepsy. Significance and phenomenology. *Arch Neurol* 1986;43:766–770.

86. Engel J Jr, Ackermann RF, Caldecott-Hazard S, Chugani HT. Do altered opioid mechanisms play a role in human epilepsy? In: Fariello RG, Morselli PL, Lloyd K, Quesney LF, Engel J Jr, eds. *Neurotransmitters, seizures, and epilepsy. II.* New York: Raven Press, 1984;263–274.

87. Hong JS, Gillin JC, Yang HYT, Costa E. Repeated ECS and the brain content of endorphins. *Brain Res* 1979;177:273–278.

88. Hong JS, Wood PL, Gillin JC, Yang HYT, Costa E. Changes of hippocampal metenkephalin content after recurrent motor seizures. *Nature* 1980;285:231–232.

89. Vindrola O, Briones R, Asai M, Fernandez-Guardiola A. Amygdaloid kindling enhances the enkephalin content in the rat brain. *Neurosci Lett* 1981;21:39–43.

90. Belluzzi JD, Stein L. Enkephalin may mediate eurphoria and drive reduction reward. *Nature* 1977;266:556–558.

91. Kline NS, Li CH, Lehmann HE, Lajtha A, Laski E, Cooper T. Beta-endorphine-induced changes in schizophrenic and depressed patients. *Arch Gen Psychiatry* 1977;34:1111–1113.

92. Holaday JW, Belenky GL. Opiate-like effects of ECS in rats: a differential effect of naloxone on nociceptive measures. *Life Sci* 1980;27:1929–1938.

93. Post RM, Putnam F, Contel NR, Goldman B. Electroconvulsive seizures inhibit amygdala kindling; implications for mechanisms of action in affective illness. *Epilepsia* 1984;25:234–239.

94. Engel J Jr, Caldecott-Hazard S, Bandler R. Neurobiology of behavior: anatomic and physiologic implications related to epilepsy. *Epilepsia* 1986;27(Suppl 2):S3–S13.

95. Frost JJ, Mayberg HS, Fisher RS, Douglass

KH, Dannals RF, Links JM, Wilson AA, Ravert HT, Rosenbaum AE, Snyder SH, Wagner HN. Mu-opiate receptors measured by positron emission tomography are increased in temporal lobe epilepsy. *Ann Neurol* 1988;23:231–237.

96. Hitzemann JR, Hitzemann BA, Blatt S, Meyerhoff JL, Tortella FC, Kenner JR, Belenky GL, Holaday JW. Repeated electroconvulsive shock: effect on sodium dependency and regional distribution of opioid-binding sites. *Mol Pharmacol* 1987;31:562–566.

97. Caldecott-Hazard S, Mazziotta J, Phelps M. Cerebral correlates of depressed behavior in rats, visualized using ^{14}C-2-deoxyglucose autoradiography. *J Neurosci* 1988;8:1951–1961.

98. Katz JR, Roth KA, Carroll BJ. Acute and chronic stress effects on open field activity in the rat: implications for a model of depression. *Neurosci Biobehav Rev* 1981;5:247–251.

99. Gundmoundsson G. Epilepsy in Iceland. *Acta Neurol Scand [Suppl 25]* 1966;43:1–124.

100. Ounstead C, Lindsay J. The long-term outcome of temporal lobe epilepsy. In: Reynolds EG, Trimble MR, eds. *Epilepsy and psychiatry.* London: Churchill Livingstone, 1981;185–215.

101. Stevens JR. An anatomy of schizophrenia. *Arch Gen Psychiatry* 1973;29:177–189.

102. Maynert EW. The role of biochemical and neurohumoral factors in the laboratory evaluation of antiepileptic drugs. *Epilepsia* 1969;10:145–162.

103. Landolt H. Electroencephalographic investigation in noncatatonic schizophrenia. Preliminary report. *Schweiz Z Psychol* 1957;16:26–30.

104. Stevens JR, Livermore A. Kindling of the mesolimbic dopamine system: animal model of psychosis. *Neurology* 1978;28:36–46.

105. Sato M, Ogawa T. Abnormal behavior in epilepsy and catacholamines. In: Fariello RG, Morselli PL, Lloyd KG, Quesney LF, Engel J Jr, eds. *Neurotransmitters, seizures, and epilepsy. II.* New York: Raven Press, 1984;1–9.

106. Efron R. Post-epileptic paralysis: theoretical critique and report of a case. *Brain* 1961;84:381–394.

107. Pinel JPJ, Treit D, Rovner LI. Temporal lobe aggression in rats. *Science* 1977;197:1088–1089.

108. Caldecott-Hazard S, Ackermann RF, Engel J Jr. Opioid involvement in postictal and interictal changes in behavior. In: Fariello RG, Morselli PL, Lloyd K, Quesney LF, Engel J Jr, eds. *Neurotransmitters, seizures, and epilepsy. II.* New York: Raven Press, 1984;305–314.

109. Caldecott-Hazard S, Engel J Jr. Limbic postictal events: anatomical substrates and opioid receptor involvement. *Prog Neuropsychopharmacol Biol Psychiatry* 1987;11:389–418.

110. Carroll MN, Lim RKS. Observations on the neuropharmacology of morphine and morphine like analgesia. *Arch Int Pharmacodyn* 1960;75:383–403.

111. Caldecott-Hazard S, Yamagata N, Hedlund J, Camacho H, Leibeskind JC. Changes in simple and complex behaviors following kindled sei-

zures in rats: opioid and nonopioid mediation. *Epilepsia* 1983;24:539–547.

112. Bandler R. Brain mechanisms of aggression as revealed by electrical and chemical stimulation: suggestion of a central role for the midbrain periaqueductal gray region. In: Epstein A, Morrison A, eds. *Progress in psychobiology and physiological psychology,* vol 13. New York: Academic Press, 1988;67–153.
113. Flynn JP. Neural basis of threat and attack. In: Grenell RG, Gabay S, eds. *Biological foundation of psychiatry.* New York: Raven Press, 1976;273–295.
114. Siegel A, Pott CB. Neural substrates of aggression and flight in the cat. *Prog Neurobiol* 1988;31:261–283.
115. Bandler R, Carrive P. Integrated defence reaction elicited by excitatory amino acid microinjection in the midbrain periaqueductal gray region of the unrestrained cat. *Brain Res* 1988;439:95–106.
116. Bandler R, Carrive P, Zhang SP. Somatic and autonomic integration in the midbrain of the cat: a second pattern evoked by excitation of neurones in the subtentorial part of the midbrain periaqueductal gray. *Neurosci Lett* [*Suppl*] 1989;34:S56.
117. Carrive P, Dampney RAL, Bandler R. Excitation of neurones in a restricted portion of the midbrain periaqueductal gray elicits both behavioural and cardiovascular components of the defense reaction in the unanesthetised decerebrate cat. *Neurosci Lett* 1987;81:273–278.
118. Carrive P, Bandler R, Dampney RAL. Somatic and autonomic integration in the midbrain of the unanaesthetized decerebrate cat: a distinctive pattern evoked by excitation of neurones in the subtentorial portion of the midbrain periaqueductal gray. *Brain Res* 1989;483:251–258.
119. Goodchild A, Dampney RAL, Bandler R. A method for evoking physiological responses by stimulation of cell bodies, but not axons of passage, within localized regions of the central nervous system. *J Neurosci Methods* 1982;6: 351–363.
120. Goodman RR, Snyder SH, Kuhar MS, Young WS III. Differentiation of delta and mu opiate receptor localizations by light microscopic autoradiography. *Proc Natl Acad Sci USA* 1980;77:6239–6243.
121. Moss MS, Glazer EJ, Basbaum AI. The peptidergic organization of the cat periaqueductal gray. I. the distribution of immunoreactive enkephalin-containing neurons and terminals. *J Neurosci* 1983;3:603–616.
122. Reiching DB, Kwait GC, Basbaum AI. Anatomy, physiology and pharmacology of the periaqueductal gray contribution to antinociceptive controls. In: Fields HL, Besson J-M, eds. *Pain modulation. Prog Brain Res* [*Special Issue*] 1988;77:31–46.

123. Shaikh MB, Shaikh AB, Siegel A. Opioid peptides within the midbrain periaqueductal gray suppress affective defense behavior in the cat. *Peptides* 1988;9:999–1004.
124. Brutus M, Zuabi S, Siegel A. Effects of D-Ala²-Met⁵-enkephalinamide microinjections placed into the bed nucleus of the stria terminalis upon affective defense behavior in the cat. *Brain Res* 1988;473:147–152.
125. Siegel A, Edinger H. Neural control of aggression and rage behavior. In: Morgane PJ, Panksepp J, eds. *Handbook of the hypothalamus,* vol 3, Part B. New York: Marcel Dekker, 1981;203–240.
126. Siegal A, Brutus M, Shaikh MB, Edinger H. Effects of temporal lobe epileptiform activity upon aggressive behavior in the cat. *Int J Neurol* 1985/1986;19/20:59–72.
127. Adamec RE, Stark-Adamec C. Limbic kindling and animal behavior—implications for human psychopathology associated with complex partial seizures. *Biol Psychiatry* 1983;18:269–293.
128. Engel J Jr, Bandler R, Caldecott-Hazard S. Modification of emotional expression induced by clinical and experimental epileptic disturbances. *Int J Neurol* 1985/1986;19/20:21–29.
129. Griffith NC, Cunningham AM, Goldsmith RF, Bandler R. Alterations in CSF GABA in an animal model of temporal lobe epilepsy. Submitted for publication.
130. Griffith N, Engel J Jr, Bandler R. Ictal and enduring interictal disturbances in emotional behaviour in an animal model of temporal lobe epilepsy. *Brain Res* 1987;400:360–364.
131. Bohlen P, Huoit S, Palfreyman MG. The relationship between GABA concentrations in brain and cerebrospinal fluid. *Brain Res* 1979;167:297–305.
132. Loscher W. GABA in plasma, CSF and brain of dogs during acute and chronic treatment with gamma-acetylenic GABA and valproic acid. In: Okada Y, Roberts E, eds. *Problems in GABA research from brain to bacteria.* Amsterdam: Excerpta Medica, 1982;102–112.
133. Bandler R, Depaulis A, Vergnes M. Identification of midbrain neurones mediating defensive behavior in the rat by microinjections of excitatory amino acids. *Behav Brain Res* 1985;15: 107–119.
134. Depaulis A, Vergnes M. Elicitation of intraspecific defensive behaviors in the rat by microinjection of picrotoxin, a GABA antagonist, into the midbrain periaqueductal gray matter. *Brain Res* 1986;367:87–95.
135. Di Scala G, Schmitt P, Karli P. Flight induced by infusion of bicuculline methiodide into periventricular structures. *Brain Res* 1984; 309:199–208.
136. Shaikh MB, Siegel A. GABA-mediated regulation of feline aggression elicited from midbrain periaqueductal gray. *Brain Res* 1990;507:51–56.

Advances in Neurology, Vol. 55, edited by
D. Smith, D. Treiman, and M. Trimble,
Raven Press, Ltd., New York © 1991.

7

Behavioral Correlates of Interictal Spikes

C. D. Binnie,* S. Channon,† and D. L. Marston*

*The Maudsley Hospital, London SE5 8AZ, England; and †The Middlesex Hospital,
London WC1, England*

Although the occurrence of episodic abnormal neuronal discharges has long been fundamental to concepts of epilepsy, there is continuing uncertainty concerning the possible clinical effects of epileptiform electroencephalographic (EEG) discharges occurring in the intervals between overt seizures. The finding of spike-and-wave activity during seizures was one of the first discoveries in clinical electroencephalography (1), but it was rapidly followed by the realization (2) that similar discharges could occur without concomitant overt clinical manifestations. Such EEG events have variably been described as "larval," "subclinical," or "interictal" discharges. It soon became necessary to reconsider their nature when Schwab (3) demonstrated, by the use of a simple reaction time task during EEG recording, that subclinical discharges may in fact be accompanied by subtle decrements in cognitive function. Without the occurrence of any obvious absence seizure, he found that the patient often failed to respond to a stimulus presented during generalized spike-and-wave discharge or exhibited an increase in reaction time.

Since Schwab's classical study, upwards of 40 other investigations have, with a single exception (4), confirmed the occurrence in some 50% of patients with subclinical discharges of a momentary cognitive deficit, to which Aarts et al. (5) attached the name of "transitory cognitive impairment" (TCI). This phenomenon calls into question the description of the accompanying discharges as "subclinical," but for purposes of the present communication the term "subclinical discharges" will continue to be used to describe those epileptiform events (spikes or spike-and-wave activity), whether focal or generalized, which are not accompanied by epileptic seizures recognizable by overt behavioral changes, without the use of cognitive testing. Unfortunately, most authors gloss over the problem of distinguishing overt seizures with a global unresponsiveness or involuntary acts from the more subtle qualitative changes of TCI. Only a minority of studies document behavior during the investigation (6–12). Even fewer are restricted specifically to patients who exhibited no overt seizures during the investigation (13) or include people not considered to suffer from epilepsy (14). Only the investigation of Aarts et al. (5) and some subsequent studies have made use of continuous video monitoring to document behavior during testing. It is difficult, therefore, to determine to what extent the early literature relates to TCI or merely describes the neuropsychological features of the absence seizure. Prior to the report of Aarts et al. (5), all studies—with the exception of those of Kooi and Hovey (7) and of Prechtl et al. (4)—had been concerned only with generalized discharges. One investigation including focal discharges showed no effect but also was unique in failing to demonstrate TCI during generalized spike-and-wave activity (4). The other investigation suggested that focal discharges disrupted performance less consistently than did those which were generalized (7).

TESTS USED FOR DETECTION OF TCI

It is clear that the probability of demonstrating TCI in a particular patient is related to the nature of the test employed:

1. *Simple Reaction Time*. Reaction time is increased in many subjects, but not necessarily during every discharge (8,11,15–19). There may be a total failure to respond throughout the duration of the discharge, as shown by some of the patients of Schwab (3); however, Tizard and Margerison (20) found a response to the majority of stimuli during spike-and-wave discharges, even in the presence of overt absences. The sensory modality of the stimulus does not appear to affect the sensitivity of simple reaction time tasks to TCI.

2. *Choice Reaction Time*. All the subjects of Tizard and Margerison (20) showed an increased choice reaction time during generalized spike-and-wave activity, whereas none of those studied by Prechtl et al (4) did so. The findings of Lehmann (21) are unique in that he showed a reduced choice reaction time in the second preceding the occurrence of a discharge. The elegant investigation of Hutt et al. (22) showed a linear regression of choice reaction time with respect to the information content of the stimulus (log to the base 2 of the number of equiprobable stimuli) and that the regression coefficient increased during epileptiform discharges, more dramatically during spike-and-wave than during less typical epileptiform activity.

3. *Signal Detection Tasks*. Tizard and Margerison (20) obtained somewhat inconsistent results with an auditory digit detection task, and Mirsky and Van Buren (23) also observed marked fluctuations in the incidence of demonstrable TCI during a continuous performance task. Hutt (24) was able to show that the incidence of demonstrable TCI increased with rate of gain of information. Hutt et al. (25) used an auditory detection task to compare performance of photosensitive subjects during trials, with or without photic stimulation used to induce subclinical discharges. Subjects were required to report the presence or absence of a tone during each trial. Signal detection theory (26) was used to analyze the results in order to distinguish between changes in the perceptual threshold and

changes in reporting bias. The investigators found no elevation in perceptual threshold, but subjects' decision criteria to report the presence or absence of the light appeared to become more conservative.

4. *Simple Motor Tasks*. Both extremely simple repetitive tasks such as tapping, key pressing, or string pulling (6,8,9,16,23,27) are relatively insensitive to the effects of subclinical discharges, as indeed are those with some very limited processing of sensory information, such as operating a pursuit rotor (12) and the drawing test of Guey et al. (10).

5. *Tests of Attention and Recall*. Digit retention tests (9,24,28) are fairly sensitive to TCI. Serial sevens, backward counting, mental arithmetic, and finger counting have also been used, demonstrating TCI during about one-third of discharges and in two-thirds of patients (6,9,14,29). Mirsky and Van Buren (23), using a delayed identification task, showed that the effects of discharges were greatest when they occurred during the stimulus. Milstein and Stevens (30) showed no effect of discharges on verbal learning or on conditioned avoidance.

6. *General Tests of Intelligence*. Using various subtests of Wechsler and the Halstead–Reitan battery, Chatrian et al. (16) found no effect of subclinical discharges, whereas Kooi and Hovey (7) claimed never to have obtained an "adequate solution to a problem during continuous bilaterally synchronous" spike-and-wave activity. Siebelink et al. (31) found impairment during discharges on four out of six subtests of the shortened Revised Amsterdamse Kinder Intelligence Test [a Dutch test battery resembling the Wechsler Intelligence Scale for Children (WISC)].

7. *Ad Hoc Clinical Tests*. During routine EEG recording, many departments employ simple ad hoc tests to demonstrate impairment during discharges, asking patients to read or recite aloud, repeat random words spoken by the technologist during the discharge, or count simultaneously on the fingers of both hands.

TIMING AND NATURE OF DISCHARGE

In general, TCI is most likely to be demonstrated during generalized, symmetrical, regular spike-and-wave activity at about 3/sec and becomes decreasingly probable the more the discharge pattern departs from this. Thus, irregular spike-and-wave or paroxysmal delta bursts have less effect (7,9,12,15,17,23). Until recently, effects of focal discharge had been claimed only by Kooi and Hovey (7) in three subjects. It is unclear whether these effects were statistically significant, but they were less marked than those of generalized discharges. Most investigators found TCI to be most probable during long discharges but found it to be rare during spike-and-wave activity lasting less than 3 sec (9,12,17,20,23). In contrast, Browne et al. (15) found no effect of discharge length. Within the discharge, a "trough of consciousness" may be found; that is, TCI progressively increases over the first 3 sec of the discharge and disappears 1–2 sec before its end (6,11,12,32). Some tests demonstrate maximum TCI early in the course of the discharge (15,20,23). Effects before or after the discharge do not generally seem to be present (33), although Lehmann (21) reported reduced reaction time in the second preceding the discharge.

NATURE OF THE COGNITIVE DEFICIT

Tizard and Margerison (20) somewhat speculatively explained the effects of subclinical discharges and the differential sensitivities of the various tasks in terms of information theory, and Hutt et al. (25) more rigorously showed that the effects of subclinical discharges on the choice reaction time were interpretable in terms of reduced channel capacity.

Impairment of working memory appears to be a factor in the failure to perform some types of task and may explain the selective effects of discharges during the stimulus (23) preventing retention of the material. The occurrence of a discharge while information is being presented serially is most likely to impair recall of the most recent item (13), a result explicable in terms of reduced capacity of working memory. Binnie et al. (34), using short-term memory tasks, found TCI predominantly when the discharge fell during, or in the 2 sec preceding, the stimulus. Discharges during response were without effect on er-

rors, but speed of response was not assessed. In contrast, Kooi and Hovey (7) claimed that retention was generally unimpaired; the patients often hesitated, perseverated, or gave an inadequate answer during the discharge, responding correctly after the discharge had ended.

DETECTION OF TCI FOR CLINICAL PURPOSES

The overwhelming majority of patients who have taken part in research studies of TCI have been unusual in that the discharge rate under test conditions was so high as to permit sufficient numbers of events to be captured during performance of fairly brief psychological tests. If it is considered that cognitive disturbances during subclinical discharges may be clinically relevant (as will be argued below), then assessment for possible TCI should be available as a routine service. It is, however, difficult to carry out such testing in the wider, less selected population of patients who exhibit interictal discharges on routine EEG examination. The tasks generally used in research studies are too tedious to be performed continuously for more than a few minutes, and attending to the task may in any event reduce the discharge rate.

Discussing the problem, if not its solution, Binnie (35) suggested that a routine clinical test for TCI should fulfill the following criteria:

1. The task must not suppress discharges so strongly that a sufficient number cannot be captured during a reasonable period of testing.

2. Conversely, the task must be acceptable for administration over a period sufficiently long for the number of discharges captured, to be sufficient to permit tests of statistical significance to be applied to the results. Much of the literature of TCI concerns across patients pooled data and fails to establish a significant effect in any individual.

3. The difficulty should be adaptive to the patient's own level of performance. Tasks which the subject finds easy are relatively insensitive to TCI (22,24) but overly difficult tasks may decrease, or occasionally increase, the amount of epileptiform activity (20,24).

4. The task should be, as far as possible, continuous; if it is intermittent, the number of discharges falling during testing will be reduced. A solution which has been suggested to this problem is the use of automated discharge recognition to trigger the test procedure (11,36). This, however, is open to the theoretical objection that discharge probability is influenced by state of awareness and that discharges may occur preferentially when the patient is already inattentive. Although any method of testing is open to this objection, the problem would seem to be less if the test is continuous and performance during each discharge may therefore be compared with that immediately preceding or following it.

5. The task should have face validity. An important and as yet unresolved aspect of TCI is determining its relevance to everyday life. Impairment of a practical everyday skill is more readily accepted as clinically relevant than is a decrement in execution of some recherché test of a hypothetical psychological function.

6. Ideally the tests employed should selectively distinguish between disturbances of different psychological functions, so as to permit conclusions about the nature of any cognitive deficit and possibly to relate this to the type and the distribution of EEG discharges.

Aarts et al. (5) described a task which they claimed met, to a large degree, the criteria set out above. This was a short-term memory test presented in the form of a television game and bearing some resemblance to Corsi's Block Tapping Test. An array of blocks was presented on the screen, some of which flashed on and off in a sequence which the subject was then required immediately to reproduce by pointing at the blocks with a light pen. A similar task employing verbal material presented a sequence of four-letter words on the screen which the subject was then required to point out in sequence from the list. Both tasks were adaptive, the difficulty (sequence length) being adjusted such that the subject responded correctly to 50% of trials. The tasks were made more entertaining by the use of color and sound effects, and it was found that most subjects above a mental age of 6 years were able and willing to work at them

for periods of up to 1 hr. Over this prolonged period of testing there was usually rapid habituation of any initial suppression of discharges by the task; in the series studied by Aarts et al. (5), it was possible to capture sufficient discharges to draw some conclusions about the presence of TCI in 90% of cases. Continuous video monitoring was carried out during testing, and any patients showing overt seizures during the investigation were excluded. It was found that the application of this criterion virtually eliminated any subjects with generalized symmetrical spike-and-wave activity of more than 3 sec duration, since these individuals invariably exhibited clinical signs. Nevertheless, despite the exclusion of just those subjects in whom the literature indicated that TCI was most likely to be detected, an effect statistically significant within each individual was found in 50% of those considered testable. Indeed, the sensitivity of the tasks was sufficient to demonstrate TCI not only in the presence of generalized discharges, but also with equal frequency during asymmetrical or focal discharges.

SPECIFICITY OF COGNITIVE DEFICITS

This last finding of an effect of focal epileptiform activity led to a novel and important observation, namely that the two tasks, spatial and verbal, responded differentially to the effects of right- or left-sided discharges. Cognitive impairment was thus more likely to be demonstrated during right-sided discharges using the spatial task and during left-sided paroxysms with the verbal version. Rugland et al. (37) have replicated these findings, and Shewmon and Erwin (38) showed lateralized effects of focal discharges on reaction times to stimuli presented in the contralateral visual field or on responses made with the contralateral hand.

The theoretical implications of these findings are far reaching: TCI is not merely the result of a nonspecific global impairment of awareness as apparently assumed by most investigators, nor is it even a general reduction in channel capacity as proposed by Tizard and Margerison (20) and by Hutt et al. (22); instead, the phenomenon apparently shows some degree of specificity to the neuropsychological functions of the brain region involved by the discharge. This, in turn, has implications for the interpretation of neuropsychological deficits found in people with epilepsy.

COGNITIVE DEFICITS IN EPILEPSY

Neuropsychological functioning in children and adults with epilepsy has been the subject of much attention in the literature. Studies have examined a wide range of seizure disorders from the viewpoint of cognitive functioning, although comparisons between the publications from different centers are limited by (a) variability in the tests employed, (b) the methods of interpretation used, and (c) the heterogeneous samples studied. The accurate assessment of cognitive impairment in epileptic subjects is particularly difficult in view of the threat to reliability of measurement posed by the potential effects of seizure activity and anticonvulsant medication on cognitive functioning.

Studies of intellectual functioning have demonstrated a wide range of abilities in patients with epilepsy, but a number of these studies have concluded that there is a reduced I.Q. level in many patients as compared to that in age-matched normal control subjects (39). Attempts to relate discrepancies in performance between the verbal and nonverbal tests of the Wechsler Adult Intelligence Scale (WAIS) to the lateralization of the lesion or neurophysiological focus have not been entirely successful. Thus, patients with left-sided (dominant hemisphere) lesions should show verbal deficits relative to nonverbal, and the converse for right-sided (nondominant) lesions. Some studies of patients with temporal lobe lesions have confirmed this prediction (40), whereas others have failed to find laterality effects (41). This may be due, in part, to differences between the scales other than the verbal/nonverbal distinction, since the nonverbal tests are all scored on speed as well as accuracy, and thereby readily affected by psychomotor slowing, whereas the verbal tests are not reaction time-dependent.

Research has also focused on the memory and learning abilities of patients with epilepsy; unfortunately, few reports have used comparable tests, and different aspects of memory and learning have been assessed in the various studies. Patients with temporal lobe lesions have aroused the greatest interest with respect to these abilities, since striking deficits have been reported in the surgical literature on temporal lobectomy for the relief of intractable seizures. Scoville and Milner (42) described in detail the global amnesic syndrome which resulted from the bilateral removal of temporal lobe structures in a single case. Their patient, H.M., showed a severe retrograde amnesia for events occurring after his operation, although he had unimpaired intellectual function and short-term memory and also retained procedural learning ability. Unilateral temporal lobectomy has been associated with material-specific deficits: Dominant hemisphere lesions have resulted in impaired verbal memory, and nondominant lesions have produced impaired visuospatial memory (43,44). While many studies have reported memory deficits in seizure patients without gross cerebral damage, the evidence for material-specific differences is less clear. Thus, Glowinski (45) and Loiseau et al. (46) failed to find significant relationships between laterality of lesion and impairment of verbal and nonverbal memory. A large number of studies have investigated a range of cognitive abilities in epilepsy, and a full review is beyond the scope of this chapter. However, it is reasonable to expect that any deficits found will vary according to the characteristics of the samples studied, and the careful delineation of these factors is likely to be more useful than are attempts to make general statements about a set of heterogeneous disorders.

A number of studies have attempted to relate cognitive deficits associated with epilepsy to features such as the type and frequency of the seizures, the age of onset, and the duration of the epilepsy. There are, of course, a number of other pertinent factors such as the site and extent of underlying brain lesions, anticonvulsant medication, and emotional state, which will not be dealt with here. Links between features of the seizures and cognitive deficits are of interest, since the processes operating may be similar to those which produce the impairments in performance noted in TCI.

Frequent seizures over long periods may produce impairments in cognitive functioning both directly, through the temporary disturbance of consciousness (46), and indirectly, by producing cerebral damage due to repeated seizures (47). While the precise mechanisms are poorly understood, many of the studies which have investigated these factors have found evidence of a relationship between seizure patterns and impairment of functioning. Thus, twin studies carried out by Dodrill and Troupin (48) found that the twin with more frequent seizures performed worse on tests of cognitive function, although this may have reflected more extensive underlying brain damage causing the seizures. Farwell et al. (39) reported a negative correlation between intelligence and duration of seizure disorder in children. A more detailed review is provided by Besag (49).

The evidence for a relationship between neuropsychological deficits and type of seizure activity is less straightforward, and it is partially confounded by differences in the samples included in the various studies and by the diagnostic criteria used. Comparisons of intellectual performance between subjects with generalized and partial seizures have produced mixed results. O'Leary et al. (50) reported lower I.Q. results in children with early-onset generalized seizures than in those with early-onset partial seizures. Patients with partial seizures were found to perform better on a range of I.Q. subtests than did those with generalized seizures, regardless of whether they had primary or secondary generalized seizures (51). Lower-than-average I.Q. was found to be associated with almost all the seizure types studied by Farwell et al. (39), including generalized and partial seizures, minor motor seizures, and atypical absences, with the exception of those with classic absence seizures alone. There have been some suggestions that it may be the number of different seizure types experienced that is the determining factor in producing intellectual impairment (52).

POSSIBLE SIGNIFICANCE OF TCI FOR NEUROPSYCHOLOGICAL FINDINGS

Because of the large number of factors which can impair cognition in epilepsy, it is often difficult to determine which are responsible for the disabilities of any individual. TCI could perhaps be an exception if it were possible to demonstrate unequivocally that this is contributing to the impaired performance when discharges occur during testing. The finding that TCI may selectively affect particular psychological functions lends credence to this view; and because the deficits found in epilepsy are not uniform and global, particular subtests appear to be differentially affected, with performance on short-term memory tasks being especially poor (53). Moreover, it has been established that abnormalities of neuropsychological test patterns increase with the amount of interictal epileptiform EEG activity and are greater with generalized discharges than with focal activity (54,55). The following question must therefore arise: Does the association between neuropsychological dysfunction and interictal discharges simply reflect a common relationship to general biological factors such as the type or severity of epilepsy, or does it have a closer causal relationship, with the psychological deficits being, at least in part, manifestations of "subclinical neurophysiological disturbances" (54)?

Apart from the investigation briefly reported by Kooi and Hovey (7), only one study appears to have been undertaken to address this possibility. Siebelink et al. (31) applied a battery of six subtests to a group of school children with epilepsy, under continuous EEG and video monitoring. Test performance was scanned item by item to determine the possible effects of discharge occurrence on error rates. There was significant impairment of performance in association with discharges on four of the six subtests. Overall, the group performed particularly poorly on a test of short-term memory, as previously reported. However, this effect was shown only by those children who exhibited discharges during presentation of this particular test, whereas the others exhibited no deficiency of short-term memory in comparison with the performance on other material. The short-term memory test in those exhibiting subclinical discharges while carrying it out was particularly sensitive to TCI. These findings do, therefore, support the contention that selective neuropsychological deficits in people with epilepsy may be due, in part, not to static cerebral pathology nor to the ongoing effects of medication, but to the intermittent cognitive impairment produced by subclinical EEG discharges.

This has implications for preoperative assessment in patients being considered for surgical treatment of epilepsy, where it is conventionally assumed that neuropsychological localization of cerebral dysfunction is independent from, and may be used to corroborate, electrographic findings. The subsequent removal of a discharging focus may possibly lead to an improvement of test performance, possibily mitigating cognitive deficits caused by the surgery. This could perhaps account for, or contribute to, the lack of memory disturbance, or indeed improvement in cognitive function, seen particularly after selective amygdalohippocampectomy (56).

If the neuropsychological deficits shown by many patients with epilepsy are due, if only in part, to TCI, then they may be open to amelioration by suitable therapy to suppress the discharges.

ELECTRICAL BRAIN STIMULATION

Most studies of TCI are dependent on the occurrence of discharges, which may be unpredictable and do not tend to fall neatly between the onset and offset of stimulus or response. This places considerable constraints on the questions which can be experimentally addressed. An exception to this has been the work of Hutt et al. (22), described above; these investigators have used experimentally controlled light stimulation to induce discharges in photosensitive epileptic subjects. However, this technique has a limited applicability because the majority of patients with epilepsy do not respond to light stimulation.

Useful information about the effects of transient disruption of brain activity on cognitive functioning can be gained from studies of electrical stimulation of the cortex and subcortical structures, carried out under local anesthesia (57). This offers a flexible research tool, since the timing of the stimulation and the intensity and duration can be experimentally controlled to compare different anatomical sites, although there are methodological limitations. Moreover, brain stimulation is clearly an invasive procedure which can only

be justified when it facilitates clinical decision-making. This is usually in relationship to surgery for the relief of intractable seizures, when electrical stimulation may be used to give more information about the location and nature of neurophysiological dysfunction and to identify areas of functional importance which should be spared in the resection. The degree to which findings on epileptic populations can be generalized to the normal brain is unknown. Nevertheless, electrical stimulation is a powerful tool which can considerably extend our knowledge of the relationship between cognitive functioning and transient brain dysfunction.

It is questionable to what extent the dysfunction induced by an alternating electrical current is directly comparable to that produced by naturally occurring subclinical epileptic discharges. Both excitatory and inhibitory effects may be produced (58), and the precise physiological events which will be produced in an individual case cannot be fully specified in advance. The level of current should be such that an afterdischarge is not produced, in order to limit the effect of the stimulation to the point in time when the current is terminated and, as far as possible, to the stimulated site (59). The extent of the area affected by the current is difficult to predict and must be established empirically (59). Nevertheless, the effect of stimulation has been likened to that of a temporary lesion or, in certain circumstances, a local seizure (59).

Studies of brain stimulation have identified localized sites relating to language and memory functions (59–62). The application of an electrical current has been shown to selectively disrupt task performance momentarily, depending upon the nature of the task and the locus of the stimulation. Ojemann (59) reported considerable between-subjects variability in the anatomical location of cortical sites relating to language and memory functioning, and some within-subjects variability with repeated testing has also been described (63).

Ojemann (59) commented on the striking specificity of the functional effects produced by electrical stimulation, since a functional deficit such as naming errors may reliably be produced at a particular site on every trial, whereas stimulation with the same current at a nearby site, perhaps 0.5 cm away, might have no detectable effect on the same function. Ojemann (59) reported that stimulation mapping of language and memory functions tended to give stable data over time in a few cases where repeated testing was carried out some months apart. The validity of data obtained by electrical stimulation mapping of language sites was confirmed by Ojemann and Dodrill (62), who demonstrated that the presence or absence of naming errors at cortical sites within the surgical resection were useful indices of the severity of postoperative language impairment. Ojemann and Dodrill (64) also found that the extent of any language and memory deficits following cortical resection was related to the degree to which the resection removed lateral sites implicated in those functions, as determined by stimulation mapping.

The strategy adopted by Ojemann and his colleagues to map cortical sites was to (a) measure each chosen function during three stimulation trials and (b) compare error rates in performance with the error rate produced in a large number of similar trials presented without stimulation. This procedure would be repeated at a range of anatomical sites for each patient, so that a detailed functional map could be drawn up (59). Tests were devised to measure naming, reading of simple sentences, short-term memory, mimicry of orofacial movements, and phoneme identification. The findings revealed that often only one of the language functions tested was altered at a particular site.

A slightly different technique was reported by Halgren et al. (65), who studied patients with depth electrodes implanted in the temporal lobe to investigate the origin of their seizures. Stimulation was applied bilaterally to sites at the amygdala, anterior hippocampus, and middle hippocampus simultaneously in order to produce a transient widespread medial temporal lobe disruption without an afterdischarge. The effects of stimulation on memory functioning were examined by presenting a series of slides of complex scenes for brief periods of 100–200 mscc. After a brief intervening task, subjects were asked to distinguish between slides they had already seen and distractor slides by pressing a "Yes" or "No" key. Stimulation was delivered to all the sites simultaneously during the slide presentations in the initial and test phases. Subjects showed impaired recognition memory for the slides, provided that the gap between the initial presentation and the recognition phase was more than 2 sec. The deficit was restricted to memory, since subjects were able to make perceptual discriminations and execute responses despite memory impairment. Unilateral medial temporal lobe stimulation was also found to disrupt memory functioning in four of the nine patients tested, but only when it was applied to the hemisphere contralateral to the suspected lesion. When stimulation during the acquisition phase alone and the test phase alone were compared, Halgren (65) found that deficits in recognition performance could result from either one but were less than the deficit resulting from stimulation during both the acquisition and test phases.

The findings from brain stimulation studies provide a framework of reference for examining the possible mechanisms operating in TCI. A relationship between the side of focal discharges and selective task impairment has been reported in the TCI literature (5). Clearly the nature of any transient cognitive deficit produced will be determined by the site of the discharge and the extent of spreading of the epileptic activity. Brief focal subclinical discharges which remain localized may be difficult to detect on a wide range of cognitive tasks, yet they may produce severe impairment of a particular function. Stimulation studies which have compared functioning at a range of single neighboring sites (59,64) suggest that functional task disruption shows a high degree of anatomical specificity, at least at certain sites in the temporal cortex.

In this context the increasing use of depth electrodes and the recent introduction of minimally invasive intracranial recording through the foramen ovale have highlighted the frequency in people with epilepsy of subclinical discharges not detectable at scalp electrodes. It is interesting to consider the implications for cognitive function. In the classical studies of TCI, cognition was shown to be impaired during scalp discharges—in contrast to performance when these were absent. However, during the control periods it may be presumed that in many patients, unrecognized discharges were occurring in deep structures. If these had any marked cognitive effects, TCI during discharges in the scalp EEG would not have been distinguishable. Our own preliminary results suggest that TCI is not an invariable concomitant—and possibly not even a common concomitant—of discharges confined to deep structures.

EFFECTS OF COGNITIVE ACTIVITY ON DISCHARGES

The complex interactions of cognitive activity and EEG discharges became apparent from early telemetric studies (e.g., see refs. 10 and 66). Different discharge rates were found during everyday activities as varied as reading, eating, and playing a musical instrument. Here it is necessary to observe a distinction between nonspecific effects of cognitive activity on epileptiform EEG activity and the reflex epilepsies. Discharges or seizures may be precipitated by simple sensory stimuli (flicker, linear patterns, touch) or complex cognitive tasks (reading, calculation, playing chess, etc.). Patients with highly specific reflex epilepsies may attract medical interest and appear in the literature as rarities. However, Altafullah and Halgren's (67) report on a patient with mesial temporal discharges precipitated by routine administration of memory tasks during depth recording raises the possibility of many patients being susceptible to triggering of discharges by specific activities, the effects of which may not be recognized.

Whatever the prevalence of stimulus-specific reflex epilepsies, nonspecific effects of cognitive activity on discharge rate are probably common. During a variety of psychological tests, Kooi and Hovey (7) found suppression of generalized discharges but observed less consistent effects of focal activity. In contrast, two patients studied by Aarts et al. (5) showed such a marked increase in discharges (with associated myoclonus) during a memory task as to be untestable. Within the performance of a single task, different cognitive activities may have different effects on discharges. Thus, against the background of a general reduction in epileptiform activity during testing, Kooi and Hovey (7) found the discharge rate to be least while the patients were responding and greatest in the interval between response and the next question. Using the spatial and verbal memory tasks described by Aarts et al. (5), Binnie et al. (34) captured at least 30 discharges during the spatial test in 19 subjects and during the verbal version in 15. Sixteen and six, respectively, showed a statistically significant difference in discharge rate between different phases of the task. There was, however, no between-subjects consistency: stimulus, stimulus–response interval, or response could be associated with maximum discharge rate. In the series of Kooi and Hovey (7) there was one patient who differed from the others by showing the highest discharge rate while responding during all items of a test battery.

Clearly there is a complex interaction between cognition and discharges: Cognitive activity affects discharge rate, whereas the epileptiform phenomena affect cognition. These relationships have not been formally studied, but it was, for instance, interesting to observe during the study of Siebelink et al. (31) that the task which the children performed most poorly, and which they presumably experienced as most difficult, was accompanied by the highest discharge rate and was particularly susceptible to the effects of TCI. Under some circumstances a positive feedback may thus be established: TCI increases perceived task difficulty, thereby leading to a greater discharge rate and further cognitive disruption.

PRACTICAL IMPLICATIONS

TCI has been extensively studied as an interesting subject of scientific inquiry, but there has been little consideration on its possible practical consequences. Conversely, epileptiform EEG abnormalities, particularly in children with educational problems, appear to be regarded as prima facie evidence of cerebral dysfunction and are sometimes treated by means of antiepileptic drugs. Such a practice is generally deplored by experienced neurologists and pediatricians who may accuse its advocates as indulging in "EEG cosmetics" or who insist that they will treat patients for epilepsy only if they have seizures and not on account of EEG abnormalities. While the clinical attitudes reflected by such statements may seem wholly commendable, the phenomenon of TCI calls in question the definition of a seizure. Indeed a brief cognitive change accompanying an intermittent cerebral dysrhythmia would seem to meet contemporary definitions of an epileptic seizure and should satisfy any clinician who is properly reluctant to treat the EEG in the absence of clinical manifestations.

Ignoring the semantic arguments, the point at issue is whether cognitive disturbances accompanying EEG discharges adversely affect the patient's psychosocial functioning in daily life. A first step towards such a demonstration was made by Kasteleijn-Nolst Trenité et al. (68), who carried out EEG and video monitoring of children with epilepsy while they performed reading and math tests. Reading was closely monitored; and hesitations, repetitions, interpolations, and misreadings were noted on a copy of the text, as was the timing of any epileptiform EEG discharges. The occurrence of discharge was associated with an increased rate of errors per word read, although (paradoxically) the actual reading speed was also increased during the discharges. Thus the subclinical discharges did not simply cause an interruption of reading, which might easily be recognized by a teacher; rather, they produced faster, inaccurate reading. Because the learning of reading skills and their subsequent use as a general means of acquiring information represent major daily activities of school children, it may be claimed that this study provides a direct demonstration of impairment by TCI of a practical social skill.

To highlight the relevance of TCI to daily life, Kasteleijn-Nolst Trenité et al. (69) also undertook a study of the effects of subclinical discharges on driving an automobile. They deliberately avoided the use of any form of simulation; the subjects drove a dual-control car (accompanied by qualified instructors) in light traffic on motorways for distances of over 310 miles. All subjects had a current driving license, and all had suffered from epilepsy. The majority held their license legitimately, having been seizure-free for more than 2 years; others held their license illegally, having failed to declare their epilepsy. The vehicle was equipped with a variety of transducers to monitor driving performance, and

the EEG was monitored and stored on magnetic tape. Half the patients showed a statistically significant increase in variation of lateral position on the road (i.e., they either swerved from side to side or failed properly to follow the contours of the road) when discharges were present. It was not the purpose of this study to draw any conclusions concerning the significance of subclinical discharges for fitness to drive, and the investigators pointed out that there are many other, probably more important, causes of unsafe driving (such as psychopathy and fatigue) which fall outside legal control. However, the study did represent a compelling demonstration of the possible significance of seemingly subclinical discharges for performance of an everyday skill.

At present, it would not be possible to sustain a claim that all people with subclinical EEG discharges suffer transitory cognitive impairment which adversely affects their psychosocial function. The most sensitive method of testing used to date was probably that employed by Aarts et al. (5), but even this approach succeeded in demonstrating TCI in only 50% of a group of patients with subclinical discharges, despite the fact that those with overt seizures during testing had been screened out by video monitoring. Failure to demonstrate TCI does not, of course, indicate that it is absent: The number of discharges captured may have been insufficient, or the nature of the task may have been inappropriate. Thus the findings of Aarts et al. (5) can be regarded only as a conservative estimate of prevalence of TCI in this particular type of patient. Moreover, the population at risk may be substantially greater if people who have subclinical discharges but who are not known to have epilepsy are considered. In children without epilepsy, some 10% may exhibit phenomena regarded as epileptiform (70). One study of TCI (14) included children with subclinical discharges without known epilepsy; in some of these children, TCI was in fact demonstrable. At the present time it would certainly be unsafe to assume that all people with epileptiform EEG discharges suffer from TCI; however, the presence of frequent discharges, particularly in a person with problems of social or cognitive functioning, could be regarded as an indication for carrying out appropriate testing to determine whether TCI is present.

TREATMENT

When TCI is demonstrable in a person with problems of psychosocial function, the question of treatment must arise; the use of antiepileptic drugs (AEDs) would seem to be the most obvious approach. However, apart from generalized 3/sec spike-and-wave activity in absence seizures, which readily responds to effective medication (71,72), epileptiform EEG discharges are generally difficult to suppress by chronic AED administration (see refs. 73 and 74 for reviews). Indeed it is striking that some AEDs may produce a deterioration in the EEG (75,76). Despite good evidence of acute effects of AEDs on EEG discharges (77,78), along with a handful of reports of suppression of focal discharges with chronic medication (79,80), most reports suggest that interictal discharge rates bear little relationship to seizure frequency (81), except in absences, and are little affected by most AEDs. Some current experimental AEDs such as lamotrigine (82) may even produce a reduction of focal EEG discharges; otherwise, attempts to suppress interictal discharges may need to be confined to the use of (a) valproate and ethosuximide for generalized spike-and-wave activity and (b) benzodiazepines for other types of discharge. All established AEDs (and the benzodiazepines in particular) readily produce cognitive impairment, and the trade-off between TCI and drug side effects may not necessarily be to the advantage of the patient. At an anecdotal level, patients have been reported [e.g., by Aarts et al. (5)] whose psychosocial function was manifestly improved by suppression of subclinical discharges with AEDs. Rugland et al. (37) are performing an open prospective study of children with TCI, with careful checks on possible cognitive effects of medication. Rugland (*personal communication*) claims to have found dramatic benefits of treatment; however, in view of the known effects of therapeutic actions on the expectations and reports of teachers and parents, rigorous controlled trials will be necessary to justify the routine use of AEDs for suppression of TCI.

Other therapeutic possibilities should not be overlooked. An important feature of TCI is its intermittence, and this may be taken into account in selecting teaching methods. Children showing this phenomenon may easily miss the flow of verbally presented material, and it is to be expected that they would be considerably helped by teaching material with a high level of redundancy and by making full use of visual aids.

CONCLUSION

For the electroencephalographer, TCI presents an intriguing paradox. Having learned to avoid overinterpretation of the EEG, and having persuaded colleagues that spikes are not equivalent to epilepsy and are generally a poor guide to its severity, control, or prognosis, one is then forced to adopt a diametrically opposed position and point out that subclinical EEG discharges may occasionally be of practical clinical significance. Perhaps one should not be greatly surprised: Considering the dramatic changes in cerebral electrical activity often seen during these phenomena which we have learned to call subclinical, it would surely be remarkable if sensitive testing did not show adaptive brain function to be adversely affected.

Certainly, based on present evidence there can be no justification for postulating TCI due to discharges not detectable in the scalp EEG as an explanation for cognitive dysfunction in people with epilepsy.

The possible consequences of TCI for the everyday function of those who show it, the criteria and methods for its recognition, the possibilities of its control by medication, and the indications for its treatment should provide fertile fields for future study.

REFERENCES

1. Berger H. Über das Elektrenkephalogramm des Menschens: siebente Mitteilung. *Arch Psychiatr Nervenkr* 1933;100:301–320.
2. Gibbs FA, Lennox WG, Gibbs EL. The electroencephalogram in diagnosis and in localization

of epileptic seizures. *Arch Neurol Psychiatry* 1936;36:1225–1235.

3. Schwab RS. A method of measuring consciousness in petit-mal epilepsy. *J Nerv Ment Dis* 1939;89:690–691.

4. Prechtl HFR, Boeke PE, Schut T. The electroencephalogram and performance in epileptic patients. *Neurology (Minneap)* 1961;11:296–302.

5. Aarts JHP, Binnie CD, Smith AM, Wilkins AJ. Selective cognitive impairment during focal and generalised epileptiform EEG activity. *Brain* 1984;107:293–308.

6. Shimazono Y, Hirai T, Okuma T, Fukuda T, Yamamasu E. Disturbance of consciousness in petit mal epilepsy. *Epilepsia* 1953;2:49–55.

7. Kooi KA, Hovey HB. Alterations in mental function and paroxysmal cerebral activity. *Arch Neurol Psychiatry* 1957;78:264–271.

8. Yeager CL, Guerrant JS. Subclinical epileptic seizures. *Calif Med* 1957;86:242–247.

9. Davidoff RA, Johnson LC. Paroxysmal EEG activity and cognitive motor performance. *Electroencephalogr Clin Neurophysiol* 1964;16:343–354.

10. Guey J, Tassinari CA, Charles C, Coquery C. Variations du niveau d'efficience en relation avec des décharges épileptiques paroxystiques. *Rev Neurol* 1965;112:311–317.

11. Porter RJ, Penry SK, Dreifuss FE. Responsiveness at the onset of spike–wave bursts. *Electroencephalogr Clin Neurophysiol* 1973;34:239–245.

12. Goode DJ, Penry JK, Dreifuss FE. Effects of paroxysmal spike–wave and continuous visual motor performance. *Epilepsia* 1970;11:241–254.

13. Hutt SJ, Gilbert S. Effects of evoked spike–wave discharges upon short-term memory in patients with epilepsy. *Cortex* 1980;16:445–457.

14. Ishihara T, Yoshii N. The interaction between paroxysmal EEG activities and continuous addition work of Uchida–Kraepelin psychodiagnostic test. *Med J Osaka Univ* 1967;18:75–85.

15. Browne TR, Penry SK, Porter RS, Dreifuss F. Responsiveness before, during and after spike–wave paroxysms. *Neurology (Minneap)* 1974; 24:659–665.

16. Chatrian GE, Lettich E, Miller LH, Green JR, Kupfer C. Pattern-sensitive epilepsy, Part 2. Clinical changes, tests of responsiveness and motor output, alterations of evoked potentials and therapeutic measures. *Epilepsia* 1970;11: 151–162.

17. Schwab RS. The influence of visual and auditory stimuli on electroencephalographic tracing of petit-mal. *Am J Psychiatry* 1941;97:1301–1312.

18. Grisell JL, Levin SM, Cohen BD, Rodin EA. Effects of subclinical seizure activity on overt behaviour. *Neurology (Minneap)* 1964;14:133–135.

19. Tuvo F. Contribution à l'étude des niveaux de conscience au cours des paroxysmes épileptiques infracliniques. *Electroencephalogr Clin Neurophysiol* 1958;10:715–718.

20. Tizard B, Margerison JH. Psychological functions during wave–spike discharges. *Br J Soc Clin Psychol* 1963;3:6–15.

21. Lehmann HJ. Präparoxysmale Weckreaktion bei pyknoleptischen Absencen. *Arch Psychiatr Nervenkr* 1963;204:417–426.

22. Hutt SJ, Newton S, Fairweather H. Choice reaction time and EEG activity in children with epilepsy. *Neuropsychologica* 1977;5:257–267.

23. Mirsky AF, Van Buren HM. On the nature of the "absence" in centrencephalic epilepsy: a study of some behavioural electroencephalographic and autonomic factors. *Electroencaphalogr Clin Neurophysiol* 1965;18:334–338.

24. Hutt SJ. Experimental analysis of brain activity and behaviour in children with 'minor' seizures. *Epilepsia* 1972;13:520–534.

25. Hutt SJ, Denner S, Newton J. Auditory thresholds during evoked spike–wave activity in epileptic patients. *Cortex* 1977;12:249–257.

26. Green DM, Swets JA. *Signal detection theory and psychophysics*. New York: Wiley, 1966.

27. Hauser F. *Perception et réponses motrices au cours des paroxysmes de pointes-ondes*. Paris: Foulon, 1960.

28. Geller MR, Geller A. Brief amnestic effects of spike-wave discharges. *Neurology (Minneap)* 1970;20:380–381.

29. Jus A, Jus K. Retrograde amnesia in petit mal. *Arch Gen Psychiatry* 1962;6:163–167.

30. Milstein V, Stevens JR. Verbal and conditioned avoidance learning during abnormal EEG discharge. *J Nerv Ment Dis* 1961;132:50–60.

31. Siebelink BM, Bakker DJ, Binnie CD, Kasteleijn-Nolst Trenité DGA. Psychological effects of sub-clinical epileptiform EEG discharges in children: general intelligence tests. *Epilepsy Res* 1988;2:117–121.

32. Goldie L, Green JM. Spike and wave discharges and alterations of conscious awareness. *Nature* 1961;191:200–201.

33. Tizard B, Margerison JH. The relationship between generalized paroxysmal EEG discharges and various test situation in two epileptic patients. *J Neurol Neurosurg Psychiatry* 1963; 26:308–313.

34. Binnie CD, Kasteleijn-Nolst Trenité DGA, Smit AM, Wilkins AJ. Interactions of epileptiform EEG discharges and cognition. *Epilepsy Res* 1987;1:239–245.

35. Binnie CD. Detection of transitory cognitive impairment during epileptiform EEG discharges: problems in clinical practice. In: Kulig BM, Meinardi H, Stores G, eds. *Epilepsy and behaviour, 1979*. Lisse: Swets & Zeitlinger, 1980; 91–97.

36. Binnie CD, Lloyd DSL. A technique for measuring reaction times during paroxysmal discharges. *Electroencaphalogr Clin Neurophysiol* 1973;35:418.

37. Rugland AL, Bjøæs H, Henrikson O, Løyning A. The development of computerized tests as a routine procedure in clinical EEG practice for the evaluation of cognitive changes in patients with epilepsy. *17th Epilepsy International Congress: Abstracts* 1987;P10.2.

38. Shewmon DA, Erwin RJ. The effect of focal interictal spikes on perception and reaction time.

II. Neuroanatomic specificity. *Electroencephalogr Clin Neurophysiol* 1988;69:338–352.

39. Farwell JR, Dodrill CB, Batzel LW. Neuropsychological abilities of children with epilepsy. *Epilepsia* 1985;26:395–400.
40. Blakemore CB, Ettlinger G, Falconer MA. Cognitive abilities in relation to the frequency of seizures and neuropathology of the temporal lobes in man. *J Neurol Neurosurg Psychiatry* 1966;29:268–272.
41. Camfield PR, Gates R, Ronen G, Camfield C, Ferguson A, MacDonald GW. Comparison of cognitive ability, personality profile, and school success in epileptic children with pure right versus left temporal lobe EEG foci. *Ann Neurol* 1984;15:122–126.
42. Scoville WB, Milner B. Loss of recent memory after bilateral hippocampal lesions. *J Neurol Neurosurg Psychiatry* 1957;20:11–21.
43. Milner B. Visually-guided maze learning in man: effects of bilateral hippocampal, bilateral frontal, and unilateral cerebral lesions. *Neuropsychologia* 1965;3:317–338.
44. Milner B. Memory and the medial temporal regions of the brain. In: Pribram KH, Broadbent DE, eds. *Biology of memory*. New York; Academic Press, 1970;29–50.
45. Glowinski H. Cognitive deficits in temporal lobe epilepsy. An investigation of memory function. *J Ment Nerv Dis* 1973;137:129–137.
46. Loiseau P, Strube E, Signoret JL. Memory and epilepsy. In: Trimble MR, Reynolds EH, eds. *Epilepsy, behaviour and cognitive function.* Chichester: Wiley, 1987.
47. Reynolds EH, Elwes RDC, Shorvon SD. Why does epilepsy become intractable? Prevention of chronic epilepsy. *Lancet* 1983;ii:952–954.
48. Dodrill CB, Troupin AS. Seizures and adaptive abilities. *Arch Neurol* 1976;33:604–607.
49. Besag FMC. Cognitive deterioration in children with epilepsy. In: Trimble MR, Reynolds EH, eds. *Epilepsy, behaviour and cognitive function.* Chichester: Wiley, 1987;113–127.
50. O'Leary DS, Lovell MR, Sackellares JC, Berent S, Giordani B, Seidenberg M, Boll TJ. Effects of age of onset of partial and generalised seizures on neuropsychological performance in children. *J Nerv Ment Dis* 1983;171:624–629.
51. Giordani B, Berent S, Sackellares JC, Rourke D, Seidenberg M, O'Leary DS, Dreifuss FE, Boll TJ. Intelligence test performance of patients with partial and generalised seizures. *Epilepsia* 1985;26:37–42.
52. Bourgeois BFD, Prensky AL, Palkes AL, Talent BK, Busch SG. Intelligence in epilepsy: a prospective study in children. *Ann Neurol* 1983;14:438–444.
53. Dodrill CB. A neuropsychological battery for epilepsy. *Epilepsia* 1978;19:611–623.
54. Parsons OA, Kemp DE. Intellectual functioning in temporal lobe epilepsy. *J Consult Psychol* 1960;24:408–414.
55. Wilkus RJ, Dodrill CB. Neuropsychological correlates of the electroencephalogram in epileptics. I. Topographic distribution and average rate of epileptiform activity. *Epilepsia* 1976;17:89–100.
56. Wieser HG. Selective amygdalohippocampectomy: indications, investigative technique and results. In: Symons L, ed. *Advances and technical standards in neurosurgery,* vol 13. Vienna: Springer, 1985;39–133.
57. Penfield W, Jasper H. *Epilepsy and the functional anatomy of the human brain*. Boston: Little, Brown, 1954.
58. Ranck J. Which elements are excited in electrical stimulation of mammalian central nervous system. A review. *Brain Res* 1975;98:417–440.
59. Ojemann GA. Brain organisation for language from the perspective of electrical stimulation mapping. *Behav Brain Sci* 1983;6:189–230.
60. Penfield W, Roberts L. *Speech and brain mechanisms*. Princeton, NJ: Princeton University Press, 1959.
61. Fedio P, Van Buren J. Memory deficits during electrical stimulation of speech cortex in conscious man. *Brain Lang* 1974;2:78–100.
62. Ojemann GA, Dodrill C. Predicting post-operative language and memory deficits after dominant hemisphere anterior temporal lobectomy by intraoperative stimulation mapping. In: *Abstracts, American Association of Neurological Surgeons, 50th Annual Meeting,* 1981;76–77.
63. Van Buren J, Lewis D, Schutte W, Whithouse W, Ajmone Marsan C. Flurometric monitoring of NADH levels in cerebral cortex: preliminary observations in human epilepsy. *Neurosurgery* 1978;2:114–121.
64. Ojemann GA, Dodrill C. Verbal memory deficits after left temporal lobectomy for epilepsy: mechanism and intraoperative prediction. *J Neurosurg* 1985;62:101–107.
65. Halgren E, et al. Dynamics of the hippocampal contribution to memory: stimulation and recording studies in humans. In: Seifert W, ed. *Neurobiology of the hippocampus*. New York: Academic Press, 1983;529–572.
66. Vidart L, Geier S. Enregistrements teleencéphalographiques chez des sujets épileptiques pendant le travail. *Rev Neurol (Paris)* 1967;117:475–480.
67. Altafullah I, Halgren E. Focal medial temporal lobe spike–wave complexes evoked by a memory task. *Epilepsia* 1988;29:8–13.
68. Kasteleijn-Nolst Trenité DGA, Bakker DJ, Binnie CD, Buerman A, van Raaij M. Psychological effects of sub-clinical epileptiform discharges: scholastic skills. *Epilepsy Res* 1988;2:111–116.
69. Kasteleijn-Nolst Trenité DGA, Riemersma JBJ, Binnie CD, Smit AM, Meinardi H. The influence of subclinical epileptiform EEG discharges on driving behaviour. *Electroencephalogr Clin Neurophysiol* 1987;67:167–170.
70. Eeg-Olofsson O, Petersén I, Selldén U. The development of the electroencephalogram in normal children from the age of 1 through 15 years: paroxysmal activity. *Neuropädiatrie* 1971;2:375–404.
71. Villarreal HJ, Wilder BJ, Willmore LJ, Bauman AW, Hammond EJ, Bruni J. Effect of valproic

acid on spike and wave discharges in patients with absence seizures. *Neurology (Minneap)* 1978;28:886–891.

72. Bruni S, Wilder BS, Bauman AW. Clinical efficacy and long-term effects of valproic acid therapy on spike-and-wave discharges. *Neurology (NY)* 1980;30:42–46.

73. Gram L, Drachmann Bentsen K, Parnas J, Flachs H. Controlled trials in epilepsy: a review. *Epilepsia* 1982;23:491–519.

74. Van Wieringen A, Binnie CD, De Boer PTE, Van Emde Boas W, Overweg J, De Vries J. Electro-encephalographic findings in six antiepileptic drug trials *Epilepsy Res* 1987;1:3–15.

75. Pryse-Phillips WEM, Jeavons PM. Effect of carbamazepine (Tegretol) on the electroencephalograph and ward behaviour of patients with chronic epilepsy. *Epilepsia* 1970;11:263–273.

76. Wilkus RJ, Dodrill CB, Troupin AS. Carbamazepine and the electroencephalogram of epileptics: a double blind study in comparison to phenytoin. *Electroencephalogr Clin Neurophysiol* 1978;51:186–191.

77. Milligan N, Oxley MJ, Richens A. Acute effects of intravenous phenytoin on the frequency of interictal spikes in man. *Br J Clin Pharmacol* 1983;16:285–289.

78. Binnie CD. Preliminary evaluation of potential anti-epileptic drugs by single dose electrophysiological and pharmacological studies in patients. *J Neural Trans* 1988;72:256–259.

79. Wilkus RJ, Green JR. Electroencephalographic investigations during evaluation of the antiepileptic agent sulthiams. *Epilepsia* 1974;15:13–25.

80. Kellaway P, Frost JD, Hrachovy RA. Relationship between clinical state, ictal and interictal EEG discharges, and serum drug levels: partial seizures/phenobarbital. *Ann Neurol* 1978;4:197.

81. Gotman J, Marciani MG. Electroencephalographic spiking activity, drug levels and seizure occurrence in epileptic patients. *Ann Neurol* 1985;17:597–603.

82. Binnie CD, Beintema DJ, Debets RMC, Van Emde Boas W, Meijer JWA, Meinardi H, Peck AW, Westendorp A-M, Yuen WC. Seven day administration of lamotrigine in epilepsy: add-on trial. *Epilepsy Res* 1987;1:202–208.

Advances in Neurology, Vol. 55, edited by
D. Smith, D. Treiman, and M. Trimble,
Raven Press, Ltd., New York © 1991.

8

Acute Behavioral Symptomatology at Disappearance of Epileptiform EEG Abnormality

Paradoxical or "Forced" Normalization

Peter Wolf

Epilepsy-Centre Bethel, 4800 Bielefeld 13, Federal Republic of Germany

In an early electrophysiological study of psychiatric aspects of epilepsy, Heinrich Landolt, then medical head of the Swiss Epilepsy Center at Zurich, recorded the electroencephalograms (EEGs) of institutionalized patients with epilepsy during episodes of disturbed behavior and in the nonsymptomatic interval, and then he compared them. He expected to find increased abnormalities during the abnormal episodes, and in some cases he found that this was true. He was amazed, however, to discover a quite different group, for whom the EEG looked less pathological when the behavior was deteriorated and for whom nonspecific and epileptiform dysrhythmias could disappear.

In his first report of this puzzling observation (1), he indicated that it could be due to an excess of inhibition. In his later work, however, he wanted to avoid such a definite pathogenetic statement, since it did not seem to be sufficiently established. To describe this seemingly paradoxical observation, he would instead use the terminology "forcierte Normalisierung," which he considered as merely descriptive and not implying any definite pathogenetic hypothesis. This, however, has frequently been misunderstood, since it was not sufficiently clear [especially in his only paper written in English (2)] why he chose the term. In the papers in his native language,

there is much less ambiguity, since it is clear that the two components of the composite term are heterogenous. "Normalization" refers to the aspect of the scalp EEG; in addition, it is helpful to remember that in those early stages of electroencephalography, scalp recordings were more readily taken at their face value and mock "normality" such as in alpha coma was unheard of. In reality, Landolt's report is one of the earliest observations intentionally indicating that not all that looks normal in the EEG is normal. Unfortunately, the additional term he suggested—forciert—was less clear. It is not self-explanatory, and Landolt did not explain it. "Forciert" is an uncommon German word which sounds less suggestive of a definite "force" in German than it does in English, and translation of the composite term as "overnormalization" would come nearer to the original meaning than would the direct translation "forced normalization."

"Normalization" rather than "normality" implies a development, and the diagnosis thus requires a comparison of at least two recordings in different clinical conditions. Still, nothing specific in the aspect of the EEG was pointed out as suggesting that the normalization was "forced." This had to be inferred from the observation of a clinical deterioration accompanying the normalization of the

EEG aspect. The term is thus a clinical–EEG hybrid. If Landolt had chosen to talk about "paradoxical" or "spurious" normalization, he probably would have been more widely understood.

This is not what happened. The knowledge of this curious issue remained largely confined to German- and perhaps French-speaking epileptologists, whereas most English-speaking authors seemed to hesitate whether paradoxical normalization (PN)—as I intend to call it throughout this chapter—belonged to the realm of medical science or, rather, medical mythology. I very much suspect that this was mainly a consequence of the unfortunate English terminology, because the existence of the counterpart of PN—remission of psychosis following seizures or electroconvulsive therapy—was undoubted.

In a paper on the concept of biological antagonism and epileptic psychosis (3), Trimble and I have tried to improve this somewhat unsatisfactory state of information, and we discussed in some historical detail the relation between PN and convulsive antipsychotic treatment. Recently, and for perhaps the first time in the New World, the subject was taken up by an article (4) and an editorial (5) in the *Archives of Neurology,* followed by an exchange of letters (6,7) which documented the

interest which these publications had generated.

This chapter will discuss the phenomenology, pathogenesis, and possible pathophysiology of paradoxical normalization.

PARADOXICAL NORMALIZATION IN THE ELECTROENCEPHALOGRAM

"Normalization" as it is discussed here refers to the disappearance of epileptiform discharge from the scalp EEG, as demonstrated by a series of routine recordings in the wake state including hyperventilation.

It has never been discussed if and how PN can be diagnosed if the routine EEG of a patient with epilepsy never shows epileptiform discharge, which is far from uncommon. It would indeed be difficult to establish a guideline for this situation, since there do not seem to exist any rules concerning the background EEG activity of these cases. In one patient with juvenile absences (8) who developed delusions of reference with complete control of absences and spike-and-wave discharge by ethosuximide but not with equally complete clinical and EEG control by valproic acid, we have been able to compare PN with uncomplicated normalization in the EEG (9). In PN,

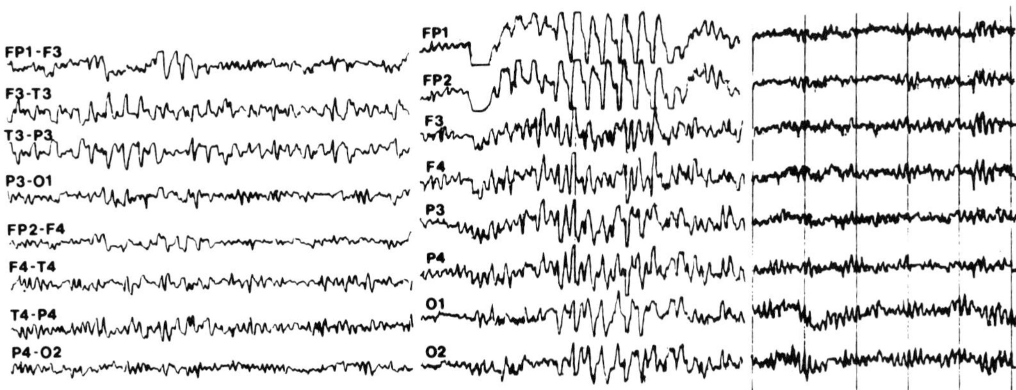

FIG. 1. Patient 1. **Left tracing:** Left temporal focus of slow and sharp waves. Slightly abnormal background activity with irregular alpha and interspersed theta waves. Carbamazepine monotherapy, serum level 8.5 μg/ml. **Middle tracing:** Paroxysms of irregular 3-Hz spike wave, precipitated by eye closure, after 5 min of hyperventilation. Drug levels: carbamazepine 6.6 μg/ml, phenobarbital 5.9 μg/ml, desmethyl-mesuximide 7.0 μg/ml. **Right tracing:** Background activity in paradoxical normalization. Antiepileptic drug levels: carbamazepine 4.5 μg/ml, phenobarbital 5.8 μg/ml, desmethyl-mesuximide 26.3 μg/ml.

TABLE 1. *Epileptiform discharges in the sleep EEGs of two patients who developed PN during ES monotherapy for absences*[a]

	Patient A		Patient B	
	Unmedicated	In PN	Unmedicated	In PN
NREM				
Stage 1	0.14	0.02	0.07	0.15
Stage 2	3.6	0.61	0.14	0.04
Stage 3	3.8	2.32	0.11	0
Stage 4	15.0	1.57	0.03	0.01
REM	0.07	0	0.1	0.03
WASO	0	0	1.5	0.5

[a]Discharge rate is given as *N* spike-and-wave paroxysms per minute of all-night registration. Length of spike-and-wave paroxysms was not considered. In both patients, a significant reduction of spike-and-wave activity was found with PN, but epileptiform discharge did not disappear completely. The distribution on the different sleep stages remained essentially unchanged, although in patient B there is a relative increase in light NREM sleep. The sleep charts of patient A have been published (ref. 31, Fig. 8.1). PN, paradoxical normalization; REM, sleep with rapid eye movements (paradoxical sleep); NREM, non-REM (orthodox or slow-wave sleep, stages according to Rechtschaffen and Kales); WASO, wake after sleep onset (interspersed wake phases during night).

the alpha rhythm was less prominent and less well organized, of smaller amplitude, and more restricted to the posterior leads, but there was more interspersed slow activity. Without direct comparison of the recordings, however, the background activity in PN would still have been considered as perfectly normal, and the differences might reflect nothing more than insufficient relaxation during the psychotic state.

Figure 1 shows EEG recordings of a patient who presented her most normal background activity ever in a state of florid delusions during PN.

Thus, if the disappearance of epileptic activity from the routine scalp EEG, together with behavioral deterioration, sufficiently establishes a diagnosis of PN, the question remains whether epileptic discharge has completely vanished in this condition or whether it could still be detected with more sophisticated procedures. No spontaneous sleep recordings during PN seem to have been published, but there is a report on six such patients (10) who were given propanidide, a short-acting barbiturate derivative (11). Generalized spike-and-wave patterns were provoked in one, and focal slow and steep waves (probably not epileptiform activity in the strict sense) were provoked in the other five. In our own studies on the influence of various antiepileptic drugs (AEDs) on sleep, two patients experienced an episode of PN, and their

night sleep was monitored. In both, a considerable decrease but not complete disappearance of spike-and-wave discharge was observed (Table 1).

More specifically, in his stereotaxic intracerebral EEG studies, Wieser (12) has been able to demonstrate restricted focal subcortical seizures without alteration of the scalp recording in conditions which would probably have been diagnosed as PN without knowledge of the subcortical findings. This has, of course, some importance for the theory of PN.

Magnetoencephalography could be helpful for the noninvasive detection of such activity, but it seems to not yet have been applied in such a situation.

CLINICAL APPEARANCES OF PARADOXICAL NORMALIZATION

Alternative Psychosis

The term "forced normalization," as will be remembered, was mostly concerned with the EEG but included awareness of some clinical deterioration, especially the development of a psychotic condition. Some years following Landolt's report, the term "alternative psychosis" was introduced by Tellenbach (13) in a paper entitled "Epilepsy as a Seizure Disorder and a Psychosis. On Alternative Epileptic Psychosis with 'Forced Normalization' (Landolt) of the EEG of Patients with Epilepsy." There were two reasons why Tellenbach introduced this additional term. The first was that it was awkward to always have to refer to "epileptic psychosis with forced normalization of the electroencephalogram," and clearly a shorter term was desirable. Secondly, as was pointed out above, the term "forced normalization" was considered primarily an EEG phenomenon, whereas the new term paid more attention to the presence or absence of seizures.

The concept was not altogether new. Glaus (14) had already (in 1931) stated "that in the cases of combinations of epilepsy and schizophrenia an alternating relationship is the rule," and Wyrsch (15) had discussed the "syndromatic antagonism" of these disorders, concluding that it was not permissible to assume, from the syndromatic antagonism, an "antagonism of the basic disorders."

These were the ideas under the influence of which Meduna (16) developed the convulsive therapy of psychoses. Tellenbach, however, when he used the term "alternative," referred to a paper by Landolt (17), in which it was suggested that the efficiency of modern AEDs had demonstrated the limits of epilepsy therapy and placed the physician before the alternative: mental illness or epilepsy, seizures or madness. Regardless of which of these two traditions is referred to, the term "alternative psychosis" seems to imply that, in such cases, the cessation of seizures does not signify cure or even inactivity of the underlying disease. This, however, was not discussed in detail, and Tellenbach did not present any pathogenic hypothesis.

He did discuss the psychopathology of alternative psychosis, which he found to be (to a certain extent) similar to schizophrenia. It differed from schizophrenia by a much lower propensity to systematized delusions and by a peculiar coexistence of two realms of experience ("Erlebniswelten"): the real one and the psychotic one. Tellenbach was impressed to see that in his patients the delusions were, to an unusual degree, concerned with the role of the parents, especially the father. The psychotic syndrome could resemble various types of lucid productive psychoses, but a paranoid delusion as the presenting symptom seemed to be most common.

We also found this to be true in our material on 19 alternative productive psychotic episodes, 12 of which were paranoid or paranoid–hallucinatory, four catatonia-like or ecstatic, two coenesthetic, and one a delusion of parasitosis (18).

RELATED SYNDROMES

Prepsychotic Dysphoria (Praepsychotische Verstimmung)

Tellenbach (13) had pointed out that in many instances of paradoxical normalization, the development of psychotic symptomatology was preceded by premonitory symptoms. The most important of these seemed to be insomnia, anxiety, and feelings of oppression, accompanied by a most characteristic behavior of withdrawal from other people and from usual activities. This has much interested the present author because of the implications which such premonitory events may have for the prevention of alternative psychosis (19).

We have pointed out that the administration of a benzodiazepine-type tranquilizer at the development of such symptomatology may prevent the evolution into psychosis if insomnia is controlled (19). As a consequence of this therapeutic guideline, instances of isolated "prepsychotic" dysphoria not followed by psychosis have become the second most important manifestation of forced normalization in our studies.

Hysterical and Hypochondriacal States

In five of our 36 patients with forced normalization (18), this presented as a hysterical episode (hysterical seizures in three patients, an abasia in one, and regressive symptomatology mimicking a twilight state in the last one). The patient with psychogenic abasia had several episodes of this as well as forced normalization with paranoid delusions. In the latter, the abasia would occur as a premonitory sign of the psychosis. It seems that in this patient the hysterical symptomatology was an exact parallel of the prepsychotic dysphoria of others.

In two of these patients, the episode of hysteria was further accompanied by hypochondriacal complaints, and one of these with several episodes of forced normalization presented at another occasion as a hypochondriacal episode. Two additional patients had episodes characterized by hypochondriacal symptomatology. In one of these, there was a complaint of physical weakness very close to hysterical abasia. There seemed to be no clear border between the two conditions, and their strict diagnostic separation would thus be inadequate.

Affective Disorders

In four of our patients, forced normalization presented as an affective disorder (two depressive and two manic). The depressive cases corresponded to the criteria of vital psychotic depression, and the manic disorders were severe and included flight of ideas and uncontrolled expansive behavior—in one case, delusions of grandeur and reference; in the other, a suicide attempt.

It was remarkable that in these four patients the symptomatology corresponded well with their primary personality. In one of the depressed patients there was a family predisposition for depressive illness. This is different from patients with paranoid alternative psychoses, where there was no such correlation with the primary personality. It may be remembered that paranoid delusion is one of the most nonspecific of psychiatric symptoms.

Miscellaneous

More unusual presentations of forced normalization in our studies were a twilight state, an episode of depersonalization and derealization, and dysphoric states with a symptomatology different from that of "prepsychotic" dysphoria, with irritability, unrest, and emotional upset.

In several patients, PN occurred repeatedly, sometimes with a similar symptomatology but in other instances with a different one, so that a total of 44 different syndromes were found in 36 patients (18). Since 1984, some additional observations have been added to our body of information, but they were of limited significance.

A recent observation will illustrate some of the features of PN: Patient 1 is a 33-year-old housewife who has seven brothers and sisters, and the child of one had febrile convulsions. The patient's only daughter, who is 11 years old, had also suffered febrile convulsions at age 2. The patient's seizure disorder started in her second year. It is not known whether the onset was also with febrile convulsions, but she has had generalized tonic–clonic and complex partial seizures ever since. She has always received AED treatment but was never seizure-free for any considerable period. She did not finish regular school and had to give up training as a sales assistant, but she worked as a sales assistant in a store until age 22, at which time her only child was born. At 28, she had an early abortion. There were no other important diseases. Her physical examination was unremarkable except for slight obesity. She is of slightly subnormal intelligence, but her appearance does not indicate this. It troubles her, however, that she is unable to help her child with her schoolwork, and it appears that she had to suffer some rather offensive teasing on her dullness from her husband's side of the family. This is her weak point and her concern. Otherwise, she lives quietly with her husband (who is a technical employee in their hometown) and daughter.

At age 30, she was psychiatrically hospitalized for a month with a diagnosis of depression. She had never been depressed before, and neither the symptomatology nor the pathogenesis had been included in the hospital report. But it may be noteworthy that the depression developed at the end of a period of several months with considerably increased seizure frequency, which troubled her sufficiently to make her change her neurologist. Some months later, she was admitted to our department with a request to optimize her AED treatment. She was then on carbamazepine (CBZ) with trough serum levels of 8–11 μg/ml and had, in one month, six simple and three complex partial seizures.

Her computerized tomography (CT) and magnetic resonance imaging (MRI) scans were unrevealing. The EEG (Fig. 1, left and middle tracings) demonstrated a left temporal focus of slow and occasional sharp waves along with some irregular bilateral spike-and-wave discharge during hyperventilation, sometimes provoked by eye closure (20). The background activity was slightly abnormal (alpha of about 8 Hz, with increased interspersed theta).

She proved to be resistant to a maximal tolerated CBZ dose, and she was discharged with a CBZ (1200 mg)–phenobarbital (PB; 150 mg) combination (serum levels of approximately 7 and 32 µg/ml, respectively) which made her complain of drowsiness, nausea, and edema of the lower extremities. She still had several simple partial seizures per month. A 300-mg dose of mesuximide (MS) was then added, which reduced her clinical seizures to one or two short epigastric sensations per month (serum level 13.3 µg/ml). Subsequent decrease of PB dose to 50 mg (serum level 11.3 µg/ml) stopped her complaints of sedation and nausea. There was still a tendency to develop edema, and an attempt was made to withdraw CBZ. At 450 mg, however, complex focal seizures reappeared, and it was decided to proceed with 600 mg CBZ slow release, 30 mg PB, and an increased dose of 600 mg MS. In the following 4 months, she had only three isolated epigastric auras, and her EEG became, for the first time, completely normal (Fig. 1, right tracing). Her serum levels were CBZ 4.5, PB 5.8, and desmethyl-MS 26.3 µg/ml. She was, however, gravely insomnic and was also in a depressive mood. She had delusions of reference, stating that our hospital report on her had been published in the journal of the German self-help groups for epilepsy and that her case had been discussed in a plenary of the Chamber of Physicians so that all physicians of the region were informed on how stupid she was and had detailed instructions on how to deal with her.

MS had to be withdrawn, which made her complex partial seizures reappear and led to rapid recovery from psychosis.

It should be noted that the MS level was in the medium range and that the psychotic state could not be explained by intoxication. The drug level was, however, sufficient to provide seizure control and EEG "normalization."

PARADOXICAL NORMALIZATION, TYPE OF EPILEPSY, AND EPIDEMIOLOGY

There is a widespread belief that psychosis in epilepsy involves the temporal lobe or, more specifically, the left temporal lobe. Population-based studies of relatively unselected material, however, have failed to establish such a relationship (21–23). The abundant literature on this is deplorably devoid of discussion of such problems as unilateral or bilateral temporal lobe involvement, combinations of focal and generalized epileptiform discharges, and the differentiation of frontal and temporal lobe complex partial seizures. Differences in seizure type or the different pathogenetic types of psychosis have rarely been considered.

What is known in this respect about psychoses with PN? Patient 1 has focal seizures and a family background of febrile convulsions, and she probably also has a personal history of febrile convulsions. Her EEG shows generalized epileptiform discharges independently of left temporal sharp waves. Thus, her epilepsy is not clearly classifiable as partial or generalized [group 3.1 of the International Classification of Epileptic Syndromes (8)]. In a retrospective study, Bruens (24) found that patients with a combination of temporal lobe epilepsy (TLE) and bilateral synchronous spike-and-wave discharge had the highest risk of developing epileptic psychosis. His study included patients with PN but also included those with other psychoses. This finding seemed to confirm a hypothesis of Tellenbach (13).

Landolt (2) had first described PN in patients with TLE. Later, however, the picture changed, and in 1963 Landolt (17) reported: "The relation turned towards the generalized epilepsies. This was clearly correlated with progress in the treatment of petit mal. When we, in 1954, introduced the succinimide drugs there was an immediate increase in cases of forced normalization . . . in petit mal."

Many case reports of PN are indeed not found in the literature on psychosis and epilepsy but have been found in papers about succinimide treatment, which were reviewed by Roger et al. (25). Patients receiving this treatment and responding to it can be expected to suffer from absences and thus belong to the group of patients with generalized epilepsies.

In our studies on psychoses in epilepsy, there is a significant correlation between generalized idiopathic epilepsies and psychoses with forced normalization, in contrast to that between other epilepsies and other types of psychoses (3).

In her recent brilliant epidemiological study, Schmitz (26) looked at many aspects of psychosis in epilepsy in the outpatient population of a neurological university hospital. Although some bias towards difficult cases in such a secondary referral facility can be expected, she found in a total of 697 patients with epilepsy only 28 (4%) with at least one psychotic episode of any type. This lifetime prevalence is very low considering that all psychoses, including acute organic syndromes (but not depressive syndromes), were included.

Of the 28 psychoses, only three were classified as alternative psychoses with PN. To these, four instances of PN with nonpsychotic related syndromes (*vide supra*) could be added. This confirms that PN is rare and explains why it seems to have escaped the attention of even experienced investigators.

Of the seven patients with PN, four had a diagnosis of generalized epilepsy whereas three were diagnosed as having a localization-related epilepsy. None of them had an epilepsy with both focal and generalized features, unlike Patient 1 of this chapter.

A similar distribution was found for psychoses in general, and of all the epileptic syndromes in the ILAE classification (8), pyknolepsy or childhood absence epilepsy was the only one with an increased risk for psychoses. Analysis with respect to the seizure types, however, resulted in some remarkable observations, since it revealed that in generalized epilepsy a combination of both convulsive and nonconvulsive seizures was a prerequisite for a psychotic development. In localization-related epilepsies, this finding was not reproduced, but when three classes of focal nonconvulsive seizures—complex partial, simple partial involving the limbic system (Table 2), and simple partial not involving the limbic system—were formed, it turned out that there was a high correlation with complex focal seizures but not with simple partial limbic or nonlimbic seizures. This suggests that the still unsubstantiated impression that psychosis is particularly frequent in TLE may be due to the frequency of complex partial seizures [i.e., partial seizures with impairment of consciousness (27)] in this type of epilepsy.

TABLE 2. *Types of simple partial seizures considered as probably related to the limbic system[a]*

Autonomic (including epigastric)
Affective
Dysmnesic
Olfactory
Gustatory
Auditory
Complex hallucinations

[a]Simple partial auditory seizures have been included but are not per se indicative of limbic involvement, because they often seem to spread to limbic structures—especially in the case of complex auditory hallucinations.

There was no left versus right difference.

PN was not apparently different from psychoses and related syndromes of other pathogenesis, but of course the numbers are small in this study.

Thus, the common denominator for both generalized and localization-related epilepsies seems to be that, as a double prerequisite for the development of psychoses, an epileptic brain must be able to produce limited seizure discharge, but there must also be a history of ictal impairment of consciousness. This, again, is of interest for the discussion on pathogenesis.

PARADOXICAL NORMALIZATION AND ANTIEPILEPTIC DRUGS

The first observations of Landolt concerned episodes of PN which developed spontaneously. These, however, seem to be the exception. Much more frequently, the condition develops following control of seizures and epileptic EEG discharge by medication. It appears that more or less all AEDs, including benzodiazepines such as clonazepam and clobazam, have been charged with the precipitation of mental symptoms accompanying the therapeutic effect. Of the drugs in contemporary use, it is especially ethosuximide (ES) that has been reported to produce PN. Other drugs for absences of much less practical importance, such as MS and the oxazolidines, do not seem to differ significantly from ES (e.g., as with patient 1). The specific influence of this drug in absence patients was highlighted after the introduction of an equally effective, but pharmacologically quite different, drug for absences, namely valproic acid (VPA). This was quantitatively studied by Wolf et al. (28), who reported the psychiatric complications observed in 229 adolescents and adults who at the onset of therapy in a neurological seizure clinic still suffered from absences. PN was observed in 18 (7.8%; 8 psychotic, 10 nonpsychotic). ES was involved in the therapy of 17, and MS was involved in that of the remaining one. A comparison of regimens, including the various drugs for absences, revealed that ES is a highly significant risk factor for PN whereas VPA is not.

This remarkable relation to one specific drug seems not to be due to toxicity, since PN has been reported even at low doses and apparently subtherapeutic ES serum levels (29). A possible pathogenic factor could be an arousal effect produced by ES. Many patients report sleep disturbances with this drug, in contrast to what is reported for VPA. As mentioned above, insomnia is often an early sign of PN. This seems to be especially true for PN in patients with generalized idiopathic epilepsy (18). In a study comparing the effects of the two drugs on the sleep of patients with epilepsy, Röder and Wolf (30) have been able to demonstrate deep-sleep deprivation and increase of light sleep with ES, along with an increase of interspersed stage 1 in, and in close vicinity to, rapid-eye movement (REM) phases. Both these effects could be of some relevance for the PN. Later in that study, PN with ES has been observed in a 14-year-old patient with absences. His sleep charts revealed considerable deterioration of his sleep quality, and this may have been an important unspecific pathogenic factor (31). For his spike-and-wave discharge, see Table 1.

A highly interesting point is the time aspect of the development of drug-induced PN, as is demonstrated by the following case histories:

Patient 2 is a 39-year-old single female school teacher who has no familiar antecedents and whose epilepsy started at age 8 with generalized tonic–clonic seizures mostly in the morning and late afternoon. She is not quite sure if her absences manifested at the same time, since nobody ever paid any attention to these. Antiabsence drugs were never part of her AED regimen, although she has always been in treatment, and generalized spike-and-wave discharge was always present on her EEG. When she was questioned, she was also aware of short lapses of consciousness. Her seizures were never controlled in spite of constant therapy with a variety of AEDs as monotherapy or in combination.

When we first saw her, she was on 1000 mg primidone (PR; serum level of 8.3 μg/ml with a PB level of 27.5) and 800 mg CBZ slow release (CBZ SR 4.3 μg/ml, CBZ-epoxide 1.3 μg/ml) and her EEG contained several 3- to 4-hz spike-and-wave paroxysms which, during hyperventilation, lasted up to 9 sec, without concomitant clinical symptomatology (Fig. 2). In the temporal leads, these presented with alternate lateralization. Photosensitivity could not be ruled out. She was having infrequent generalized tonic–clonic (GTC) seizures, and only on direct interrogation did she admit to having experienced absences.

There seemed to be little hope for better control as long as the absences were neglected, and stepwise replacement of CBZ by VPA was recommended. This, however, did not have the expected effect, since the patient had two severe GTC seizures at a short interval, the absences did not decrease, and the EEG remained more or less unchanged even with VPA trough levels of 70–90 μg/ml.

The patient was hospitalized for closer observation on September 14, 1988; on her own account, she had re-started CBZ and was presently taking 1000 mg PR, 1200 mg CBZ SR, and 1200 mg VPA. On the morning of September 15, she had a GTC seizure. On September 22, VPA was reduced by 300 mg, and 250 mg ES was started; on September 25, another 300 mg VPA was replaced by 250 mg ES, and on September 28 the ES dose was increased to 750 mg. No absences were reported or observed. On the morning of September 29, an EEG control was, for the first time, completely free of spike-and-wave paroxysms. When I broke the good news to her, she said: "Doctor, first of all I wish to know what game is going on, who are the real nurses and patients on this ward, and who are the fakes who are there under disguise to observe me." Until the day before, no such idea had transpired.

The patient was taken off ES, and the psychotic symptoms remitted slowly. It was only

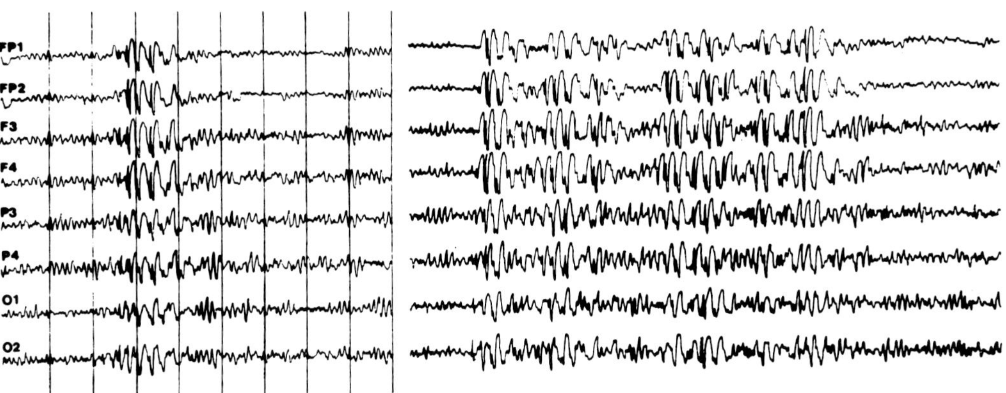

FIG. 2. Patient 2. **Left tracing:** Short, generalized 3.5-Hz spike-and-wave paroxysm in resting condition. **Right tracing:** With hyperventilation, prolonged slightly discontinuous spike-and-wave discharge, subclinical. Antiepileptic drug levels: phenobarbital 27.5 μg/ml, carbamazepine 4.3 μg/ml.

then that we came to know that 6 years earlier, she had suffered an episode with delusions following a cluster of GTC seizures.

We have repeatedly observed this type of rapid development, but there are also examples of a quite different time course.

Patient 3 is an example of an extremely slow psychotic development with PN. He suffered from idiopathic generalized epilepsy, probably with an unobserved onset of simple absences. At age 14, bilateral myoclonic seizures in full consciousness and GTC seizures on awakening became manifest. His EEG showed 3-Hz spike-and-wave discharges. At age 24, his seizures were completely controlled following adjustment to 750 mg PR and 1000 mg ES, which at first he seemed to tolerate well. His EEG was repeatedly free of epileptic discharges.

During the following 3 years, he developed a slowly progressive delusional system around his father, whom he accused of attempted murder. It finally involved most family members, his neurologist, and still other people. Twice he moved in panic to another town when he thought his father had discovered where he was hiding from him.

When we saw him at this stage we did not believe that this was a case of PN, because the time relationship between the seizure, the spike-and-wave control, and the psychosis was unconvincing and also because his relationship with his father had always been most problematic, which indicated an autochthonic

psychotic development. There was a family history of psychiatric disorders (including cases of schizophrenia), and his delusional system seemed to indicate schizophrenia because it was much more stable and well-organized than is usually seen in epilepsy psychoses (13). Furthermore, the patient was deeply convinced of this delusion, whereas in epilepsy psychosis the patient can often be talked out of it temporarily (32).

We stopped his ES medication mainly because we wanted to do something, and the patient was unwilling to accept any other suggestions. VPA (1200 mg) was given instead. Shortly after this change, he experienced some absences which disappeared again with VPA (1500 mg) and PR (500 mg).

Immediately after the withdrawal of ES, the psychotic symptoms lost some of their acuity, and over the next 4 months the psychosis faded off into complete remission. The patient moved back home, and then he successfully took his final examination after having long postponed it when still psychotic. We have been able to follow him for more than 5 years, and he has remained asymptomatic. It could be discussed whether this was a toxic rather than an alternative psychosis. This is, however, unlikely. Although ES serum levels were, at that period, not measured, the dose was low average, and no elevated levels would have been expected. More importantly, a toxic psychosis would have emerged acutely when ES levels had reached their steady state, which is a matter of few days with this drug. A slow time course is much more compatible with a complex multifactorial pathogenesis, as we shall discuss with regard to PN (see below).

PSYCHOSOCIAL FACTORS

We have just mentioned the possible contribution of an untoward family situation in the development of psychoses with PN. Another psychosocial factor could be the lack of independence, since the patient had not completed his professional training. We have been interested for a long time in psychosocial influences on the clinical symptomatology of PN which seems to be apparent in many case histories.

In a first approach, we looked at possible differences between patients with alternative psychosis and with alternative prepsychotic dysphorias (33) and found only one significant difference. The majority of patients who became psychotic were vocationally disintegrated, having no job or no professional training. For the dysphoric patients, this was not true. This was reconfirmed in 1986 (31), when our study consisted of nine patients with prepsychotic dysphorias, seven of whom were employed and two in training at the time of PN. Of 18 patients with alternative psychosis, only six were employed, eight in training, and four unemployed ($p<0.05$).

Two hypotheses can be formed to explain the differences:

1. Social integration is a stabilizing factor in a potentially psychotogenic situation.
2. Better social integration is an indictor of a more stable primary personality, which is more able to cope with such a situation.

We have suggested (34) a simple way of interaction for such factors. A very important means of prevention of alternative psychosis seems to be early control of insomnia (usually by transitory administration of a tranquilizer). This will usually require that the patient quickly reports the onset of insomnia or similar prepsychotic symptoms. To wait until the next routine appointment at the clinic may be too long a wait for the prevention of psychosis. Several of our patients with a prepsy-chotic symptomatology saw us urgently because they did not feel well, whereas others presented at the routine appointment with psychotic symptoms that had been preceded by premonitory signs of a similar order to which, however, these patients had not reacted. Patients of inadequate social adjustment may be more reluctant to leave their routine. To take an extra step and ask for an urgent appointment requires a minimum of social versatility that some patients do not seem to possess. This may prove deleterious in such a situation.

Psychosocial aspects of epilepsy-related psychoses in general (i.e., not restricted to PN) have been discussed elsewhere (34) on the basis of a controlled retrospective investigation of our data. Some substantial differences were found in patterns of everyday life between the families of the patients with epilepsy and psychoses and matched controls. During adolescence, the psychotic patients were less often (or at a later age) allowed to adopt certain new roles and perform them according to their own interests. This restrictive practice was supported by a prevailing pattern of physical punishment. No relationship between these family characteristics and indexes of social class could be found. The families of patients with psychoses comparatively more often adhered to religious minority groups. Further studies should look more closely at the significance of this factor for the everyday life of the families. In the families of patients with psychoses, there is a higher uncertainty about issues such as sexuality and the meaning of the member's epilepsy for the family. This may result in uncertainty with regard to the adoption of social roles in general and could be linked to the indices of social instability in adulthood that were apparent in patients with psychotic episodes as reported above.

Our findings, however, must be taken with the reserve appropriate for retrospective studies. Particularly, the psychotic experience may have influenced the patients' recall of their own history.

Schmitz (26) reconfirmed the correlation of psychosis and lack of professional qualification, especially in patients who had successfully finished their scholastic career. From an intercorrelation analysis, however, she added the caveat that such a social situation was especially found in patients who had other risk factors of psychosis, such as (a) a combination of GTC and absence seizures in generalized epilepsy or (b) an insufficient response to AED treatment.

RELATION OF PN AND OTHER EPILEPSY PSYCHOSES; DISCUSSION OF PATHOGENESIS

In the previous sections, psychoses (and related syndromes) with PN have repeatedly been discussed indiscriminately along with other psychoses. This may appear inconsiderate and requires an explanation. A more superficial reason is that numbers, even in rather extensive studies such as the one of Schmitz (26), remain small; moreover, many aspects could not be analyzed if many subgroups were formed. But there is a more serious and philosophical reason. The various types of psychosis—ictal, postictal, alternative, episodic, and chronic, with and without impairment of consciousness—are much less easily separable in practice than in theory. Especially, it would be impossible to assign every patient of a study to one of these categories because, in the course of time, many of them will have experienced various varieties. Thus in the study of Schmitz, of 43 patients, 30 suffered more than one episode; in 11 of these the relapses belonged to a diagnostic category other than that of the first manifestation (26). Elsewhere, we have reported two examples of this (34), and patients 1 and 2 of this chapter are further examples of a sequence of different types of behavioral disorder caused by (a) increased seizures in the first instance and (b) PN in the second instance.

In the extensive literature on epilepsy-related psychoses, this aspect has received remarkably little attention, probably because most patients were not studied longitudinally and also because their presenting psychiatric manifestation was considered in isolation. This is obviously inadequate for a more comprehensive understanding of psychoses in epilepsy. A psychotic episode, even if not experienced in full consciousness and apparently remitting without residue, seems not to become extinguished but to remain part of the patient's history and indentity. Remarkably, longitudinal observations such as those just mentioned indicate that such experiences may be reactivated both by physical and psychosocial pathogenic factors. Delusions once experienced seem to become part of a person's (and a brain's) disposable pattern of behavior and may serve as a response to various extreme conditions. A discussion on pathogenesis and pathophysiology of PN should include the aforementioned considerations and should also develop hypotheses which are compatible with them.

MECHANISMS

The subject of an alternative relationship between seizures and psychoses has given rise, over the years, to many theoretical considerations and hypotheses. The most important ones will be discussed here.

1. Alternation of seizures and psychoses is just one of several examples of a psychotic reaction to the sudden termination of a severe and chronic disease. Well-known examples are psychoses following surgical cure of such different conditions as congenital blindness or disabling heart disease. This viewpoint can be traced back to Esquirol (35) and was renewed by Ferguson and Rayport (36), the latter not surprisingly referring to patients with operative therapy of focal epilepsy. They described the deep life crisis of patients who are suddenly expected to function like healthy people after they have learned to look at themselves as disabled. It is, however, questionable whether their findings can be applied to the less suddenly and spectacularly achieved seizure control by an efficient medication. This hypothesis cannot explain a rapid onset of psychosis as in our case 2, nor can it explain the different responses to equally efficient but chemically unrelated drugs.

2. There is a "biological antagonism" between seizures and psychoses (16). This historical hypothesis was initially unspecified and open but has stimulated more detailed theories (see Chapter 3).

Reynolds (37) has reviewed the reports indicating that folate deficiency was frequent in medicated patients with epilepsy, and that it was correlated with mental symptoms. The significance of these findings for PN, however, remains to be determined. Folate deficiency has been demonstrated in patients receiving phenytoin, phenobarbital, or primidone, whereas succinimide-treated patients seem not to have been studied as yet.

In the same paper Reynolds has reviewed other biochemical data which seem to support the concept of antagonism. Most of these are based on the effects of some substances (AEDs, phenothiazines, folic acid, methionine, and methionine-sulfoximine) which seem to alleviate psychotic symptoms and induce seizures, or vice versa. A similar situation seems to exist with dopamine agonists and antagonists (38) (see Chapter 6).

The possible influence of pharmacological and toxicological factors is probably limited to certain patient groups, which is obvious because alternative syndromes do not necessarily require any pharmacological influences. They had been known long before the introduction of active AEDs (35,39,40), and Landolt's first observation (1) of PN involved spontaneously alternating behavior.

Biochemical hypotheses will have to allow for slow developments as well as sudden drastic changes, both with a possibility of full reversal. Because these hypotheses tend to turn into transmitter hypotheses, they will perhaps converge with the neurophysiological hypotheses discussed below.

3. If an epileptic aura is not terminated by a convulsive seizure, it may go on for a considerable time as an "epileptic equivalent" which may present as paranoid psychosis (41). This hypothesis assumes that alternative psychosis (AP) occurs only when GTC seizures are suppressed, and it does only apply for focal seizures. Both assumptions have subsequently been disproved. Still, in the case of focal discharge, this hypothesis is reassumed in the observation of Wieser (12) that the aspect of the scalp EEG in PN may be similar to the desynchronization which can be seen during local critical discharge in the allocortex so that a "bioelectrically strictly confined limbic status epilepticus" could be at the bottom of PN. Positive confirmation of this hypothesis by investigations of patients in PN is, however, missing and will not easily be obtainable.

4. The fact that the patient does not become asymptomatic at cessation of seizures and EEG discharges strongly suggests that the generator of epileptic discharge is still active and that only the usual pathways of propagation are blocked. It can be assumed that the discharge spreads along different pathways and that this spread causes the psychotic symptoms (42). This hypothesis can of course be, and has been refined by, the assumption of kindling processes.

Both hypotheses 3 and 4 propose that AP is a special variant of ictal psychosis similar to continuous aura (43), with strictly subcortical discharge. The difference is that hypothesis 3 suggests only a prolongation of the habitual discharge but that hypothesis 4 suggests, in addition, a spread along unusual pathways. It has been suggested that this altered spread comprises parts of the limbic as well as the ascending reticular system (24). Hypothesis 4 is more probable because although some symptoms of AP may be recognizable derivatives of seizure symptoms, the great majority are not. The weakness of both hypotheses is that no cases have been reported in which a psychosis developed in a clearly recognizable stepwise manner out of a continuous aura or simple partial status. Thus the hypothesis of AP caused by focal status activity has a missing link.

5. AEDs influence only the seizures but not the underlying metabolic disturbances. These are usually critically readjusted by the seizure. If no seizure occurs, the metabolic disorder increases and produces a psychosis (44). The dated theory of epilepsy which forms the basis of this hypothesis is out of fashion, but not necessarily forever; for example, it could be turned into a neuroendocrinological theory. The observation that AP sometimes is terminated by a GTC seizure is in favor of this hypothesis.

6. PN is due to the reaction of the healthy parts of the brain against the epileptic focus. For unknown reasons, this reaction is, in the case of PN, excessive and thus becomes pathogenic. This is approximately the statement of Landolt (45) in the paper where he is most specific about his theories of PN.

7. Improved seizure control and EEG normalization are due to activation of the wake system of the reticular formation, which, if

excessive, may produce a psychosis (46). This was the spontaneous reaction of Hess to hypothesis 6.

8. The reticular formation is inhibited by hippocampal structures. A temporarily decreased hippocampal activity (by exhaustion after a status epilepticus, or due to pharmacological action) may increase reticular activity through disinhibition (47). This further embellishment of hypotheses 6 and 7 is attractive because it proposes a mechanism which could be active in epilepsy-related psychoses of different pathogeneses. Its weaknesses are that postictal psychoses after status epilepticus do not suggest hypervigilant states and that it is confined to TLE.

9. In another attempt to expand on the ideas of Landolt (45) and Hess (46), we have discussed the possible role of sleep withdrawal in the pathogenesis of AP (31).

Hypotheses 7 to 9 are closely related through the possible role attributed to increased arousal which would be a nonspecific factor in epileptic psychoses. Apart from the fact that increased arousal can have many causes and that we look for processes with variable possible causes, there is another argument in favor of this line of thought: AP is phenomenologically very similar to amphetamine psychosis, which is due to excessive arousal (33,48–50).

10. Another response to Landolt's theories was the proposal of Christian (51) that the falsely normal aspect of the EEG resulted from the interaction between an increased epileptic activity and its equally increased inhibition. The electrobiological homeostasis was renewed on an increased level of tension. This increased tension would be responsible for the psychosis. The new aspect of this hypothesis was that it introduced considerations on the energetic background of AP, because the "tension" in this theory is an energetic concept resulting from the assumption of increased levels of both excitation and inhibition. A similar concept is proposed by Meldrum (see Chapter 2, *this volume*). Probably, Christian came to think along these lines because the psychosis of his patient was heralded by a severe grand mal seizure after a long period with only nonconvulsive seizures and also because observations of this kind, which are by no means uncommon in PN,

clearly indicate that PN is something quite different from true normalization.

11. The patient described by Christian (51) gave rise to a quite different, anthropological hypothesis which is distant from neurophysiological thinking but nonetheless fascinating. According to Bilz (52), the abnormal EEG of patients with epilepsy in a state of psychic equilibrium indicates a phylogenetic immaturity of the nervous system, an "archaic" state not adapted to our contemporary environment. The psychosis resulting from compulsory normalization of the EEG activity constitutes an environment of "archaic savagery" which corresponds to the state of maturity of the nervous system. Whereas Christian (51) stressed the formal aspect of energy, Bilz (52) addressed an interesting formal aspect of the psychotic contents which is usually considered from the psychodynamic–biographic aspect only. Here, an archaic experience inventory is assumed which is latently present in the brain of modern man, where it may be activated in certain conditions, and perhaps more easily in the presumably immature brain of persons with epilepsy.

CONCLUSION

The hypotheses on PN and AP which have just been reviewed are not necessarily mutually exclusive but may be combined into an attempt at a comprehensive hypothesis. This would basically assume that in PN the epilepsy is still active through subcortical, restricted neuronal discharge or through pathological metabolic or transmitter activity. At the same time, powerful inhibitory processes seem to be active. If the GTC seizure is taken, in the traditional sense, as the prototype of a "complete," unrestricted, or insufficiently inhibited seizure, a history of less completely developed seizures (both simple and complex partial as well as nonconvulsive generalized seizures) would indicate that, in a given case, the brain possesses efficient inhibitory mechanisms which are able to prevent a more extensive ictal development. The finding that [in keeping with our earlier observations (53)] a history of partial or of nonconvulsive generalized seizures is one of two prerequisites of epilepsy psychosis (26) is therefore strongly in favor of this argument.

The epileptic activity, apart from providing energy, may contribute some direct symptoms such as abnormal emotions or hallucinations. Novel symptoms produced by epileptic discharge are also possible because of its presumed altered spread or an altered interplay of excitation and inhibition. Massive inhibition of the epileptic activity by specific drugs (such as the succinimides) or by an increased arousal level, or by both, result in insomnia and, perhaps, a hypervigilant state. This results in a critical clinical symptomatology characterized most often by a peculiar dysphoric state. A risk of psychosis is impending, but its manifestation still depends on several factors, including general risk factors of psychosis, genetic background, premorbid personality, and psychotic or related experiences of whatever etiology in the past, social competence, present life situation, and so on.

It may well be that the second prerequisite of psychosis in epilepsy, a history including ictal impairment of consciousness (26,53), is one of these factors. I am not very much inclined to believe that this is a factor of value in terms of neurophysiological implications, since it does not seem to contribute to the understanding of AP and PN, which are defined by restriction and not by expansion of epileptic activity. I am rather inclined to consider this as a biographic factor which has to do with the complete loss of control experienced in seizures when consciousness is lost or gravely impaired. A person suffering from seizures with abnormal sensations or movements but with preserved consciousness learns that funny things may happen with one's own body. In the course of time, the patient will become familiar with these experiences even if they remain disturbing or even uncanny. A person who repeatedly suffers seizures with loss of consciousness acquires the much more threatening experience that anything in life, even the most dangerous, can happen at any time. Such an experience challenges the notion of reliability of the natural matter of course ("natürliche Selbstverständlichkeit"), the loss of which has been found to be a central experience early in the development of schizophrenic psychoses (54).

It is suggested that in PN there is ongoing epileptic activity just as in other psychotic conditions in epilepsy. The differences seem not to be fundamental but gradual. It could be that ictal psychosis is characterized by a direct expression of epileptic activity, whereas in postictal psychosis a momentum of exhaustion is added; moreover, in PN the prevailing pathogenic factor is increased arousal or an abnormally high level of balance between excitatory and inhibitory processes.

SUMMARY

Paradoxical or "forced" normalization of the EEG of patients with epilepsy was first described by Landolt in 1953. It refers to conditions where disappearance of epileptiform discharge from the routine scalp EEG is accompanied by some kind of behavioral disorder. The best known of these is a paranoid psychotic state in clear consciousness, which is also known as "alternative" psychosis. Thus, the issue is related to much older observations which indicated a "biological antagonism" between productive psychotic symptomatology and epileptic seizures, which led to the therapy of psychoses with artificially induced convulsions. Apart from psychotic episodes, the clinical manifestations of PN comprise dysphoric states, hysterical and hypochondriacal syndromes, affective disorders, and miscellanea.

PN can be observed in both generalized and localization-related epilepsies as a rare complication. A subset where it is more frequently seen are in adults with persistent absence seizures when the latter become finally controlled by succinimide therapy. These seem to be the drugs with the highest hazard of precipitation of PN, but all other AEDs have also been suspected. Sleep disturbance by succinimide treatment may play a crucial role, but a variety of other factors are also involved, including psychosocial factors.

The pathogenesis of this condition has given rise to some debate but remains still unresolved. Eleven of the most important hypotheses have been discussed and seem to converge into a more comprehensive hypothesis which basically assumes that, during PN, the epilepsy is still active subcortically, perhaps with spread of discharge along unusual pathways. This activity is supposed to provide energy and, possibly, some of the symptoms included in the psychotic syndrome. A critical clinical condition results, usually with a dysphoric symptomatology, where a development towards psychosis is impending but still depends on the presence or absence of a variety of risk factors. Along with neurophysiological factors such as powerful inhibition of the spread of epileptic discharge, these may also include biographic factors such as the repeated experience of ictal sudden, unexpected loss of consciousness.

Because during PN there presumably is ongoing epileptic activity, the differences with respect to other psychotic conditions in epilepsy are probably subtle rather than fundamental. Thus, it could be that ictal psychosis is characterized by a direct expression of epileptic activity, whereas in postictal psychosis a momentum of exhaustion may be added; moreover, in PN the prevailing pathogenic factor could be an abnormally high level of balance between excitatory and inhibitory processes.

ACKNOWLEDGMENT

Dr. Ute-Ulrike Röder-Wanner (Berlin) was kind enough to provide the data in Table 1 which form part of a paper in preparation.

REFERENCES

1. Landolt H. Some clinical electroencephalographical correlations in epileptic psychoses (twilight states). *Electroencephalogr Clin Neurophysiol* 1953;5:121.
2. Landolt H. Serial electroencephalographic investigations during psychotic episodes in epileptic patients and during schizophrenic attacks. In: Lorentz de Haas AM, ed. *Lectures on epilepsy.* Amsterdam: Elsevier, 1958;91–133.
3. Wolf P, Trimble MR. Biological antagonism and epileptic psychosis. *Br J Psychiatry* 1985;146: 272–276.
4. Pakalnis A, Drake ME, John K, Kellum JB. Forced normalization. Acute psychosis after seizure control in 7 patients. *Arch Neurol* 1987; 44:289–292.
5. Schiffer RB. Epilepsy, psychosis and forced normalization. *Arch Neurol* 1987;44:253.
6. Vaillancourt PD. Forced normalization. *Arch Neurol* 1988;45:138.
7. Pakalnis A, Drake ME, John K, Kellum JB. In Reply. *Arch Neurol* 1988;45:138–139.
8. Commission on Classification and Terminology of the ILAE. Proposal for revised classification of epilepsies and epileptic syndromes. *Epilepsia* 1989;30:389–399.
9. Wolf P. Psicopatologia dell'epilessia: aspetti generali e problemi farmacologici. *Boll Lega Ital Epil* 1981;21–28.
10. Hajnšek F, Faber B. Erfahrungen mit Propanidid bei der Provokation im EEG. *Z EEG-EMG* 1975;6:88–91.
11. Hajnšek F, Faber B. Further experience with Epontol in EEG activation. *Electroencephalogr Clin Neurophysiol* 1973;34:771–772.
12. Wieser HG. 'Psychische Anfälle' und deren stereo-electroenzephalographisches Korrelat. *Z EEG-EMG* 1979;10:197–206.
13. Tellenbach H. Epilepsie als Anfallsleiden und als Psychose. Über alternative Psychosen paranoider Prägung bei 'forcierter Normalisierung' (Landolt) des Elektroenzephalogramms Epileptischer. *Nervenarzt* 1965;36:190–202.
14. Glaus A. Über Kombinationen von Schizophrenie und Epilepsie. *Z Gesamte Neurol Psychiatry* 1931;135:450–500.
15. Wyrsch J. Über Schizophrenie bei Epileptikern. *Schweiz Arch Neurol Psychiatr* 1933;31:113–132.
16. Meduna L von. Versuche über die biologische Beeinflussung des Ablaufs der Schizophrenie. I. Campher- und Cardiazolkrämpfe. *Z Gesamte Neurol Psychiatr* 1935;152:235–262.
17. Landolt H. Die Dämmer- und Verstimmungszustände bei Epilepsie und ihre Elektroenzephalographie. *J Neurol* 1963;185:411–430.
18. Wolf P. The clinical syndromes of forced normalization. *Jpn J Psychiatry Neurol* 1984;38: 187–192.
19. Wolf P. The prevention of alternative psychosis in outpatients. In: Janz D, ed. *Epileptology.* Stuttgart: Thieme, 1976;75–79.
20. Guirao Bringas IP, Behl I, Wolf P. Epileptic discharge after eye closure: relation to epileptic syndromes. In: Wolf P, Dam M, Janz D, Dreifuss FE, eds. *Advances in epileptology,* vol 16. New York: Raven Press, 1987;255–258.
21. Small JG, Milstein V, Stevens JR. Are psychomotor epileptics different? *Arch Neurol* 1962;7: 187–194.
22. Small JB, Small JF, Hayden MP. Further psychiatric investigations of patients with temporal and nontemporal lobe epilepsy. *Am J Psychiatry* 1966;123:303–310.
23. Stevens JR. Psychiatric implications of psychomotor epilepsy. *Arch Gen Psychiatry* 1966;14: 461–471.
24. Bruens JF. Zur Frage der kausalen Beziehung zwischen Psychose und Epilepsie. In: Penin H, ed. *Psychische Störungen bei Epilepsie.* Stuttgart: Schattauer, 1973;67–74.
25. Roger J, Grangeon H, Guey J, Lob H. Incidences psychiatriques et psychologiques du traitement par l'éthosuccinimide chez les épileptiques. *Encéphale* 1968;57:407–438.
26. Schmitz B. *Psychosen bei Epilepsie. Eine epidemiologische Untersuchung.* PhD thesis, West Berlin, 1988.
27. Commission on Classification and Terminology

of the ILAE. Proposal for revised clinical and electroencephalographic classification of epileptic seizures. *Epilepsia* 1981;22:489–501.

28. Wolf P, Inoue Y, Röder-Wanner UU, Tsai JJ. Psychiatric complications of absence therapy and their relation to alteration of sleep. *Epilepsia* 1984;25:S56–S59.

29. Wolf P. The role of antiepileptic drugs in epileptic psychosis. In: Majkowski J, ed. *Posttraumatic epilepsy—pharmacological prophylaxis.* Warsaw: Polish Chapter ILAE, 1977;248–255.

30. Röder UU, Wolf P. Effects of treatment with dipropylacetate and ethosuximide on sleep organization in epileptic patients. In: Dam M, Gram L, Penry JK, eds. *Advances in epileptology,* vol 12. New York: Raven Press, 1981;145–157.

31. Wolf P. Forced normalization. In: Trimble MR, Bolwig TG, eds. *Aspects of epilepsy and psychiatry.* London: Wiley, 1986;101–112.

32. Wolf P. Zur Kritik des Begriffs schizophrenie-ähnliche Psycose bei Epilepsie. In: Wolf P, Köhler GK, eds. *Psychopathologische and pathogenetische Probleme bei Epilepsie.* Bern: Huber, 1980:77–83.

33. Wolf P. *Psychosen bei Epilepsie.* PhD thesis, West Berlin, 1976.

34. Wolf P, Thorbecke R, Even W. Social aspects of psychosis in patients with epilepsy. In: Whitman ST, Hermann BP, eds. *Psychopathology in epilepsy: social factors.* New York: Oxford University Press, 1986;269–283.

35. Esquirol JED. *Esquirol's allgemeine und specielle Pathologie und Therapie der Seelenstörungen.* Frei bearbeitet von K. C. Hille. Leipzig: Hartmann, 1827.

36. Ferguson SM, Rayport M. The adjustment to living without epilepsy. *J Nerv Ment Dis* 1965; 140:26–37.

37. Reynolds EH. Biological factors in psychological disorders associated with epilepsy. In: Reynolds EH, Trimble MR, eds. *Epilepsy and psychiatry.* Edinburgh: Churchill Livingstone, 1981; 264–290.

38. Trimble MR, Meldrum BS. Monoamines, epilepsy and schizophrenia. In: Obiols J, Ballus E, Gonzales M, Pujol J, eds. *Biological psychiatry today.* Amsterdam: Elsevier, 1979;470–475.

39. Flemming CF. *Pathologie und Therapie der Psychosen.* Berlin: Hirschwald, 1859.

40. Hoffmann H. *Beobachtungen und Erfahrungen über Seelenstörungen und Epilepsie.* Frankfurt: Rütten, 1859.

41. Korzeniowski L. Les problèmes diagnostiques concernant les psychoses paranioiaques schizophreniformes en épilepsie. *Ann Med Psychol (Paris)* 1965;123/I:35–42.

42. Wolf P. Zur Pathophysiologie epileptischer Psychosen. In: Penin H, ed. *Psychische Störungen bei Epilepsie.* Stuttgart: Schattauer, 1973;51–65.

43. Scott JG, Masland RL. Occurrence of continuous symptoms in epilepsy patients. *Neurology* 1953;3:297–301.

44. Ditfurth H von. Zur Problematik der modernen Epilepsiebehandlung, zugleich ein kasuistischer Beitrag zur Frage der sog. Epilepsiepsychosen. *Nervenarzt* 1953;24:348–349.

45. Landolt H. Über Verstimmungen, Dämmerzustände und schizophrene Zustands-bilder bei Epilepsie. *Schweiz Arch Neurol Psychiatr* 1955; 76:313–321.

46. Hess R. Diskussionsbemerkung. *Schweiz Arch Neurol Psychiatr* 1955;76:102–107.

47. Karbowski K. Status psychomotoricus. Klinische und elektroenzephalographische Aspekte. In: Karbowski K, ed. *Status psychomotoricus und seine Differential-diagnose.* Bern: Huber, 1980;39–72.

48. Zutt J. Über die polare Struktur des Bewußtseins. Durch psychiatrische Erfahrungen mit Pervitin angeregte Gedanken. *Nervenarzt* 1943; 16:145–162.

49. Ellinwood EH. Amphetamine psychosis. *J Nerv Ment Dis* 1967;144:273–283.

50. Griffith JD, Cavanaugh J, Held J, Oates JA. Dextroamphetamine. Evaluation of psychomimetic properties in man. *Arch Gen Psychiatry* 1972;26:97–100.

51. Christian W. EEG-Befund bei einem Fall von epileptischer Halluzinose. *J Neurol* 1957;176: 693–700.

52. Bilz R. *Paläanthropologie.* Frankfurt: Suhrkamp, 1971.

53. Wolf P. Psychic disorders in epilepsy. In: Canger R, Angeleri F, Penry JK, eds. *Advances in epileptology,* vol 11. New York: Raven Press, 1980;159–160.

54. Blankenburg W. *Der Verlust der natürlichen Selbstverständlichkeit. Ein Beitrag zur Psychopathologie symptomarmer Schizophrenien.* Stuttgart: Enke, 1971.

Advances in Neurology, Vol. 55, edited by
D. Smith, D. Treiman, and M. Trimble,
Raven Press, Ltd., New York © 1991.

9

Interictal Psychoses of Epilepsy

Michael R. Trimble

*Department of Psychological Medicine, The National Hospital for Neurology, London WC1N
3BG, England*

Although associations between psychiatric illness and epilepsy may be found in some of the earliest medical writings, it was the continental authors of the 19th century who made the first substantial contributions (1). Morel (2) and Falret (3) both drew attention to the mental state of patients between seizures. Falret (3) recognized peri-ictal psychiatric disorders (namely, those associated in time with the seizure) and those that were interparoxysmal. He also acknowledged that there was a group of patients who entered a prolonged delirium, the so-called "folie epileptique" (epileptic insanity proper).

British views at this time were found to vary. Investigators such as Reynolds (4) were unable to accept that there was any special mental state related to epilepsy, whereas Jackson (5) recognized epilepsy as a cause of insanity in 6% of cases, identifying in his writings mainly the ictal variety. In seeking explanation for a link, Clouston (6) suggested that the area of brain which when disturbed leads to epilepsy might also be responsible for the abnormal mental state. Turner (7) reported on paroxysmal psychoses which either preceded, succeeded, or replaced convulsive episodes and which could include hallucinatory, delusional, maniacal, melancholic, or psychasthenic states. He also noted that a number of patients with epilepsy passed eventually into a state of continued delusional insanity requiring asylum treatment.

One consequence of the contributions was that "Epileptic Insanity" held a separate place in the majority of classifications of insanity that were put forward at that time, as

distinctive, for example, as "General Paralysis of the Insane." Although this was, in part, linked with ideas of hereditary degeneration which were prevalent in neurological and psychiatric circles towards the end of the last century, it also reflected the bias of referral populations that these various investigators examined. The psychiatrists, especially the alienists, saw institutionalized patients and thus were more inclined to comment on the longer-term alteration of the mental state in patients with intractable seizures, whereas others, such as Jackson (5), dealt more with the acute paroxysms as were seen on a neurological inpatient ward.

In the early part of this century, the relationship between epilepsy and psychosis attracted little attention, and indeed the pendulum swung to suggest that, if anything, epilepsy and psychosis were less often found together than would occur by chance (8) such that an antagonism between the two conditions was suggested.

It was the increasing use of the electroencephalogram (EEG), along with the identification of temporal lobe epilepsy, which led to a recrudescence of the idea that psychiatric disorders were more common in patients with epilepsy, but this time the association was more with focal temporal lobe epilepsy (9). Other investigators commented on a chronic paranoid hallucinatory state in epilepsy, referring to it as a definitive entity and suggesting that patients with this condition usually had temporal lobe epilepsy with typical complex auras (10). The psychotic episodes began several years after the onset of the seizures, and they often occurred in the setting of a diminishing seizure frequency, with similar findings being reported by Hill (11) and Slater and Beard (12). The latter investigators were most influential with their report on 69 patients with epileptic psychosis, who they referred to as being "schizophrenia-like." They also commented that the psychoses tended to develop a number of years after the seizure disorder had started, and that the majority of patients had temporal lobe abnormalities and were diagnosed as having temporal lobe epilepsy. They were referred to as "schizophrenia-like" because many of them had classical first-rank symptoms of Schneider, but differences between this epileptic psychosis and a process of schizophrenia were acknowledged. These included the maintenance of a warm affect, the presentation often with intense affective symptoms, and the absence of any clearly defined premorbid personality style such as the schizoid personality. They further emphasized the lack of genetic predisposition to schizophrenia.

CLASSIFICATION

A simple classification of the relationship between seizures and psychoses is shown in Table 1. It acknowledges the earlier division into ictal and interictal states, and it distinguishes between episodic and chronic forms of the condition. It is arguably overinclusive, and many psycho-organic episodes and con-

fusional states do not present with typical psychotic symptoms. Peri-ictal disturbances are clearly related to abnormal electrical activity in the brain and can be seen on the EEG if it is recorded at the time of the behavior disturbance—in contrast to the interictal disturbances, which are seen between seizures and not clearly interlinked with an observed acute neurophysiological disturbance. However, this does not mean that abnormal electrical activity is not ongoing somewhere in the central nervous system, which is directly linked to the psychotic picture (see below).

The most frequent peri-ictal disturbance is an acute organic brain syndrome which occurs shortly after partial or generalized seizures. In these cases, patients in a state of confusion may appear psychotic and sometimes report hallucinations or delusions. A patient may wander in a confused fashion, but he or she is rarely aggressive unless inappropriately handled. In some cases, particularly following several bouts of seizures, a prolonged organic psychosyndrome can ensue which goes on for hours of occasionally days. Certainly, if during a seizure, anoxic brain damage or severe head injury has occurred, then a prolonged psychosis may rarely emerge which again reflects the organic brain syndrome and for which further investigation is mandatory.

Complex partial and absence seizures may present as a form of status epilepticus. While rare, these probably occur more frequently than suspected, and appropriate EEG moni-

TABLE 1. *Suggested outline of the psychoses associated with epilepsy*

		Disturbance of consciousness	EEG; most common disturbances
Episodic:	Postictal automatism	+	Slow waves
	Petit mal status	+	Three-per-second spike-and-wave
	Complex partial seizure status	+	Continuous temporal lobe abnormality
	Confusional states	+	Generalized abnormality
	Psycho-organic episodes	+	Very abnormal EEG with slow dysrhythmia
	Forced normalization states	−	Normal
Chronic:	Paranoid states	−	Temporal lobe abnormalities
	Schizophrenic-like states	−	Temporal lobe abnormalities (left side)
	Manic–depressive states	−	Temporal lobe abnormalities (?)

toring at the time of the disturbance is mandatory to make the diagnosis. In both, consciousness is clouded and the patient shows overt confusion and difficulty in manipulating cognitive tasks which may, however, particularly with complex partial seizure status, be subtle. Such episodes can continue for many days, and the patient may present with a variety of psychopathological phenomena, including hallucinations, delusions, and affective symptoms. The absence status is less likely to be associated with clearly defined psychotic manifestations than is temporal lobe status, with the patient often appearing in a prolonged twilight state with fluctuating levels of arousal and periodic bursts of rapid eyeblinks or myoclonic jerks. However, hallucinations are sometimes reported as part of the clinical picture.

In contrast, interictal psychoses occur between seizures and cannot directly be linked to the ictus. However, clinically there are some patients who develop a psychosis following an increase in seizure frequency and who, when their seizures resolve, continue to display psychotic symptoms for a prolonged period of time. In one variety, patients usually, after a bout of seizures, have a lucid interval of some 24–48 hr and then switch into a psychotic state of overactivity, elation and dysphoria, delusions, illusions, and hallucinations, often with a marked aggressive or religious content. Clouding of consciousness may be seen if the appropriate clinical testing is carried out and the EEG is abnormal. This condition may last days or even weeks, slowly resolving into a chronic, often well-encapsulated psychotic state or gradually dissipating. This clinical picture emphasizes the close relationship between the peri-ictal disturbances and interictal states as commented on by Ferguson and Rayport (13). Thus, in these patients it is difficult in the later stages of the psychosis to be certain that the psychotic phenomena, which may not be accompanied by surface EEG abnormalities, are not related to continuing electrophysiological disturbances in deep structures. Certainly the evidence is strong that many patients with psychosis and *no* epilepsy may show spike-and-wave disturbances in various regions of the limbic system when they have electrodes

implanted in these areas (14). In addition, psychotic symptoms can be provoked by stimulation of limbic system structures in experimental circumstances.

Clinically, the interictal disturbances are seen as chronic psychotic states with a fairly typical psychiatric picture. Manic–depressive psychoses, presenting with fluctuating states of overactivity, flight of ideas, and pressure of speech in which the patient is euphoric, irritable, and aggressive, are seen, but sudden mood swings are not uncommon, and often, on close questioning, patients describe a dysphoria rather than a euphoria. True cyclical manic–depressive illness seems rare, although depressive illness with a psychotic, especially paranoid flavoring is common. These latter patients demonstrate a classical paranoid state with vigilance, overt hostility, and suspiciousness with over sensitiveness towards their environment. Delusions may occur which have a persecutory content, and in chronic states patients may accumulate vast amounts of documentary information supporting their contentions and grievances. The schizophreniform psychoses have the form of a schizophrenic illness, although some differences have been already noted and were reported by Slater and Beard (12). Persecutory and religious delusions are often reported, although hebephrenic deterioration and catatonic phenomena are rare. The long history of religiosity in association with epilepsy was reviewed by Dewhurst and Beard (15), who presented a number of cases of their own, all of which were diagnosed as having temporal lobe epilepsy.

One study has recently used intensive monitoring in a group of seizure patients with psychotic episodes. Ramani and Gumnit (16) monitored 10 patients with video telemetry. Sixty-five percent of their group had complex partial seizures. Twenty-six percent of those had secondary generalized seizures. The patients all had long-standing epilepsy (average duration 17.9 years), and their psychosis had been present for a mean of 12.3 years. Nine patients were diagnosed as having a schizophrenia-like presentation, and in no patient did the episode of psychosis last longer than about 3 weeks. One patient showed a striking reduction of the spikes on EEG during the psychotic phase; two others showed a tendency towards aggravation of psychosis, with a reduction of seizure frequency brought about by prescription of anticonvulsants. In all patients, interictal paroxsymal abnormalities were reported. Eight had bilateral or generalized discharges. This comprehensive study of peri-ictal psychosis confirms that schizophrenia-like states can occur in association with epilepsy, and that a reciprocal link between the seizures and psychotic symptoms occurs in some cases.

THE ANTAGONISM BETWEEN EPILEPSY AND PSYCHOSIS

Thus, closely allied to the ictally related psychoses, but interictal in nature and often of brief duration and paroxysmal in presentation, are short-lived psychotic bouts in which there is some form of antagonism between either seizure frequency or abnormal EEG discharges and the psychotic symptoms. Landolt (17) recorded changes in the EEG during pre-seizure dysphoric episodes and limited periods of overt psychosis lasting days or weeks. During these he noted improvement in previously abnormal EEGs and referred to this phenomenon as "forced normalization." At the end of the psychotic episodes the EEGs again were abnormal. In the extensive collection reported by Dongier (18), EEG data on 536 psychotic episodes that occurred in 516 patients were reported. EEG abnormalities disappeared during the psychosis in 78 cases, and in 53% of these there was no obvious clouding of consciousness. Delusions were particularly frequent in patients in whom a preexisting focal discharge disappeared, and in these patients the episode lasted a particularly long time, sometimes several weeks. Both Landolt (17) and Dongier (18) suggested that paranoid and schizophreniform states were more likely to be seen following the suppression of focal (particularly temporal focal), as opposed to generalized, discharges.

The theme has been taken up more recently by Wolf and Trimble (19,20). It has been pointed out that the term "forced normalization" was poorly translated into English, implying in that language some form of active force, which in German was not the intention;

for Landolt it was purely descriptive. Although Landolt initially concentrated on partial seizures, in his later writing he also recognized forced normalization to occur with generalized attacks, particularly following the introduction of the succinimide drugs. These observations are supported by the studies of Wolf (19). In addition, Wolf points out that forced normalization may result in a number of differing clinical patterns that are not necessarily psychotic. He includes such phenomena as pre-psychotic dysphoria, which may herald a psychotic state, but he also includes hypochondriacal states, episodes of hysterical symptomatology, depressive states, manic states, and twilight states.

The term "alternative psychosis" was introduced by Tellenbach (21) to provide a shortened term which paid more attention to the presence or absence of seizures than to EEG phenomena. It implied that in some cases the control of seizures did not mean cure of the clinical problem or even inactivity of any underlying disease process, and that psychoses may flower as a result.

THE AFFINITY BETWEEN EPILEPSY AND PSYCHOSIS

Prevalence

There are few careful epidemiological studies of psychopathology in patients with epilepsy, and therefore estimating the incidence of psychosis is difficult. In Pond and Bidwell's study (22) nearly 30% of their patients had "psychological difficultes," with 7% having been in a psychiatric hospital before or during the survey year. A temporal lobe group had a higher rate of hospitalization to psychiatric hospitals and a higher rate of severe personality change and psychosis. Gudmundsson (23), in a survey of the population of Iceland, was able to compare the prevalence rates for psychiatric illness in epilepsy with those without epilepsy. In the epilepsy population some 8% were psychotic, again being greater in his temporal lobe sample. In a similar extensive survey, Zielinski (24) provided further data on nonselected patients with epilepsy from a population in Poland. Fifty-eight percent showed some "mental abnormality," and approximately 3% had psychotic symptoms. In that survey, psychopathology was overrepresented in those with temporal lobe epilepsy and secondary generalization.

In spite of these data, a number of investigators still question whether psychosis is more likely to occur in epilepsy than, for example, in other chronic disorders, and they also question whether there is a link to temporal lobe epilepsy. An important investigation was carried out by Hermann and Whitman (25). As part of a review of the literature on epilepsy and behavior, they examined (by means of meta-analysis) psychopathology as rated by the Minnesota Multiphasic Personality Inventory (MMPI) in a large number of patients with epilepsy using chronic non-neurological or neurological disorders as controls, taken from published findings in the literature. When they examined those patients with psychopathology, the epilepsy group showed a significantly higher rate of psychosis than did the neurological controls, who in turn showed a higher rate than did the chronically medically ill controls. They thus suggested that if a special type of psychopathology was manifest in patients with epilepsy, there was a higher probability that this was a psychotic disorder.

In summary, there does appear to be evidence that patients with epilepsy may be more prone to the development of psychosis, stemming from several different investigations. Some investigators suggest either (a) an overrepresentation of temporal lobe epilepsy or (b) temporal lobe epilepsy where the seizures secondarily generalize.

Risk Factors

It is obvious that most patients with temporal lobe epilepsy do not develop psychosis, and therefore attempts to clarify those who may be more at risk have been carried out. Hermann and Whitman (25) have listed some of these as determined from the literature. They include (a) a past history along with present findings suggestive of organicity, (b) being left-handed or ambidextrous, (c) having automatisms or secondary generalized seizures, (d) having a lower frequency of complex partial seizures, (e) showing focal spike

activity in medial as opposed to lateral temporal cortical recording leads, and (f) showing more independent spike foci and a higher frequency of maximal spike foci at such leads and bilateral mesiobasally located spike abnormalities. They also note poorer social adaptation and more psychosexually disturbed relationships.

Hermann et al. (26), again using the MMPI, made a significant contribution when comparing patients with temporal lobe epilepsy with those with generalized epilepsy by separating out a temporal lobe group that had an aura of fear, in contrast to those who had different auras. The fear group displayed pathological elevations on several MMPI scales, especially for schizophrenia. Since ictal fear results from activity of the medial temporal lobes, especially the amygdala and hippocampus (27), these data reinforce suggestions that medial temporal lesions (i.e., those with more clearly identified limbic system lesions) may be more associated with the likelihood of development of psychosis.

Another important factor which seems to be emerging is the relationship not between temporal lobe epilepsy per se and psychosis, but between complex partial seizures that secondarily generalize and psychopathology, suggesting either (a) a more widespread epileptic disturbance or (b) a greater propensity for seizures to generalize through limbic system structures. This has emerged from several studies, including (a) that of Rodin et al. (28), who noted that most mental disturbances in temporal lobe epilepsy occurred in those that had more than one seizure type, and (b) that of Bruens (29), who noted that the highest incidence of psychosis was in patients who had a temporal lobe EEG focus and bilateral spike-and-wave activity and who were suffering from both psychomotor and generalized seizures.

The studies of Taylor (30) identified the possible importance of (a) "alien tissue lesions" in temporal lobe structures and (b) age of onset of seizures after the age of 10. This latter factor has been examined in more detail by Hermann et al. (31), who examined MMPI scales in patients with epilepsy in relationship to age of onset and type of seizures. An adolescent onset with temporal lobe epilepsy was associated with the highest scores on the schizophrenia scale. In general, a group with generalized epilepsy of adolescent onset scored lower on most of the scales than did the group with temporal lobe epilepsy, suggesting an age–seizure-type interaction.

Phenomenology

A criticism of much of the work in this field is that the term "psychosis" has been used without definition by most investigators and that little attempt has been made to specify the precise phenomenology of the patients who are examined. It is noteworthy that the British investigators who have written on this subject tend to use the concepts of Kurt Schneider for the diagnosis of a schizophrenia-like illness, relying in particular on the presence of first-rank symptomatology. The importance of being precise is emphasized by more recent techniques that have used standardized and validated methods for quantifying psychopathology in the psychoses of epilepsy (32).

Using such methodology, it has been possible to compare as objectively as possible the presentation of psychosis in epilepsy with process schizophrenia, in the absence of epilepsy. In the first report of this kind, Perez and Trimble (32), using the Present State Examination (PSE) of Wing, presented data on 24 patients with epilepsy and psychosis prospectively referred. The psychosis occurred in the setting of clear consciousness, and it was present for at least a month. This technique, which allowed for diagnosis of the psychosis to be made by the Catego computer program, gave a PSE syndrome profile for the group with epilepsy which was compared with non-epileptic schizophrenic controls. In this study, 50% of the patients with epilepsy and psychosis were categorized as having schizophrenic psychosis, with 92% having a profile of nuclear schizophrenia based on the first-rank symptoms of Schneider. The syndrome profile of the patients with schizophrenia and epilepsy, when compared with that of the patients with schizophrenia, showed few significant differences, thereby emphasizing the similarity of the clinical presentation of these two disorders. Toone et al. (33), in a retrospective study also using the PSE, have reported similar findings. These data thus suggest that in a group of patients with psychosis and epilepsy a significant number will have a schizophrenia-like presentation that is very similar to the presenting symptoms of schizophrenia in the absence of epilepsy. However, the differences between the two (notably the preservation of affective warmth and failure of personality deterioration in the majority of schizophrenia-like psychoses of epilepsy), highlighted by Slater and Beard (12), have stood the test of time.

Perez and Trimble (32) further examined in their sample the differences in presentation between psychotic patients with temporal lobe epilepsy and those with generalized epilepsy. All patients who were diagnosed by the Catego as having nuclear schizophrenia had temporal lobe abnormalities on their EEG and received a clinical diagnosis of complex partial seizures. Patients with psychosis and generalized epilepsy had a variety of psychopathological presentations, which included (a) schizophrenia without first-rank symptoms and (b) manic and depressive psychoses. This study was thus a confirmation of the direct link between certain types of epilepsy and certain patterns of clinical presentation, suggested by others dating back to the early reports of Hill (11) and Pond (10).

These recent studies clarify some of the rather obscure issues which have perplexed some nonmedical investigators on the subject of psychosis and epilepsy. Thus, the link between temporal lobe epilepsy and psychosis has provoked considerable argument, almost as vociferous as that which relates to the link between temporal lobe changes and personality disorder, in spite of the fact that, in general, most investigators who have looked at this issue do find an overrepresentation of temporal lobe abnormalities in their psychotic group. It is pointed out that patients with temporal lobe epilepsy tend to be overrepresented in populations presenting to hospitals; furthermore, it is emphasized that nonclinical studies (using, for example, rating scales such as the MMPI), or even some clinical studies, fail to note differences between patients with temporal lobe seizures and those with other types of seizure (25). However, there are exceptions, such as the data from Hermann et al. (26). It appears that a link emerges be-

tween a certain nuclear form of schizophrenia-like illness and temporal lobe epilepsy.
This does not mean that patients with other
forms of epilepsy may not also develop psychosis, although the clinical presentation of it
may well be different. It is unfortunate that in
much of the literature in this field the investigators make accurate attempts to note epileptic variables but show considerable laxity in
precision with regard to psychiatric variables.

LATERALITY

A further important consideration was introduced by Flor-Henry (34). He suggested
that left-sided temporal lobe lesions in particular were associated with a schizophreniform
presentation, contrasting with the right-sided
abnormality linking with a manic–depressive
picture. The hint of this laterality difference is
noted further in the work of Taylor (30), Pritchard et al. (35), and the earlier work of Sherwin (36). In the follow-up study of Ounsted
and Lindsay (37), in which unselected patients earlier diagnosed as having temporal
lobe epilepsy were reassessed 13 years later,
nine patients developed a schizophreniform
psychosis with first-rank symptoms of
Schneider, seven had a left-sided focus, and
two had bilateral discharges. Perez and Trimble (32), using EEG criteria for lateralization
of focus, studied the PSE syndrome profiles
of psychotic temporal lobe epilepsy patients
with left-sided foci and compared them to the
profiles of patients with right-sided lesions. In
their study, eight patients had consistent left-
sided EEG abnormalities, two had bilaterally
independent foci, four had right-sided abnormalities, and two patients had a unilateral focus (one left and one right) in all EEG recordings except their most recent. The left-sided
patients had a significantly higher incidence
of nuclear schizphrenia and ideas of reference
than did the right-sided patients.

Although in these studies the clinical documentation of patients was as precise and objective as possible, it is clear that evaluation
of laterality from surface EEG recordings is
open to criticism. In order to circumvent this
difficulty, Sherwin (38) carried out several
studies of patients who, while awaiting temporal lobe surgery, had the laterality of their

focus established by depth recording of ictal episodes; following temporal lobectomy,
these patients experienced cessation of seizures. Again he was able to conclude that patients with left-sided temporal lobe epileptogenic lesions were at special risk for the
development of the schizophrenia-like psychoses, and that psychosis was a rare complication in patients with other focal (nontemporal) lesions.

Toone et al. (39), in a retrospective study
using the syndrome check list (SCL) derived
from the PSE, have also examined the question of laterality using computerized axial tomography (CAT). Fifty-seven patients with
psychosis and epilepsy were examined, and a
tendency towards an excess of left-sided abnormalities in schizophreniform cases was reported. Unlike the studies using EEG techniques, this difference was not significant,
although hallucinations were seen exclusively
in the patients with bilateral or left-sided lesions.

Taken together, these data would suggest
that a pattern of psychosis, resembling nuclear schizophrenia, does occur more commonly in patients with temporal lobe epilepsy
than in those with other forms of epilepsy;
these data also suggest that this pattern, when
present, is much more likely to be associated
with a left-sided or predominantly left-sided
lesion. Moreover, since the studies using the
EEG have been more convincing in demonstrating this relationship than were those using the CAT scan data, the evolution of the
clinical pattern would seem more likely to be
dependent on functional, as opposed to
strictly structural, abnormalities. Further evidence for this suggestion derives from a second recent study of CAT scan data in patients
with schizophreniform psychoses of epilepsy.
Trimble and co-workers (40) quantitatively
evaluated the CAT scans of 10 patients with
epileptic psychosis and nuclear first-rank
symptoms, 10 patients with non-nuclear psychoses of epilepsy, and eight patients with
schizophrenia who did not have epilepsy. All
these psychotic groups had high values for the
bilateral septum caudate distance, and the
sizes of the third and fourth ventricles when
compared with the expected normal data;
however, no laterality differences were noted
with regard to these indices, nor were they

noted with regard to measures of cortical abnormalities.

Three additional points should be made. The first is that several investigators have failed to detect a relationship between the laterality of focus and presentation of the psychosis (see e.g., refs. 41 and 42), although such investigators have also failed to use precise diagnostic criteria as outlined above. The second is that there is a growing and now extensive literature on laterality in non-epileptic psychiatric patients which points in a similar direction—namely, to abnormalities of left hemisphere function in schizophrenia (43). Finally, the literature on the link between manic–depressive illness and right-sided lesions is less substantial, and to date this second hypothesis emerging from Flor-Henry's data has yet to be confirmed.

MECHANISMS

Further questions may be asked with regard to the mechanism of the development of psychosis. A number of different explanations have been put forward, and the majority take as their starting point the now established relationship between the temporal-lobe–limbic system and affective experiences. There are two main contrasting hypotheses. The first is that the schizophrenia-like illnesses are seizure-related phenomena and should be referred to as "epileptic psychoses." The second is that they are a manifestation of organic neurological damage and are thus not specific for epilepsy. The former view has been most strongly expressed by Flor-Henry (34). Criticizing the absence of a control population in some of the earlier studies, he noted in his series, as reported by others (see, e.g., refs. 10 and 11), an inverse relationship between the frequency of psychomotor seizures and the presence of psychosis in some patients. Support for this suggestion comes from other studies in which depth electrodes have been implanted in psychotic patients who do not have epilepsy. Abnormal electrical activity in the deep temporal structures is shown to be associated with suppression of surface cortical activity; furthermore, when patients display psychotic behavior, abnormal spike-and-wave activity may be detected in these deep areas—notably the septal region, which is not seen with conventional surface electrodes (14).

The alternative position was taken by Slater and Beard (12). They noted that a significant proportion of the psychotic patients had a defined organic basis for their epilepsy, and that the onset of the psychosis seemed to be linked to the duration of the epilepsy. Their conclusion stressed the importance of an underlying structural lesion in the temporal lobe. A similar view was taken by Kristensen and Sindrup (41). Kiloh (44) made the point that almost any diffuse brain disease may occasionally be associated with a similar clinical picture, and epilepsy is often not present. He suggested that psychoses were a reflection of a certain stage of what, in the long run, was a dementing process. Follow-up studies of such patients do not, however, lend support to this view (12).

Bruens (29) put forward the idea that both the organic and the psychodynamic events potentiate each other. The patient is unable to protect himself against the vicissitudes of life except by using pathological defense mechanisms, which result in psychosis. Pond (10) suggested that the abnormal experiences associated with temporal lobe epilepsy which gradually become integrated into a person's psychic life eventually lead to the development of psychosis. However, these explanations do not account for the laterality findings and, as Slater and Beard (12) point out, do not take into account the volitional disturbances, thought disorder, and hebephrenic symptoms noted in some of the patients.

Symonds (45) pointed to the "epileptic disorder of function." He suggested that it was not the loss of neurons in the temporal lobe that was responsible for the psychosis, but the disorderly activity of those that remain. A similar view was stressed by Taylor (30), who stated: "Perhaps it is better, from the point of view of avoiding psychosis, for the [temporal] lobe to be nonfunctional rather than dysfunctional." Another possibility that has been suggested is that of kindling, such that chronic subictal activity leads to a kindling process within dopaminergic pathways, overactivity of which leads to the development of abnormal behavior patterns and psychosis. To date, the evidence from human studies that such mechanisms exist is negligible, and the role of kindling in behavioral changes must remain speculative (46).

Further information on mechanism derives from recent studies of Trimble and co-workers (47) using positron emission tomography (PET) with radioactivity labeled oxygen to measure cerebral blood flow (rCBF) and metabolism (rCMRo$_2$) in humans. These studies confirmed that patients with temporal lobe epilepsy, interictally, had hypometabolic areas in association with the site of the epileptic focus, which were extensive, affecting temporal, frontal, and basal ganglia regions on the side of the focus. Psychotic patients have the more extensive changes on the left side, especially in the temporal regions. Since none of their patients had severe epilepsy (patients mainly experienced infrequent partial seizures), these findings imply that any explanation for the development of interictal psychosis must take into consideration the "down-regulation" of activity in certain brain structures, especially those linked to the basal ganglia and the limbic system.

These changes are not accompanied by major identifiable structural alterations. Using magnetic resonance imaging, Trimble and co-workers (48) have failed to note differences in T_1 relaxation times when epilepsy patients with and without psychosis were compared, with the exception of increased T_1 times in the area of the left temporal white matter in the hallucinatory psychotics.

Finally, the possible role of anticonvulsant drugs should be considered. There has now accumulated considerable evidence that polytherapy, and perhaps certain of the older anticonvulsant compounds such as phenobarbitone and phenytoin, can be interlinked with psychopathology of epilepsy (for review see ref. 49). However, apart from some idiosyncratic reactions, the phenomenon of forced normalization, and the production of an organic brain syndrome with gross toxicity, the link between chronic anticonvulsant drug therapy and the provocation of psychosis has never been substantiated, even by those investigators who have looked at this question (12).

In summary, at the present time the evidence for a functional, as opposed to a structural, change in limbic system struc-

tures—both within the temporal lobes and downstream in forebrain limbic structures—may be the most useful hypothesis to follow with regard to understanding the development of at least some of the psychoses of epilepsy. Alternative mechanisms, including recurrent brain damage with anoxia or head injury, may, along with polytherapy, be responsible for cognitive dulling and the development of a dementia-like picture. In the older texts this was confused with the picture of psychosis, but our thinking and methodologies have progressed considerably since that time. Animal models, particularly the kindling model with accompanied behavior alterations, behavior observed following other temporal lobe lesions in animals and humans, and the EEG abnormalities recorded in association with psychosis in the absence of epilepsy in limbic system structures, also point in this direction.

REFERENCES

1. Berrios GE. Insanity in the 19th century. In: Roth M, Cowie V, eds. *Elliot Slater: a tribute.* London: Gaskel Press, 1979;161–171.
2. Morel BA. *Traité des maladies mentales.* Paris: 1860.
3. Falret J. De l'état mental des épileptiques. *Arch Gen Med* 1860;16:661–679.
4. Reynolds R. *Epilepsy.* London: John Churchill, 1861.
5. Jackson JH. On temporary mental disorders after epileptic paroxysms. In: Taylor J, ed. *Selected writing of John Hughlings Jackson,* vol. 1. London: Staples Press, 1875;119–134.
6. Clouston TS. *Clinical lectures on mental diseases.* London: J & A Churchill, 1887.
7. Turner WA. *Three lectures on epilepsy.* Edinburgh: Mackenzie, 1910.
8. Glaus A. Uber Combination von Schizophrenie und Epilepsie. *Z Dieg Neurol Psychiatr* 1931; 135:450–550.
9. Gibbs FA. Ictal and nonictal psychiatric disorders in temporal lobe epilepsy. *J Ment Dis* 1951;133:522–528.
10. Pond DA. The schizophrenia-like psychosis of epilepsy—discussion. *Proc R Soc Med* 1962;55: 311.
11. Hill D. Psychiatric disorders of epilepsy. *Med Press* 1953;229:473–475.
12. Slater E, Beard AW. The schizophrenia-like psychoses of epilepsy. *Br J Psychiatry* 1963;109: 95–150.
13. Ferguson SM, Rayport M. Psychosis and epilepsy. In: Blumer D, ed. *Psychiatric aspects of epilepsy.* Washington, D.C.: APA Press, 1982; 229–270.

14. Heath RG. Subcortical brain function correlates of psychopathology and epilepsy. In: Shagass C, Gershon S, Friedhoff AJ, eds. *Psychopathology and brain dysfunction*. New York: Raven Press, 1977;51–68.

15. Dewhurst K, Beard AW. Sudden religious conversions in temporal lobe epilepsy. *Br J Psychiatry* 1970;117:497–507.

16. Ramani V, Gumnit RJ. Intensive monitoring of inter-ictal psychosis of epilepsy. *Ann Neurol* 1982;11:613–622.

17. Landolt H. Serial electroencephalographic investigations during psychotic episodes in epileptic patients and during schizophrenia attacks. In: Lorantz de Haas AM, ed. *Lectures on epilepsy*. Amsterdam: Elsevier, 1958;91–133.

18. Dongier S. Statistical study of clinical and EEG manifestations of 536 psychotic episodes occurring in 516 epileptics between clinical seizures. *Epilepsia* 1959;601;117–142.

19. Wolf P. The clinical syndromes of forced normalisation. *Folia Psychiatr Neurol Jpn* 1984;38:187–192.

20. Wolf P, Trimble MR. Biological antagonism and epileptic psychosis. *Br J Psychiatry* 1984;146:272–276.

21. Tellenbach H. Epilepsia als Anfallsleiden und als Psychose. *Nervenarzt* 1965;36:190–202.

22. Pond DA, Bidwell BH. A survey of epilepsy in 14 general practices. *Epilepsia*. 1959;1:285–299.

23. Gudmundsson G. Epilepsy in Iceland. *Acta Neurol Scand* 1966;43:1–124 (Supp. 25).

24. Zielinski JJ. *Epidemiology and medical–social problems of epilepsy in Warsaw*. Warsaw, Poland: Warsaw Psychoneurological Institute, 1974.

25. Hermann BP, Whitman S. Behavioural and personality correlates of epilepsy. *Psychol Bull* 1984;95:451–493.

26. Hermann BP, Dickman S, Schwartz MS, Karnes WE. Inter-ictal psychopathology in patients with ictal fear: a quantitative investigation. *Neurology* 1982;32:7–11.

27. Gloor P. Temporal lobe epilepsy: its possible contribution to the understanding of the functional significance of the amygdala and its interaction with neocortical–temporal mechanisms. In: Eleftherio NB, ed. *The neurobiology of the amygdala*, vol. 1. New York: Plenum Press, 1972;423–457.

28. Rodin EA, Katz M, Lennox K. Differences between patients with temporal lobe seizures and those with other forms of epileptic attacks. *Epilepsia* 1976;17:313–320.

29. Bruens JH. Psychoses in epilepsy. Historic concepts and new developments. In: Canger R, Angeleri F, Penry JK, eds. *Advances in epileptology: XIth Epilepsy International Symposium*. New York: Raven Press, 1980;161–166.

30. Taylor DC. Factors influencing the occurrence of schizophrenia-like psychosis in patients with temporal lobe epilepsy. *Psychol Med* 1975;5:531–544.

31. Hermann BP, Schwartz MS, Karnes WE, et al. Psychopathology in epilepsy: relationship of seizure type to age at onset. *Epilepsia* 1980;21:15–23.

32. Perez MM, Trimble MR. Epileptic psychosis—a diagnostic comparison with process schizophrenia. *Br J Psychiatry* 1985;146:155–163.

33. Toone BK, Garalda ME, Ron MA. The psychosis of epilepsy and the functional psychoses: a clinical and phenomenological comparison. *Br J Psychiatry* 1982;141:256–261.

34. Flor-Henry P. Psychosis and temporal lobe epilepsy. *Epilepsia* 1969;10:363–395.

35. Pritchard PB, Lombroso CT, McIntyre M. Psychological complications of temporal lobe epilepsy. *Neurology* 1980;30:227–232.

36. Sherwin I. Psychosis associated with epilepsy: significance of laterality of the epileptogenic lesion. *J Neurol Neurosurg Psychiatry* 1981;44:83–85.

37. Ounsted C, Lindsay J. The long-term outcome of temporal lobe epilepsy in childhood. In: Reynolds EH, Trimble MR, eds. *Epilepsy and psychiatry*. Edinburgh: Churchill Livingstone, 1980;185–215.

38. Sherwin I. The effect of location of an epileptogenic lesion on the occurrence of psychosis in epilepsy. In: Koella WP, Trimble MR, eds. *Temporal lobe epilepsy, mania, schizophrenia and the limbic system*. Basel: Karger, 1982;81–97.

39. Toone BK, Dawson J, Driver MV. Psychoses of epilepsy. A radiological evaluation. *Br J Psychiatry* 1982;140:244–248.

40. Perez MM, Trimble MR, Reider I, Murray NM. Epileptic psychosis, a further evaluation of PSE profiles. *Br J Psychiatry* 1985;146:155–163.

41. Kristensen O, Sindrup EH. Psychomotor epilepsy and psychosis. *Acta Neurol Scand* 1978;57:361–370.

42. Jensen I, Larsen JK. Psychoses in drug-resistant temporal lobe epilepsy. *J Neurol Neurosurg Psychiatry* 1979;42:948–954.

43. Gruzelier JH. Cerebral laterality and psychopathology. Fact or fiction. *Psychol Med* 1981;11:219–227.

44. Kiloh LG. Psychiatric aspects of epilepsy. In: Winton RR, ed. *Geigy symposium on epilepsy*. Sydney: Geigy, 1971.

45. Symonds C. The schizophrenia-like psychoses of epilepsy—discussion. Proc R Soc Med 1962;55:311.

46. Bolwig TG, Trimble MR. *The clinical relevance of kindling*. Chichester: John Wiley & Sons, 1989.

47. Gallhofer, B, Trimble MR, Frackowiak R, Gibbs J, Jones T. A study of cerebral blood flow and metabolism in epileptic psychosis using positron emission tomography and oxygen-15. *J Neurol Neurosurg Psychiatry* 1986;48:201–206.

48. Conlon P, Trimble MR, Rogers D, Callicott C. MRI in epilepsy. *Epilepsy Res* 1988;2:37–43.

49. Thompson PJ, Trimble MR. Anticonvulsant drugs and cognitive functions. *Epilepsia*. 1982;23:532–544.

Advances in Neurology, Vol. 55, edited by
D. Smith, D. Treiman, and M. Trimble,
Raven Press, Ltd., New York © 1991.

10

Behavioral Consequences of Epilepsy in Children

Developing a Psychosocial Vocabulary

David C. Taylor and Moira Lochery

*Department of Child and Adolescent Psychiatry, University of Manchester,
Swinton M27 1FG, England*

Epilepsy, as a general term, essentially only describes a social categorization. Although the medical implications of epileptic behavior are substantial, they are also variable and so diverse as to be weak predictors of social functioning if epilepsy is the only deviation. However, the social impact of the categorization can be judged from the continuing validity of the summary by Bridge (1) [quoted by Corbett and Trimble (2)]: "The most serious handicap to happy and satisfactory living that most epileptic children have to face is not their seizures, but the failure to adapt themselves psychologically to their disease and its accompanying circumstances."

Although we will argue with many aspects of Bridge's summary, it is true that being found wanting in social skills and social performance, being the butt of jokes and teasing, and searching (with family and school support) for secrecy to avoid shame are still principal basic components in the presentation of children with epilepsy to physicians. The fear of seizures adversely affects not only their medical condition but also their social status, in the sense that they betray membership of a minority group which is associated with many negative stereotypes. The essence of these negative images, which are extensively maintained throughout the social fabric, is that they are sufficiently nourished on a sporadic (intermittent re-enforcement) basis as a result

of the unhappy fate of occasional individuals and the generally poor prognosis of certain forms of epilepsy. The negative stereotype is both betrayed and sustained through the exhibition of behaviors which are considered unacceptable, and these range beyond seizure phenomena. Indeed, being "epileptic" may be confessed to or claimed as a means of explaining a behavioral deviance which might otherwise be regarded as either willful or crazy. There is thus the paradox that epilepsy can be a stigmatizing categorization but also a category that may be claimed to explain behavioral deviance rather than having the deviance be thought by others to be an aspect of one's self. In a sense, even a book such as this, dedicated to the general notion that epilepsy is a proper unifying rubric, actually perpetuates both the social use of the term "epilepsy" and some of its negative aspects. We concede that there are some positive aspects of such conventions—not the least of which is the fact that no one sees, or studies exclusively in sufficient numbers, sufferers from any one given subgrouping which does have medical validity.

Graham (3) depicts the particular and different behavioral implications of various chronic handicapping conditions such as Down's and Turner's syndromes, phenylketonuria, hypothyroidism, and XYY syndrome, most of which would also fit under the rubric "mental handicap." From the sorts of issues that he discusses, it becomes apparent that labels such as "mental handicap" are administrative labels and that they serve social, rather than medical, purposes. This is also true of the term "epilepsy," which is an administratively convenient rubric provided that we are only considering its social purpose.

Furthermore, even considering so finely limited an abnormality as "Down's syndrome," which is now specified to a detailed genetic level, it is evident that in behavioral or in psychological terms there will be huge variations in the degree of its effect, in impact, and in outcome in any given individual. These will be determined not only by variations in the real chromosomal effects both known and unknown, but also by a host of psychological and intellectual endowments dependent upon other genes and also a whole series of possible contingencies. These arise from the moment of conception, and they include how the pregnancy was experienced, sickness in baby or mother, what the shock of discovery of the condition revealed, and whether evocation of self-blame or anger at others was involved. All this will occur within, and will partly determine, both a family system and a social environment or niche. These components of sickness were called the "predicament" by Taylor (4).

Childhood epilepsies are by no means as closely specified as Down's syndrome, though some individual diseases which give rise to epilepsy are (not excluding Down's syndrome itself). It is therefore necessary to specify as closely as possible all that can reasonably be known about a patient. This requires a biographical approach, including autobiography where possible. Scientifically, it requires that the most careful possible forms of categorization are arrived at as bases for study.

Seizure disorders of quite similar etiology and general character may express themselves at different moments in time in development, and the different stages of development may well modify further any behavioral consequences. The quality of management before medical intervention was first made, and also from that time to the time of its being the subject of scientific study, will also affect reported results. Furthermore, the vocabulary of psychiatric nosology is extraordinarily limited, particularly so for children's disorders, not only in its descriptive range but in its total construction.

In this chapter, however, we shall experiment with less conventional descriptions while hoping to maintain an understandable and credible discourse. Our purpose is to expand the psychosocial vocabulary rather than to constrain it within inappropriate limitations. It deserves mention that, probably unwittingly, people with epilepsy have been denied description within large tracts of the DSM nosology as far as we understand it. There are preclusive statements such as "not due to any organic mental disorder," which research workers have to either set aside or take seriously. The vocabulary given for the description of organic brain syndromes, on the other hand, is so coarse as to suppose that cerebral pathology limits the potential range of expression of psychopathology rather than being a likely basis of it (5). Something better is needed now to match the quantum leap in investigating potential afforded by neuroimaging, neurochemistry, and neurophysiology.

The categories of behavioral deviation which arise from case research are not necessarily those which doctors have chosen. Parents, having come to terms with seizures, are then concerned with the day-to-day management of their child, and their preoccupations are psychosocial rather than medical (6,7). When given the opportunity to express them, the concerns of children with epilepsy are not necessarily the concerns of their parents or of their doctors. The fabric of much of our conventional discourse follows from pursuing an issue from a particular perspective. Sometimes it helps to change that perspective.

PATIENT REFERRAL AND SOURCES

The patients discussed in this chapter are those children who have seizure-related problems and who were referred to a child and adolescent psychiatry clinic at the Royal Manchester Children's Hospital. These are almost exclusively "tertiary" referrals; that is, they came via other hospital consultant pediatricians or pediatric neurologists, either directly or indirectly or for second opinion as requested by their own general practitioner. Referrals are achieved as a resultant between the forces applied by the parents and those applied by their local consultant, acting, as it were, against various prejudices inherent in the system which tend to militate against referral. These include: parents' unwillingness to see a psychiatrist and to deal with the labeling that is involved; a certain unwillingness by former physicians to concede that much has been left undone or untried; and a social and medical structure which tends to be prejudiced against people with epilepsy and to prefer low-cost solutions. The result is a highly variable filter. Referral depends upon knowledge of the existence of such a clinic and upon the level of expertise of former consultants. The whole process constrains our cases towards being both chronic and severe. We can have no epidemiological aspirations, and we would not wish to generalize our findings. However, the clinic does reveal (a) the sorts of phenomena involved, such as "severity" and "chronicity," (b) the range of psychological presentations, which are often repeated, and (c) the sorts of predicaments in which families find themselves. Ultimately, what medical science aspires to is to equip physicians with precise and rational bases for treatment choices. We take the view that many of the treatment options are available in the social system and that much fewer are in the biosystem of the patient. Because deviant behavior is the product of the interaction between sociosystem and biosystem, and also because it is of a reverberating, self-perpetuating character, it makes practical sense to intervene in both systems and to monitor both systems when making an intervention to one or another.

SAMPLE AND OUTLINE FINDINGS

We reviewed 50 consecutive epilepsy patients who were seen in the special psychiatry clinic at the Royal Manchester Children's Hospital and whose mean age at interview was 12 years. Onset of epilepsy usually occurred at age 4, and the typical age at diagnosis was approximately 5. Some etiology could be entertained for only half the sample.

About half the cases were admitted for inpatient investigation and treatment. Seventy percent were male.

"Severity" was as often as not a psychosocial phenomenon, but 40% suffered seizures more than once per week; 30% were of average intelligence, and about half the sample was in normal school at the time of referral.

Problems within the psychosocial sphere were not the only reason for referral but occurred in 70% of the sample. About half the patients experienced mood-related disorders, and about half were considered "aggressive." We distinguished between "attack" behavior and "rage," though these often occurred in the same children. Aggression was almost entirely limited to males (85%). About one-third of children had experienced uncontrolled "voiding" of feces or urine in their attacks.

A brief "case vignette" was written describing the key components of the child's presentation, and these vignettes were used to illustrate deficiencies in a group of key "behaviors" deemed necessary to support the child's functioning in society. These behaviors are as follows:

Sleeping	Talking	Relating
Eating	Thinking	Working
Voiding	Learning	Sexual behavior
Walking	Socializing	

The perspective of our work with epileptic children deserves to be made clear, since the descriptive study that follows stems from that perspective.

1. *Epilepsy betokens a cerebral problem.* This may be secondary or primary, trivial and transient, or chronic and severe. The significance of the seizure disorder may even become lost in the totality of the handicap.

2. *The cerebral problem will have other manifestations.* The more overt these other manifestations, the more problematic for the neuropil to sustain normal social function and behavior. However, severe deviations in social performance may not correlate with cerebral abnormality at our present level of knowledge (8).

3. *Seizures and cerebral problems may have behavioral consequences.* They may di-

rectly affect the behaviors noted above, but they may also enhance the risk of developing serious psychiatric disorder, albeit via a complex and probabilistic system (9).

4. *"Seizure prone" is a social category.* It declares minority status which is negatively evaluated. Furthermore, it is an involuntary and "visible" declaration (10).

5. *Individuals enter the category with different resources.* Some individuals enjoy many years of normal life and acquire many contingent skills from normal development before suffering from epilepsy, whereas others do not; the development of the latter individuals is impaired as a result of lesion, seizures, handicaps, and stigma (1).

6. *The psychosocial aspects are manifest in an environment and from the experience of prior environments.* Human social behavior is interactive with others, and others may contribute very much to the quality of that behavior. Behavior is learned and guided and can be misdirected.

7. *The "predicament" of suffering epilepsy.* That predicament generated by becoming seizure-prone will be ascribed a personal meaning and will acquire a meaning to others in the immediate social system. These meanings will influence behavior (12).

8. *Impaired cerebral function.* Impaired cerebral function provides the common basis for the most general characteristics seen in children with epilepsy. Impaired function leads to regressions towards more infantile thinking, action, and response and also leads to limitation of the behavioral repertoire. A schema of psychosocial development, such as that based on the work of Erikson (cited in ref. 13), provides the most helpful explanatory models, though these are woefully underresearched (but see refs. 14 and 15).

SPECIFIC "BEHAVIORS" AND EPILEPSY

Sleeping

Sleep is the principal state of the newborn, a proportion of time which is gradually reduced with development and which may become minimal in old age. Sleep and seizures are so clearly related that it is inevitable that their mechanism will prove to be largely coextensive. But the relationship between sleeping and epilepsy is not limited to coextensive physiological mechanisms; instead, it includes the whole question of biorhythms and circadian rhythms and secondary psychological effects.

In the past, organic psychosyndromes were often morally evaluated, and negative attributions were given to the children; in other instances, poor management by the parents was cited as being the basis of the child's "behavior."

Several instances of tonic seizures in sleep provide serious problems for families hoping to either control, help, or give succor or comfort during prolonged hours of nocturnal seizuring. These cases were a rich source of misdiagnosis of "hysterical elaboration," because they were exquisitely sensitive to environmental changes and also because the retention of partial awareness during the tonic seizure struggle led to negative labeling of the behavior.

R.H.

This patient was first seen in a psychiatric clinic at age 17 because her neurologist and her psychologist had given up on her; the presumptive diagnosis was hysterical seizures.

However, she was a child of precocious development until the onset of epilepsy at the age of 3½ in the Far East, and her illness was associated with vertigo. Her daytime routine electroencephalograms (EEGs) mostly showed no abnormality at all. She was a sweet but moralizing girl, was very old-fashioned, and had no friends.

When asked to illustrate the sort of fits that went on for hours at night with threshings about and falling out of bed, the girl illustrated Charcot's "Arc en Cercle." Our diagnosis oscillated between the genuine and the hysterical, depending upon the flamboyance of the recent reports. However, neuropsychological testing showed a verbal I.Q. of 93 and a performance I.Q. of 58, and despite the total absence of seizures by day over a period of 4 years in our care, we accepted that this was a purely nocturnal epilepsy when this was confirmed during her admission to an epilepsy center at our request.

State-relatedness of seizures is most prominent in young children, but various confluences of events which precipitate any given seizure probably involve states which will vary with mood. In medicating against seizures it is possible to actually promote as a side effect just that state in which seizures are more probable for that individual; somnolence is the most common case.

In pediatrics, fear of sleep occurs in certain children who experience ictal phenomena on the edge of sleep. Children thus prone must avoid "dropping off" during the day if they are to retain secrecy.

Night terrors and nightmares in children are sometimes so intense as to raise the suggestion that they are seizures, or seizure equivalents. Management depends upon the precise circumstances. Some sleep disorders are simply mismanagement by parents overwhelmed by their situation.

Postictal sleep is a component of many seizures, often quite disproportionate in length or in degree of need with respect to the manifest seizure which precipitated it; the recovery phase can create problems at school. Clearly there are parallels with those seizures which give rise to incontinence. However, postparoxysmal sleep is a prominent component of paroxysmal displays of whatever provenance (16), especially orgasm and labor. In contrast, the imminence of a paroxysmal display tends, in itself, to be arousing. Extreme and sudden external arousals (e.g., the telephone, the patter of feet, the shouted forename) will sometimes inhibit the paroxysmal behavior. Sudden emergence from a seizure because of such a change of arousal sometimes leads children to be thought of as "faking it."

Eating

Eating is a major focus of family behavior and is often a more direct and intimate place of confrontation than any other. Eating has to do with giving and receiving, with the acknowledgment of gift (17) and of status; certain protocols, table positions, and feeding orders are observed. It is also an opportunity of group conviviality, mutuality, and close observation. It is commonplace for certain seizure disorders to be first observed during feeding or at the table, and it is also commonplace for the mealtime to become a further focus of observation and to be an opportunity to check on the ingestion of medication.

The manner in which family eating proceeds usefully reflects the social dynamics of the family, and indeed it may expose familial disintegration more clearly than would most other situations. Father absenteeism, idiosyncracies of diet, self-removal, or dismissal from the eating group are among the more obviously evident behaviors.

It would be interesting to know whether the association between mealtimes and seizures was purely social, or was precipitated by relaxation to another state, or was mediated by oral activity and food stimulation. Jackson's (18) attention was particularly drawn to "the taste region of Ferrier" (19) by the oral, chewing automatisms with which certain seizures were associated and which Jackson showed were likely to have temporal lobe origins.

Vomiting at some stage of a seizure was a common problem in our patients. The more extreme use of vomiting as an expression of the social impact made by the expulsion of vileness was publicized in the movie "The Exorcist," which purported to represent temporal lobe seizures. Ictal vomiting summates the paroxysmal displays and combines their unacceptability. Vomiting adds the danger of inhalation of vomitus in a seizure to the lethal potential of seizures.

K.S.
This patient was seen at the age of 10 when her right temporal solid lesion was diagnosed and removed. Her initial behavioral presentation with epilepsy was by vomiting at 18 months. She would turn aside from the meal table and vomit copiously and then turn to resume her meal. These sporadic attacks persisted until they merged with urinary incontinence and circumoral pallor by the age of 2½ years and were then diagnosed as epilepsy.

Vomiting is a high-impact social behavior which is highly aversive and forms a component of the aversive nature of seizure disorders.

Voiding

In some doctors' minds, especially in emergency departments, as evidence of bona fide epilepsy, the involuntary passage of urine and feces remains a "rite of passage." Thus it could be a disadvantage in that situation not to experience these behaviors which in other circumstances are so seriously incommoding. In some cases the absence of these traits (including tongue biting) has been taken as evidence favoring a diagnosis of hysterical seizures or of hysterical elaboration of a seizure tendency. Voiding of urine is the more common and was seen in 35% of our patients. It was occasionally psychologically devastating.

L.C.
Aged 11 on entry to senior school, this girl's first public seizure was in the dining queue where at least 100 fellow pupils saw her urine running from her as she stood stock still in her "absence" attack. The impact of her social catastrophe led to school avoidance and depressive loss of self-esteem.

Voiding is also associated nonspecifically with epilepsy through mental retardation and poor habit learning.

Disorders of sleeping, eating, and voiding, along with disorders of sexual behavior, can be taken as presumptive of direct involvement by the seizure with limbic components, though this may occur by secondary spread rather than originating there. Some clue may be gained by the precise point at which the behavior occurs in the whole sequence of behaviors that make up the typical fit.

Walking

Walking is expected between 12 and 14 months in Europe, but it is expected earlier in the United States. The pattern of emergence over time of the sequence of behaviors leading to walking is evidence of the degree of integration of the central nervous system. Walking may reveal developmental delay and anomaly, hemiparesis, clumsiness, weakness, and a propensity to collapse attacks.

The essential initial separation of the "psychomotor" seizure is evident in its infantile presentation (described in the Hippocratic writings) as a subjective experience, usually of fear, which leads to a search for, or dash towards, adult security before the seizure generalizes.

G.J.
A 12-year-old boy suffering complex partial seizures experienced relationship problems in school. His illness dated from septicemia at 5 months. From the age of 3 he would wander vacantly towards his mother, staring at her strangely. When he was a little older he would also complain of "a headache in my tummy" at these times. Epilepsy was not diagnosed until he was 6 years old.

Talking

Abnormalities in speech cannot be evident before the time in development when speech is expected to emerge in the ethogram. The ethogram is a good model of certain epoch-related problems, conveying their unpredictability and leading to the expectant policy which creates delays of diagnosis and exacerbates problems. Speech delays are another index of cerebral malfunction in higher-order skills; furthermore, a whole range of language-related problems are seen in children with epilepsy, from total lack of language to idiosyncratic usage and a certain relentlessness in discourse which has led to the use of epithets such as pedantic, religious, and boring. Recently, some such children have been recognized as showing Asperger's syndrome (20,21), which some see as kindred to autism but which is perhaps a different level of expression of a similar defect. Social deficit in interpersonal exchanges, eccentricity, motor clumsiness, and hobbies that are curious, rather unusual, and all-absorbing are components of the diagnosis.

Autism, especially with handicap, is one association of infantile spasms, in a sense paralleling the schizophrenic association with certain cases of temporal lobe epilepsy seen at a later developmental epoch. Epilepsy supervening in children already suffering from Asperger's syndrome or higher functioning autism is usually of a psychomotor type with some major seizures and is relatively mild.

There are a variety of degrees to which speech may be suddenly lost with the onset of early-childhood seizures that are rather broader in scope than the Landau–Kleffner syndrome. Speech may be lost permanently or temporarily.

T.S.
At the time of incoming of speech, this little girl suffered a severe episode of convulsions which was associated with massive speech regression; on emergence from this, she exhibited rather wild behavior with

rather frantic non-speech vocalizations. Her capacity for receptive language improved within a year or two, but expressive speech lags significantly behind.

Ictal-speech automatisms (i.e., stereotyped repeated utterances within a seizure) are seen in children but are reported less often than in adults. Serafetinides and Falconer (22) were able to show that ictal-speech automatisms were more common when the focus of origin was in the nondominant lobe. Ictal-speech arrests, arising from dominant-hemisphere foci, are difficult to identify in children who seem to find it hard to distinguish between a train of thought and the urge to speak it.

S.N.

This 15-year-old boy's epilepsy started at the age of 5 with blank stares. These persist, but in more extended seizures he annexes speech from a concurrent context and repeats it in the seizure. After having recently watched "The Mercenaries" on TV, his eyes glazed, his lips went blue, his face distorted, and he uttered "USA or USSR!; USA or USSR!" repeatedly.

For this boy, however, the most incapacitating part of suffering epilepsy was his overwhelming postictal sleep even after the briefest of psychomotor seizures.

Thinking

Poverty of language and slowness in thinking have been prominently reported in people with epilepsy and have led to the concept of an epileptic dementia. The curious quality of thought in which long time-delays between question and answer are evident was termed "ixophrenia." The precisely correct answer may be delivered so far removed in conversational time from the question that it then seems a meaningless interjection.

Several features of thought in children with epilepsy are also seen in people with schizophrenia. Slowing may seem like poverty of thought or thought block. In certain psychomotor seizures, two lines of thought are reported (19); and in certain utterances, sound grammar may disintegrate during a partial seizure. Complex aura onsets are similar to forced thinking or thought insertion (23). Recent research studying the children of schizophrenic parents has shown that such children experience much above average rates of developmental difficulties of the sort which abound in children with epilepsy. The prepsychotic traits during the childhood of those people with epilepsy who become schizophrenic are not known.

S.C.

A retarded boy of 14 expresses marked paranoid persecutory ideas and attempts to "escape" or run away from his current situation in the prodrome of his psychomotor seizures. Epilepsy began with two prolonged episodes of status epilepticus at the age of 9 months and 15 months. Persistent stereotyped psychomotor seizures with a prominent aura of terror began by 3 years and still persist. Except in the prodrome of his complex seizures which then generalize, he is a limited and obtunded boy with no evidence of psychosis. The implication is that his ictal state provides the experience of terror which he interprets as emanating from his immediate situation (24).

Learning

Not surprisingly, subsidiary language skills such as reading both for accuracy and especially for comprehension are characteristically rather severely affected. In this study, 73% of those whose reading level had been assessed were reading at least 1 year behind their chronological age.

In turn, certain educational difficulties associate very closely with behavioral difficulties described in the "conduct" or "conduct and emotional" categories of conventional diagnostic schedules. Children with epilepsy who are also experiencing educational problems are more prone to conduct disorders. Boys prominently outnumber girls in such categories (25).

D.K.

Referred at the age of 17 because of progressive personality problems, this boy had suffered stereotyped seizures since the age of 1 year. Despite his brilliant intellect, he was failing to achieve his potential in subjects other than mathematics. He was aloof, friendless, and prone to make chillingly accurate but inappropriate remarks about people. A solid lesion of the left temporal lobe was diagnosed and removed. Seizures ceased, and his rehabilitation was successful enough for him to go on to college.

Socializing

Marked impairment of the capacity for forming good social relationships characterizes the majority of the children in this sample, but often, as has been shown from obvious and stigmatizing aspects of their disorder, there are additional children whose difficulties stem from (a) a direct incapacity to form adequate social relationships, (b) a sort of social imperception, (c) an inability to read the state of mind of others, and (d) a lack of awareness of the effect that their behavior may have on those with whom they are trying to socialize. These children are notable for their rejection by their peer groups, their unacceptability to their teachers, and their tendency to alienate themselves from their parents, but they fall short of the "Asperger" category.

T.T.

This boy's left temporal lesion was recognized when he was 7 but was operated upon when he was 17, when a radical excision was deemed impossible. It was an oligoastrocytoma. The seizures were heralded by macrusia and dysphasia, tachycardia, and a needle-sharp pain in the right antecubital fossa. Ictal automatisms or finding a safe spot led to many seizures not being witnessed. The whole dynamic of the boy's life was towards social avoidance; he went from a special language unit to a special school for children with emotional disorders and relationship problems. His reticence and inappropriateness contributed considerably to the delay in surgical treatment because of the underestimate of his seizure frequency.

Relating

Children, whose general levels of socialization and understanding of social interactions may be perfectly adequate, may have great difficulties in relating because of their tendency towards aggression and attack behaviors. The capacity for maintaining relationships may also be impaired by intercurrent phenomena such as depressive illnesses and also by prolonged periods spent in an obtunded state during status of minor epilepsy. These children differ from children with primary impairments of socialization by their capacity to maintain good relationships when they are not actually aggressive or unwell. These children are most frequently described by their parents as having "Jekyll and Hyde" characters.

E.A.

A 7-year-old girl experiences several auras each day, and she also experiences weekly seizures which are visible to witnesses. Her first seizure was status epilepticus at 11 months in the context of a roseola infantum infection. After an aura of fear, nausea, and tachycardia, her behavior changes dramatically to be oppositional, angry, reckless, and stubborn. Other children fear these sudden changes. Her parents respond by being oversolicitous, guarding the child 24 hr a day, responding instantly to her expressions of fear, and sleeping alongside her. The parents resent being caught up in this degree of commitment but cannot extricate themselves.

S.T.

A 17-year-old mentally handicapped girl with limited speech regressed from her busy, cheerful self. She wet herself several times daily, tore her clothing, did not respond to requests, and was difficult about eating. On the threshold of doors she started to give a piercing scream. Her seizure frequency was unchanged. The house staff of her home overlooked a significant loss of a love relationship; they had regarded it as infantile, but it was in fact the basis of this depressive regression.

Working

The capacity to work and the availability of work are crucial to maintenance of a place in the social fabric and the maintenance of self-esteem. Work history was an important part of psychiatric history-taking (26), but constraints on work availability and early retirement have increasingly made its significance less clear. However, it remains true that people with handicaps and the already marginally adjusted are more likely to suffer unemployment. The jobless are also economically deprived and experience more problems with obtaining adequate health care. People with continuing seizures, especially those suffering concurrent problems, are particularly likely to be discriminated against in the work market. In their follow-up study, Taylor and Harrison (27) showed what were then considered to be relatively high unemployment rates in survivors, and they also showed depressed achievement in those who worked despite continuing epilepsy. A more detailed study by Sillanpaa (28) confirmed these findings.

G.C.

A boy of 16 left school to find work and chose to be a "roofer," one of the building trade's most hazardous activities. His seizures began at 11, onsetting with an aura of nausea; his seizures also included jargon dysphasia and rotatory movements. Family life was chaotic and he was noncompliant with treatment, though attacks occurred only once or twice a year. Regular appointments for investigation, treatment, and rehabilitation were planned but were sabotaged by the patient, whose behavior and personality traits suggested a frontal lobe lesion. He fathered a child and committed criminal offenses. However, it was also clear that he was terrified of his epilepsy, had no hopes from his family, and simply lived for the moment. There was evidence of a frontal focus in one of the EEGs, and eventually his frontal lesion was proved by magnetic resonance imaging (MRI) scanning. His personality structure was also preventing his physicians from making adequate investigations to treat him appropriately. His checkered work career is contributed to by his personality as a result of both his lesion and his real, as well as prejudicial, anxiety about his safety at work.

SUMMARY

In this chapter we have described some of the experiences of a special psychiatric clinic for children with epilepsy, drawing our examples from a series of 50 children. The behavioral consequences of epilepsy cannot be adequately described within the limited nosology available for classifying the behavior disorders of children. As an alternative, a series of behaviors which children actually require in order to maintain their social existence have been identified; furthermore, impairments of those behaviors have been pointed to, and consequences of these behavioral impairments have been outlined. The behavioral consequences of epilepsy are often multiple and are sometimes mutually interactive. The extent to which these behavioral deviations depend both upon the exhibition of seizures and the presence of structural abnormalities in the brain is made most evident by the marked changes in behavior which can be achieved when epilepsy is relieved and a lesion is removed. Unfortunately, such a strategem is not available to the majority of children with epilepsy. For the time being, their cerebral impairment and the continuation of their epilepsy have to be taken for granted, and intervention then consists of the best possible management of their impairments and their distressing behaviors. Such management clearly requires psychiatric and psychological skills, although these skills do not necessarily lead to greater success than does the use of anticonvulsants or the use of surgery. Success is not an adequate measure of the appropriateness of the endeavor.

It goes without saying that not all children with epilepsy suffer behavioral consequences along these lines, and indeed behavioral disturbances were not universal even in this highly selected series. Some children were seen merely as a way of improving their medical status or achieving surgical treatment. These more traditional medical maneuvers are easier to undertake and are more understandable to parents than are complex strategies of psychiatry. In any event, parents deserve considerable support.

The language of psychiatry for children with organic cerebral impairments is extremely limited; this chapter has been an attempt to improve our vocabulary, which will be a necessary underpinning in order to improve the quality of our classification.

Finally, we return to Bridge's statement. Firstly, we do not regard epilepsy as a disease any more than we would regard cough as a disease, and we find that orientations in that direction are likely to thwart our attempt at piece-by-piece dismantling of the many sorts of disease which might be associated with seizures. This is abundantly evident in our mere 50 cases: It is not even likely that there is a single "seizure mechanism" at a level which will have clinical meaning.

Secondly, it is more than likely that seizures do generate most of the childrens' problems directly or through their behavioral concomitants. As with most medical problems, a direct attack which cures will also preempt most of the endeavors of psychosocial scientists.

Thirdly, Bridge imputes the failure of adaptation in a way which suggests a moral fault in the child. This is an easy and common error; it is a projection onto the child of grownups' inability to be more helpful.

REFERENCES

1. Bridge EM. *Epilepsy and convulsive disorders in children.* New York: McGraw–Hill, 1949.
2. Corbett JA, Trimble MR. Epilepsy and anticonvulsant medication. In: Rutter M, ed. *Developmental neuropsychiatry.* Edinburgh: Churchill Livingstone, 1984.
3. Graham PJ. Specific medical syndromes. In: Rutter M, ed. *Developmental neuropsychiatry.* Edinburgh: Churchill Livingstone, 1984.
4. Taylor DC. The components of sickness: diseases, illnesses and predicaments. In: Apley J, Ounsted C, eds. *One child.* London: Spastics International Medical Publications/Heinemann Medical Books, 1982.
5. Beran RG, Flanagan PJ. Psychosocial sequelae of epilepsy: the role of associated cerebral pathology. *Epilepsia* 1987;28:107–110.
6. Coulter DL, Koester BS. Information needs of parents of children with epilepsy. *Dev Behav Pediatr* 1985;6:334–338.
7. Lochery, 1986. (Personal Communication.)
8. Hodgman CH, McAnarney ER, Myers GJ, et al. Emotional complications of adolescent grand mal epilepsy. *J Pediatr* 1979;95:309–312.
9. Hoare P. Development of psychiatric disorder among schoolchildren with epilepsy. *Dev Med Child Neurol* 1984;26:3–13.
10. Goffman E. *Stigma: notes on the management of spoiled identity.* New York: Prentice–Hall, 1964.
11. Lindsay J, Glaser G, Richards P, Ounsted C. Developmental aspects of focal epilepsies of childhood treated by neurosurgery. *Dev Med Child Neurol* 1984;26:574–587.
12. Taylor DC. Epilepsy: a model of sickness. In: Sander M, ed. *Psychopharmacology of anticonvulsants.* Oxford: Oxford University Press, 1982.
13. Taylor DC. Psychiatry and sociology in the understanding of epilepsy. In: Gelder MG, Mandlebrote BM, eds. *Psychiatric aspects of medical practice.* London: Staples, 1971.
14. Viberg M, Blennow G, Polski B. Epilepsy in adolescence: implications for the development of personality. *Epilepsia* 1987;28:542–546.
15. Garyfallos G, Manos N, Adamopoulou A. Psychopathology and personality characteristics of epileptic patients: epilepsy, psychopathology and personality. *Acta Psychiatr Scand* 1988;78:87–95.
16. Ounsted C. Some aspects of seizure disorders. In: Gairdner D, Howle D, eds. *Recent advances in paediatrics*, 4th ed. London: J & A Churchill, 1971.
17. Mauss M. *The Gift: forms and functions of exchange in archaic societies.* London: Cohen & West, 1969.
18. Jackson JH. On a particular variety of epilepsy ("intellectual aura"). One case with symptoms of organic brain disease. *Brain* 1880;11:179–207.
19. Taylor DC, Marsh SM. Hughlings Jackson's Dr. Z: the paradigm of temporal lobe epilepsy revealed. *J Neurol Neurosurg Psychiatry* 1980;43:758–767.
20. Asperger H. Die 'autistischen Psychopathen' im Kindesalter. *Arch Psychiatr Nervenkr* 1944;117:76–136.
21. Wing L. Asperger's syndrome: a clinical account. *Psychol Med* 1981;11:115–129.
22. Serafetinides EA, Falconer MA. Speech disturbances in temporal lobe seizures: a study in 100 epileptic patients submitted to anterior temporal lobectomy. *Brain* 1963;86:333–346.
23. Taylor DC, Lochery M. Temporal lobe epilepsy: origin and significance of simple and complex auras. *J Neurol Neurosurg Psychiatry* 1987;50:673–681.
24. Hermann BP, Dikmen S, Schwartz MS, Karnes WE. Interictal psychopathology in patients with ictal fear: a quantitative investigation. *Neurology* 1982;32:7–11.
25. Hoare P. Psychiatric disturbance in the families of epileptic children. *Dev Medicine Child Neurol* 1984;26:14–19.
26. Mayer-Gross W, Slater E, Roth M. *Clinical psychiatry.* London: Cassell & Co., 1960.
27. Taylor DC, Harrison RM. Childhood seizures: a 25 year follow-up. *Lancet* 1976;1:948–951.
28. Sillanpaa M. Social functioning and seizure of young adults with onset of epilepsy in childhood: an epidemiological 20-year follow-up study. *Acta Neurol Scand [Suppl]* 1983;96:68.

Advances in Neurology, Vol. 55, edited by
D. Smith, D. Treiman, and M. Trimble,
Raven Press, Ltd., New York © 1991.

11

Evocation and Inhibition of Seizures

Behavioral Treatment

Peter Fenwick

The Maudsley Hospital, London SE5 8AZ, England

The view of epilepsy as a simple medical condition is one that has been current for many years. The accepted model of seizure genesis is that seizures arise as a result of abnormal brain discharges, usually caused by a damaged area of brain tissue or as a result of a change in the physiology of the brain. Although it is becoming recognized that this model is too simple, it is not generally appreciated that there must, of necessity, be a close relationship between (a) ongoing cerebral activity and (b) the capacity of those cells involved in that activity to be diverted into a seizure process. There is a close link between brain activity, the psychic life of the individual, and the genesis of the seizure activity.

In reductionist terms, mind and brain are synonymous, and all aspects of mind are determined entirely by alterations in brain states. When brain function is abolished, so too is mind. It does not matter whether we wish to describe the subjective experience of our perceived worlds in terms of the alteration of the flow of neural impulses in different cerebral circuits or whether we wish to describe it in terms of emotion, intellect, and volition. Reductionist science, by definition, is unable to draw a distinction between these two.

Because the reductionist viewpoint is not properly understood, the sciences of psychiatry and neurology are seen as fundamentally different. This has led to a division within the clinic. The neurologist defines epilepsy as a pathological brain state and tries to rectify it with physical treatments (usually drugs),
whereas the psychiatrist sees the seizure as being influenced by the patient's state of mind and therefore uses counseling, analysis, and behavioral treatment as well as physical treatments (drugs).

Epilepsy is therefore a bridge between these two disciplines. The neurologist sees the pathological seizure discharge as arising in a particular structure and spreading through distinct brain areas. The psychiatrist sees the aura (which is the beginning of the seizure discharge) as an experience which is followed by an alteration in the subjective world of the sufferer as the epileptic discharge sweeps through his brain. Within the seizure discharge is the synthesis of neurology and psychiatry. The discharge is a pure demonstration of the precise linking of mind (subjective experience) and brain. It also emphasizes the point that a true understanding of a patient and his seizures requires both the neurological and the psychiatric points of view.

SEIZURE GENESIS

Lockard (1) proposed an elegant model of seizure genesis in focal epilepsy. She used aluminum hydroxide paste to produce focal epileptogenic lesions in the cortex of monkeys. She then implanted this epileptogenic area with microelectrodes and defined two populations of epileptogenic cells which she called group 1 and group 2.

Group 1 neurons were situated at the center

of the focus, were partially damaged, and always fired in an epileptic, bursting mode. These cells were pacemaker cells, and they fired abnormally all the time. Their activity was not modified to any significant extent by surrounding brain activity. Group 2 cells were partially damaged neurons surrounding the focus, and they could fire in both the bursting, epileptic mode and in a normal mode. Their activity could therefore be modified by surrounding brain activity. When a seizure occurred, group 1 cells, which were continually discharging, recruited group 2 cells into the seizure discharge. The spreading out of abnormal discharges within the group 2 cells was a focal seizure. If group 2 cells recruited cells in the normal brain surrounding the abnormal focus, then the focal seizure would spread throughout the brain and become secondarily generalized.

This model clearly shows that there are two points in the evolution of a seizure when ongoing brain activity can either increase or decrease the likelihood of the seizure developing. The first is between group 1 and group 2 neurons, and the second is between group 2 and normal brain neurons. If this model is correct, then the background activity of surrounding populations of cells would be of crucial importance in determining whether or not a seizure is likely to occur, and whether or not it is is likely to spread. If behavior can be described in terms of excitation and inhibition of populations of neurons surrounding and influencing the focus, then it follows that behavior must be extremely important in the genesis of seizure activity.

SPIKE-AND-WAVE SEIZURES

A new model of spike-and-wave seizures, based on the effect of penicillin on the cortex of the cat, has been proposed by Musgrave and Gloor (2) and Avoli and Gloor (3) from the Montreal Neurological Institute. Injected penicillin induces generalized spike-and-wave activity. The underlying mechanism is thought to be the reduction of inhibition by penicillin, leading to hyperexcitability of cortical neurons. Gloor and co-workers (2,3) have convincingly showed that spike-and-wave generation is predominantly cortical, al-

though it can be modified by reticular formation stimulation. The thalamus in this model plays only a secondary role. Thus, a complete description of the seizure generator is probably reticulocortical. If this model is correct for humans [there is sufficient indirect evidence that this may be so (4)], then it would be expected that overall changes in reticular activity would be likely to lead to either the genesis or inhibition of seizure discharges. Reticular activity, like cortical activity, varies as a function of behavior; thus, again, behavior could be expected to have a direct effect on seizure frequency.

It is becoming clear that reticular formation activity may have a direct effect on seizure genesis, and so its role in the control and inhibition of seizures is likely to be more important as this work advances. It has been shown that there are zones within the brain that control seizure spread. For example, the spread of kindling discharges from limbic structures in animal models can be inhibited by the pars reticulata of the substantia nigra. Such controlling zones may also be involved in humans, and thus seizure control is likely to be spread throughout several brain areas.

SPIKE ACTIVITY

Spike activity is thought to be caused by the synchronization of populations of group 1 neurons (1). The exact reason for this synchronization is not clear, but in this model the spikes are seen as excitatory. Engel et al. (5) have suggested an alternative significance for epileptic spikes, postulating that epileptic spikes may be inhibitory in nature. They point to, amongst other evidence, the commonly observed fact that spike activity usually slows and then ceases before the development of a grand mal seizure. Whichever model is used, it is likely that changes in spike frequency can be related either directly or indirectly to seizure frequency.

Lockard (6) has also shown that the numbers of spikes occurring at any one time can be modified by, amongst other things, psychosocial processes. In an elegant experiment, she carried out spike counts on her epileptic monkeys before, during, and after an epileptic monkey low on the social hierarchy was exposed to a more dominant monkey. This exposure significantly increased spike firing and presumably increased the likelihood of seizures.

CORTICAL EXCITATION AND BEHAVIOR

The contingent negative variation (CNV) is a slow negative potential shift which arises on the surface of the cortex in a forewarned reaction time task. The CNV has been called the "readiness potential," because it is thought to indicate cortical priming occurring before physical or mental activity. It is only one of a number of negative potential shifts which occur prior to activity For example, the bereitschaftspotential occurs over the motor cortex, just prior to a movement. These potentials are believed to increase the likelihood of neuronal firing, thereby facilitating the action. More recent work has shown that the CNV can be activated asymmetrically over the right or left cortex, and that this activation is related to specific tasks (7,8). For example, right temporal tasks (e.g., the classifications of line diagrams) activate the right temporal region more than the left, whereas the classification of line-drawn pictures by a verbal category activates the left temporal region more than the right. Additional evidence suggests that there are differences in CNV amplitude related to personality factors (9). Other studies have shown electroencephalographic (EEG) differences for personality and intelligence (10). All these studies point to an interaction between behavior, personality, intelligence, and cerebral excitability.

Recent measurement of scalp DC (or very low frequency waves) potentials carried out at the University of Tubingham Department of Psychology has shown that there is a rapid increase in the scalp negativity in the seconds before a seizure occurs. This change is also paralleled by slow magnetic field changes. These changes could be due to the onset of the seizure discharge in the depths, or they could be due to a generalized recruitment process which just antedates the seizure.

If the facilitatory negative shifts occur in close proximity to the epilepsy focus, they will increase the likelihood of abnormal cerebral discharges. Alterations of behavior, by enhancing the activity of neighboring popula-

tions of cells through these widely distributed negative shifts, will thus alter the probability of seizure occurrence.

EVOKED SEIZURES

Terminology

The precipitation of seizures by specific external stimuli has been called "reflex epilepsy." Gowers (11) described the precipitation of seizures by external stimuli and formalized the idea of reflex epilepsy in 1901. In 1925, Hughlings Jackson (12) also recognized the term. Since then, with the advance of physiology, the term "reflex epilepsy" has fallen into disrepute. "Evoked seizures" was the term preferred by Symonds (13), whereas Penfield and Erickson (14) preferred the term "sensory precipitation epilepsy." However, as Merliss (15) points out, the term "sensory" would exclude many seizures that may be triggered by emotional or other nonsensory components. The term "evoked seizures," as used by Symonds, will be used here for those epilepsies which have a specific external precipitant.

Mechanism of Seizure Spread

Photosensitive epilepsy is a good example of the way that external stimuli can trigger a seizure. The precise mechanism has been studied in detail by many workers. The clearest account and model is that of Wilkins et al. (16,17) and Binnie et al. (18). Rhythmic driving of the retina produces rhythmic stimulation of cells in the visual cortex. Provided that sufficient cells are stimulated, the discharges will spread from the driven cells to the surrounding normal cells, and a generalized seizure may occur. Both spatial and temporal summation of a stimulated population of cells are thought to be required before a critical mass of excited cells is reached. These investigators, as well as others (19,20), have shown that a simple way to prevent photic seizures is to close one eye. This reduces the population of cells within the visual cortex which are being directly stimulated by the light flashes, so that the critical mass of excited cells is never reached.

Photosensitive epilepsy is only one example in which rhythmic stimulation of the sensory input to the body may lead to an evoked seizure. It is a general property of the central nervous system that in susceptible individuals, any form of appropriate (usually rhythmic) peripheral stimulation may evoke a seizure.

Evoked seizures are said to occur in about 5% of people with epilepsy (13), though higher rates may occur, particularly in hospital populations. Fenwick (21) has suggested that the rate may be nearer 25% in those epilepsy patients attending the Maudsley Hospital. Reading, eating, stimulation of the skin, movement, sounds, and smells can all trigger seizures (15,21). The mechanism is presumed to be similar to that of photic stimulation. The current concept is that peripheral stimulation raises the level of activity within a damaged area of the cortex, by rhythmic driving of the cells, and thus allows seizure discharges to spread within this area. Alternatively, using the model of Lockard mentioned above, peripheral activity would so greatly increase the level of excitation within a population of neurons that group 1 neurons would be able to recruit group 2 neurons and thus allow a focal seizure discharge to develop. In Lockard's model the opposite can also occur: An alteration in the level of excitation in that area of damaged cortex where the epileptic focus is located will prevent seizure activity from arising and spreading. This point will be discussed in greater detail below.

PSYCHOGENIC EPILEPTIC SEIZURES

In 1981, Fenwick (21) proposed a classification of seizures generated by an action of mind. He called these seizures "psychogenic epileptic seizures," indicating that they arose as a consequence of mental activity. He divided psychogenic epileptic seizures into primary and secondary. Primary psychogenic epileptic seizures are those produced by the direct action of will—the patient deliberately attempts to induce a seizure. Secondary psychogenic epileptic seizures (also called the "thinking epilepsies") are those which occur when the subject is thinking or "feeling" but not trying to induce a seizure, and they are caused by ongoing activity of the mind (22).

The word "psychogenic" was introduced into psychiatry in 1894 by Robert Sommer (23). He referred to "morbid states which are evoked by ideas and can be influenced by ideas." The original definition was intended to refer to a group of cases forming part of the hysterical spectrum. Kraeplin (24) considered psychogenic to refer "not only to hysteria but also to other forms of degenerative insanity." Campbell (25) draws attention to progressively less selective application of the term over the years "so that it becomes synonymous with 'mental' or 'psychological,' or something they distill." Within the field of epilepsy there has been a tendency to use the term "psychogenic" to refer to pseudoseizures (hysterical seizures): "The most frequently encountered of non-epileptic seizures are psychogenic seizures, also called hysterical [seizures] or pseudoseizures" (26). This is unfortunate, because it has given the word "psychogenic" a pejorative flavor that it does not deserve. Sonnen (27) draws attention to possible confusion: "Psychogenic seizures are seizures provoked by some psychic event and both epileptic and hysterical attacks can be provoked in this way." We are concerned here with cases of "true" epilepsy where individual seizures may be precipitated or provoked by acts of will or specific functions of the mind, and they can therefore be described as "psychogenic seizures" in a literal sense of the term. Thus, the thinking epilepsies of Ingvar and Nyman (28) would be included in the term "psychogenic seizures."

Primary Psychogenic Epileptic Seizures

Primary psychogenic epileptic seizures are those seizures which the patient attempts to precipitate deliberately by an act of will. He has usually learned by experience that by thinking specific thoughts or feelings he is able to generate a seizure at will. Thus, by a willed action the patient alters neuronal activity in brain areas surrounding his epileptogenic focus, thereby allowing a seizure to arise. Psychogenic epileptic seizures are common; some examples may be helpful.

Case 1
A young man aged 36 had suffered from complex partial seizures since the age of 4 years, following an attack of meningitis.

His seizures commenced in his left temporal lobe and were accompanied by an epigastric aura and a feeling of sadness. He had discovered, when an adolescent, that thinking sad thoughts could cause an aura which would then go on to trigger a secondary generalized seizure. At the time of his father's death, when the patient was in his late teens, he would frequently use his seizures to blot out his miseries and unhappiness. He could generate his own seizures by encouraging feelings of unhappiness to arise within him.

Case 2

A 40-year-old woman suffered from brain damage at birth, resulting in focal motor adversive seizures arising in her right frontal lobe. These seizures would start with her head and eyes turning slowly to the left, followed by secondary generalization and a tonic–clonic grand mal seizure. She discovered, again in her teens, that she could generate these seizures herself by slowly moving her head in the direction that it was moved by the aura, while at the same time deliberately looking out of the left-hand corner of her eyes. She found that the seizures were even more likely to occur if this procedure was accompanied by chomping movements of her jaws. She too, as an adolescent, would carry out this maneuver to produce seizures when her mother had upset her.

Patients with either absence attacks or primary grand mal seizures are also able to generate their own seizures.

Case 3

A 19-year-old boy had suffered from petit mal epilepsy since the age of 7. His mother had suspected for many years that when she was cross and scolded him he would have a shower of absence attacks. However, he had always denied it. In the clinic he told me how he achieved it. He did this by an alteration of his attention. While listening to his mother scolding him, he would suddenly swing his attention to the periphery of his visual attentional field, so as in some way to produce a split in his concentration. This would automatically induce a small absence seizure. He retained this ability right up to the age at which he finally lost his absence attacks.

Case 4

A 22-year-old man with a strong family history of epilepsy had had tonic–clonic seizures from the age of 9. There was no evidence of any brain damage either in his history or in his investigations. His seizures commenced with his losing consciousness without a warning and had no focal features. He discovered that he could generate his seizures by lying on the bed and deliberately holding his mind empty and blank for a number of minutes. This would lead to a grand mal seizure; he would then awake in a postictal state, confused and disoriented—a sensation that he quite enjoyed. Not infrequently he would do this on weekends whenever he was bored and disgusted.

Both these patients with generalized seizures were able to generate their attacks by manipulating their attention. It thus seems clear that primary psychogenic epileptic seizures may be produced either by activating specific brain areas (in the case of focal seizures) or by using the mechanism of attention and thus altering arousal levels throughout the brain (in the case of generalized seizures).

In a recent survey of 76 patients attending the epilepsy clinic at the Maudsley Hospital, 22.4% (Fig. 1) answered "Yes" to the question, "This may seem a strange question, but some people with epilepsy have at some time, by a conscious wish, caused a seizure to occur. Have you ever done this?" (pseudosei-

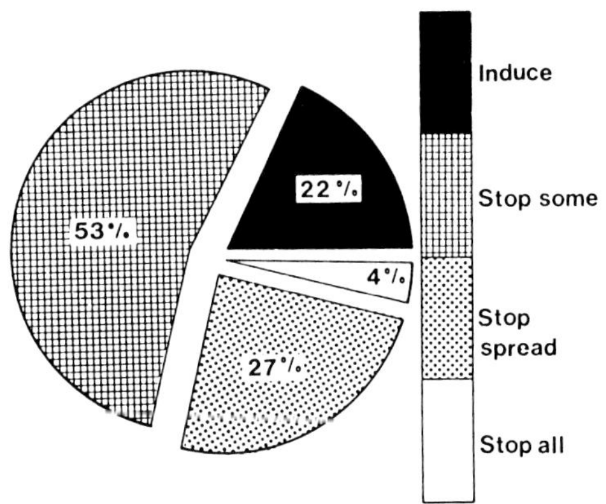

FIG. 1. In a recent study of 76 patients at the Maudlsey Hospital Epilepsy Clinic, carried out by Dr. Loza, 22% could voluntarily induce their seizures; 53% could sometimes stop their seizures; 27% were able to stop their seizures from spreading; and only 4% were always able to inhibit their seizures once they had started. (From ref. 128, with permission.)

zures were carefully excluded). In answer to the question, "Have you ever, when feeling upset in some way, encouraged a seizure to come?", 15.6% said that they had. However, when asked, "Can you describe what you need to do to make a seizure occur?", 28.6% were able to do so. These percentages suggest that between one-quarter and one-third of patients attending a psychiatric epilepsy clinic are able to generate their own seizures at will, which may seem high. However, Dahl et al. (29) report that 16% of their children "can elicit seizure on demand," suggesting that the Maudsley figures are likely to be correct.

It is well known that patients describe having a higher frequency of seizures in certain situations. In the Maudsley survey, over 50% of the patients said that they had seizures when they were tense, depressed, or tired, and over 30% had them when they were angry, excited, or bored (Fig. 2). In 1984, Tempkin and Davis (30) studied the effect of major life events, and of more minor stresses and strains, on the likelihood of patients having seizures. In a prospective design using 12 patients with severe epilepsy, they monitored the occurrence of seizure and stress over a 3-month period. They found that high stress lev-

els and stressful events were associated with more frequent seizures for most patients. Negative events were the most powerful, whereas positive events seldom correlated with an increase in seizure frequency. This paper confirms our observation from the Maudsley Epilepsy Clinic that happiness is a very powerful anticonvulsant. Only 4% of patients said that they had seizures when they were happy. Dahl et al. (29) reported that 66% of the children in their study could "identify a low-risk situation for seizure occurrence." There is thus a very fine line between deliberate induction of seizures and allowing oneself the luxury of a mental state that you know is likely to induce a seizure.

Secondary Psychogenic Epileptic Seizures— The "Thinking" Epilepsies

Just as stimulation of the brain by a peripheral input will in certain cases cause seizures, so too will activity within the brain caused by thinking or emotional feelings. Seizures brought on by thinking, calculating, and other mental acts have been called the "thinking epilepsies" by Ingvar and Nyman (28), Fenwick (21), and Merliss (15). Mental activity, such as multiplication or addition, can precipitate seizure activity (13,31–36). Wilkins et al. (37) reported the case of a patient with a parietal lobe lesion who had an absence attack whenever he carried out a mathematical calculation. Wilkins gave the subject the Wechsler Adult Intelligence Scale (WAIS) test while measuring his EEG, and he found that the subtests which tested predominantly spatial abilities produced excessive amounts of spike-and-wave activity. Block design was the test that produced the greatest increase. Wilkins was able to show that tests which specifically activated the parietal region were the most effective in producing spike-and-wave activity. Thus, there is little doubt that specific stimuli, either mental or physical, can produce seizures by changing levels of excitation in epileptogenic zones.

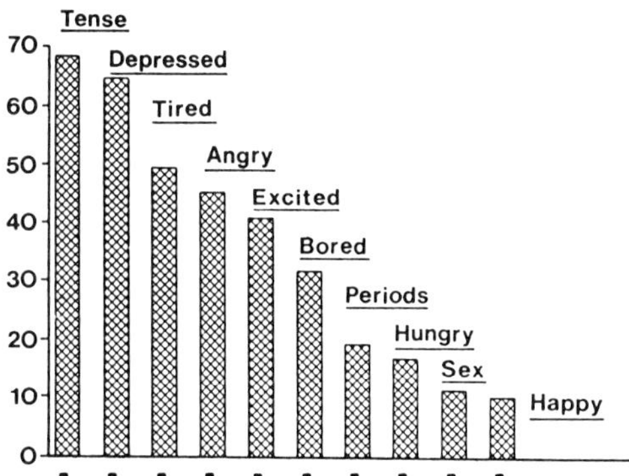

FIG. 2. In a recent survey at the Maudsley Hospital, patients (*N* = 76) were asked which mental states tended to precipitate seizures. The above graph shows the most important factors. It is interesting that nearly 70% of patients had more seizures when they were tense or depressed but that only 7% had more seizures when they were happy. It would seem that happiness is a powerful anticonvulsant. (From ref. 128, with permission.)

SEIZURE INHIBITION

Seizure inhibition, like seizure generation, consists of both primary and secondary components. Primary seizure inhibition is the direct inhibition of seizures by an act of will; secondary seizure inhibition is the inhibition of seizures by an action of mind or behavior which interferes with seizure generation but which is not deliberately intended to do so (38).

Primary Inhibition

The use of external stimulation to inhibit seizure occurrence is already well-reported (39–42). Most patients will admit to having a mental mechanism which they use to try to inhibit their seizures. A study of 70 outpatients at the Maudsley Hospital has shown that 36.4% claimed that they could sometimes stop their seizures. In answer to the question, "Do you sometimes make yourself have fewer seizures?", 33.8% said "Yes." When asked the question, "Can you sometimes stop your seizures from happening?", 36.4% said "Yes." In response to the question, "Can you stop your seizures from spreading?", 27.3% said "Yes" (Fig. 1).

These mental mechanisms do not always succeed: Clearly, patients do have seizures which they cannot stop. In response to the question, "Can you always stop seizures if you try?", only 3.9% said "Yes." However, the removal of specific precipitants can be very valuable.

Case 1
A 42-year-old woman had her first grand mal seizure at the age of 16, when she then came to medical attention. Since the age of 6 or 7 she had had feelings of déjà vu which had at times been associated with feelings of guilt. She mentioned one occasion when her vicar called and she had not done her typing for the church magazine. She felt very guilty and immediately had a seizure. Her therapy, in part, consisted of helping her deal with her guilt. She has stated that the most powerful anticonvulsant that she has ever received was, firstly, the recognition that guilt brought on her seizures and, secondly, to be taught a method of dealing with this guilt.

This patient had a right temporal lesion, with a right temporal focus on EEG. It is likely that it was a medial surface lesion, because she had dilatation of her right temporal

horn. Thus the group 1 neurons were probably situated in the hippocampus and amygdala, and these areas were involved in her feelings of guilt. It is thus likely that when she felt guilty she was activating this area. When seizures arise from a different area of cortex, different inhibitory strategies will be needed.

Case 2
A 28-year-old man had been suffering from focal motor seizures for 2 years. These seizures were confined to his left leg, and they consisted of rhythmical jerking of the leg, lasting from a few seconds to a minute, with practically no impairment of consciousness. He found that walking down an incline or walking into a large room was likely to precipitate an attack. In each case, the feeling of unsteadiness was the trigger. In the case of the incline, unsteadiness was due to poor balance; in the case of the room, however, unsteadiness was caused by a sudden change in visual cues. His seizures were considerably helped by telling him to keep his gaze fixed on a point when walking down an incline or when entering a wide open space. He reported that after dong this he experienced fewer seizures in those situations.

Although it is not possible to be certain why this strategy succeeded, it is known that with routine movements such as stepping and walking, the task-related fusimotor drive—the "set"—is operated at a low level as well as being static. However, when motor actions are difficult or unpredictable, the dynamic gamma-motor neuronal drive is turned on at full force, and there is enhanced feedback from the muscle spindles (43). It is possible that this change in feedback in some way alters the excitability of the cortex, thus altering the ability of cells to be recruited into the seizure discharge. Further evidence for this comes from magnetic stimulation of the brain. It is known that the threshold of the motor cortex controlling a limb is considerably reduced if the limb is taking part in, or is about to be used in, a voluntary movement. This suggests that the excitability level of motor neuron pools is susceptible to the anticipation of conscious movement. It is possible that by getting this patient to fix his gaze on a specific point (thereby stabilizing his walking), he did not have to bring into action his dynamic fusimotor drive; furthermore, the motor cortex threshold was not significantly changed, since no complex movements were required.

Efron (39) described a patient with temporal lobe epilepsy who experienced an unusually prolonged and stereotyped aura, beginning with depersonalization and proceeding through phases of forced thinking, olfactory hallucinations, and auditory hallucinations and resulting in adversive head movement and a tonic–clonic seizure. Smelling an unpleasant odor prior to the phase of forced thinking aborted a seizure, but it did not reduce the overall frequency of auras. Presumably the stimulus altered the excitability of cells surrounding the focus in some nonspecific way, thus preventing further spread of the seizure discharge. Later, it was possible to condition the patient to a visual stimulus (a bracelet which was present at the same time as the smell) so that seizures could be aborted by looking at the bracelet alone. It was fortuitously discovered that a similar effect occurred if the patient thought about the bracelet instead of actually looking at it. Following this, there was a decline in seizure frequency until the patient eventually considered herself cured. On the model that is being put forward, it would have to be argued that thinking about the conditioned stimulus changed neuronal excitability in the area of the brain from which seizures were arising. Some support for this is provided by both (a) blood flow studies, which show that blood flow is increased in the expected cortical areas during thinking, and (b) recent EEG brain mapping work, which indicates a change in EEG frequencies over the active area of cortex.

Indirect Primary Inhibition

Indirect primary inhibition of seizures occurs when the patient carries out a set of actions (either physical or mental) which are designed to stop the seizure from occurring or generalizing but which act in a nonspecific way.

Although it is convenient to think of both scizure induction and inhibition as being capable of altering the level of cortical excitability surrounding an epileptic focus, and thus either facilitating or inhibiting the spread of seizure discharges, there are cases where this model does not seem to fit so well. Penn and Wada (44) described the case of a woman with a right temporal lesion and an aura of déjà vu who was able to inhibit her complex partial seizures by singing. She was being assessed for temporal lobectomy, and the intracarotid sodium amytal test showed that her cerebral dominance for speech was located in the left hemisphere, with her dominance for music being located in the right hemisphere. Humming was found not to inhibit seizure activity, although singing did so. Unfortunately, it is now known whether verbal activity on its own would be as effective as singing. What this case showed was that left hemisphere involvement was essential (the words of the song and not just the tune) if her seizures were to be inhibited.

Because the excitability of the brain can be altered in a global fashion by changes in reticular formation activity, many nonspecific strategies make use of this mechanism to inhibit seizures. Mostofsky and Balaschak (45) give examples of different strategies which have been found to be effective in stopping seizures (see below). The main mechanism of action is the alerting of the patient in some way, thereby altering the level of cortical excitability in a nonspecific way. Patients whose seizures have focal onsets will commonly say "no" to themselves, or else they will try to attend to something different at the onset of the aura.

Case 3

A 35-year-old woman with focal motor seizures starting in her arm would, immediately after they started, walk about the room or in some other way alert herself. By doing this she was sometimes able to stop the seizures from spreading.

Case 4

A young man would hit his arm at the seizure onset, and this would sometimes prevent the seizure from generalizing. Whether this functioned by nonspecific arousal or by local stimulation of the arm, thereby indirectly changing cortical motor excitability, is debatable.

The modification of focal cortical epileptogenic discharges by afferent impulses has been described by Prince (46) and Tassinari (47).

Deliberate alerting in boring situations has been known to produce a reduction in petit mal seizures. Jung (48) showed that seizure frequency fell in a patient with petit mal epilepsy when he was kept interested. In another single case study, Ounsted et al. (49) described the case of a girl with petit mal absences who was subjected to a burst of photic stimulation (described by her as being mildly unpleasant) whenever a spike-and-wave paroxysm occurred on her EEG during the experimental sessions. After having been severely incapacitated by frequent absence seizures, the patient improved and had only occasional seizures. These investigators speculated that repeated photic bombardment raised the total level of physiological arousal, and analysis of background EEG data supported this by showing a decrease in slow-wave components.

Pritchard et al. (50) found that about 10% (7 of 71) of their patients with complex partial seizures were able to reduce their seizure frequency. Those who could reduce and limit their seizures had attained higher educational status, better social and vocational adjustment, and better psychological adjustment than those who could not. They were also more likely to have right-hemisphere EEG abnormalities. None of 18 patients with simple partial seizures were able to reduce seizure frequency. The strategies which individual patients used were highly idiosyncratic. Four patients used a mental relaxation technique, two used physical measures, and one used a combination of the two. One patient who had an EEG taken during his relaxation exercise showed a reduction in interictal spiking for 3 min during practice.

Dahl et al. (29) reported that in a group of 18 children, about 40% were "at some time able to counteract seizure." The methods the children used are not described. However, the figure of 40% is very close to that of the Maudsley figure of 36.4%. Clearly, more studies are required in this area: firstly, to determine the actual strategies the patients use and, secondly, to find how frequently patients employ these methods of seizure limitation.

Secondary Inhibition

Secondary inhibition occurs when a patient behaves or thinks in such a way as to produce a reduction in seizure frequency by an alteration in cortical activity surrounding the focus, without deliberately intending to do so. Maintenance of interest or alertness are such measures. A recent study (51) measured the number of seizures that children had in the art room when soothing music was played, and the children were kept interested in painting and modeling. Their seizure frequency was compared with an ordinary class when there was no music and no special attempt was made to keep the childrens' interest. During the interesting and relaxed art class, the children had significantly fewer seizures.

It is usual for patients to state that there are situations in which they seldom, if ever, have seizures. This varies from patient to patient and also varies with the type of epilepsy. Some patients will have a greatly reduced seizure frequency, or even no seizures, when they are on vacation. Others say that they are unlikely to have seizures at the theater–that is, in situations in which their interest is held. Yet other patients report that a low-key lifestyle, with regular and habitual activity, is the one way in which they can keep themselves seizure-free (see above).

There is now some evidence that if psychological variables are targeted in treatment programs, there is a consequent decrease in seizure frequency. Davis et al. (52) studied the effect of a cognitive-behavioral program on the depressive symptoms of 13 clinically depressed epilepsy patients. They counseled the patients in 2-hr weekly sessions over a period of 6 weeks. At the end of the study the group is reported as being much improved (see section behavioral treatments, below).

Although it is not known why these particular strategies work for particular people, it does seem that certain types of activity tend to enhance the possibility of seizure occurrence, whereas others tend to prevent it. The final common pathway for all such activity in those patients who have focal seizures is the stimulation of group 2 neurons, so that they become sufficiently excited to take part in the seizure discharges. A reduction in the excitability levels of this pool of neurons will lead directly to seizure inhibition. Interest or boredom in a task also leads to changes in reticular formation activity and thus leads to the modification of excitability in pools of group 2 neurons, thereby altering the likelihood of seizure discharges.

SEIZURE BEHAVIOR

Patients who have focal seizures, particularly those whose seizures are followed by complex automatisms, show a very wide range of behavior during the seizure itself, as well as during the period of automatic activity. In these patients there is frequently an interaction between the patient, his mental content at the time his seizure starts, and his environment. Patients who have generalized tonic–clonic seizures show stereotyped behavior consisting of (a) loss of consciousness, (b) falling to the ground, and (c) tonic–clonic jerking movements and a postictal confusional state. Because of the complete and total disruption of brain activity, there is no integration between the seizure behavior and the patient's environment.

The time course of an automatism can be divided into three parts:

1. *The initial phase.* This phase lasts only a few seconds and usually consists of staring or simple mouthing and chewing movements.
2. *The intermediate phase.* This phase consists of more complex behavior which is still stereotyped and repetitive, such as fumbling with objects, picking at clothes, or standing up and turning. This lasts a few seconds or minutes.
3. *The final phase.* In this phase, behavior is most complex and may range from the stereotyped into the normal. Complex movements of turning and standing may progress to searching, handling, and walking, which then merge imperceptibly into normal behavior (53).

Memory is always impaired during an automatism, because for the automatism to arise there must have been a bilateral spread of the seizure discharge into the periamygdaloid–hippocampal structures. Jasper (54) has shown, in stimulation experiments at operation, that automatisms arise when the bilateral involvement of the amygdaloid–hippocampal structures spreads to the mesial diencephalon and temporoparietal cortex. Automatisms usually arise in patients with temporal lobe lesions, but they are also seen in discharging lesions of the frontal lobe and of the orbitofrontal and parietal regions of the mesial surface of the hemisphere (55,56). Consciousness is also interfered with during an automatism, so that actions are poorly directed and executed. The patient appears to be confused, dazed, and disoriented. Aggressive acts are very rare, but they are more common out of hospital than in hospital. Most automatisms are brief. Knox (57) found that 80% last less than 5 min, 12% less than 15 min, and the remaining 8% less than 1 hr. In a study of 40 patients with 163 complex partial seizures, 14% lasted less than 30 sec, with the ictal phase ranging from 3 to 343 sec (mean 54 sec) and the postictal phase ranging from 3 to 767 sec (mean 89 sec) (58).

There is always some interaction between the patient and his environment during a complex partial seizure: The form the automatism takes is at least partly determined by the patient's thought content and surroundings before a seizure begins. Forster and Liske (59) quote the case of an organist who had a seizure while playing a hymn. He stopped during the aura and then played a few bars of jazz before recommencing the hymn again. Thus, if during an epileptic automatism a crime is committed, it is possible that some elements of the action may appear purposive.

Because the seizure discharges activate structures which are already involved in ongoing behavior, the later phases of the automatism contain some of this activity. Thus, patients who have complex partial seizures on the pavement seldom walk into the road, and patients who have seizures on station platforms seldom fall onto the track. Although both these do happen, they happen less frequently than might be expected.

PSYCHOLOGICAL METHODS FOR TREATMENT OF EPILEPSY

Because of the close relationship between seizure activity and the ongoing patterns of excitation and inhibition in the neuronal pools which surround the epileptogenic focus, it would be expected that if these neuronal patterns could be modified by a change in behavior, this would also result in an alteration in seizure activity. Thus, it would be predicted that standard methods of behavior modification would alter seizure activity. Two major reviews in this area are those by Mostofsky and Balaschak (45) and by Mostofsky (60). This section will concentrate on more recent work in this area, and readers are referred to the above reviews for an account of the early studies. The classification system used by Mostofsky and Balaschak (45) defines three areas: reward management, self-control, and psychophysiological treatments. Many of the cases reported in the literature are single case studies without proper controls. Indeed, as pointed out by Mostofsky and Balaschak, in most of these studies it is not clear whether the experimenters have successfully isolated any single treatment variable. These methodological points were also raised by Krafft and Poling (61) in their critical review of 11 studies that used operant or respondent conditioning procedures in the treatment of seizure disorders.

It must also be recognized that there is likely to be more than one therapeutic factor in a conditioning program. For example, the success of the program will improve the patient's self-image and will enhance their self-esteem. Any consequent drug reduction will improve the patient's alertness and sense of well-being, and this may lead to employment being obtained. All these factors will then tend to accelerate a positive behavioral change and will thus reduce seizure frequency (see above).

Reward Management

Overt Reward

Reward programs aim to positively reinforce seizure-free periods. The rewards can be either (a) an increase in privileges or (b) tokens allowing the purchase of privileges (62–65). Cataldo et al. (66), in line with previous work, treated a 5-year-old boy suffering from frequent myoclonic seizures (occurring 50–400 times a day) and occasional grand mal seizures (occurring two to six times a week) by giving him sweets, contingent upon non-seizure activity following a progressive schedule. The results showed an elimination of his grand mal seizures and also showed a great reduction in myoclonic activity, although there was some reversal of the trend upon removal of the reward.

Cinciripini et al. (67), in a complex behavioral program involving both restraint and reward, significantly reduced seizure frequencies in a 7-year-old child who suffered from petit mal seizures and who had both spontaneous seizures and precipitated seizures by self-stimulation with his hand in front of a light. Treatment consisted of (a) holding his hand and (b) differential reinforcement distracting his attention. The differential reinforcement consisted of (a) praise for using his hands appropriately at a task or (b) praise for keeping them flat on the table and attending to his classroom work. There was a rapid improvement in all target symptoms during the program, and the effects were well maintained at an 8-month follow-up.

Covert Reward

Covert reward is the giving of a reward in fantasy rather than reality. The usual procedure is for the patient to imagine situations in which seizures may occur, and then to fantasize about (a) the nonoccurrence of seizures and (b) the positive gains that would follow. Usually, the imagined occurrence of seizures is included, and this is followed by imagined punishments (non-reward). These fantasy sessions are usually carried out as part of a relaxation program, so it is possible that the mechanism involved is covert desensitization rather than covert reward (see below). However, no study has yet tried to disentangle these two aspects (68, 69).

Denial of Reward

Seizures evoke in other people a humane response and a wish to help. This natural response often leads to involvement and overprotection by the patient's caregiver. Because there is a close relationship between behavior and seizure activity (as we have already seen), this natural response may inadvertently reinforce behaviors leading to seizures. The seizure then becomes a powerful method of controlling the patient's relationships. Dahl et al. (29) noted that 50% of the children in their study "reported mainly positive consequences associated with seizures." The psychological strategy of denial of reward is a direct attempt to break this cycle. Gardner (70) reported the abolition of seizures in a 10-year-old girl after her parents were instructed to ignore their daughter's seizures. (It's not entirely clear whether these were pseudoseizures or true seizures). A second study is that of Daniels (69).

Punishment Program

Penalty Program

This strategy involves intervention (following a seizure) by either withdrawal of privileges or placing the patient in a time-out room (65,71).

Punishment Program

The aim of a punishment program is to follow a seizure immediately with an unpleasant stimulus such as a foul odor, electric shocks, shouting, or hitting the patient (64,71–74).

Relief Avoidance

In relief avoidance paradigms, the occurrence of seizure activity, either electrically or behaviorally, invokes the onset of an unpleasant stimulus. This stimulus then continues until there is either a reduction in seizure behavior or an improvement in electrical seizure activity.

Clearly, this strategy is very close to overt punishment. However, it would seem to be classifiable as a distinct entity, since the punishment is discrete and continuous until there is an alteration in seizure activity (49,75,76).

Self-control Strategies

The aim of self-control procedures is to allow the patient, by cognitive processes, to gain control of his seizure activity. Patients normally use a wide range of self-control strategies to avoid having seizures. It must also be recognized that in some patients similar strategies are used to induce seizures. Self-control strategies are thus aimed at the elimination of seizure induction and the reinforcement of seizure inhibition.

Self-Control

Self-control strategies have already been specifically mentioned in the discussion of primary and secondary psychogenic seizures and of primary and secondary inhibition of seizures. It is clear that most patients with epilepsy have cognitive strategies that they use to inhibit seizure activity, both by avoiding circumstances that they know are likely to cause seizures and by attempting to abort seizures once they have begun (22,38,77; also see above).

Relaxation and Desensitization

Relaxation training usually involves progressive relaxation using the method of Wolpe (78). The patient is taught deep muscular relaxation and is then encouraged to reproduce these feelings of relaxation if a seizure seems imminent. Wells et al. (79) carried out such a study in a group of patients with psychomotor seizures. They were taught how to relax, and they could induce this feeling of relaxation when they felt a seizure was about to occur. The training generalized well from a hospital to a home situation, and the investigators reported a reduction of seizures in their cases.

Rousseau et al. (80) studied 15 patients with epilepsy, only eight of whom completed the investigation. They took into account the methodological criticisms of Krafft and Poling (61) and Mostofsky and Balaschak (45). The patients were suffering mainly from complex partial seizures, with and without secondary generalization. The groups were split into two. Group 1 had baseline assessment followed by a period of treatment and then a second period of treatment. Group 2 had baseline assessment followed by sham treatment and then a period of active treatment. The treatment consisted of progressive relaxation using the differentiation training tape of Goleman

(81). The sham treatment consisted of being told to sit quietly for 20 min twice a day and then being told to "relax as best they could."

The results of the study showed an overall significant decrease in seizure frequency for the treatment conditions. However, there was also a significant decrease in two of the four patients in the sham treatment group. Of interest was one subject who showed a reduction from 77 to 38 seizures during the sham treatment but who returned almost to baseline during the real treatment. The second subject showed a decrease in the sham sessions but showed a further decrease in the real sessions. This could suggest that nonspecific factors play an important part in any study of this nature, but because the sham and treatment procedures are so similar, it may simply mean that the sham condition was a weaker form of therapy, a result not without interest.

An extension of this method is relaxation and covert desensitization. In this method the patient carries out a protocol of relaxation and, while relaxed, imagines both (a) the occurrence of a seizure and (b) the anxiety that having a seizure produces. Desensitization to the occurrence of a seizure is thought to result in reduction in seizure frequency (38,82–87). The Swedish group, Melin and Dahl, have published widely in this area. Their first study (88), which involved four single subjects with different seizure types, determined the effect of contingent relaxation on epileptic seizures. These investigators showed a significant fall in seizures in all their patients. In their latter two cases they tried a short period of reversal when the subjects were instructed not to relax themselves on the cue of a seizure occurring. There is some suggestion that seizures may have increased in this period. Follow-up continued for 6 months, during which time seizure reduction continued. This study showed that psychomotor seizures and auras respond more than do grand mal seizures, and that relaxation is necessary. Although nonspecific controls were not used, the study is encouraging.

A later study determined whether or not children were able to predict the likelihood of a seizure and detect its onset (29). The children were instructed in the characteristics of their seizure onset and were asked to undergo avoidance behavior therapy of many different types. Eighteen children entered the study.

All 18 were able to predict their seizures; three could elicit them on demand, and 12 were able to identify situations at a low risk for seizure occurrence. The 18 children were split up into three groups of six: The first one was an active treatment group whose members were taught the early signals concerning their seizure onset and were then taught a method of relaxation to counteract this; the second one was an attentional control group whose members were given the same amount of attention by the psychologist; the third one was a control group who were not specifically treated during the study. The results were of interest because they showed that the children were able to discover preseizure cues and also because the use of a relaxation technique significantly reduced seizure frequency. Nonspecific attention did not have this effect. This study is important because it clearly showed the benefit of the identification of seizure cues and also showed the possibility of their modification by behavioral techniques.

In 1987, Dahl et al. (89), in a more sophisticatedly controlled study, looked at a group of 18 adults with refractory seizures. In phase 1 of the study, patients were divided into three groups: a relaxation group, a control group given attention, and a no-treatment group. The relaxation treatment was a standard training in muscle relaxation, which the patients were taught to carry out during their everyday life. They were asked to use this particularly in situations of high risk when they were likely to have a seizure. The attentional control group received professional attention in the form of supportive therapy, and the number of sessions attended was equal to that of the treatment group. An additional waiting-list control group was added. Results of the study showed that those patients who were given relaxation therapy achieved a significant reduction in the number of seizures. The attentional group, surprisingly, showed an increase in the number of seizures, probably because these patients were required to focus on seizure behavior. The study also showed that patients were able to determine the early onset of their seizures and were then able to abort them with the relaxation procedure. However, not all seizures could be stopped this way, and the investigators could find no clear predictors as to those seizures which could or could not be stopped. After the end of the study, patients reported increased confidence and greater control over their epilepsy.

Dahl et al. (90) and Dahl and Brorson (91) further investigated subjects' ability to modify their seizures once preseizure cues had been fully identified. In three children with severe refractory seizures, they first studied the effect on the frequency of seizures once the children had been taught to discriminate the early effects of paroxysmal activity and/or the sensations preceding seizures. This information did not affect the children's seizure frequency. However, when an intervention technique consisted of an adapted countermeasure (e.g., the moving of an arm in the direction opposite to that caused by seizure onset), then both seizure frequency and paroxysmal EEG activity were significantly reduced. Because of the design of the study and the improvement brought about by this intervention technique, no further improvement was noted after subsequent contingent relaxation therapy or after positive reinforcement for correct responses. What this paper does show is that it is not sufficient just to identify preseizure behavior but that there must also be an active intervention, and it is the result of this intervention which stops seizures from spreading and reduces seizure frequency.

The method of flooding—that is, exposing the patient to the situation in which a seizure is likely to be evoked—has been used by Pinto (92) in one patient, with some success.

Psychotherapy

Individual or group psychotherapy has been tried by different investigators. The aim of the psychotherapy is usually directed towards allowing the patient to gain an understanding of himself and of the relationship between his seizures and his difficulties in life. Group psychotherapy not only has these aims, but also modifies the patient's relationship with other peer members and gives further insight into how other patients with epilepsy deal with their personal problems and with their seizures. It is likely that psychotherapy works at many different levels. Better life adjustment leads to greater relaxation and a sense of fulfillment (both powerful anticonvulsants), together with, in some patients, the reduction of covert seizure induction. Discussion of cognition surrounding the seizures leads to enhanced strategies of self-control (93,94). That this is not always successful is shown in a report of Correa (95), who attempted to change the locus of control of 13 children with epilepsy. Despite an education program, no significant changes in the locus of control measures were noted, nor were there any significant changes in seizure frequency.

Tan and Bruni (96) studied a group of patients undergoing cognitive behavior therapy and supportive counseling and compared them with a waiting-list, no-treatment control group. Twenty-seven patients were assigned to one of these conditions. The aim of the study was to produce an alleviation of psychosocial problems, along with a reduction of seizure frequency. The cognitive behavior therapy group received a total of eight 2-hr sessions of group cognitive behavior therapy each week. The supportive counseling group had a similar number of sessions, but discussion within the group was related to a clarification of feelings, with no specific control behaviors being taught. The results showed no significant differences in terms of seizure frequency and patients' complaints between any of the three groups. However, a global rating of psychological adjustment was found to be improved for the two therapy groups but not for the waiting-list control. The investigators comment that, overall, little support was found for the efficacy of group cognitive behavior therapy for the reduction of psychosocial difficulties or seizures.

Helpfulness and resourcefulness in coping with epilepsy were studied by Rosenbaum and Palmon (97). They argued that the emotional sequelae of epilepsy are a joint function of the severity of the epilepsy and the repertoire of individual self-control skills. They therefore postulated that there should be a relationship between seizure frequency and resourcefulness. The patients were divided into two groups: highly resourceful and less resourceful. The significant finding was that in the medium and low categories of seizure frequency, the highly resourceful subjects were significantly less depressed and anxious and coped better with their disability as compared to the less resourceful subjects. However, in the high-frequency range of seizures, the highly resourceful and less resourceful epilepsy patients showed equally low levels of emotional adjustment. These data suggest that patients with less severe epilepsy are influenced by their ability to cope with personal and social circumstances.

An interesting variation was the technique of Feldman and Paul (98), who showed the patients videotapes of their seizures during the treatment sessions. They reported significant seizure reduction in all five patients who were treated. Although the investigators claim that the improvement was due to "the conscious awareness of the association between the specific emotional stimulus and the seizure" [as Mostofsky and Balaschak (45) point out], several other psychological mechanisms could have been involved.

PSYCHOPHYSIOLOGICAL METHODS FOR TREATMENT OF EPILEPSY

One of the most interesting concepts related to epilepsy is that seizures are capable of being precipitated in a classical Pavlovian conditioning paradigm. This has been demonstrated by Forster (99) in brain-damaged cats as well as by Gastaut in humans. The conditioning of seizures is a fragile process, and the establishment of the conditioned response could be obliterated by one grand mal seizure. However, the important point is not the fragility of the response but that the principle has been shown. Forster (100) is the major investigator in the field of applying the classical methods of habituation and extinction to the control of epilepsy. The aim of this method is to extinguish the abnormal cortical discharges which are evoked by a specific stimulus, by continually exposing the subject to the stimulus until habituation occurs. This has been tried in the visual, auditory, and sensory modalities, with some success (41,101–104).

Biofeedback

Anticonvulsant Rhythms

There was a vogue in the 1970s, started by Sterman (105), for using biofeedback training to increase the 12- to 16-Hz sensorimotor rhythm (SMR) in humans, in the belief that this could have powerful anticonvulsant properties. This work was taken up by several different investigators, with varying degrees of success (106–109). Tansey (110) reported a single case study of sensorimotor training in a significantly undermedicated 14-year-old girl with petit mal epilepsy. After 21 training sessions, her absence seizures ceased, her emotional problems and sudden rages improved, and her physicians were able to discontinue her medication. Of interest is the 30% increase in her SMR rhythm on withdrawal of her medication, accompanied by the marked improvement in her quality of life. However, there was no control period in this report, and again this case could simply reflect nonspecific changes, although this is an unlikely explanation.

Some investigators reported no success, and they attributed any reduction in seizure frequency to nonspecific factors rather than to enhancement in SMR training (111–113), although Kuhlman (114) was able to show that biofeedback training for a 9- to 14-Hz SMR was effective in reducing seizures in 60% of the epilepsy subjects tested. Kuhlman was able to exclude both placebo and relaxation effects, because both random feedback and yoked control procedures were included. Although this experiment again showed the effectiveness of biofeedback procedures, compared to relaxation and placebo, it still left unanswered the specificity of the SMR. A study by Quy et al. (115) showed no clear reduction in seizure frequency that could be specifically attributed to the SMR group (for a review see ref. 21).

Sterman and Shouse (116) extended their observations by investigating the difference between fast activity and SMR feedback by treating eight 18- to 35-year-old patients with an 8- to 24-year history of psychomotor seizures. Patients were given 10 laboratory feedback sessions; half of the patients received rewards for producing SMR activity (12–15 Hz), and the other half were given fast activity feedback (18–23 Hz). The two groups were then reversed, so that each received the alternative type of feedback. Some home practice was also given, using portable feedback units. Significant seizure reduction occurred in both the SMR and the 18- to 23-Hz sessions. The effect of the sessions could also be seen in the patients' sleeping records, when there was an excess of the conditioned EEG frequencies. During the training sessions, there was also a reduction in delta activity and in faster frequencies (20–23 Hz). This led the investigators to conclude that SMR feedback training is nonspecific, that other EEG frequencies are effective, and that EEG feedback training tended to normalize the EEG outside recording sessions. However, in both groups the investigators did note a change in SMR quantity which correlated with seizure reduction. But because many rhythms in the non-SMR feedback group change, it is still not clear whether the SMR change is specific.

A later study by Lantz and Sterman (117) using the same paradigm as that of Sterman and Shouse (116) looked at the neuropsychological changes in 24 patients who were undergoing feedback training. In summary, these investigators found that subjects who showed the greatest seizure reduction performed better on tests of general problem solving ability (but not on other cognitive tests) and were more intact psychosocially. They were, however, worse on tests involving strong motor components. The successful subjects tended to take fewer drugs than did the less successful subjects. Following the training, cognitive and motor functioning improved only in those subjects who showed the greatest seizure reduction; this was confined to those who had undergone active feedback, since it was not seen in subjects whose seizures had fallen during the control conditions. Although there were changes in Minnesota Multiphasic Personality Inventory (MMPI) scores, which tended to improve, this was found in all groups and was not specific to feedback.

Current opinion now supports the view that the SMR change may contain components specific to the reduction of seizures.

Nonspecific EEG Biofeedback

It was to be expected that once Sterman et al. (118) had shown that SMR biofeedback could apparently reduce seizure frequency, other investigators would try the effect of conditioning different rhythms. Cabral and Scott (83) used conventional occipital rhythm biofeedback training, whereas Whyler et al. (119) used biofeedback training to increase fast low-voltage activity and suppress slow-wave activity surrounding the epileptic focus. Both these groups reported some success, as did Kaplan (120) and Kuhlman and Allison (112) using augmentation of mu activity. Lubar et al. (121) reported a well-controlled study containing a nontreatment baseline and noncontingent feedback baseline. They taught eight patients with different seizure types, refractory to medication, either to suppress slow activity at 3–8 Hz or to enhance 12- to 15-Hz activity. A third group simultaneously suppressed 3- to 8-Hz activity while enhancing 11- to 19-Hz activity ("A" phase). These conditions were compared to the enhancement of slow activity (3–8 Hz) ("B" phase). Both neuropsychological testing and EEG analysis were carried out before, during, and after training. The investigators found that there was a reduction of 21% and 15%, respectively, in seizure frequency for the two A conditions of the A–B–A design. The B portion did not result in an increase in seizures, but there was a leveling off of seizure reduction. There was little or no change in psychological test results. This study adds further evidence of the nonspecific nature of EEG operant feedback.

Lockard et al. (122) have extended biofeedback techniques to their alumina-gel monkey model of epilepsy, with some change in seizure frequency, although this was not consistently beneficial. An interesting experiment is that of Pasata (123), in which electrodes were implanted in the caudate nucleus of epileptic cats; 5-Hz stimulation was given to this structure on the occurrence of an interictal cortical spike. Spike depression occurred instantly after the onset of feedback stimulation; this depression became stable after 3–4 days of operant training, and it persisted with very little reinforcement in a daily training schedule. The investigators postulated that by stimulating the caudate nucleus at the time of abnormal spiking, there is a recovery of function of recurrent, inhibitory, caudatocortical loops, which contributes to the stabilization and normalization of cortical excitability.

The reduction of seizure activity through the conditioning of other EEG frequencies is most likely to be due to a nonspecific effect rather than to the direct alteration of cerebral rhythms (for a review see ref. 21).

Feedback of Other Physiological Parameters

An interesting study by Fried et al. (124) argued that seizures could be caused by high cerebral arterial blood carbon dioxide tension ($Paco_2$). They based their work on the findings of Lennox et al. (125), Holmberg (126), and Swanson et al. (127), who showed the relationship between EEG frequencies, abnormal cerebral activity, and $Paco_2$. They argued that patients who showed a high end-tidal CO_2 were likely to have more seizures. If the end-tidal CO_2 could be reduced by training in breathing, then seizure frequency could be expected to fall, and cerebral rhythms normalize. Twenty-two patients (ranging in age between 10 and 42 years) with an abnormal breathing pattern and a wide range of seizure disorders were admitted to the study. Each patient was taught a method of diaphragmatic respiration which would result in (a) a lowering of percent end-tidal CO_2 and (b) a normalization of respiration. The value of percent end-tidal CO_2 was shown to them in a biofeedback form on a video monitor. Both EEG and electrocardiographic (ECG) variables were measured. Eighteen treatment sessions were given. The results of this study showed that respiratory pattern, end-tidal CO_2 levels, and respiratory rate, together as a composite measure, were normalized in the patient group. Their EEG power spectrum "normalized," and their seizure frequency was significantly reduced. This paper suggested that modification of physiological variables other than the EEG by biofeedback methods could be helpful in leading to seizure reduction. However, whether the changes seen were due to a placebo effect or to the active treatment is not yet known.

SUMMARY

These behavioral studies provide abundant evidence of the close interrelation between seizure activity and behavior. They reaffirm the point already made several times in this chapter: Seizures do not occur in a behavioral vacuum. They also strengthen the theoretical framework which provides for behavioral treatment of patients with epilepsy. With the detailed knowledge that we now have of the epilepsy focus and the way that it is connected to the surrounding cerebral mechanisms, it really is not surprising that seizure control is significantly influenced by altering the outlook and behavior of the patient with epilepsy.

Seizures should not be thought of as arising randomly. They occur, in the case of focal seizures, when the pools of group 2 neurons are sufficiently excited for seizure activity to spread. Generalized seizures occur when the level of cortical excitability or of corticoreticular excitation has reached a point at which thalamic recruiting volleys generalize and start to spread.

In the case of the focal epilepsies, a detailed clinical history should be taken as to the nature and characteristics of the aura; the history should also include details regarding the form that the seizure generalization or spread may take. This information allows the accurate location of the seizure focus, as well as of the cerebral structures through which the seizure discharge passes. The position of the focus will determine the relationship between the individual and his epilepsy. It will define those aspects of the psychic life or behavior of a patient which will both trigger and inhibit seizure activity.

Detailed discussion of this information with the patient will help him to understand that his seizures are not part of a random process but are, instead, intimately related to how he feels, what he is doing, and what he is thinking. A complete treatment of epilepsy is not just the administration of drugs; rather, it also includes (a) teaching the patient about his brain and its functioning and (b) how the patient's feelings, thinking, and behavior can all be used in the control of his epilepsy.

REFERENCES

1. Lockard JS. A primate model of clinical epilepsy: mechanisms of action through quantification of therapeutic effects. In: Lockhard JS, Ward AA, eds. *Epilepsy: a window to brain mechanisms.* New York: Raven Press, 1980, pp. 11–49.
2. Musgrave J, Gloor P. The role of the corpus callosum in bilateral interhemispheric synchrony

of spike and wave discharge in feline penicillin epilepsy. *Epilepsia* 1980;21:369–378.

3. Avoli M, Gloor P. Role of the thalamus in generalised penicillin epilepsy: observations on decorticate cats. *Exp Neurol* 77(2):386–402.

4. Fenwick P. The EEG. In: Reynolds E, Trimble M, eds. *Epilepsy and psychiatry*. London: Churchill Livingstone, 1981, 242–263.

5. Engel J, Alzerman R, Caldecott-Hazard F, Kuhl D. Epileptic activation of antagonistic systems may explain paradoxical features of experimental and human epilepsy: a review. In: Wada J, ed. *Kindling*, vol 2. New York: Raven Press, 1981.

6. Lockard JS. Social primate model of epilepsy. In: Lockhard JS, Ward AA, eds. *Epilepsy: a window to brain mechanisms*. New York: Raven Press, 1980, 165–190.

7. Brown D, Fenwick P, Howard R. CNV asymmetries in response to a task of right or left temporal lobe activation. Manuscript in preparation.

8. Anderson E, Fenwick P. CNV used as an indicator of temporal lobe damage in patients with TLE. Manuscript in preparation.

9. Howard R, Fenton G, Fenwick P. *Event related brain potentials and personality in psychopathology: a Pavlovian approach*. Chichester, England: Research Studies Press (John Wiley & Sons, 1982, p. 75.

10. Gasser T, et al. Correlating EEG and IQ: a new look at an old problem using computerised EEG parameters. *Electroencephalogr Clin Neurophysiol* 1983;55:493–504.

11. Gowers W. *Epilepsy and other chronic convulsive disorders: their causes, symptoms and treatment*. London: Churchill, 1901;29.

12. Jackson JH. *Neurological fragments*. Oxford: Oxford University Press, 1925.

13. Symonds C. Excitation and inhibition in epilepsy. *Brain* 1959;82(2):133–146.

14. Penfield W, Erickson TC. *Epilepsy and cerebral localisation*. Springfield, IL: Charles C Thomas, 1974, Ch. 25.

15. Merliss JK. Reflex epilepsy. In: *Handbook of neurology, vol 15: The epilepsies*. 1974.

16. Wilkins AJ, Binnie CD, Darby CE. Visually-induced seizures. *Prog Neurobiol* 1980;15:85–117.

17. Wilkins AJ, Binnie CD, Darby CE. Interhemispheric differences in photosensitive epilepsy I: pattern sensitivity thresholds. *Electroencephalogr Clin Neurophysiol* 1981;52:461–468.

18. Binnie C, Findlay J, Wilkins A. Mechanisms of epileptogenesis in photosensitive epilepsy implied by the effects of moving patterns. *Electroencephalogr Clin Neurophysiol* 1985;61:1–6.

19. Jeavons P, Harding G. *Photosensitive epilepsy: review of the literature and a study of 460 patients*. London: Heinemann, 1975.

20. Newmark ME, Penry AK. *Photosensitivity and epilepsy: a review*. New York: Raven Press, 1979.

21. Fenwick P. Precipitation and inhibition of seizures. Reynolds E, Trimble M, eds. In: *Epilepsy and psychiatry*. London: Churchill Livingstone, 1981, pp. 306–321.

22. Fenwick P, Brown S. Evoked and psychogenic epileptic seizures. *Acta Scand Neurol* 1989;80:535–540.

23. Lewis A. "Psychogenic": a word and its mutations. *Psychol Med* 1972;3:209–215.

24. Kraeplin E. *Psychiatrie*, 5th ed. Leipzig: Bath, 1896.

25. Campbell PG. Psychogenesis. In: Russell G, Hersov, L, eds. *Handbook of psychiatry, vol 4: The neuroses and personality disorders*. Cambridge, England: Cambridge University Press, 1983.

26. Porter RG. *Epilepsy—100 elementary principles. Major problems in neurology, series 12*. Eastbourne: Saunders, 1984.

27. Sonnen AEH. Psychogenic seizures. *Br J Clin Pract* [*Suppl*] 1982;18:53–56.

28. Ingvar DH, Nyman GE. A new psychological trigger mechanism in a case of epilepsy. *Neurology* 1962;12:282.

29. Dahl J, Melin L, Brorson L, Schollin J. Effects of a broad-spectrum behaviour modification treatment programme on children with refractory epileptic seizures. *Epilepsia* 1985;26:303–309.

30. Tempkin N, Davis G. Stress as a risk factor for seizures among adults with epilepsy. *Epilepsia* 1984;25(4):450–456.

31. Bingel A. Reading epilepsy. *Neurology* 1957;7:752–756.

32. Gomez GL, Escueta AV. In: Forster FM, ed. *Reflex epilepsy, behavioural therapy and conditional reflexes*. Springfield, IL: Charles C Thomas, 1977.

33. Ch'en H, Ch'in C, Ch'u C. Chess epilepsy and card epilepsy. *Chin Med J* 1965;84:470–474.

34. Forster FM, Richards JF, Panitch HS, Huisman RE, Paulsen RE. Reflex epilepsy evoked by decision making. *Arch Neurol* 1975;32:54–56.

35. Forster FM. Epilepsy evoked by higher cognitive functions; decision-making epilepsy. In: Forster FM, ed. *Reflex epilepsy, behaviour therapy and conditioned reflexes*. Springfield, IL: Charles C Thomas, 1977;124–134.

36. Cirignotta F, Cicogna P, Lugaresi E. Epileptic seizures during card games and draughts. *Epilepsia* 1980;21:137–140.

37. Wilkins AJ, Zifkin B, Anderman F, McGovern E. Seizures induced by thinking. *Ann Neurol* 1981;11:608–612.

38. Brown S, Fenwick P. Seizure inhibition. *Acta Scand Neurol* 1989.

39. Efron R. The effect of olfactory stimuli in arresting uncinate fits. *Brain* 1956;79:267–281.

40. Forster FM, Paulsen W, Baughman F. Clinical therapeutic conditioning in reading epilepsy. *Neurology* 1969;19:71–77.

41. Forster FM. Behavioral therapy of reflex epilepsy: maintenance or reinforcement of ther-

apy. *Reflex epilepsy, behaviour therapy and conditioned reflexes.* Springfield, IL: Charles C Thomas, 1977;242–255.

42. de Weerdt CJ, van Rijn AJ. Conditioning therapy in reading epilepsy. *Electroencephalogr Clin Neurophysiol* 1975;39:417–420.

43. Prochazka A, Hulliger M, Zangger P, Appenteng K. "Fusimotor set": new evidence for alpha-independent control of gamma-motor neurones during movement in the awake cat. *Brain Res* 1985;339(1):136–140.

44. Penn A, Wada J. Differential effects of singing and dressing/undressing on complex partial seizures originating in the speech non-dominant hemisphere. *Epilepsia* 1986;27:590–650.

45. Mostofsky DI, Balaschak BA. Psychobiological control of seizures. *Psychol Bull* 1977;84:723–759.

46. Prince DA. Modification of focal cortical epileptogenic discharges by afferent impulses. *Epilepsia* 1966;7:181–201.

47. Tassinari CA. Suppression of focal spikes by somato-sensory stimuli. *Electroencephalogr Clin Neurophysiol* 1969;25:574.

48. Jung R. Blocking of petit mal attacks by sensory arousal and inhibition of attacks by an active change in attention during the epileptic aura. *Epilepsia* 1962;3:435.

49. Ounsted C, Lee D, and Huth SJ. Electroencephalographic and clinical changes in an epileptic child during repeated photic stimulation. *Electroencephalogr Clin Neurophysiol* 1966;21:388–391.

50. Pritchard P, Holmstrom V, Giacinto J. Self-abatement of complex partial seizures. *Ann Neurol* 1985;18(2):265–267.

51. Brown S. Personal communication. David Lewis Centre for Epilepsy, Alderly Edge, Cheshire, U.K., 1988.

52. Davis GR, Armstrong HE, Donovan DM, Tempkin NR. Cognitive-behavioural treatment of depressed affect among epileptics: preliminary findings. *J Clin Psychol* 1984;40:930–935.

53. Fenton GW. Epilepsy and automatism. *Br J Hosp Med* 1972;7:57–64.

54. Jasper H. Some physiological mechanisms involved in epileptic automatism. *Epilepsia* 1964;5:1–20.

55. Geier S, Bancaud J, Talairach J, Bonis A, Szikla G, Enjelvin M. Automatisms during frontal lobe epileptic seizures. *Brain* 1976;99:447–458.

56. Geier S, Bancaud J, Talairach J, Bonis A, Szilkla G, Emjelvin M. The seizures of frontal lobe epilepsy. *Neurology* 1977;27:951–958.

57. Knox S. Epileptic automatisms and violence. *Med Sci Law* 1968;8:96–104.

58. Theodore W, Porter R, Penry K. Complex partial seizures: clinical characteristics and differential diagnosis. *Neurology* 1983;33:1115–1121.

59. Forster FM, Liske E. Role of environmental clues in temporal lobe epilepsy. *Neurology (Minneap)* 1963;13:301–305.

60. Mostofsky DI. Recurrent paroxysmal disorders of the central nervous system. In: Turner S, ed. *Handbook of clinical behaviour therapy.* 1981, pp. 447–473.

61. Krafft KM, Poling AD. Behavioural treatments of epilepsy: methodological characteristics and problems of published studies. *Appl Res Ment Retard* 1982;3:151–162.

62. Flannery RB Jr, Cautela JR. Seizures: controlling the uncontrollable. *J Rehabil* 1973;39:34–36.

63. Balaschak BA. Teacher-implemented behaviour modification in a case of organically based epilepsy. *J Consult Clin Psychol* 1976;44:218–223.

64. Zlutnick SI, Mayville WJ, Moffat S. Behavioural control of seizure disorders: the interruption of chained behaviour. In: Katz RC, Zlutnick SI, eds. *Behaviour therapy and health care: principles and applications.* Elmsford, NY: Pergamon Press, 1975.

65. Iwata BA, Lorentzson AM. Operant control of seizure-like behaviour in an institutionalised retarded adult. *Behav Ther* 1976;7:247–251.

66. Cataldo MF, Russo CC, Freeman JM. A behaviour analysis approach to high rate myoclonic seizures. *J Autism Dev Disord* 1979;9:413–427.

67. Cinciripin PM, Epstein LH, Kotanchik NL. Behavioural intervention of self-stimulatory, attending and seizure behaviour in a cerebral palsied child. *J Behav Ther Exp Psychiatry* 1980;11.

68. Cautela JR. Covert extinction. *Behav Ther* 1971;2:192–200.

69. Daniels LK. The treatment of grand mal epilepsy by covert and operant conditioning techniques: a case study. *Psychosomatics* 1975;16:65–67.

70. Gardner JE. Behaviour therapy treatment approach to a psychogenic seizure case. *J Consult Psychol* 1967;31:209–212.

71. Adams KM, Klinge V, Keiser TW. The extinction of a self-injurious behaviour in an epileptic child. *Behav Res Ther* 1973;11:351–356.

72. Wright L. Aversive conditioning of self-induced seizures. *Behav Ther* 1973;4:712–713.

73. Zlutnick SI. The control of seizures by the modification of pre-seizure behaviour: the punishment of behavioural chain components. Ph.D. thesis, Utah State College. *Diss Abstr Int* 1972;33:6B (University Microfilms No. 72-31, 182).

74. Bandler R, Kaufman I, Dykens J, Schleifer M, Shapiro L. Seizures and the menstrual cycle. *Am J Psychol* 1957;113:704–798.

75. Stevens JR. Endogenous conditioning to abnormal cerebral electrical transience in man. *Science* 1962;137:974–976.

76. Dorcas RM, Schaffer GW. *Textbook of abnormal psychology,* 3rd ed. Baltimore: Williams & Wilkins, 1945, pp. 247–262.

77. Fenwick P. The significance of a seizure. In: Trimble MR, Reynolds EH, eds. *Bridge*

between neurology and psychiatry. London: Churchill Livingstone, 1988.

78. Wolpe J. *The practice of behaviour therapy*. Elmsford, NY: Pergamon Press, 1969.

79. Wells K, Turner S, Bellack A, Hersen M. Effects of cue-controlled relaxation on psychomotor seizures. *Behav Res Ther* 1978;16:51–54.

80. Rousseau A, Herman B, Whitman S. Effects of progressive relaxation on epilepsy: analysis of a series of cases. *Psychol Rep* 1985;57:1203–1212.

81. Goleman D. *Deep relaxation*. New York: Psychology Today, Cassette, 1976.

82. Ince LP. The use of relaxation training and a conditioned stimulus in the elimination of epileptic seizures in a child: a case study. *J Behav Ther Exp Psychiatry* 1976;7:39–42.

83. Cabral RJ, Scott DF. Effects of two desensitization techniques, biofeedback and relaxation, on intractable epilepsy: follow-up study. *J Neurol Neurosurg Psychiatry* 1976;39:504–507.

84. Muthen J. Psychological treatment of epileptic seizures. Ph.D. thesis, Institute of Applied Psychology, Uppsala University, Sweden, 1978.

85. Mostofsky DI. Teaching the nervous system. *NYU Ed Q* 1975;Spring: 8–13.

86. Standage KF. Treatment of epilepsy by reciprocal inhibition of anxiety. *Guys Hosp Rep* 1972;121:217.

87. Parrino JJ. Reduction of seizures by desensitization. *J Behav Ther Exp Psychiatry* 1971;2:215–218.

88. Melin L, Dahl J. Effects of contingent relaxation on epileptic seizures. *J Psychiatr Treatment Eval* 1981;3:201–207.

89. Dahl J, Melin L, Lund L. Effects of a contingent relaxation treatment programme on adults with refractory epileptic seizures. *Epilepsia* 1987;28(2):125–137.

90. Dahl J. Melin L, Leissner P. Effects of a behavioural intervention on epileptic seizure behaviour and paroxysmal activity: a systematic replication of three cases of children with intractable epilepsy. *Epilepsia* 1988;29(2):172–183.

91. Dahl J, Brorson L. The behaviour analysis of epilepsy: in theory and practice. *Scand J Behav Ther* 1983;12:195–209.

92. Pinto R. A case of movement epilepsy with agarophobia, treated successfully by flooding. *Br J Psychiatry* 1972;121:287–288.

93. Gottschalk LA. Effects of intensive psychotherapy on epileptic children. *Arch Neurol psychiatry* 1953;70:361–384.

94. Williams DT, Spiegel H, Mostofsky DI. Neurogenic and hysterical seizures in children and adolescents: differential diagnostic and therapeutic considerations. *Am J Psychiatry* 1978;135:82–86.

95. Correa S. Locus of control in children with epilepsy. *Psychol Rep* 1987;60:9–10.

96. Tan S, Bruni J. Cognitive-behaviour therapy with adult patients with epilepsy: a controlled outcome study. *Epilepsia* 1986;27(3):225–233.

97. Rosenbaum M, Palmon N. Helplessness and resourcefulness in coping with epilepsy. *J Consult Clin Psychol* 1984;52(2):244–253.

98. Feldman RG, Paul NL. Identity of emotional triggers in epilepsy. *J Nerv Ment Dis* 1976;162:345.

99. Forster FM. IBID ref. 100.

100. Forster FM. Classification and conditioning treatment of the reflex epilepsies. *Int J Neurol* 1972;9:73–86.

101. Booker HE, Forster FM, Klove H. Extinction factors in startle (acoustico-motor) seizures. *Neurology* 1965;15:1095–1103.

102. Forster FM, Campos GB. Conditioning factors in stroboscopic-induced seizures. *Epilepsia* 1964;5:156–165.

103. Forster FM, Ptacek LJ, Peterson WG, et al. Stroboscopic-induced seizure discharges: modification by extinction techniques. *Arch Neurol* 1964;11:603–608.

104. Forster FM, Ptacek LJ, Peterson WG. Auditory clicks in extinction of stroboscope-induced seizures. *Epilepsia* 1965;6:217–225.

105. Sterman MB. Neurophysiological and clinical studies of sensori-motor EEG biofeedback training: some effects of epilepsy. In: Birk L, ed. *Biofeedback: behaviour medicine*. Boston: Grune & Stratton, 1973;507–526.

106. Siefert AR, Lubar JF. Reduction of epileptic seizures through EEG biofeedback training. *Biol Psychol* 1975;3:156–184.

107. Lubar JF, Bhaler JF. Behavioural management of epileptic seizures following EEG biofeedback training of the sensori-motor rhythm. *Biofeedback Self Regul* 1976;1:77–104.

108. Lubar JF. Electroencephalographic methodology and the management of epilepsy. *Pavlov J Biol Sci* 1977;12:147–185.

109. Finlay WW, Smith HA, Etherton MD. Reduction of seizures and normalisation of the EEG in a severe epileptic following sensorimotor biofeedback training: preliminary study. *Biol Psychol* 1975;2:189–203.

110. Tansey MA. The response of a case of petit mal epilepsy to EEG sensorimotor rhythm biofeedback training. *Int J Psychophysiol* 1985;3:81–84.

111. Finlay WW. Operant conditioning of the EEG in two patients with epilepsy. Methodological and clinical considerations. *Pavlov J Biol Sci* 1977;12:93–111.

112. Kuhlman WM, Allison T. EEG feedback training in the treatment of epilepsy: some questions and answers. *Pavlov J Biol Sci* 1977;12:112–122.

113. Sterman MB. Effects of sensorimotor EEG feedback training on sleep and clinical manifestation of epilepsy. In: Beatty J, Legewie H, eds. *Biofeedback and behaviour*. New York: Plenum Press, 1977;167–200.

114. Kuhlman WN. EEG feedback training of epileptic patients: clinical and electroencephalographic analysis. *Electroencephalogr Clin Neurophysiol* 1978;45:699–710.

115. Quy RJ, Hut SJ, Foresst S. Sensorimotor

rhythm feedback training in epilepsy. *Biol Psychol* 1979;9:129–149.

116. Sterman MB, Shouse MN. Quantitive analysis of training, sleep EEG and clinical response to EEG operant conditioning in epileptics. *Electroencephalogr Clin Neurophysiol* 1980;49:558–576.

117. Lantz D, Sterman MB. Neuropsychological assessment of subjects with uncontrolled epilepsy: effects of EEG feedback training. *Epilepsia* 1988;29(2):163–171.

118. Sterman MB, Macdonald LR, Stone RK. Biofeedback training of the sensorimotor EEG rhythm in man: effects on epilepsy. *Epilepsia* 1974;15:395–416.

119. Whyler AR, Lockard JS, Ward AA, Finch CA. Condition EEG desynchronisation and seizure occurrence in patients. *Electroencephalogr Clin Neurophysiol* 1976;41:501–512.

120. Kaplan BJ. Biofeedback in epilepsy: equivocal relationship of reinforced EEG frequency to seizure reduction. *Epilepsia* 1975;16:477–485.

122. Lockard JS, Wyler AR, Finch CA, Hulbert KE. EEG operant conditioning in a monkey model. 1. Seizure data. *Epilepsia* 1977;18(4):471–479.

123. Psatta DM. Control of chronic experimental focal epilepsy by feedback caudatum stimulation. *Epilepsia* 1983;24:444–454.

124. Fried R, Rubin SR, Carlton RM, Fox MC. Behavioural control of intractable idiopathic seizures. 1. Self regulation of end-tidal CO_2. *Psychosom Med* 1984;46(4):315–331.

125. Lennox WG, Gibbs FA, Gibbs EL. The relationship in man of cerebral activity to blood flow and blood constituents. *J Neurol Psychiatry* 1938;1:221–225.

126. Holmberg G. The electroencephalogram during hypoxia and hyperventilation. *EEG Clin Neurophysiol* 1953;5:371–376.

127. Swanson AG, Stavney LS, Plum F. Effects of blood pH and carbon dioxide on cerebral electrical activity. *Neurology* 1958;8:787–792.

Advances in Neurology, Vol. 55, edited by
D. Smith, D. Treiman, and M. Trimble,
Raven Press, Ltd., New York © 1991.

12

Epilepsy and Disorders of Mood

Dietrich Blumer

*Neuropsychiatry Program, Epicare Center, Baptist Memorial Hospital,
Memphis, Tennessee 38104*

Since the studies of Morel and Falret in the mid-19th century, characteristic mood changes were described by psychiatrists as prime mental symptoms in epilepsy (1). As outlined in a relatively recent psychiatric textbook (2), they were known to occur as either (a) prodromal moods of depression or irritability which may be relieved by the occurrence of the seizure, or (b) postictal moods lasting for some days after the seizure. Independent of seizures, sudden variations of mood were described among patients with epilepsy, distinct from those observed among manic–depressives by their sudden onset and by their brief duration. Moods of irritability, to the degree of violent anger, were considered as perhaps the most prevalent moods in patients with epilepsy. Until recently the modern debate about the psychiatric disorders associated with epilepsy had centered on personality and behavior changes (including irritability) and on psychoses, rather than on mood disorders in the narrower and current clinical sense of the term.

It is probable that the presence of depression among patients with epilepsy was simply viewed as a reaction to a difficult chronic illness. We will not focus here on reactive depressive *feelings,* such as the grief over the diagnosis or over the handicaps associated with intractable epilepsy, which require support and counseling. Rather, we will discuss mood *disorders* occurring among patients with epilepsy which appear to be endogenous and which often require pharmacologic intervention.

Modern evidence suggests that mood changes represent the most important mental disorders related to epilepsy and cannot be viewed as disorders secondary to difficult life situations. Depressive episodes are frequently associated with the interictal phase of certain seizure disorders (3–5) and carry a heightened risk for suicide (6,7). Those mood changes, which in some patients are clearly associated with the ictal phase of their seizure disorder, demonstrate with particular clarity the relationship of temporolimbic discharges to mood disorders and need to be reviewed first.

ICTAL AND PERI-ICTAL MOOD CHANGES

Among about 2000 patients with epilepsy living normal home lives, Williams (8) found a group of 165 who had complex feelings in the epileptic attack; he studied 100 of this group who felt an emotion as part of their customary seizure. Fear was the leading emotion, reported by 61 patients, with depressive mood being the next common. The depressive mood reported by 21 patients ranged from the experience of "feeling very sad" to the sudden onset of acute depression with a vaguely remembered thought about "death and the world" and with a compulsive urge to commit suicide.

The opposite sense of pleasure, reported by nine patients, ranged from the experience of "satisfaction" to a feeling of "extreme well-being involving all senses." All patients with a pleasurable aura reported a simultaneous visceral sensation. Finally, Williams (8) reported an ictal sensation of "unpleasure" among nine patients, ranging from "a picture which is unpleasant" to the sickening hallucination, associated with deepest horror, of the body appearing disfigured.

Of particular interest is the observation by Williams (8) that in all his patients with ictal depression, their mood would persist beyond the attack for 1 hr to 3 days, even in cases when a secondarily generalized seizure had taken place. A prolonged depressive state following complex partial seizures can be documented even in patients whose ictal experience does not include a depressed mood, as illustrated by a case of our own study.

Case 1
A 21-year-old female with borderline mental retardation suffered from frequent and intractable complex partial seizures since age 10. The attacks occurred without warning and were at times followed by secondary generalization. Surgical treatment was not carried out because of the presence of bitemporal spike discharges. Intermittent depression had remained a significant problem over the years, and suicidal ideation had been reported. Prior to a seizure she often experienced a racing of her thoughts for about 2 hr.

When first seen she was friendly and animated, but then she experienced a complex partial seizure consisting of a sudden cry, torsion of the body, and clonic limb movements lasting about 1 min and followed by a brief period of confusion. Thereafter, she remained in a severe depressive state marked by lack of any initiative, minimal responsiveness, and a mood of utter dejection.

It became evident that not only did she suffer from prolonged depressive episodes of various durations, but that her seizures specifically were followed by marked depression for 24 hr. When carbamazepine was raised to a maximum tolerated level and imipramine was added and gradually increased to 125 mg daily, her seizures became shorter, their frequency improved significantly, and all her depressive episodes improved markedly.

Three of 19 patients reported in our series of epilepsy patients treated for psychiatric complications (cases 4, 15, and 16) suffered from a postictal depressive state lasting from several hours to a few days (9). Postictal

depression is not a rare event, but it tends to be mistaken as ordinary postictal fatigue and prostration. This emotional aftermath of a complex partial seizure persists beyond the well-known after-effects, and its depressive nature is clearly identified by the patients themselves. Some patients may experience hypomanic states following their complex partial seizures (10), but this appears to be a rare finding.

Many patients with epilepsy, perhaps 10–20%, experience preictally an unpleasant prodrome consisting of a depressive–irritable mood; this is sometimes accompanied by headaches, anxiety, tension, or restlessness. Rarely, the prodrome consists of an elated mood. An unusual fixed relationship between seizures and a bipolar mood change is illustrated in a case from our own study.

Case 2
A truck driver, of average intelligence and married with two children, was recognized as having complex partial seizures at age 34. He had to move to a job in the truck plant, and then at age 40 he became disabled as a result of very frequent seizures. He was evaluated for surgical treatment of the epilepsy at age 45. It was learned that he had a history of meningitis at age 2, and that at age 13 he had begun to experience simple partial seizures described as "a flushed feeling in the head, as one would have with an orgasm"; these attacks had not been recognized as epileptic in nature.

For several years prior to the evaluation, he would experience, about every 2 weeks, clusters of 7–8 seizures daily for 2–3 days. For several days prior to each cluster of seizures he would feel energetic and elated, would play with the children, and have sexual relations with his wife at least once daily. Throughout the 2–3 days of frequent seizure activity, he would then experience a depressed mood, accompanied by excessive guilt, hopelessness and suicidal ideation, frequent awakenings at night, decreased appetite, lack of smell and taste, listlessness, and absence of libido. Irritability was marked during the same phase, particularly right after each seizure. After termination of each seizure cluster, for about 12–48 hr, he would experience increased libido with persistent decrease in energy level and a resolution of his depressive mood. In between the described phases, for about 2 weeks per month, he was well adjusted and had sexual intercourse about twice a week.

Recording of seizures by subdural strip electrodes demonstrated a right temporal onset, and consequently a right temporal lobectomy was carried out. He returned to work in a factory 1 month later; on follow-up over 9 months after the operation, it was evident that he had regained full health. He was free of any type of seizure, had gained 20 pounds, was free of any depression and entirely even in his mood, was stable in his energy level, and enjoyed sexual relations two or three times per week.

As is well known from scalp and depth recordings, the interictal phase is characterized by irregular subclinical seizure discharges, not by normal neuronal activity, and the moods of many patients may be profoundly affected. The interictal mood disorders are, in general, of much greater clinical significance than those associated with the ictal phase.

INTERICTAL MOOD CHANGES

As indicated initially, psychiatric observers had emphasized the sudden onset and short duration of the mood changes among patients with epilepsy. Morel (11), prior to the use of anticonvulsant drugs, had listed the "periodic alternation of depression and excitement" as a leading symptom of the psychiatric disorder of epilepsy, and Kraepelin (12) stated: "The moods of patients with epilepsy are labile—despondent or morose, then joyful and contented." Betts (13), speaking from 15 years of experience with mentally ill people with epilepsy, stated: "When an endogenous type of depressive illness presents itself in someone with epilepsy it tends to be of sudden onset and sudden departure and may also fluctuate quite markedly whilst it is present." Contemporary investigators have not focused on these rather striking longitudinal mood changes; instead, they have tended to take a cross-sectional approach in studying the presence of mood disorders among patients with epilepsy. In further contrast to the investigators who took the traditional psychiatric approach, few modern investigators have aimed to gain a comprehensive view of the setting of the mood changes within the full range of

mental changes which may be associated with epilepsy.

The more recent studies have been reviewed by Robertson (14). Many clinical investigators have reported that depression is common in both adult and child patients with epilepsy (3,15–22). Robertson (14) cites a number of studies employing the Minnesota Multiphasic Personality Inventory (MMPI) or various schedules or inventories, all of which found that patients with epilepsy had higher depression scores than did controls.

In contrast, manic psychoses are rarely reported in the literature. Wolf (23) found only nine case studies of mania in patients with epilepsy, but he reported six cases of his own with manic syndromes. Toone et al. (24) found only three patients with evidence of bipolarity among 69 patients with epilepsy and psychosis. Robertson et al. (25) reported only two patients with bipolar illness in a series of 66 patients with epilepsy and depression. Robertson (14) cited the antimanic effect of anticonvulsants as a possible reason for the relative absence of manic mood swings among patients with epilepsy, but she also considered the fact that they may be less often documented.

Several studies indicated that patients with left-sided foci scored higher on depression scores than did patients with right-sided foci (4,15,25–29), whereas some studies did not support any laterality hypothesis (30,31). Several investigators noted a decrease in seizure frequency prior to the onset of the depressive illness (3,32–34).

Robertson et al. (25) studied 66 patients with epilepsy who fulfilled criteria for major depressive disorder and found that 13 were psychotic as defined by mood congruent hallucinations or delusions; only two patients had a history of bipolar disorder. Attendant features of the depression were high state anxiety, high neuroticism, and high hostility, especially the intropunitive scores of self-criticism and guilt. The longer the history of epilepsy, the more severe was the depression.

Mendez et al. (4) carried out a rather comprehensive study of depression in epilepsy. They investigated the prevalence of depression in comparably disabled outpatients and found that nearly twice as many outpatients with epilepsy (55%) reported depression when compared with matched disabled controls (30%); the prevalence of prior suicide attempts among the epilepsy patients (30%) was more than four times higher than among the controls (7%). The phenomenology of depression was studied in 20 depressed inpatients from a VA Hospital and was found to be characterized by "endogenous" rather than "neurotic" features, accompanied by more psychotic traits, paranoia, and underlying chronic dysthymia. Ten of 11 patients with a lateralized electroencephalographic focus had foci lateralized to the left hemisphere. Between major depressive episodes, epilepsy patients furthermore tended to manifest significantly more irritability, emotionality, and humorlessness than did controls. The investigators concluded that their study suggested the existence of a specific epileptic psychosyndrome among patients with epilepsy in the form of an atypical endogenous depression.

In an effort to investigate the mood changes peculiar to patients with temporal lobe epilepsy (TLE), we studied 15 outpatients with TLE referred for psychiatric complications and compared them to a matched control group of patients with chronic pain on a depressive basis [(dysthymic pain disorder (DPD)] (35). The Hamilton Depression Rating Scale (HDRS) and the Questionnaire for Pain Syndromes (QPS) were used for assessment of the depressive manifestations. A scale developed to assess mood shifts, paranoid–hallucinatory events, anxiety, and various other mental changes (Himmelhoch-Blumer Mood Scale [HBMS]) was used to measure traits reportedly associated with the interictal phase of TLE; also used in this regard was the Bear–Fedio Inventory (BFI). The findings are listed in Table 1. Both groups scored high on the HDRS, and only two patients with TLE reported no significant depressive events. Surprisingly, the prevalence of protracted pain was nearly even. However, in six patients with TLE the pain was only episodic. In the DPD group, 13 had chronic depressive mood and none had marked mood swings, whereas in the TLE group, 12 had marked mood shifts and only one was chronically depressed.

Significant episodes of euphoric mood occurred in six patients with TLE for an average duration of 4 hr at an average frequency of

TABLE 1. *Mental changes in 15 patients with temporal lobe epilepsy and in 15 patients with dysthymic pain disorder[a]*

| | Similarities | | |
Disorder	HDRS mean scores	Depression (HBMS)	Pain (QPS)
TLE	26.3	13	14
DPD	21.0	15	15

| | Dissimilarities | |
	Chronic depression (HBMS)	Episodic depression (HBMS)
TLE	1	12
DPD	13	—

	Chronic pain (QPS)	Episodic pain (QPS)
TLE	8	6
DPD	15	—

| | | Schizophreniform traits (HBMS) | | Anxiety (HBMS) | | |
	BFI mean scores	Paranoid	Hallucinatory	Chronic	Episodic	Paroxysmal
TLE	47.5	10	8	3	9	9
DPD	27.5	3	2	5	6	2

[a]TLE, temporal lobe epilepsy; DPD, dysthymic pain disorder; HDRS, Hamilton Depression Rating Scale; QPS, Questionnaire for Pain Disorders; HBMS (Himmelhoch-Blumer Mood Scale).

three times per month, whereas the dysphoric moods of the majority of patients with TLE lasted for 12 hr and occurred five times per month, on the average. Furthermore, a majority of TLE patients and very few of the DPD patients reported paranoid and/or hallucinatory experiences. Chronic anxiety was more often reported by patients with DPD, whereas episodic anxiety (particularly paroxysmal bouts of anxiety) was more prevalent among the TLE group. The TLE group scored almost twice as high on the BFI than did the DPD group. The findings confirm the high prevalence of depressive symptomatology among patients with TLE who required referral to a psychiatrist. Striking was the almost ubiquitous presence of chronic pain in the TLE group. The psychopathology, however, was clearly more variable and polysymptomatic (pleomorphic) in the TLE group, with the admixture of schizophreniform traits, episodic anxiety, and a variety of the interictal behavioral traits measured by the BFI.

The findings of an atypical and pleomorphic psychopathology, with predominant depressive traits, among patients with epilepsy confirm the findings of Mendez et al. (4) and, in addition, point at the highly variable or episodic nature of the psychopathology among these patients. The complexity of the mental changes that may be associated with seizure disorders requires a comprehensive and detailed analysis of each individual case.

We have reported a series of 19 patients with epilepsy referred for treatment of their psychiatric complications; the report includes a synopsis of every case (9). All patients were thoroughly evaluated, most patients were seen on many occasions, and follow-ups were obtained for at least 1 year from the beginning of treatment. In view of the wealth of significant mental changes displayed by the patients at various times (Table 2), categorization by traditional psychiatric diagnosis was not possible. Seventeen patients had suffered from episodic (12) or protracted (6) depression, nine of them with suicidal tendencies; five of the patients with depressive disorder had also experienced manic-like episodes; one patient suffered from a persistent hypomanic state without any depression. Thirteen patients had experienced episodes of marked anger, and 12 patients had displayed

TABLE 2. *Significant mental changes in a series of 19 patients with epilepsy referred for psychiatric treatment*

Mood disorders	
Depression	17
Maniform episodes	5
Hypomania	1
Irritability	13
Schizophreniform changes	12
Anxiety	7
Substance abuse	7
Dysthymic pain	6
Confusional–amnestic episodes	2
	70

schizophrenia-like (paranoid, delusional, hallucinatory) symptomatology. Nine patients had both mood changes and schizophrenia-like symptoms; eight had both mood disorders and angry-irritable behavior; five patients had shown all three of the most prevalent mental changes. Only one patient was monosymptomatic (episodes of explosive anger). Of the major symptoms listed in Table 2, there were an average of 3.7 symptoms per patient. Furthermore, the patients averaged a score of 47.5 on the BFI, suggesting the presence of a wealth of subtle interictal personality and behavior traits.

In their study of the schizophrenia-like psychoses of epilepsy, Slater and Beard (36) had commented on the presence of affective components among their patients. When careful mental state evaluations were carried out on psychotic patients with epilepsy, the presence of a mixed kind of psychosis was confirmed (37). Betts (13) pointed out: "It can be very difficult to tell sometimes whether one is seeing a depressive illness in which schizophrenic symptoms are also occurring, or whether one is seeing a true schizophrenic illness in which there is a large depressive component." Betts reported the interesting observation that in patients who showed depressive and schizophrenic symptoms simultaneously, there was often a concomitant increase in attack frequency around the time of the onset of the psychotic experience, with control of the epilepsy sometimes leading to a resolution of the psychosis. Mendez et al. (4) have reported a similar finding.

MOOD CHANGES AS THE PRIME SYMPTOMS OF THE NEUROBEHAVIORAL DISORDER OF EPILEPSY

It is evident that seizure disorders may be associated with a complex mixture of psychopathology. Most prominent are rapid shifting moods with predominant depression, episodic irritability with occasional explosive anger, and schizophrenia-like episodes with paranoid, hallucinatory, or delusional symptoms. Recurrent attacks of anxiety, symptoms of a somatization disorder, amnestic–confusional episodes, and indeed symptoms reminiscent of any psychiatric disorder may also be present secondary to a seizure disorder.

Though highly complex and seemingly heterogeneous, the mental symptoms associated with epilepsy tend to present in a characteristic pattern: They are *atypical* for the psychiatric disorder they resemble; they tend to occur in a highly *episodic* form, often with sudden onset and termination; and they tend to be *pleomorphic* in a given patient, presenting simultaneously as a mixed state or in succession. In addition, a range of relatively stable but often subtle traits, termed "interictal personality and behavior changes (core traits)," may be present among patients with seizure disorder. These traits tend to be complex by themselves, and they may be grouped under the headings of hyperemotionality, viscosity, and hyposexuality [inverse Klüver–Bucy syndrome (38)]. Finally, organic mental changes such as amnestic–confusional episodes may be present. The broad term "neurobehavioral disorder of epilepsy" is suggested to embrace the full range of complex psychopathology which tends to be present. Table 3 represents a suggested listing of diagnostic criteria for the disorder, in the style of the APA's *Diagnostic and Statistical Manual.* The term "neurobehavioral" refers to an underlying organic substrate but does not claim a specific anatomic basis as implied by synonymous terms such as "temporal lobe syndrome" or "limbic mental syndrome."

The symptoms characteristic of the neurobehavioral syndrome of epilepsy may be present in patients without any clinical seizures, as was first described by B. A. Morel in 1860 (11). Such patients tend to present with evidence of some cerebral impairment (e.g.,

TABLE 3. *Neurobehavioral disorder of epilepsy*

Mood disorder   (dysphoric, euphoric, rapid-cycling, mixed)
Irritable–impulsive disorder
Schizophreniform disorder   (paranoid, delusional, hallucinatory)
Anxiety disorder   (panic, phobic, generalized)
Amnestic–confusional disorder
Somatoform disorder   (pseudoseizures, pain)
Personality disorder   (hyperemotional, viscous, hyposexual)
Compound   (more than three categories)
Not otherwise specified

head injury, encephalitis, cerebrovascular accident, paroxysmal electroencephalogram) and/or a family history of epilepsy or migraine (39). The term "paroxysmal neurobehavioral disorder" is proposed for this group of patients. The term "paroxysmal" denotes the sudden on-and-off presentation that is characteristic of many of the mental symptoms, and it refers to the presumed substrate of sudden, irregular, and excessive neuronal activity. As an alternative name for the paroxysmal neurobehavioral disorder, the term "Morel's disorder" is suggested for historical reasons.

It should not be surprising to find the neurobehavioral disorder of epilepsy associated with a more chronic seizure disorder (i.e., with TLE). Even very chronic forms of TLE, however, may be completely free from any traits of the neurobehavioral disorder. On the other hand, it is not unusual to find a patient with primary generalized epilepsy suffering from a significant neurobehavioral disorder. In such cases we assume a secondary involvement of limbic structures, and we have been impressed that such patients may respond particularly well to our pharmacologic intervention (9). We have postulated that this may be due to the absence of an active temporolimbic focus.

ANTICONVULSANTS AND MOOD CHANGES

The beneficial effects of anticonvulsant monotherapy, as well as the choice of proper anticonvulsant for the quality of life of the patients, have been widely recognized. A number of studies document what the alert clinician can observe on a regular basis—that is, that anticonvulsants may have significant effects on the mood of the patient with epilepsy. The studies of the effects of anticonvulsant drugs on cognitive function and behavior have been recently reviewed by Trimble (40).

Shorvon and Reynolds (41) reduced polytherapy to monotherapy in a series of chronic patients with epilepsy and reported an improvement of alertness, concentration, drive, mood, and sociability. Thompson and Trimble (42,43) showed that a group of patients who had their polytherapy rationalized showed significant improvements on rating scales of mood, in particular for anxiety and depression. A second group of patients had carbamazepine substituted for one or all of the drugs they had been receiving, and they subsequently rated themselves less anxious and more lively; those who had high depression scores before the medication change showed significant improvements following the change to carbamazepine. A control group showed no changes of mood.

The psychotropic effects of carbamazepine have been noted since its earliest use over 25 years ago (44). Over the past 10 years, the increasingly wide use of carbamazepine for patients with a variety of psychiatric diagnoses in the absence of any seizure disorders has established the psychotropic effects of carbamazepine beyond any doubt (45). Carbamazepine tends to be prescribed for patients who have not responded to traditional psychotropic medications, particularly for those with lithium-resistant manic syndromes; a more precise range of indications has not been established. Post et al. (46) have reported that carbamazepine is particularly effective for patients who have rapid-cycling mood disorders and who also have dysphoria, anxiety, and no family history of affective disorders. The drug has only moderate antidepressant effects (47). Valproate and, to a lesser degree, clonazepam have been increasingly prescribed by psychiatrists with a similar wide range of indications (48). Carbamazepine, valproate, and clonazepam are listed by Schatzberg and Cole (49), together with lithium, as mood stabilizers. There is evidence that the excellent responders to carbamazepine among psychiatric patients may suffer from atypical, highly

episodic, and pleomorphic syndromes of organic origin which may be considered to be formes frustes of epilepsy; we have referred to these syndromes as "paroxysmal neurobehavioral disorders" or "temporal lobe syndrome" (39).

In an early survey of 40 investigations on over 2000 patients with epilepsy, a psychotropic effect of carbamazepine was reported in about 50%; the anticonvulsant appeared to be beneficial for (a) slowness and viscosity, (b) emotional intensity and lability, and (c) apathy, depressed mood, and anxiety (50).

A few controlled studies of the effects of carbamazepine on the mood of patients with epilepsy have been carried out. Marjerrison et al. (51) noted that patients on carbamazepine as compared to phenytoin were less retarded and less unhappy. Robertson et al. (52) studied patients with epilepsy and major depression and found that patients on phenobarbital were more likely to record higher depression scores, whereas patients on carbamazepine rated themselves as less depressed and had lower anxiety scores. Andrewes et al. (53) started half of a group of 42 patients on monotherapy with phenytoin, and they started the other half on monotherapy with carbamazepine; at follow-up, higher carbamazepine levels corresponded to lower rating scale scores for anxiety, fatigue, and depression. Brent et al. (54) compared the psychopathology in 15 children with epilepsy treated with phenobarbital and 24 children treated with carbamazepine. Those treated with phenobarbital showed a much higher prevalence of major depressive disorder (40% versus 4%) and suicidal ideation (47% versus 4%), as determined by semistructured psychiatric interviews. The differential prevalence of depression between the two medication groups was only noted in those with a family history of a major affective disorder among first-degree relatives.

The high prevalence of depressive features among children treated with phenobarbital had been documented earlier by British investigators (55). Brent (56), in an evaluation of 131 consecutive suicide attempts made by 126 children and adolescents seen at a Children's Hospital over the period of 5 years, found that nine of the patients had epilepsy (an incidence 15 times higher than expected) and that eight of the nine patients were treated with phenobarbital.

In summary, patients with epilepsy and a mood disorder need to have any sedative anticonvulsants (phenobarbital, primidone) removed and should have a modern anticonvulsant regimen established (i.e., monotherapy with carbamazepine or valproate). Mood-stabilizing effects of valproate for patients with epilepsy, while not as well documented as those of carbamazepine, are supported by clinical experience as well as by the experience in patients with mental disorders without epilepsy. Patients with epilepsy and mood disorder who are treated with phenytoin may need to be switched to carbamazepine or valproate.

TREATMENT OF THE MOOD DISORDERS OF EPILEPSY

The pharmacologic treatment of psychiatric disorders has been described in a series of patients treated and followed over a prolonged period of time (9). Of prime importance for the treatment of mood disorders associated with epilepsy is the establishment, if possible, of a modern anticonvulsant monotherapy, preferably with carbamazepine (for simple or complex partial seizure disorders) or valproate (for primary generalized seizure disorders). Even marked psychiatric disturbances may respond to this approach alone. If the psychiatric disorder does not remit upon optimal anticonvulsant treatment, the addition of an antidepressant or lithium at a modest dose is indicated.

We prefer to add a tricyclic antidepressant at a dose of 75–125 mg daily. Imipramine prescribed at bedtime can be highly effective, but if a patient lacks energy and has no problem with insomnia, the use of desipramine in divided doses may be preferable. A marked insomnia may require the prescription of a more sedative antidepressant (amitriptyline or doxepin) at bedtime. Trazodone tends to be less effective, but monoamine-oxidase (MAO) inhibitors (phenelzine or tranylcypromine) or fluoxetine may serve as alternative and more effective adjuncts to the anticonvulsant, in some cases. Lithium may be used as comedication in place of an antidepressant.

A lowering of the seizure threshold with the prescription of modest doses of a tricyclic antidepressant is very rarely of clinical significance. The seizure threshold appears to be chiefly affected upon rapid introduction of the drug and by doses of over 200 mg daily (57).

The pharmacologic treatment of the mood disorders of epilepsy tends to be very effective, and its principles are basically simple. However, it may require patience to establish both the optimal level of anticonvulsant and the most effective psychotropic comedication. The treatment does not differ if schizophrenia-like traits or explosive anger or anxiety or any other mental changes are present. Neuroleptics are not useful in the majority of cases; however, they may occasionally be effective as adjuncts, in small doses. The relative simplicity of the biologic treatment of the complex and multiform psychopathology of epilepsy strongly suggests that we have to deal with a disorder which is homogeneous in nature.

The following case history from our treatment series (9) illustrates how significant mood changes may occur a long time before the diagnosis of epilepsy is ever made. The follow-up is updated, and it documents a lasting remission from a complex neurobehavioral disorder.

Case 3
Seizure history. A 43-year-old male executive had experienced two febrile convulsions at age 2 or 3. At age 32, he began to experience brief stereotyped sensations ("like an ocean wave through the head together with a smell of ether") that were particularly bothersome because he would be depressed for hours or days after they occurred. Two months prior to our evaluation, one of his peculiar sensations became more intense and was followed by a generalized tonic–clonic seizure. The diagnosis of epilepsy was now made, and treatment with phenytoin and carbamazepine was initiated. Both the electroencephalogram and the computed tomography scan were negative.

Psychiatric history. At age 25, he began to suffer from marked mood swings (3 months of hypomania, 3–6 months of depression, a few months of normal mood) and from intestinal problems. For 2 years he had been in psychotherapy, and for a few months doxepin (75 mg daily) had been prescribed with only transient success. For episodes of anxiety he would take 7.5 mg clorazepate as needed. He was highly meticulous and persistent in minor matters and was very conscientious, and he also could be temperamental; he tended to write down his personal experiences; his sexual desire was decreased for the past 10 years—markedly so for the past 3 years. Thus, subtle personality and behavioral changes characteristic for the interictal phase were clearly present by the time of evaluation, and the mood swings, which had preceded the seizures by 7 years, had been the first manifestation of the neurobehavioral disorder.

Treatment. On evaluation, he was a precise, articulate, and intense individual. He scored 50 on the BFI (his wife gave him a score of 27). He was asked to resume 75 mg doxepin at bedtime; the carbamazepine was increased, whereas the phenytoin was gradually phased out. His recovery was delayed by the phasing out of the phenytoin and by the substitution of Tegretol with a generic brand of carbamazepine by his pharmacist, resulting in a lower blood level and a recurrence of psychic seizures. Ten months after initiation of treatment, while on 2100 mg of carbamazepine daily in four doses (with a blood level of 11 μg/ml) and 75 mg doxepin at bedtime, he reached a full remission. At follow-up, 8 months later, he was taking desipramine (50 mg daily) in place of the doxepin because the doxepin had exerted too much of a sedative effect. Every 6–8 weeks or so, he had a very mild psychic seizure without any depressive after-effects, his mood swings and irritability had vanished, and his regular sexual arousal was reestablished. He felt far better than he had felt for some 20 years. For an occasional anxiety state, he still took some clorazepate, perhaps once a month. At last follow-up (which was more than 2 years after he had achieved remission), he continued to do very well while taking the same medication and seeing his neurologist twice a year.

CONCLUSION

The peculiar mental events that recur in a stereotyped fashion as the aura of many seizures include a wide range of experiences—from fear, sadness, pleasure, hallucinations, illusions, paranoia, delusions, and forced thinking to sexual arousal. In the peri-ictal phase, before and after a seizure, more protracted and less stereotyped mental events may take place, which tend to be essentially dysphoric in nature. Postictal depression is not a rare occurrence, and it appears to follow invariably upon the ictal experience of sadness—suggesting an underlying intimate relationship between ictal and postictal events.

The interictal phase of many patients with epilepsy is characterized by a marked vulnerability for mood changes. Depressive phenomena are the most predominant; they range from depressed mood, feelings of guilt and worthlessness, listlessness, inability to enjoy pleasure, diminished ability to concentrate, insomnia, sleep disturbance, loss of appetite, and protracted pain to suicidal preoccupation. Though in some patients a depressive baseline persists, the mood typically fluctuates markedly. Brief euphoric episodes with flight of ideas, talkativeness, overactivity, and little need for sleep may be interspersed. The mood changes of epilepsy are distinct from manic–depressive illness, not only by their rapid-cycling nature and by their sudden onset and termination, but moreover by the admixture of disparate mental changes; irritability, anxiety, paranoia, delusions, hallucinations, hysteriform or confusional states may be variously present as well. Any events that may be manifest at the time of a limbic ictus may also appear during the interictal phase, in the form of atypical phenocopies of functional psychiatric disorders.

For the atypical, episodic, and pleomorphic mental changes characteristic of epilepsy, the conventional assessments by schedules designed to measure a certain trait at a certain point in time are particularly inadequate. A systematic assessment of complex changes requires a likewise complex methodology that is capable of recording (as accurately as possible) atypical features, changes over time, and the simultaneous or successive presence of a multitude of mental changes.

Suicide is a serious risk in the depressed patient with epilepsy, and early recognition and treatment of the mental disorders associated with epilepsy is of exceptional importance. Modern use of anticonvulsants, combined with the adjunct employment of modest amounts of an antidepressant drug, can be highly effective. The relative simplicity of the pharmacologic treatment of the mental changes of epilepsy, which appear so heterogeneous on the surface, suggests a basic homogeneity of the disorder we have termed "the neurobehavioral disorder of epilepsy."

REFERENCES

1. Blumer D. The psychiatric dimension of epilepsy: historical perspective and current significance. In: Blumer D, ed. *Psychiatric aspects of epilepsy.* Washington, DC: APA Press, 1984;1–65.
2. Slater E, Roth M. *Clinical psychiatry,* 3rd ed. London: Baillière & Tindall, 1969.
3. Betts TA. A follow-up study of a cohort of patients with epilepsy admitted to psychiatric care in an English city. In: Harris P, Maudsley C, eds. *Epilepsy: proceedings of Hans Berger centenary symposium.* Edinburgh: Churchill Livingstone, 1974;326–338.
4. Mendez MF, Cummings JL, Benson DF. Depression in epilepsy: significance and phenomenology. *Arch Neurol* 1986;43:766–770.
5. Robertson MM, Trimble MR. Depressive illness in patients with epilepsy: a review. *Epilepsia* 1983;24(Suppl 2):S109–S116.
6. Zielinski JJ. Epilepsy and mortality rates and causes of death. *Epilepsia* 1974;15:191–201.
7. Matthew WS, Barabas G. Suicide and epilepsy: a review of literature. *Psychosomatics* 1981;22:515–524.
8. Williams D. The structure of emotions reflected in epileptic experiences. *Brain* 1956;79:29–67.
9. Blumer D, Zielinski JJ. Pharmacologic treatment of psychiatric disorders associated with epilepsy. *J Epilepsy* 1988;1:135–150.
10. Barczak P, Edmunds E, Betts T. Hypomania following complex partial seizures. *Br J Psychiatry* 1988;152:137–139.
11. Morel BA. D'une forme de délire, suite d'une surexcitation nerveuse se rattachant à une variété non encore décrite d'épilepsie (épilepsie larvée). *Gaz Hebd Med Chir* 1860;7:773–775, 819–821, 836–841.
12. Kraepelin E. *Psychiatrie,* vol 3, 8th ed. Leipzig: Johann Ambrosius Barth, 1923.
13. Betts TA. Depression, anxiety and epilepsy. In: Reynolds EH, Trimble MR, eds. *Epilepsy and psychiatry.* New York: Churchill Livingstone, 1981;60–71.
14. Robertson MM. Epilepsy and mood. In: Trimble MR, Reynolds EH, eds. *Epilepsy, behavior and cognitive function.* New York: John Wiley & Sons, 1988;145–157.
15. Dominian J, Serafetinides EA, Dewhurst M. A follow-up study of late onset of epilepsy: II. Psychiatric and social findings. *Br Med J* 1963;1:431–435.
16. Currie S, Heathfield KWG, Henson RA, Scott DF. Clinical course and prognosis of temporal lobe epilepsy: a survey of 666 patients. *Brain* 1971;94:173–190.
17. Taylor DC. Mental state and temporal lobe epilepsy: a correlative account of 100 patients treated surgically. *Epilepsia* 1972;13:727–765.
18. Serafetinides EA. Psychosocial aspects of neurosurgical management of epilepsy. In: Purpura DP, Penry UK, eds. *Advances in neurology,* vol 8. New York: Raven Press, 1975;323.
19. Gunn J. *Epileptics in prison.* London: Academic Press, 1977.
20. Toone BK, Driver NV. Psychosis and epilepsy. *Res Clin Forums* 1980;2:121–127.
21. Mellor DF, Lowit I, Hall DJ. Are epileptic children behaviourally different from other children? In: Harris P, Maudsley C, eds. *Epilepsy: proceedings of the Hans Berger centenary symposium.* Edinburgh: Churchill Livingstone, 1974;313–316.
22. Pazzangia P, Frank-Pazzangia L. Record in grade school of pupils with epilepsy: an epidemiological study. *Epilepsia* 1976;17:361–366.
23. Wolf P. Manic episodes in epilepsy. In: Akimoto H, Kazamatsuri H, Seino M, Ward AA, eds. *Advances in epileptology: 13th epilepsy international symposium,* New York: Raven Press, 1982;237–240.
24. Toone BJ, Garralda MF, Ron MA. The psychoses of epilepsy and the functional psychoses: a clinical and phenomenological comparison. *Br J Psychiatry* 1982;141:256–261.
25. Robertson MM, Trimble MR, Townsend HRA. The phenomenology of depression in epilepsy. *Epilepsia* 1987;28:364–372.
26. Deglin VL, Nikolaendo NN. Role of the dominant hemisphere in regulation of emotional states. *Fiziol Cheloveka* 1975;1:418–425.
27. Nielsen H, Kristensen O. Personality correlates of sphenoidal EEG-foci in temporal lobe epilepsy. *Acta Neurol Scand* 1981;64:289–300.
28. Perini G, Suny MD, Mendius R. Interictal emotions and behavioural profiles in left and right temporal lobe epileptics. *Abstr Psychosom Med* 1983;45:83.
29. Perini G, Mendius R. Depression and anxiety in complex partial seizures. *J Nerv Ment Dis* 1984;172:287–290.
30. Roy A. Some determinants of affective symptoms in epileptics. *Can J Psychiatry* 1979;24:554–556.
31. Camfield PR, Gates R, Ronen G, Camfield C, Ferguson A, MacDonald GW. Comparison of cognitive ability, personality profile and school success in epileptic children with pure right versus left temporal lobe EEG foci. *Ann Neurol* 1984;15:122–126.
32. Dongier S. Statistical study of clinical and electroencephalographic manifestations of 536 psychotic episodes occurring in 516 epileptics between clinical seizures. *Epilepsia* 1959/1960;1:117–142.
33. Flor-Henry P. Psychosis and temporal lobe epilepsy: a controlled investigation. *Epilepsia* 1969;10:363–395.

34. Standage KF, Fenton GW. Psychiatric symptom profiles of patients with epilepsy: a controlled investigation. *Psychol Med* 1975;5:152–160.

35. Blumer D, Heilbronn M. Depression in temporal lobe epilepsy. *Epilepsia* 1987;28:598.

36. Slater E, Beard AW. The schizophrenia-like psychoses of epilepsy. *Br J Psychiatry* 1963;109:95–150.

37. Perez MM, Trimble MR. Epileptic psychosis—diagnostic comparison with process schizophrenia. *Br J Psychiatry* 1980;137:245–249.

38. Gastaut H. Interpretation of the symptoms of psychomotor epilepsy in relation to physiological data on rhinencephalic function. *Epilepsia* 1954;3:84–88.

39. Blumer D, Heilbronn M, Himmelhoch J. Indications for carbamazepine in mental illness: atypical psychiatric disorder or temporal lobe syndrome? *Compr Psychiatry* 1988;29:108–22.

40. Trimble MR. Anticonvulsant drugs: mood and cognitive function. In: Trimble MR, Reynolds EH, eds. *Epilepsy, behavior and cognitive function*. New York: John Wiley & Sons, 1988;135–143.

41. Shorvon S, Reynolds EH. Reduction in polypharmacy for epilepsy. *Br Med J* 1979;2:1023–1025.

42. Thompson PJ, Trimble MR. Anticonvulsant drugs and cognitive functions. *Epilepsia* 1982;33:531–534.

43. Thompson PJ, Trimble MR. Comparative effects of anticonvulsant drugs on cognitive functioning. *Br J Clin Pract* 1982;18(Suppl):154–156.

44. Lorgé VM. Klinische Erfahrungen mit einem neuen Antiepilepticum Tegretol (G 32 883), mit besonderer Wirkung auf die epileptische Wesensveränderung. *Schweiz Med Wochenschr* 1963;93:1–16.

45. Post RM, Uhde TW. Anticonvulsants in non-epileptic psychosis. In: Trimble MR, Bolwig TG, eds. *Aspects of epilepsy and psychiatry*. New York: Wiley, 1986:177.

46. Post RM, Uhde TW, Roy-Byrne PP. Correlates of antimanic response to carbamazepine. *Psychiatry Res* 1987;21:71–83.

47. Ballenger JC. The clinical use of carbamazepine in affective disorders. *J Clin Psych* 1988;49(Suppl):13–19.

48. McElroy SL, Pope HG Jr. *Use of anticonvulsants in psychiatry: recent advances*. Clifton, NJ. Oxford Health Care, Inc.

49. Schatzberg AF, Cole JO. *Manual of clinical psychopharmacology*. Washington, DC: American Psychiatric Press, 1986.

50. Dalby MA. Behavioral effects of carbamazepine. In: Penry JK, Daly DD, eds. *Advances in neurology II*. New York: Raven Press, 1975;331–334.

51. Marjerrison G, et al. Carbamazepine: behavioural, anticonvulsant and EEG effects in chronically hospitalized epileptics. *Dis Nerv Syst* 1968;29:133–136.

52. Robertson MM, Trimble MR, Townsend HRA. The phenomenology of depression in epilepsy. *Epilepsia* 1987;28(4):364–372.

53. Andrewes DG, Bullen JG, Tomlinson L, Elwes RDC, Reynolds EH. A comparative study of the cognitive effects of phenytoin and carbamazepine in new referrals with epilepsy. *Epilepsia* 1986;27:128–134.

54. Brent DA, Crumrine PK, Varma RR, Allan M, Allman C. Phenobarbital treatment and major depressive disorder in children with epilepsy. *Pediatrics* 1987;80:909–917.

55. Corbett JA, Trimble MR, Nichol TC. Behavioral and cognitive impairment in children with epilepsy: the long-term effects of anticonvulsant therapy. *J Am Acad Child Psychiatry* 1985;24:17–23.

56. Brent DA. Overrepresentation of epileptics in a consecutive series of suicide attempters seen at a Children's Hospital, 1978–1983. *J Am Acad Child Psychiatry* 1986;25:242–246.

57. Dessain EC, Schatzberg AF, Woods BT, Cole JO. Maprotiline treatment in depression: a perspective on seizures. *Arch Gen Psychiatry* 1986;43:86–90.

Advances in Neurology, Vol. 55, edited by
D. Smith, D. Treiman, and M. Trimble,
Raven Press, Ltd., New York © 1991.

13

Cognitive Effects of Antiepileptic Drugs

Dennis B. Smith

*Oregon Comprehensive Epilepsy Program, Good Samaritan Hospital and Medical Center,
Portland, Oregon 97210*

> *Many physicians, in attempting to extinguish
> seizures, only succeed in drowning the finer
> intellectual processes of their patients.*
> Lennox, 1942 (1)

Throughout medical history, it has been recognized that there is an increase in behavior disorders and cognitive changes in patients with epilepsy. Estimates of the extent and prevalence of cognitive impairment and behavioral change vary, but the existence of an association is widely accepted (1–11). Trauma to the central nervous system (CNS)—whether it be metabolic or toxic, intrinsic or extrinsic, prenatal or perinatal, or generalized, widespread, or focal—may result in neurological dysfunction manifested by a wide variety of neurological symptoms, including behavioral change and seizures. Many of the known specific pathological, physiological, and neurochemical features (as well as the speculated ones) underlying both behavioral change and the production of seizures are discussed elsewhere in this volume (Chapters 1, 2, 4, and 6). This chapter will deal with the role of antiepileptic drugs (AEDs) on behavioral change in epilepsy and will review the evidence that AEDs may contribute to the cognitive decline seen in some patients with epilepsy. Speculation about possible mechanisms by which AEDs may impair cognition will be left to others; these mechanisms are alluded to in Chapters 2 and 6.

William Lennox was among the first who speculated in print about the probable contribution of AEDs to the behavioral and intellec-
tual deterioration seen in some patients with epilepsy (1,12). Until his paper in 1942, the extent of the influence of AEDs on cognition was probably underestimated, misconceptions about the mental state of patients with epilepsy were common, and the extent of CNS and psychiatric problems in this population was greatly overestimated (13). In that paper, he described the results of his study of 1245 patients with epilepsy and estimated that 15% of these patients showed mental changes that were caused, at least in part, by AEDs. Phenytoin had only recently been introduced. Most of the patients he studied were on barbiturates, although some were on bromides, either alone or in combination with phenobarbital. In later work, he adjusted his estimate of the percentage of patients showing cognitive impairment attributable to AEDs downward to 5%, perhaps in part because of the more widespread use of phenytoin and the waning use of bromides (12). The sedative effects of phenobarbital had been recognized since its introduction at the beginning of the century. The chronic effects of phenobarbital on behavior were not recognized (or at least were not reported) until the studies of Lennox were published. It is probably fair to say that his work set the stage for more recent studies, many of which have contributed significantly to our understanding of the extent and the relatively specific effects that different AEDs have on cognition and behavior.

Probably the first studies to try to quantitate the behavioral effects of AEDs were carried out on patients taking phenobarbital. In these early studies of the effect of AEDs on mental state, no attempt was made to differentiate between cognition and behavior. Trimble (14) has pointed out that cognition and behavior are two separate, but interrelated, aspects of neurological function. The distinction, however, is not always easily made. Alterations in behavior (mood, anger, anxiety) can affect cognitive abilities; conversely, the facility with which we can make decisions, recall events and facts, or understand subtleties and abstraction all affect behavior. For example, a child who cannot follow a teacher's lesson is likely to become disruptive and hyperactive, whereas a child with poor impulse control (or lack of self-confidence) and anxiety may find it difficult to sustain attention, recall facts or figures, or make decisions. Nonetheless, it is important to try to separate the effects of AEDs on higher intellectual function from effects on mood and behavior in order to define and compare the specific effects of different AEDs. Trimble (14) has provided definitions of cognition and behavior that help differentiate these two aspects of CNS function. "Cognition" is defined as the ability of a person to use information about and from the environment in an adaptive way; it is measured by standardized neuropsychological tests, including the Wechsler Adult Intelligence Scale (WAIS), the Wechsler Intelligence Scale for Children (WISC), and the Halsted–Reitan battery. In contrast, "behavior" is defined as the ability of a person to manage interpersonal relationships and is measured by arguably less exact rating scales of mood and personality, such as the Minnesota Multiphasic Personality Inventory (MMPI). This chapter will stress the effects of AEDs on cognition using this definition. In Chapter 14, Dodrill discusses the behavioral effects of AEDs.

AN INEXACT CHRONOLOGY BEGINNING WITH PHENOBARBITAL

The earliest studies on the cognitive effects of AEDs were based largely on observations of behavior and mood, subjective reports of sedation, and, in some cases, changes in global I.Q. Phenobarbital, of course, was the first drug studied in any systematic way. The sedative effects of phenobarbital were recognized in the earliest reports, but adverse effects on behavior or cognition were not examined (15). In fact, early studies reported that phenobarbital had a psychotropic effect, with patients becoming more alert and more responsive after initiation of therapy (16,17). However, the effect of seizure frequency on behavior and performance was not considered, and many patients in these studies were experiencing seizure control for the first time. An important methodologic departure in the study of the behavioral effects of AEDs was the controlled evaluation of the cognitive effects of phenobarbital reported in 1940 by Sommerfeld-Ziskind and Ziskind (18). Changes in intellectual functioning in 50 patients were examined using a battery of neuropsychological tests, including the Stanford–Binet. All patients were previously untreated and were tested before and after 1 year of treatment with phenobarbital. This group of treated patients was compared with control patients with epilepsy who remained untreated and who were matched for age and seizure duration. The group treated with phenobarbital showed no overall difference in I.Q. after 1 year when compared with the control group. A breakdown of the treatment group reveals that 10 patients had a fall in I.Q. over the year, but 12 other patients receiving phenobarbital actually showed an improvement in performance. Complicating the interpretation of this study is the fact that 79% of the treated group showed a decrease in seizure frequency, perhaps blurring any effects that phenobarbital may have had on behavior or cognition. Even though care was made to measure cognitive effects, and a control population was used for comparison, a crucial variable, seizure frequency, was not considered. Other studies on institutionalized patients also showed a tendency for improvement in I.Q. scores after receiving AEDs, but practice effects and better seizure control probably contributed to the results (16,19).

In 1956 Ingram (20) examined the effects of both phenobarbital and phenytoin on behavior and observed that 8 of 14 children on phenobarbital showed hyperactivity after exposure to phenobarbital, whereas no change was observed in 7 children given phenytoin. Duration of treatment was not specified, and although they reported that 11 children had "brain damage," it is not clear whether this group was randomly distributed. Similarly, in 1957 Lovel and et al. (19) found no change in behavior or cognition in patients with epilepsy on chronic AED therapy, and in 1961 Chaudhry and Pond (21) could find no significant effect on intellectual performance related to amount or duration of AED treatment (primarily phenobarbital). A year later, Wagner et al. (22) compared learning behavior and I.Q. before and after 6 weeks of treatment with phenobarbital. Teacher's observations were used, and seizure control was not documented. No change in behavior or intellect was observed compared with the control group.

Studies in volunteers over the same period yielded different results, and they consistently showed the adverse effects of phenobarbital on performance. An example is the study by Mirsky and Kornetsky (23) which demonstrated that phenobarbital impaired performance on tests of vigilance. Based on these results, these investigators suggested that phenobarbital may have an adverse effect on learning abilities in children. That conclusion has been criticized because they studied the acute effects of phenobarbital, and tolerance to the sedative properties of phenobarbital was not taken into consideration. Hutt et al. (24) gave volunteers phenobarbital over 12 days in doses sufficient to produce blood levels consistent with therapeutic practice, and they reasoned that initial tolerance was achieved by the time of testing. No effect of phenobarbital was found on simple, brief tests, but tasks requiring sustained effort were consistently impaired. Furthermore, tests of vigilance showed a decline proportional to serum phenobarbital levels, as did tests of verbal learning ability.

The contrast between the studies using volunteers (which uniformly demonstrated that phenobarbital had adverse effects on measures of performance) and the studies using patients with epilepsy (which generally failed to show any consistent adverse effect of phenobarbital) is remarkable. The fact that no adverse effect could be documented in the patient studies can be explained partially by (a) the confounding effects of better seizure control achieved during treatment with phenobar-

bital, (b) failure to control for practice effects, and (c) a number of other methodologic considerations. The lack of adverse effects of phenobarbital on behavior and cognition reported in these studies seems even more curious, however, in the light of studies carried out during the same decade which compared the behavioral effects of phenobarbital and the then newly introduced AED, primidone. In those studies, while seizure control was emphasized, the sedative and adverse mood effects of phenobarbital were uniformly commented upon (25–31).

In addition to the confounding effects of seizure frequency and lack of correlation with dose or blood levels of phenobarbital, the sensitivity of the performance measures used in those early studies may have contributed to their failure to consistently document any adverse effects of phenobarbital on behavior or performance. Idestrom (32), using critical flicker fusion (CFF), evaluated chronic phenobarbital usage in previously drug-naive patients and found that the CFF was depressed initially but that it tended to return to baseline after 1 1/2 to 2 months. This was really the first objective demonstration of the development of tolerance to the depressant effects of phenobarbital. Nearly two decades later, Houghton et al. (33), repeating Idestrom's paradigm but using normal volunteers, confirmed that phenobarbital in an acute setting caused a depression in CFF. In these experiments, phenobarbital was compared with a placebo; it was also compared with phenytoin, which produced no effect on CFF threshold.

Development of Tolerance

The issue of development of tolerance to the adverse effects of phenobarbital is an intriguing one. Numerous investigators in early studies reported that even though patients initially uniformly complained of sedation while on phenobarbital, they no longer complained of sedation after taking phenobarbital for several weeks. Spinks and Waring (34) found that subjective complaints of drowsiness were virtually gone by 12 days of therapy with phenobarbital. Moreover, blood level changes did not appear to account for the subjective improvements. Idestrom (32), as mentioned earlier, demonstrated the development of tolerance to a more objective measure of the adverse effects of phenobarbital: CFF threshold. Others had implied the development of tolerance, but no other study has documented the development of tolerance to the effect of phenobarbital on memory or sustained vigilance. No change in a total behavioral toxicity battery or in any specific subtest of battery was noted over 12 months in the recently completed VA study. In all chronic studies such as the VA study, the major variable seems to be blood phenobarbital level, and not the chronicity of therapy—a conclusion similar to that reached by Hutt et al. (24) more than two decades ago.

Specific Effects of Phenobarbital on Cognition

The effects of phenobarbital, specifically on cognition, have been the subject of more recent studies. In an epilepsy outpatient population, Reynolds and Travers (35) found that patients with deterioration in I.Q. and behavioral problems had significantly higher phenobarbital and phenytoin levels than did patients without mental changes, and that this change was independent of seizure frequency. Dodrill and Troupin (36) reported a very interesting study of monozygotic twins. The twins were the product of a normal pregnancy and birth, and they developed normally until the onset of seizures—one at the age of 5 and the other at the age of 6. The twins both had generalized absence and tonic–clonic seizures, and both were taking phenobarbital. One twin had a total of 37 generalized tonic–clonic seizures by the age of 19, whereas the other twin had a total of 7. When given a battery of neuropsychological tests at age 19, the twin with the greater number of seizures performed more poorly. As Lesser et al. (37) observed in their review in 1986, the poorer performance may have been related to the higher barbiturate level in the twin with the more frequent seizures (40.4 µg/ml versus 11.6 µg/ml).

Ozdirim et al. (38), in a study of 63 children with epilepsy in Turkey, compared phenobarbital and phenytoin as monotherapy with a placebo in a 3-month prospective blinded study. The children were tested prior to initiation of treatment, as well as at 3 months. Although behavior rating worsened significantly in the group taking phenobarbital compared with the group taking phenytoin or placebo ($p < 0.05$), no difference was reported on Bender–Gestalt, Peabody, or Vineland Social Maturity Scale. Review of their data, however, reveals that an improvement was seen in the placebo group at 3 months compared with pretest scores, probably reflecting a practice effect. A slight improvement was seen in the phenytoin group, but no improvement at all was seen in the group taking phenobarbital, implying that phenobarbital and possibly phenytoin had some detrimental effects on learning.

MacLeod et al. (39) looked at the specific effects of phenobarbital on memory, and they found that response times of 19 patients on a short-term memory task were remarkably slowed at high serum levels of phenobarbital (20–32 µg/ml) but were less impaired at low serum levels (8–15 µg/ml). A task requiring access to long-term memory was not significantly affected by high levels of phenobarbital.

Impairment of short-term memory could affect the ability to maintain attention (a common complaint of patients taking phenobarbital) and could lead to significant learning problems, perhaps most evident in children. In a double-blind placebo-controlled study of patients who had a single febrile seizure, Camfield et al. (40) also reported that difficulty with memory and comprehension was correlated with phenobarbital serum levels. Of interest was the fact that parents could not distinguish between phenobarbital and placebo after 12 months in the study. This observation emphasizes the subtle nature of these cognitive changes, and it also emphasizes the importance of using appropriate and sensitive measures for some of these effects to be demonstrated. This observation also emphasizes the need to discriminate between the development of subjective tolerance to the sedative properties of phenobarbital and the more persistent and insidious cognitive changes associated with chronic therapy.

Bourgeois et al. (41) identified a group of patients who had a significant fall in I.Q. which was associated with high serum levels of phenobarbital. Similar I.Q. changes were not noted in patients with high or toxic levels of phenytoin or valproate. Similarly, 312 children at a school for epilepsy were examined by Trimble and Corbett (42), who also found a trend for higher phenobarbital levels in children with lower I.Q. scores. All of these children were on polytherapy, so that it is difficult to solely incriminate phenobarbital.

Finally, Vining et al. (43) compared phenobarbital and valproate on both psychological and behavioral measures in 28 children with epilepsy using a double-blind counterbalanced crossover study design.

Each drug was given for 6 months in order to study long-term effects. Eighteen patients who were drug-naive prior to entry were studied, and a complete neuropsychological test battery was given prior to drug therapy and was then given again after 6 months on each drug. Seizure frequency was not significantly different during the two treatment periods. Few statistically significant differences emerged in the neuropsychological battery, but all differences that did occur favored valproate. Specifically, block design, performance and full-scale I.Q., and arithmetic and learning tasks were significantly more impaired by phenobarbital.

Reduction in Polypharmacy

The improvement in performance on neuropsychological tests seen with reduction in polypharmacy provides evidence for the deleterious cognitive effects of phenobarbital (and, to a lesser extent, primidone) which is almost as compelling as the evidence from the comparative studies just reviewed. Reynolds and Shorvon (44) pioneered the concept of reducing polytherapy and showed that monotherapy is effective in controlling seizures in most patients. In 1981, they reported that in 72% of 40 chronic adult patients the number of AEDs could be reduced without sacrificing seizure control. Fifty-five percent of these patients showed a marked improvement in mental function, including alertness, concentration, and psychomotor speed. Phenobarbital and primidone were the primary drugs eliminated. Much of the improvement seen was probably due to removal of barbiturates, and not due to the removal of *x* number of drugs.

The Milan Cooperative Group reported similar findings (45,46), as did Ludgate, et al. in 1985 (47). In this latter study, 12 patients whose treatment was reduced to monotherapy were analyzed. As phenobarbital, primidone, and/or phenytoin were removed from the treatment schedule, performance and full-scale I.Q. as well as block design and object assembly all showed significant ($p < 0.05$) improvement.

In Table 1, the results of reduction in polypharmacy reported by Thompson and Trimble (48) in 1982 are summarized. Only those measures that showed significant ($p < 0.05$) improvement are shown. Twenty patients on polytherapy had their number of drugs reduced. Improvement was seen in mood, anxiety, and depression, as well as in tasks of mental speed, motor speed, visual scanning, and memory. The reduction in polypharmacy was primarily the result of elimination of barbiturates (and in some cases phenytoin), lending support to the hypothesis that it is the elimination of these specific drugs that is responsible for the change.

Evidence for Cognitive Effects of Phenytoin

The toxic effects of phenytoin have been well documented since its introduction in

---

TABLE 1. *Neuropsychological measures showing improvement in performance associated with reduction in polypharmacy*[a]

Mental speed
Perceptual speed for words
Perceptual speed for pictures[b]
Decision-making for color
Decision-making for category
Motor speed
Tapping rate both hands
Visual scanning
Memory
Pictures
Immediate recall[b]
Delayed recall
Words
Immediate recall[b]
Delayed recall[b]

[a]Data were taken from ref. 48.
[b]Neuropsychological measures showing additional improvement when carbamazepine was substituted as monotherapy.

1938. Just as with phenobarbital, some of the earliest reports indicated that an improvement in performance occurred when phenytoin was given (49–52). These reports are difficult to interpret, in part because they were not controlled for (a) practice effects on neuropsychological tests, (b) dose and serum levels, or (c) the effect of improved seizure control. In addition, phenytoin was frequently substituted for phenobarbital in those studies. The elimination of the adverse effects of phenobarbital may have been responsible for the improvement seen. The conclusion that phenytoin had some psychotropic effects was probably in error.

Dilantin Encephalopathy

In addition to the more commonly described dose-related side effects of phenytoin, a confusional state or delirium can develop with chronic phenytoin therapy. Glaser (53) emphasized that this encephalopathy may not be accompanied by other signs or symptoms of toxicity such as nystagmus and ataxia. This syndrome is usually associated with high doses of phenytoin, but it can also occur with conventional "therapeutic" doses. The main feature is a gradual onset of mental deterioration and behavioral change with slowing on the electroencephalogram (EEG), with an occasional increase in seizure frequency. Increased cerebrospinal fluid (CSF) protein and a mild pleocytosis can occur. Vallarta et al. (54) described 10 patients with progressive cognitive and neurological deterioration. After discontinuation of phenytoin, the deterioration abated; in 6 of the 10, it was reversed. Kutt et al. (55) demonstrated a clear correlation between phenytoin blood levels and specific signs of toxicity: Mental changes and lethargy consistently appeared when phenytoin levels were above 40 μg/ml. Vallarta et al.'s (54) report, along with the reports by Rosen (56) and by Reynolds and Travers (35), confirm Glaser's (53) assertion that a non-dose-related Dilantin encephalopathy can develop which in some cases is not reversible.

Specific Effects on Cognitive Performance

The effects of phenytoin on cognition and behavior have been studied in both volunteers and patients with epilepsy, but few consistent results have emerged. Early studies are difficult to interpret because factors such as dose, blood level, seizure frequency, drug interactions, and duration of treatment were not consistently considered or controlled for. In volunteer studies such as those done by Smith and Lowrey in 1972 (49) and 1975 (50), claims of improvement in performance on neuropsychological tests when phenytoin was given are probably not valid. The improvement reported was, in fact, most likely due to practice effect rather than to any psychotropic effects of the drug. Booker et al. (57), in a placebo-controlled trial with 19 normal college students, found that 300 mg of phenytoin given daily for 6 days had no measurable effect on motor coordination, tactile discrimination, auditory attention, or sustained concentration. Most other studies in volunteers have shown either no effect or minimal detrimental effects on cognition. In 1972 Idestrom et al. (58) reported sedation at serum levels of 8 μg/ml, and they also reported that reaction time was longer at the higher serum levels. Houghton et al. (33) compared the effects of phenobarbital and phenytoin on CFF and found that phenytoin, in contrast to phenobarbital, had no apparent effect on CFF. The most impressive demonstration of the adverse effects of phenytoin on cognition, using volunteers, has been reported by Trimble et al. (59) and by Thompson et al. (60). In a series of experiments, volunteers were administered phenytoin or carbamazepine on a daily basis for 2 weeks in a double-blind, crossover design with a placebo control. A summary of the results of these studies is seen in Table 2.

There was a tendency for some deterioration in performance on all tests with both phenytoin and carbamazepine; but with the exception of errors of commission, the deterioration in performance reached statistical significance only for subjects taking phenytoin.

In contrast to early studies of the effects of phenytoin in patients, most studies within the last two decades have shown that phenytoin has an adverse effect on cognitive abilities. In 1974 Reynolds and Travers (35) were able to correlate higher serum phenytoin levels with intellectual deterioration in psychiatric illness. Somewhat earlier, Rosen (56) reported a remarkable overall improvement in the

TABLE 2. *Performance means and correlations between serum levels and deterioration in performance in phenytoin and carbamazepine trials*[a]

Psychologic measure (memory)	Performance means ($N = 8$)		Correlation between serum level and deterioration in performance	Performance means ($N = 8$)		Correlation between serum level and deterioration in performance
	Phenytoin ($\bar{x} = 39.4$ μmol/liter)	Placebo		Carbamazepine ($\bar{x} = 30.8$ μmol/liter)	Placebo	
Pictures						
Immediate recall	10.9	12.3	0.86[d]	12.1	12.9	−0.04
Delayed recall	10.1	12.3[c]	0.78[c]	11.1	12.3	−0.24
Recognition	39.4	39.8	—	38.6	39.8	—
Words						
Immediate recall	6.6	8.8[b]	−0.25	7.4	8.4	0.15
Delayed recall	3.4	6.0	−0.36	5.3	4.0	0.02
Errors of commission	2.3	0.9[d]	0.60	1.3	0.3[b]	−0.02
Recognition	30.6	32.4	0.02	31.5	31.6	0.23
Decision-making						
Perceptual	0.863	0.709[d]	0.71[b]	0.704	0.633	0.21
Semantic	0.926	0.773[c]	0.38	0.769	0.747	0.07

[a]Analysis based on two-tailed paired Student's *t*-tests and Spearman rank correlations. From ref. 59, with permission.
[b]$p < 0.05$.
[c]$p < 0.025$.
[d]$p < 0.01$.

WAIS, Bender–Gestalt, and other tests of intellectual function, as well as in school and work performance, in 320 patients in whom phenytoin was discontinued. In 1975 Dodrill (61) assessed the effects of phenytoin in 70 patients with epilepsy and reported that patients with high and toxic serum levels of phenytoin consistently performed more poorly on all tests than did the low and nontoxic groups. The difference, however, did not reach statistical significance except in tasks requiring a significant motor component. Similarly, Ozdirim et al. (38) reported an overall decrease in performance in patients taking phenytoin as compared with the placebo, but none of the effects reached statistical significance. Further evidence for the adverse effect of phenytoin on intellectual function comes from the study of Nolte et al. (62). They followed 20 school children with epilepsy who were treated with either primidone or phenytoin. The children were all seizure-free during the testing period. A deterioration in performance was documented in those children with high phenytoin levels, but no significant effect could be demonstrated in those children with serum phenytoin levels in the low therapeutic range.

Most recently, a study reported by Gallasi et al. (63) convincingly demonstrated adverse effects of phenytoin on specific tests of cognitive function. They studied 10 patients with epilepsy who had been seizure-free for at least 2 years on monotherapy with phenytoin. A mean blood level of 13.4 ± 6.7 was achieved. The subjects were given a complete battery of neuropsychological tests prior to withdrawal of phenytoin, which took place gradually over 1 year; serial neuropsychological evaluations were performed during the withdrawal and at 3 months and 1 year following complete cessation of therapy. A group of 10 controls matched for age and education was also used. The group taking phenytoin scored lower than the controls on all tests prior to withdrawal, but only 3 of the 13 tests reached statistical significance. In contrast, no difference from the control population was seen in patients when tested 1 year after stopping phenytoin. These findings support the conclusion that phenytoin does have an adverse effect on cognitive function, although most effects occurred in those tests requiring a significant motor component.

Other data suggesting that phenytoin has an adverse effect on cognition have emerged from studies comparing the effects of phenytoin with carbamazepine or valproate on neuropsychological test scores (48,64–66). Uniformly, those studies have shown that patients and volunteers taking phenytoin perform more poorly on a wide range of psychological tests than do patients taking carbamazepine or valproate.

A note of caution in the interpretation of all of these studies is urged, however. As Dodrill (67) has perceptively pointed out, some of the reported effects of phenytoin on higher cognitive function may be due entirely to the drug's effect on motor speed and accuracy. When Dodrill (67) factored out reaction time, he found no effect of phenytoin on other measures of cognitive function. It is very difficult to design tests of cognition that do not rely to some extent on motor performance and accuracy, and no study on the effects of phenytoin has completely controlled for that variable.

A Brief Selective Summary of the Effects of Carbamazepine on Cognition

Many of the studies which have documented the effects of carbamazepine on cognition are studies which have compared carbamazepine with either phenobarbital or phenytoin; these studies have been outlined in the two preceding sections. One of the key studies was performed by Dodrill and Troupin (65) in which phenytoin and carbamazepine were compared in a double-blind crossover study. Forty patients received both carbamazepine and phenytoin as monotherapy for 4 months in a double-blind crossover study. Results of a neuropsychological test battery which included the Halsted–Reitan battery and the MMPI were similar for each drug, though when patients were on carbamazepine (as compared to phenytoin), improvement was seen in tests of attention and problem solving. Improvements in emotional status were also reported when patients were on carbamazepine. Subjectively, patients reported less sedation while on carbamazepine. Although this report seems to favor carbamazepine, the fact that the mean phenytoin level was 31.2 mg/liter while the mean carbamazepine level was 9.3 mg/liter may have skewed the results.

Trimble et al. (59) and Thompson et al. (60) compared carbamazepine and phenytoin in normal volunteers. These studies, outlined in more detail in the preceding section, also showed that carbamazepine had little effect on the cognitive measures they used. In a more extensive study reported in 1983, Trimble and Thompson (68) evaluated the effects of four AEDs on cognition in normal healthy volunteers. They found that each of the drugs (phenytoin, carbamazepine, valproate, and clobazam) produced some negative effect on performance at "therapeutic" blood levels but that carbamazepine, valproate, and clobazam did not interfere with memory function.

The only study that directly compared the cognitive effects of carbamazepine with phenobarbital, phenytoin, and primidone was the nationwide VA cooperative study completed in 1985 (69). The importance of this study is reflected not only in the simultaneous comparison of the four most commonly used AEDs in 1985, but more importantly in the study design which avoided many of the methodologic problems of previous studies. A sufficiently large number ($N = 622$) of previously untreated or undertreated patients were entered into this study to provide for an adequate sampling and statistical analysis. A double-blind prospective study design was employed, and strict exclusion criteria limited confounding factors such as drug or alcohol abuse. All patients were given an extensive behavioral toxicity battery before receiving any AED, as well as at 1, 3, 6, and 12 months after monotherapy with one of the study drugs. The tests were designed to reflect neuropsychological functioning in four major areas, including general intellect, attention/concentration, motor skills, and mood status. When the effects of each AED on the behavioral toxicity battery was examined at 1, 3, 6, and 12 months, significant differences between the drugs were apparent (see Table 3).

The total behavioral toxicity score was derived by combining the scores of the individual subtests transformed into weighted ordinal units of change based on published norms. The higher the score on the behavioral toxicity battery, the greater the deterioration from baseline performance. A negative score (as

TABLE 3. *Total behavioral toxicity score for each drug at 1, 3, 6, and 12 months*

Month: p value:	1 0.001	3 0.002	6 NS[a]	12 0.01
Carbamazepine:	15.5	14.9	14.8	16.1
Phenytoin:	17.3	20.1	15.9	20.1
Phenobarbital:	21.3	17.2	15.8	18.5
Primidone:	17.5	18.5	16.1	18.3

[a]NS, not significant.

compared with baseline predrug test scores) indicates an improvement in performance.

None of the groups showed improvement in test scores at any of the testing periods, but carbamazepine showed the least deterioration. On subtests of the behavioral toxicity battery, carbamazepine consistently outperformed the other three drugs on tests of attention/concentration, but tests of motor performance were less discriminating. As expected, phenytoin affected motor performance most (see Table 4).

The effect of phenytoin on motor performance may partly explain the phenytoin group's poor performance on tests designed to measure attention/concentration, which also require some degree of visual–motor coordination (67).

The differential behavioral effects of the four AEDs are clearly evident from this study. Carbamazepine showed fewer adverse behavioral effects than did phenobarbital, primidone, or phenytoin. It should be emphasized, however, that even carbamazepine appeared to prevent practice effects—effects observed in a control population of 75 individuals, matched for age, sex, and education (70). These results suggest that all four drugs, including carbamazepine, have some adverse effect on motor skills, cognition, and mood.

While most studies have shown that carbamazepine has fewer adverse effects on cognition than do other AEDs (42,48,59,61,68, 69,71,72,74), some adverse effect at higher blood levels is also a consistent finding. For example, in 1986 Macphee et al. (74) demonstrated a decrement in performance on a series of psychomotor tests given to epilepsy patients on carbamazepine monotherapy who had been given a supplemental dose of 400 mg of carbamazepine. In this placebo-controlled study, free and total carbamazepine levels

TABLE 4. *Total number of best and worst scores on subtests of the behavioral toxicity battery at 1, 3, 6, and 12 months of therapy*[a]

Drug	POMS[b]	Motor	Attention/ concentration
	Best scores		
Carbamazepine	11	4	10
Phenytoin	2	1	2
Primidone	9	3	1
Phenobarbital	2	1	0
	Worst scores		
Carbamazepine	0	0	1
Phenytoin	13	4	0
Primidone	2	5	6
Phenobarbital	9	0	5

[a]"Best" and "worst" indicate scores that are significantly different from scores attained by two or more of the other groups for the same subtest at the same rating period.
[b]POMS, profile of mood states.

were monitored as was carbamazepine-10, 11-epoxide concentrations. Impairment of choice reaction time was documented at higher carbamazepine levels along with a higher sedation score. Some impairment of psychomotor tests was also found to be associated with higher blood levels of carbamazepine in patients on chronic carbamazepine therapy (75), but a direct relationship to concentration was not shown. Gillham et al. (76) did report a relationship between carbamazepine and carbamazepine–epoxide concentrations and impairment of psychomotor performance on a wide range of neuropsychological measures; these investigators suggested that the carbamazepine–epoxide concentrations, which were particularly elevated in patients on polytherapy, were the most important factor. This study did not adequately control for effects of seizure frequency even though this variable was "factored out" in analysis, and caution must be taken in interpreting these results. Nonetheless, this study and those of Macphee et al. (74) emphasize the conclusion that patients with high levels of carbamazepine do have some risk of psychomotor impairment even though it may be less than that of other currently available AEDs.

From the time of its introduction in Europe in the early 1960s, a wide range of psychotropic effects have been ascribed to carbamazepine. Evidence for a positive psychotropic effect is not consistent, as pointed out by Stores in 1975 and 1982 (77,78); further-

more, reported improvements of behavior and mental function may be partly due to improvement in seizure control in patients on carbamazepine, or to the removal of AEDs with sedative properties from the therapeutic regimen. The existence of a positive psychotropic effect from carbamazepine is discussed in more detail in Chapter 16 in this volume. Recent evidence of a possible psychotropic effect was provided by Trimble et al. (59) (see Table 2).

In an extension of a previous study in which 20 patients underwent a reduction in polytherapy, 15 additional patients were changed to carbamazepine used either as monotherapy or in combination with the existing medications. The patients who were switched to carbamazepine appeared to have an even more widespread improvement than did the group undergoing reduction in polytherapy alone. These results have been interpreted as indicating that carbamazepine has psychotropic properties. An alternative and more likely explanation is that carbamazepine simply replaced phenobarbital, primidone, or phenytoin, each of which has adverse effects on the neuropsychological measures studied.

There have been numerous other studies comparing carbamazepine with other AEDs, and the results are remarkably uniform: Treatment with carbamazepine, as compared to treatment with either phenytoin or barbiturates, tends to be associated with better scores on a wide variety of neuropsychological measures, particularly on measures of attention and problem solving. Some adverse effects on cognition do exist at higher serum levels, but the spectrum of effects on psychomotor performance is different than, and probably less than, that of other currently available AEDs—including valproate, which is also thought to have minimal effects on higher cognitive function.

Valproate, an Even Briefer Summary

Valproate, like carbamazepine, is thought to lack the sedative effects of barbiturates and possibly phenytoin. A review of the reports of sedation (and even stupor) associated with valproate therapy reveals that the sedation was probably the result of the interaction of valproate with concomitant AED therapy, and not a direct effect of valproate. Drug interaction is thought to be the explanation for reports of impaired cognitive performance (65,79,80). The results of Trimble and Thompson (81) are fairly representative of results of other volunteer trials, and they show the relative lack of adverse effect that valproate has on a variety of measures (see Table 5). In those volunteers, a valproate-induced psychotropic effect is suggested by subjective reports of increased alertness when taking valproate. While no relationship between valproate concentration and cognitive scores was seen in the volunteers taking valproate, a greater impairment was noted at higher levels of valproate in a group of patients taking valproate. Tests showing impairment at higher levels emphasized recall and concentration. Also in 1984, Gay (82), studying 129 mentally retarded patients with epilepsy, reported that valproate had no adverse effects on a variety of neuropsychological measures when compared with the control group.

A very careful double-blind crossover study of 28 children with epilepsy who had normal intelligence, comparing neuropsychological effects of phenobarbital with valproate, was reported by Vining et al. in 1987 (43). Seizure frequency was not different when patients were on valproate or phenobarbital, but the children on valproate showed a consistent tendency for better cognitive function. On most measures, however, there was no difference between the drugs. Eight of 34 measures showed statistically significant ($p < 0.01$ or 0.05) differences between valproate and phenobarbital, with patients on valproate showing superior performance; however, the patients receiving valproate tended to perform better on most of the tests.

Recent studies, carried out within the last 5 years, have uniformly demonstrated that valproate has little measurable effect on cognition when used as monotherapy. Nonetheless,

TABLE 5. *Effects of valproate on psychological measures*[a]

Measure	Volunteers	Patients (high versus low ABLs)
Memory		*
Pictures		
Words		
Concentration		
Stroop		
Visual scanning		*
Perceptual speed		
Words		
Pictures		
Decision–making		
Color	*	*
Category	*	*
Motor speed		
Tapping		

[a]Behavioral measures that showed some deterioration in performance are indicated by an asterisk. The effects noted in column 3 refer to performance measures that demonstrated greater impairment in patients with higher valproate levels. Data were taken from ref. 81.

just as with carbamazepine, higher levels are associated with more impairment, and reports of a psychotropic effect should be viewed with caution.

Other Drugs

Studies of the cognitive effects of ethosuximide have reported conflicting results: Some studies reported improvement of cognitive performance, particularly in tests of memory (83,84), whereas other studies reported no adverse effects (85). Because seizure frequency was not controlled for, and concomitant treatment with other drugs was a confounding factor, it is difficult to form any firm conclusions; however, it appears that ethosuximide, when used in usual therapeutic doses, has little effect on cognitive abilities.

There are few well-controlled studies of the selective cognitive effects of the benzodiazepines when used in the treatment of epilepsy, although sedation, behavioral deterioration, and selective memory impairment are well documented with clonazapam and diazepam (86–88). Thompson and Trimble (89), and later Cull and Trimble (90), compared both clobazam (a 1,5-benzodiazepine) and clonazapam with a placebo in normal volunteers, and they found that clonazapam produces a wide spectrum of impairment on cognitive tests, similar to the impairment produced by phenytoin, whereas clobazam showed minimal impairments at lower drug levels. Other than when used in epilepsy, the benzodiazepines are usually prescribed because of their behavioral effects. These same effects are usually considered unwanted side effects when they are used as AEDs. It cannot be denied, however, that the "tranquilizing" effects of these drugs may be useful and may even help in seizure management.

The effects of primidone are difficult to separate from its derived phenobarbital, but the results of the VA Cooperative Study (69,70,91) suggest that primidone has a different profile of behavioral effects than does phenobarbital. Specifically, patients on primidone monotherapy scored better on the profile of mood states than did patients on phenobarbital (see Tables 3 and 4). The two drugs had similar effects on tests of attention/con-centration. Impairments in tests of attention/concentration and motor functioning was apparent only at higher derived phenobarbital levels. Primidone may have some advantage over phenobarbital with respect to neurotoxicity if used as monotherapy when it is possible to achieve a primidone:phenobarbital ratio approaching 1:1. A primidone:phenobarbital ratio of 1:1 is likely to be associated with minimal cognitive impairment, and is thought to be the optimal ratio for seizure control (92).

CONCLUSIONS

While the majority of patients with epilepsy show no evidence of significant cognitive impairment or deterioration, numerous studies have shown that there is an increased incidence of cognitive impairment in the population of patients with epilepsy (1,12,93,94). Age of onset of epilepsy (41,94–97), seizure frequency (98,99), duration (100–102), seizure type (70,103–105), and AEDs have all been postulated to affect cognitive function. Evidence that factors unrelated to the effects of AEDs may contribute to the impairment of cognitive function seen in some patients with epilepsy has been provided both by the nationwide VA Cooperative Study (70) and by the study reported by Brodie et al. (106). In the VA study, a battery of neuropsychological tests was administered to 618 patients with newly diagnosed epilepsy before administration of any AED. The same test battery was given to 74 controls matched for age, sex, and education. General intellectual ability as measured by the WAIS was within normal range (100 ± 13.5). Nonetheless, significant differences in the performance on neuropsychological tests were observed between the two groups. With the exception of digit span, the patients with epilepsy, even though they were not on AEDs, did not perform as well as the control group on measures of attention/concentration or predominantly motor measures. Perhaps not surprisingly, mood scales were also depressed in the patient group.

The results of the VA study (70) and of Brodie et al. (106) suggest that some specific impairment that is related to underlying neurological dysfunction and that may also be responsible for the presence of seizures does exist in some patients with epilepsy. AEDs clearly compound these impairments. It is also clear that all currently available AEDs have some adverse effect on cognition, even when usual doses are used and when AED levels are in the usual therapeutic range. The effects are not uniform and are usually fairly subtle. The fact that the effects may be subtle, however, does not diminish their importance, nor does it diminish the need to consider these effects in the management of patients with epilepsy.

Most of the acute effects of AEDs are probably reversible with withdrawal of the drug; however, as pointed out by Hirtz and Nelson (107), the effects of chronic long-term therapy, particularly in children, are not completely understood or documented. That some chronic irreversible effect may occur is suggested by the well-documented adverse effects of phenobarbital on the developing brain; this is discussed in detail elsewhere in this volume (see Chapter 15). It is likely that phenobarbital is not the only AED that produces irreversible effects on the developing brain. Furthermore, it is now recognized that neuronal sprouting occurs in adults as well as in infants, and the possibility is therefore raised that the long-term effects of AEDs may not be limited to the developing brain. Further studies, such as those using other AEDs (see Chapter 15), are needed before definitive conclusions can be reached regarding the long-term effects of AED therapy, and regarding whether or not different AEDs affect neuronal development differently.

Even though the long-term effects of chronic treatment with AEDs have not been well documented, and despite the paucity of well-conceived, well-controlled studies of the more immediate effects of AEDs, it is clear that the currently available AEDs all have adverse effects on cognition, and that the effect of each drug is different. The barbiturates, particularly phenobarbital, have very consistent adverse effects on tests requiring sustained concentration and attention, whereas phenytoin primarily affects tasks requiring motor speed and accuracy. Phenytoin also appears to have adverse effects on tests of attention/concentration, but there remains some controversy as to the extent of this effect. Carbamazepine and valproate appear to have

the least effect on neuropsychological measures of cognitive function, but even these drugs adversely affect performance at higher blood levels.

Much has been learned and demonstrated about the effects of individual AEDs on cognition in the past several years, but a great deal of controversy regarding the specific effects of different AEDs remains. Further studies controlling for practice effects and serum AED levels and using a well-defined subject population for which normative data are available (70) are needed. For meaningful results, a control population should be included, and drugs should be assessed when used as monotherapy only. Perhaps most importantly, tests need to be used that are well standardized, sensitive, and specific and that enable us to clearly differentiate between cognitive functions of attention/concentration, motor speed and accuracy, and mood. Most studies of the cognitive effects of AEDs now recognize that these variables need to be considered, and definitive results are emerging.

REFERENCES

1. Lennox WG. Brain injury, drugs and environment a cause of mental decay in epilepsy. *Am J Psychiatry* 1942;99:174–180.
2. Lesser RP, Luders H, Wyllie E, Dinner DS, Morris HH. Mental deterioration in epilepsy. *Epilepsia* 1986;27(Suppl 2)S105–S123.
3. Gowers WR. *Epilepsy.* London: Churchill, William Wood & Co., 1985.
4. Guerrant J, Anderson WW, Fischer A, Weinstein MR, Jaros RM, Deskins A. *Personality in epilepsy.* Springfield, IL: Charles C Thomas, 1962.
5. Dodrill CB, Troupin AS. Seizures and adaptive abilities. *Arch Neurol* 1976;33:604–607.
6. Engel J, Caldecott-Hazard S, Bandler R. Neurobiology of behavior: anatomic and physiological implications related to epilepsy. *Epilepsia* 1986;27(Suppl 2):S3–S13.
7. Bruens JH. Psychoses in epilepsy. *Psychiatr Neurol Neurochir* 1971;74:175–192.
8. Ellenberg JH, Hirtz DG, Nelson KB. Do seizures in children cause intellectual deterioration? *Ann Neurol* 1985;18:389.
9. Gibbs FA. Ictal and nonictal psychiatric disorders in temporal lobe epilepsy. *J Nerv Ment Dis* 1951;113:522–528.
10. Parnas J, Korsgaard S. Epilepsy and psychosis. *Acta Psychiatr Scand* 1982;66:89–99.
11. Quadfasel AF, Pruyser PW. Cognitive deficits in patients with psychomotor epilepsy. *Epilepsia* 1955;4:80–90.

12. Lennox WG, Lennox MA. *Epilepsy and related disorders.* Boston: Little, Brown, 1960.
13. Reynolds EH. Historical aspects. In: Trimble MR, Reynolds EH, eds. *Epilepsy, behaviour and cognitive function.* New York: John Wiley & Sons, 1988;3–8.
14. Trimble MR. Anticonvulsant drugs and cognitive function. *Epilepsia* 1987;28(Suppl 3):S37–S45.
15. Barnes MR, Fetterman JN. Mentality of dispensary epileptic patients. *Arch Neurol Psychiatry* 1938;40:903–910.
16. Lennox WG. Gains against epilepsy. *JAMA* 1942;120:449–453.
17. Lennox WG. Brain injury, drugs, and environment as causes of mental decay in epilepsy. *Am J Psychiatry* 1942;99:174–180.
18. Sommerfeld-Ziskind E, Ziskind E. Effect of phenobarbital on the mentality of epileptic patients. *Arch Neurol Psychiatry* 1940;43:70–79.
19. Loveland N, Smith B, Forster FM. Mental and emotional changes in epileptic patients on continuous anti-convulsant medication. *Neurology* 1957;7:856–865.
20. Ingram TTS. A characteristic form of overactive behaviour in brain damaged children. *J Ment Sci* 1956;102:550–558.
21. Chaudhry MR, Pond DA. Mental deterioration in epileptic children. *J Neurol Neurosurg Psychiatry* 1961;24:213–219.
22. Wagner I, Thurston DL, Holowach J. Phenobarbital: its effects on learning in epileptic children. *JAMA* 1962;182:937.
23. Mirsky AF, Kornetsky C. On the dissimilar effects of drugs on the digit symbol substitution and continuous performance tests: a review and preliminary integration of behavioral and physiological evidence. *Psychopharmacology* 1964;5:161–177.
24. Hutt SJ, Jackson PM, Belsham A, Higgins G. Perceptual motor behavior in relation to blood phenobarbitone level: a preliminary report. *Dev Med Child Neurol* 1968;10:626–632.
25. Butter AJM. Mysoline in treatment of epilepsy. *Lancet* 1953;1:1024.
26. Calnan WL, Borrell YM. Mysoline in the treatment of epilepsy. *Lancet* 1953;2:42–43.
27. Handley R, Stewart ASR. Mysoline: a new drug in the treatment of epilepsy. *Lancet* 1952;1:742–744.
28. Oxley J, Hebdige S, Laidlaw J, Wadsworth J, Richens A. A comparative study of phenobarbitone and primidone in the treatment of epilepsy. In: Johannessen SI, et al., eds. *Antiepileptic therapy: advances in drug monitoring.* New York: Raven Press, 1980;237–245.
29. Smith B, Forster FM. The role of some experimental anticonvulsants, mysoline, milontin and 1461L. *M Ann District of Columbia* 1953;22:279–282.
30. Smith B, Forster FM. Mysoline and Milontin: two new medicines for epilepsy. *Neurology (Minneap)* 1954;4:137–142.
31. Smith BH, McNaughton FL. Mysoline, new anticonvulsant drug: its value in refractory cases of epilepsy. *Can Med Assoc J* 1953;68:464–467.
32. Idestrom C. Flicker-fusion in chronic barbiturate usage: a quantitative study in the pathophysiology of drug addiction. *Acta Psychiatr Neurol Scand* 1954;91:1–93.
33. Houghton GW, Latham AN, Richens A. Difference in the central actions of phenytoin and phenobarbitone in man, measured by critical flicker fusion threshold. *Eur J Clin Pharmacol* 1973;6:57–60.
34. Spinks A, Waring WS. Anticonvulsant drugs. In: Ellis GP, Went GB, eds. *Progress in medicinal chemistry,* vol 3. London: Butterworths, 1963;261.
35. Reynolds EH, Travers RD. Serum anticonvulsant concentrations in epileptic patients with mental symptoms: a preliminary report. *Br J Psychiatry* 1974;124:440–445.
36. Dodrill CB, Troupin AS. Seizures and adaptive abilities. *Arch Neurol* 1976;33:604–607.
37. Lesser RP, Luders H, Wyllie E, Dinner DS, Morris HH. Mental deterioration in epilepsy. *Epilepsia* 1986;27(Suppl 2):S105–S123.
38. Ozdirim E, Renda Y, Epir S. Effects of phenobarbital and phenytoin on the behaviour of epileptic children. In: Meinardi H, Rowan AJ, eds. *Advances in epileptology.* Amsterdam: Swets & Zeitlinger, 1977;120–123.
39. MacLeod CM, Dekaban AS, Hunt E. Memory impairment in epileptic patients: selective effects of phenobarbital concentration. *Science* 1978;202:1102–1104.
40. Camfield CS, Chaplin S, Doyle AB, Shapiro SH, Cummings C, Camfield PR. Side effects of phenobarbital in toddlers: behavior and cognitive aspects. *J Pediatr* 1979;95:361–365.
41. Bourgeois BFD, Prensky AL, Palkes HS, Talent BK, Busch SG. Intelligence in epilepsy: a prospective study in children. *Ann Neurol* 1983;14:438–444.
42. Trimble MR, Corbett J. Behavioral and cognitive disturbances in epileptic children. *Ir Med J* 1980;73(Suppl):21–28.
43. Vining EPG, Mellits E, Dorsen MM, et al. Psychologic and behavioral effects of antiepileptic drugs in children: a double-blind comparison between phenobarbital and valproic acid. *Pediatrics* 1987;80:165–174.
44. Reynolds EH, Shorvon SD. Monotherapy or polytherapy for epilepsy? *Epilepsia* 1981;22:1–10.
45. Collaborative Group for Epidemiology of Epilepsy, Milan, Italy. Adverse reactions to antiepileptic drugs: a multicenter survey of clinical practice. *Epilepsia* 1986;27:323–330.
46. Beghi E, Bollini P, DiMascio R, et al. Effects of rationalizing drug treatment of patients with epilepsy and mental retardation. *Dev Med Child Neurol* 1987;29:363–369.
47. Ludgate J, Keating J, O'Dwyer R, Callaghan N. An improvement in cognitive function following polypharmacy reduction in a group of epileptic patients. *Acta Neurol Scand* 1985;71:448–452.

48. Thompson PJ, Trimble MR. Anticonvulsant drugs and cognitive functions. *Epilepsia* 1982; 23:531–544.

49. Smith WL, Lowrey JB. The effects of diphenylhydantoin on cognitive functions in man. In: Smith WL, ed. *Drugs, development and cerebral function*. Springfield, IL: Charles C Thomas, 1972;344–351.

50. Smith WL, Lowrey JB. Effects of diphenylhydantoin on mental abilities in the elderly. *J Am Geriatr Soc* 1975;23:207–211.

51. Goldberg JB, Kurland AA. Dilantin treatment of hospitalized cultural–familial retardates. *J Nerv Ment Dis* 1970;150:133–137.

52. Millichap JG, Egan RW, Hart ZH, Sturgis LH. Auditory perceptual deficit correlated with EEG dysrhythmias. *Neurology* 1969;19:870–872.

53. Glaser GH. Diphenylhydantoin toxicity. In: Woodbury DM, Penry JK, Schmidt RP, eds. *Antiepileptic drugs*. New York: Raven Press, 1972;219–226.

54. Vallarta JM, Bell DB, Reichert A. Progressive encephalopathy due to chronic hydantoin intoxication. *Am J Dis Child* 1974;128:27–34.

55. Kutt H, Winters W, Kokenge R, et al. Diphenylhydantoin metabolism, blood levels and toxicity. *Arch Neurol* 1964;11:642–648.

56. Rosen JA. Dilantin dementia. *Trans Am Neurol Assoc* 1968;93:273.

57. Booker HE, Matthews CG, Slaby A. Effects of diphenylhydantoin on selected physiological and psychological measures in normal adults. *Neurology* 1967;949–951.

58. Idestrom CM, Schalling D, Carlquist U, Sjoqvist. Behavioral and psychophysiological studies: acute effects of diphenylhydantoin in relation to plasma levels. *Psychol Med* 1972;2:111–120.

59. Trimble MR, Thompson PJ, Huppert F. Anticonvulsant drugs and cognitive abilities. In: Canger R, Angeleri F, Penry JK, eds. *Advances in epileptology: XIth Epilepsy International Symposium*. New York: Raven Press, 1980;199–204.

60. Thompson PJ, Huppert FA, Trimble MR. Phenytoin and cognitive functions: effects on normal volunteers and implications for epilepsy. *Br J Clin Psychol* 1981;20:155–162.

61. Dodrill CB. Diphenylhydantoin serum levels, toxicity, and neuropsychological performance in patients with epilepsy. *Epilepsia* 1975;16:593–600.

62. Nolte R, Wetzel B, Brugmann G, Britzinger I. Effects of phenytoin- and primidone-monotherapy on mental performance in children. In: Johannessen SI, ed. *Antiepileptic therapy: advances in drug monitoring*. New York: Raven Press, 1980;81–90.

63. Gallasi R, Morreale A, Lorusso S, et al. Cognitive effects of phenytoin during monotherapy and after withdrawal. *Acta Neurol Scand* 1987;75:258–261.

64. Andrewes DG, Tomlinson L, Elwes RDC, Reynolds EH. The influence of carbamazepine and phenytoin on memory and other aspects of cognitive function in new referrals with epilepsy. *Acta Neurol Scand* 1984;69:23–30.

65. Dodrill CB, Troupin AS. Psychotropic effects of carbamazepine in epilepsy: a double-blind comparison with phenytoin. *Neurology* 1977; 27:1023–1028.

66. Rennick P, Keiser T, Rodin E. Carbamazepine (Tegretol): behavioral side effects in temporal lobe epilepsy during short term comparison with placebo. *Epilepsia* 1975;16:198.

67. Dodrill C. Effects of antiepileptic drugs on psychological abilities. In: Penry JK, ed. *Epilepsy and life performance*. New York: Raven Press, 1991;in press.

68. Trimble MR, Thompson PJ. Anticonvulsant drugs, cognitive function and behavior. *Epilepsia* 1983;24:S55–S63.

69. Mattson RH, Cramer JA, Collins JF, et al. Comparison of carbamazepine, phenobarbital, phenytoin, and primidone in partial and secondarily generalized tonic–clonic seizures. *N Engl J Med* 1985;313:145–151.

70. Smith DB, Craft BR, Collins J, Mattson RH, Cramer JA, and the VA Cooperative Study Group 118. Behavioral characteristics of epilepsy patients compared with normal controls. *Epilepsia* 1986;27:760–768.

71. Smith DB. Anticonvulsants, seizures and performance: the Veteran's Administration experience. In: Trimble MR, Reynolds EH, eds. *Epilepsy, behaviour and cognitive function*. Chichester: John Wiley & Sons, 1988;67–78.

72. Jacobides GM. Alertness and scholastic achievement in young epileptics treated with carbamazepine (Tegretol). Advances in epileptology—psychology, pharmacotherapy and new diagnostic approaches. In: *Proceedings of the 13th Congress of the International League Against Epilepsy, and 9th Symposium of the International Bureau for Epilepsy*, Amsterdam, 1977;114–119.

73. Schain RJ, Ward JW, Guthrie D. Carbamazepine as an anticonvulsant in children. *Neurology* 1977;27:476–480.

74. Macphee GJA, McPhail EM, Butler E, Brodie MJ. Controlled evaluation of a supplementary dose of carbamazepine on psychomotor function in epileptic patients. *Eur J Clin Pharmacol* 1986;31:195–199.

75. Brodie MJ, McPhail E, Macphee GJA, Larkin JG, Gray JMB. Psychomotor impairment and anticonvulsant therapy in adult epileptic patients. *Eur J Clin Pharmacol* 1987;31:655–660.

76. Gillham RA, Williams N, Weidmann K, Butler E, Larkin JG, Brodie MJ. Concentration–effect relationships with carbamazepine and its epoxide on psychomotor and cognitive function in epileptic patients. *J Neurol Neurosurg Psychiatry* 1988;51:929–933.

77. Stores G. Behavioral effects of antiepileptic drugs. *Dev Med Child Neurol* 1975;17:647–658.

78. Stores G. Behavioral effects of antiepileptic drugs. In: Nelson KB, Ellenberg JH, eds. *Febrile seizures*. New York: Raven Press, 1981;185–192.

79. Sommerback KW, Theilgaard A, Rasmussen KE, Lohren V, Gram L, Wulff K. Valproate sodium: evaluation of so-called psychotropic effect. A controlled study. *Epilepsia* 1977;18:159–167.

80. Bruni J, Albright P. Valproic acid therapy for complex partial seizures, its efficacy and toxic effects. *Arch Neurol* 1983;40:135–137.

81. Trimble MR, Thompson PJ. Sodium valproate and cognitive function. *Epilepsia* 1984;25(1):S60–S64.

82. Gay PE. Effects of antiepileptic drugs and seizure type on operant responding in mentally retarded persons. *Epilepsia* 1984;25(3):377–386.

83. Guey J, Charles C, Coquery C, Roger J, Soulayrol R. Study of psychological effects of ethosuximide (Zarontin) on 25 children suffering from petit mal epilepsy. *Epilepsia* 1967;8:129–141.

84. Smith WL, Philippus MJ, Guard HL. Psychometric study of children with learning problems and 14-6 positive spike S patterns, treated with ethosuximide (Zarontin) and placebo. *Arch Dis Child* 1968;43:616–619.

85. Browne TR, Dreifuss FE, Dyken PR, et al. Ethosuximide (Zarontin) in the treatment of absence (petit mal) seizures. *Neurology* 1975;25:515–525.

86. Browne TR. Clonazepam. *Arch Neurol* 1976;33:326–332.

87. Bensch J, Bleunoco G, Ferngrass H. A double blind study of clonazepam in the treatment of therapy-resistant epilepsy. *Dev Med Child Neurol* 1977;19:335–342.

88. Gastaut H. The effect of benzodiazepines on chronic epilepsy in man. In: Hindmarsh I, Stonier P, eds. *Clobazam*. Royal Society of Medicine, International Congress and Symposium, Series 43. London: Academic Press, 1981;141–150.

89. Thompson P, Trimble MR. Clobazam and cognitive function. In: Hindmarsh I, Stonier P, eds. *Clobazam*. Royal Society of Medicine, International Congress and Symposium, Series 43. London: Academic Press, 1981;33–38.

90. Cull CA, Trimble MR. Anticonvulsant benzodiazepines and performance. In: Hindmarch I, Stonier P, Trimble, MR, eds. *Clobazam: Human Psychopharmacology and Clinical Applications*. Royal Society of Medicine, International Congress and Symposium, Series 74. London: Academic Press, 1985;121–128.

91. Smith DB, Mattson RH, Cramer JA, et al. Results of a nationwide veterans administration cooperative study comparing the efficacy and toxicity of carbamazepine, phenobarbital, phenytoin and primidone. *Epilepsia* 1987;28(Suppl 3):S50–S58.

92. Smith DB. Primidone: clinical use. In: Levy R, Mattson R, Meldrum B, Penry JK, Dreifuss FE, eds. *Antiepileptic drugs*, 3rd ed. New York: Raven Press, 1989;423–438.

93. Keith HM, Ewert JC, Freen MW, Gage RP. Mental status of children with convulsive disorders. *Ped Neurol* 1955;5:419–425.

94. Harrison RM, Taylor DC. Childhood seizures: a 25 year follow-up. *Lancet* 1976;2:948–951.

95. Ellenberg JH, Hirtz DG, Nelson KB. Age at onset of seizures in young children. *Ann Neurol* 1984;15:127–134.

96. Ellenberg JG, Hirtz DB, Nelson KB. Do seizures in children cause intellectual deterioration? *Ann Neurol* 1985;18:389.

97. Bower BD. Epilepsy in childhood. *Br J Hosp Med* 1969;2:454–460.

98. Dikmen S, Matthews CG. Effect of major motor seizure frequency upon cognitive–intellectual functions in adults. *Epilepsia* 1977;18:21–29.

99. Gudmundsson G. Epilepsy in Iceland. *Acta Neurol Scand* 1966;43:64–99.

100. Mirsky AF, Primac DW, Ajmone-Marsan C, Rosvold HE, Stevens JR. A comparison of psychological test performance of patients with focal and nonfocal epilepsy. *Exp Neurol* 1960;2:75–89.

101. Dikmen S, Matthews CG, Preston Harley J. Effect of early versus late onset of major motor epilepsy on cognitive–intellectual performance: further considerations. *Epilepsia* 1977;18(1):31–36.

102. Erwin CW, Thompson EM. ECT in schizophrenia: a study of nosologic impression. In: Brady JP, Brodie HKH, eds. *Controversy in psychiatry*. Philadelphia: WB Saunders, 1978;165–182.

103. Kellaway P, Mizrahi EM. Neonatal seizures. In: Luders H, Lesser RP, eds. *Epilepsy: electroclinical syndromes*. Berlin: Springer, 1986;13–48.

104. Glaser GH. The problem of psychosis in psychomotor temporal lobe epileptics. *Epilepsia* 1964;5:272–278.

105. Hermann BP, Dikmen S, Wilensky AJ. Increased psychopathology associated with multiple seizure types: fact or artifact? *Epilepsia* 1982;23:587–596.

106. Brodie MJ, McPhail E, Macphee GJA, Larkin JG, Gray JMB. Psychomotor impairment and anticonvulsant therapy in adult epileptic patients. *Eur J Clin Pharmacol* 1987;31:655–660.

107. Hirtz DG, Nelson KB. Cognitive effects of antiepileptic drugs. In: Pedley TA, Meldrum BS, eds. *Recent advances in epilepsy*. New York: Churchill Livingstone, 1988;161–181.

Advances in Neurology, Vol. 55, edited by
D. Smith, D. Treiman, and M. Trimble,
Raven Press, Ltd., New York © 1991.

14

Behavioral Effects of Antiepileptic Drugs

Carl B. Dodrill

*Regional Epilepsy Center, Harborview Hospital; Department of Neurological Surgery,
University of Washington School of Medicine,
Seattle, Washington 98104*

Recognition that antiepileptic drugs may have effects upon behavior has existed for many years, but formal evaluations have been more recent. As used in this chapter, "behavior" refers to (a) personality and adjustment, including mood, diffuse emotional concerns, cooperativeness, hostility, irritability, attentiveness, and happiness, and (b) all aspects of psychosocial adjustment, including interpersonal concerns, vocational adjustment, etc. Cognitive effects of these medications (pertaining to various aspects of abilities) and effects which are explicitly psychiatric (pertaining to identified psychiatric disorders) are covered in other chapters of this book.

As one begins a review of this area, it is immediately evident that the area is difficult to define as well as difficult to measure. It fills the gap between the better distinguished cognitive and psychiatric domains. Also, even though the area is an important one, it is less popular and less systematically investigated. Methods of evaluating behavior in this context are also less well developed, as will become evident.

In view of the above, the present chapter will consist of two basic parts. First, studies on the behavioral aspects of antiepileptic drugs will be reviewed, with special attention given to study design. Second, the studies both in this area and in the cognitive area will be critiqued with an effort to identify ways in which further investigations in these spheres might be improved.

BEHAVIORAL EFFECTS OF ANTIEPILEPTIC DRUGS

The present review will deal with all medications chronically taken orally to stop epileptic seizures. The decision was made to include the benzodiazepines wherever they appeared in literature relevant to epilepsy, even though few are now chronically given for seizure control. The drugs reviewed include anticonvulsants (agents used to stop convulsions) as well as those medications used in connection with other forms of epilepsy. Investigations were included only if they fell within the identified domain *and* if they included some type of formal and objective measure of the phenomena of interest. Routinely, this was some type of objective test or behavioral rating scale. Studies were *not* included if they failed to include such an objective measure. Thus, papers which merely offered observations about the behavioral effects of these drugs were excluded. Unless this restriction had been applied, hundreds of studies would have been cited, the vast majority of which would have contained only casual observations about behavioral change.

Reviews of the area previously published have typically been only part of a larger literature summary which emphasized cognitive and psychiatric aspects (1–5). These reviews show that fewer studies have been done in this area than in the cognitive and psychiatric arenas, that there are significant methodological limitations (described later in this review), and that it is difficult to piece together in any detailed way the effects of these agents on a broad range of variables identified as "behavioral."

In order to systematically evaluate the investigations in the area of interest, efforts were made to unearth all those studies which met the criteria for inclusion. It was discovered that this was more difficult than was originally envisioned, since many papers meeting the criteria for inclusion had titles which emphasized topics other than assessment of behavioral effects. Frequently, a study would focus upon efficacy of seizure control of a particular drug or upon cognitive effects but then, almost as an afterthought, include a brief behavioral measure as well. Some such studies may have been missed. Studies in languages other than English or papers presented at professional meetings were included only if an abstract in English was available which gave the information essential for this review.

Using the above procedures, a total of 84 papers were found in which 90 studies were reported. In order to evaluate these studies most adequately, they were classified according to basic study design, and the results are presented in Table 1.

Several overall comments about Table 1 are in order. Of the 90 investigations cited in Table 1, 28 dealt with children and 62 dealt with adults. Although there is a definite interest in the behavioral effects of these agents on children, perhaps a reluctance to subject this group to experimental protocols has resulted in fewer studies. As Table 1 reveals, 50 (56%) employed patients with epilepsy. This is somewhat disappointing, since it is clear that only about one-half of the investigations utilized subjects from the group to which the drugs must ultimately be applied, namely, people with epilepsy. Although studies with normal volunteers are of interest, easier to do, and less likely to be contaminated by extraneous events, it is not clear whether drug response is the same as that of persons who have taken these medications for many years. In many cases the subjects in these studies were given the medications for only a few days or weeks; adjustment to the medications may take much longer (48,53). Thus, it is possible that this large group of studies may have tended to overemphasize drug effects.

TABLE 1. *Basic designs of all studies reviewed (N = 90)*

I. Studies utilizing patients with epilepsy (N = 50)
  A. Cross-sectional (N = 10)
    1. Single agents (N = 6) (refs. 6–11)
    2. Multiple agents (N = 4) (refs. 12–15)
  B. Longitudinal (N = 40)
    1. With experimentally determined drug changes (N = 35)
      a. Single agents (N = 26)
        i. Crossover designs (N = 7) (refs. 16–22)
        ii. Add-on or withdrawal-from designs (N = 10) (refs. 23–32)
        iii. Untreated patients (N = 9) (refs. 33–41)
      b. Multiple agents, multiple drug changes (N = 9) (refs. 42–50)
    2. Without experimentally determined drug changes (N = 5) (refs. 51–55)
II. Studies utilizing subjects not having epilepsy (N = 40)
  A. Single active agents versus placebo (N = 35)
    1. Benzodiazepines (N = 13) (refs. 56–68)
    2. Phenytoin (N = 8) (refs. 69–76)
    3. Barbiturates (N = 3) (refs. 63, 66, 77)
    4. Carbamazepine (N = 4) (refs. 76, 78–80)
    5. Valproic acid (N = 2) (refs. 76 and 81)
    6. Other (N = 5) (refs. 42, 73, and 82–84)
  B. Single active agents alone, not placebo-controlled, various agents (N = 5) (refs. 85–89)

To evaluate the hypothesis just advanced and to summarize the literature with respect to the behavioral effects of these agents, Table 2 was constructed. This table shows that for all drugs and all types of studies, there were 118 conclusions drawn concerning the behavioral effects of the various drugs. Of these, 45 (38%) were positive, with a given drug identified as being either (a) better than another drug in terms of behavioral effects, (b) better than placebo, or (c) better than when no drug was given at all. In 47 cases (40%), there was either no discernible behavioral impact of the drug or it was no different than the other agents being evaluated (or placebo). In 26 cases (22%), particular drugs were associated with negative behavioral effects either in an absolute sense or in comparison with other agents (or placebo).

A study of Table 2 reveals several findings of interest. First, the most positive findings are with respect to the benzodiazepines, with

TABLE 2. *Numbers of studies reporting favorable (+), neutral (0), and unfavorable (−) effects upon behavior for various antiepileptic drugs as related to general study type*

Antiepileptic medication type	Drug effects	Study type		
		Type I: Subjects with epilepsy	Type II: Subjects not having epilepsy	All studies
Benzodiazepines	+	1 (50%)	10 (67%)	11 (65%)
	0	1 (50%)	2 (13%)	3 (18%)
	−	0 (0%)	3 (20%)	3 (18%)
Phenytoin	+	2 (18%)	3 (25%)	5 (22%)
	0	5 (46%)	5 (42%)	10 (43%)
	−	4 (36%)	4 (33%)	8 (35%)
Barbiturates	+	0 (0%)	1 (20%)	1 (5%)
	0	6 (43%)	2 (40%)	8 (42%)
	−	8 (57%)	2 (40%)	10 (53%)
Carbamazepine	+	16 (47%)	4 (80%)	20 (51%)
	0	14 (41%)	1 (20%)	15 (38%)
	−	4 (12%)	0 (0%)	4 (10%)
Valproic acid	+	3 (60%)	1 (50%)	4 (57%)
	0	2 (40%)	1 (50%)	3 (43%)
	−	0 (0%)	0 (0%)	0 (0%)
Other agents	+	2 (25%)	2 (40%)	4 (31%)
	0	5 (62%)	3 (60%)	8 (61%)
	−	1 (13%)	0 (0%)	1 (8%)
Total: All drugs	+	24 (32%)	21 (48%)	45 (38%)
	0	33 (45%)	14 (32%)	47 (40%)
	−	17 (23%)	9 (20%)	26 (22%)
				Total: 118 (100%)

65% of studies reporting favorable behavioral changes. However, of the 12 studies noting such changes, only two employed patients with epilepsy (31,45). The reason for this is that in general the benzodiazepines are not used chronically as antiepileptic drugs. The only exceptions appear to be clorazepate and, outside the United States, clobazam. Diazepam is now much less commonly used chronically for seizures. Thus, although the benzodiazepines appear most positive in Table 2, their practical value appears limited as both antiepileptic drugs and agents of behavioral change.

A further review of Table 2 reveals additional findings of interest. Carbamazepine and valproic acid appear most positive, with greater than 50% of the studies reporting favorable behavioral changes. It should be noted that far more studies have been done with carbamazepine ($N = 39$) than with valproic acid ($N = 7$), and thus the conclusions are much firmer with the former than with the latter. With carbamazepine, the changes most

commonly reported are decreased anxiety and depression, increased cooperation, decreased aggression, and generally improved behavior. A distinct pattern with valproate has not yet been established, but the studies reporting positive results note increased happiness and alertness along with generally improved mood.

The barbiturates are most clearly associated with negative behavioral changes. Commonly reported are increased depression, irritability, unhappiness, inattentiveness, argumentativeness, and stubbornness. A slowing of verbal and motor responses is also frequently reported. It is of interest that the barbiturates have also been associated with the most negative cognitive effects among antiepileptic drugs (90).

With respect to phenytoin, the results are mixed. Although positive changes were occasionally seen, negative alterations have been reported just as frequently. This agrees with the fact that in the largest group of studies no changes were reported either way, and this is probably the most accurate conclusion for this agent. Again, there is a parallel with studies of cognitive effects of these medications, since the results with phenytoin are not as negative as with the barbiturates. Carbamazepine is clearly better than phenytoin with respect to behavioral effects, but in the cognitive area the difference is not as clear (90).

With respect to general type of study, a review of the data presented near the bottom of Table 2 reveals that there is a tendency for those studies identified as Type II (utilizing subjects not having epilepsy; listed under II in the outline of Table 1) to result in a greater percentage of positive inferences being made when compared to Type I studies (utilizing patients with epilepsy). Positive comments about given drugs were found in 48% of the Type II studies and in only 32% of the Type I studies. This difference was especially noticeable for carbamazepine, where there were positive behavioral changes in 80% of the Type II studies but in only 47% of the Type I studies. In the Type II studies, this agent was applied to both children and adults with behavioral/emotional lability problems, whereas in the Type I studies, it was applied to people with epilepsy. In other words, it appeared that carbamazepine more frequently had a positive behavioral effect when directly and appropriately prescribed for purposes of behavioral change than when it was prescribed primarily as an antiepileptic drug. This may be partly related to the more complex conditions found in the latter group, which included epilepsy and, in many cases, underlying brain dysfunction.

Efforts were made to relate outcome to the various subtypes of studies categorized in Table 1. This was difficult to do in a reliable manner because the number of investigations for any particular type of study was relatively small. Probably everyone would agree that studies in Table 1 under the headings I.A.2 (cross-sectional studies with the simultaneous administration of multiple agents) and I.B.2 (drug changes not experimentally determined, with multiple agents) were the least well controlled. These studies resulted in the drawing of eight conclusions about drugs: Six (75%) were positive (four carbamazepine, one sulthiame, one valproate), one (12.5%) was neutral (carbamazepine), and one (12.5%) was

negative (barbiturates). Perhaps the studies which were best controlled were longitudinal studies with experimentally determined single-agent drug changes, all of which appear under heading I.B.1.a in Table 1. Of 42 conclusions reached from these studies, eight (19%) were positive (one phenytoin, six carbamazepine, one valproate), 24 (57%) were neutral (two phenytoin, five barbiturates, 10 carbamazepine, two valproate, four other agents), and 10 (24%) were negative (three phenytoin, four barbiturates, two carbamazepine, one sulthiame). Although the number of conclusions drawn from the less well controlled studies was small, it is interesting to note that there was a statistically greater likelihood of positive findings (as opposed to all other findings) with poorly controlled studies than with well-controlled studies (Yates corrected chi-square $= 7.87$, $p < 0.01$). This is further evidence that outcome is relevant not only to type of subjects selected (patients with epilepsy show fewer positive behavioral changes), but also to degree of experimental control (tighter control is associated with fewer positive behavioral changes). In addition, negative conclusions about target drugs are less commonly discovered in studies which are poorly controlled. All of these findings are of interest, and they argue for care in the interpretation of existing studies and in the design of studies for the future.

Thus far, few comments have been offered concerning details of the types of behavior assessed. It is at this point that the studies are undoubtedly their weakest, since there is almost no agreement as to how behavioral effects are to be evaluated. For example, of the 62 studies of adults, there were 39 separate tests or procedures which were used to evaluate the behavioral effects of antiepileptic drugs. Most of these were standardized or published tests and inventories. Beyond these 39, there were also 18 rating scales which were applied (six self-ratings, 12 professional ratings), no two of which were probably identical. Thus, there were about 57 different procedures employed to evaluate behavior in 62 studies. Frequently, more than one procedure was utilized in a study. Visual analogue scales were administered on eight occasions (these were counted as a single procedure even though they varied in content from one to the next), the Minnesota Multiphasic Personality Inventory and the Mood Adjective Checklist on six, the Hamilton Anxiety Rating Scale on five, the Brief Psychiatric Rating Scale and the Washington Psychosocial Seizure Inventory on four, and the Morbid Anxiety Inventory on three. Eleven procedures were used twice, and the remaining 22 were used only once.

With respect to the 28 studies of children, there were 25 rating or testing procedures with specific names. At least some of these were standardized and published. In addition, there were 30 other rating procedures or scales (often developed for the specific studies), which were completed in 12 cases by professionals, in nine by teachers, in eight by parents, and in one case by the children themselves. In some cases the rating procedures within a study were similar for professionals, teachers, and parents, whereas in other cases they were somewhat similar and in some they were not similar at all. In a number of instances, the studies did not give definitive information on this point. On only two occasions did the evaluative procedures used with children overlap those with adults.

Overall, it is impossible to say how many unique evaluative procedures were used in the 90 studies, but it is almost certainly greater than 90. The obvious question here pertains to how progress can ever be made without determining a way to define and measure the components of the area in at least a somewhat more standardized and consistent manner. This is one of the major problems with this area, and until efforts are made to resolve it, the overall conclusions must of necessity be conservative.

CRITIQUE OF COGNITIVE AND BEHAVIORAL STUDIES OF DRUG EFFECTS

We now turn to the second major section of this chapter, which pertains to the evaluation of studies of the behavioral and cognitive effects of antiepileptic drugs. One characteristic of the literature reviews published to date is that they have tended to be uncritical summaries of the information presented in the various research reports. A critical review highlighting some of the major shortcomings is needed to help identify areas of weakness and to assist in providing improved research for the future.

This review will use as a point of departure the designs of the studies which have been completed to date. For the behavioral effects of antiepileptic drugs, a classification of these designs for 90 investigations has already been reported in Table 1. This is essentially identical to one previously presented for 78 studies on the cognitive effects of these drugs (90). A review of the research in both areas reveals a series of methodological problems that have caused investigators to incorrectly attribute behavioral and cognitive difficulties to drugs when they should instead be attributed to other factors. Four of these methodological problems will now be reviewed.

Selection Factors

In about half the studies of the cognitive effects of antiepileptic drugs, patients are studied on drug regimens which have been established solely for clinical reasons. In the most common design, patients from two or more groups are found not to differ with respect to variables such as age, sex, education, and seizure type, and it is concluded that if the groups have dissimilar performances, these dissimilarities must be due to differences in drug regimens. However, these medications are not prescribed in a random manner, and it is probable that the subject groups are intrinsically different despite the superficial resemblance of age, sex, seizure type, etc. For example, for reasons pertaining to complexity of drug regimens and presumed side effects, phenytoin may be given more frequently to less capable patients and carbamazepine may be administered to more capable persons. The groups can be easily matched for age, sex, seizure type, and other such variables, but intrinsic differences remain between the groups which are not appreciated by such variables. The result is that the groups are intrinsically different prior to the start of the drug regimens, and differences in performance may be due to this factor rather than to the medications themselves. This problem will now be illustrated with data from my own laboratory.

The neuropsychological effects of valproic acid were evaluated using a typical cross-sectional design. A broad battery of neuropsychological tests was administered to 28 adults receiving valproic acid for their seizure disorders. As is usual in studies of this type, some of the patients were receiving other medications as well. These 28 people were compared with 28 others who, in each instance, represented the next case in the neuropsychological files who was not receiving valproic acid but who had been tested in the same manner. The groups were similar on a long list of variables, including age, years of education, sex, age at onset of seizures, etiology of seizures, seizure type, seizure frequency, and total years in which antiepileptic medications had been taken. However, the groups were markedly different on a range of neuropsychological tests and on the Wechsler Adult Intelligence Scale. For example, the average Full Scale I.Q. for the valproic acid group was 87.29, and the same score for the control group (not on valproate) was 99.00. The difference was statistically significant $(t = -2.47; p < 0.02)$. Thus, one might conclude that valproic acid is detrimental to intelligence. This conclusion is incorrect, however, as can be positively proven by reference to testing conducted 5 years previously on each one of these subjects when not a single one was on valproic acid. At that time, the group which was ultimately placed on valproic acid had an average Full Scale I.Q. score of 85.36, whereas the controls average 96.69. These scores, also statistically different $(t = -2.67; p < 0.02)$, indicate that physicians had given valproic acid to patients who were duller and more difficult to manage.

It is curious how many studies have made the error just described. The result has undoubtedly been that in many cases, effects properly related to differences between subject groups have been attributed to drugs. The results of studies utilizing parallel group designs must be closely scrutinized unless there has been a random assignment of subjects. It may also be that test–retest designs are somewhat affected by this problem when drug changes have been made for clinical reasons. For example, persons complaining of toxicity on a particular drug regimen may be different than persons on the same regimen who are apparently doing well. Should conclusions based upon a subgroup of patients who are doing poorly be applied to all patients on that drug regimen?

Overall, selection factors are of great importance in evaluating studies in this area, and they are to be especially suspected when assignment of drug regimens is made on the basis of clinical needs rather than experimentally.

Statistical Factors

Statistical errors can invalidate otherwise well-executed studies. One common problem pertains to the number of statistical tests performed relative to the number of statistically significant findings reported. Often only a few differences between drug groups are noted in these papers, but they are given prominence in the reports whereas tests not producing statistically significant findings may be deemphasized or not even be mentioned as having been administered. Also, some variables which are associated with statistical findings may overlap with each other so greatly that to find a difference on several really means a difference on only one.

Another important statistical error is ignoring variability in scores when choosing statistical tests. Test data and seizure frequency data are usually not distributed normally, and special statistical procedures are required. This point is graphically illustrated by the hypothetical data presented in Table 3. After three patients were tested under both Drug A and Drug B in separate trials, statistical significance was established between the two drugs: Patients required a greater amount of time to complete the task with Drug B

TABLE 3. *Hypothetical scores (in seconds) on a test requiring motor speed under two drug conditions*

Patient	Drug A	Drug B
1	15	28
2	27	44
3	17	35
		$t = -10.47 \ (p < 0.01)$
4	21	80
		$t = -2.48$ (not significant)

($t = -10.47$; $p < 0.01$). A fourth patient confirms this hypothesis with a very bad score with Drug B, but statistical confidence is lost. The reason for this is that the standard deviation for performances with Drug B has increased dramatically, from 8.03 to 23.11. The loss of statistical significance is artifactual because of an inappropriate selection of the statistical test. The result is that a genuine drug effect is lost. Statistical significance is restored if nonparametric statistics are used or if the data are normalized before parametric analysis. The potential impact of this problem is apparent in terms of the outcome of a study reporting no differences between the groups with respect to a variable such as seizure frequency. When there is even one highly deviant patient (such as the fourth patient in Table 3) in one group and parametric statistics are used, it may be reported that seizure frequency is not relevant but that, in reality, this variable—and not the drugs at all—may be responsible for the performance differences between the groups.

One clue concerning this problem of variability in scores manifests itself when standard deviations differ substantially from one group to the next. Another tip is when standard deviations exceed means. When these conditions are found, standard parametric statistics (such as Student's t statistic or analysis of variance) should not be used without special data transformations. The reader should be suspicious of findings from such studies and from those which do not report standard deviations on test data or on important seizure history variables such as seizure frequency.

Type of Behavioral/Psychological Test Given

The lack of agreement with respect to type of test which should be used has already been emphasized with respect to the evaluation of behavioral changes. With respect to cognitive changes associated with these drugs, it should be noted that the type of test administered relates to both (a) the probability of discovering a drug effect and (b) the type of effect which is found. This is seen very clearly in Table 4. It is evident from this table that the more highly timed the test, the more often a drug

TABLE 4. *Presence or absence of drug effect as related to type of test used in studies of people with epilepsy*

Type of test	Drug effect	
	Present	Absent
Reaction time	11 (85%)	2 (15%)
Other timed tests	19 (79%)	5 (21%)
Intelligence tests	13 (59%)	9 (41%)
All other tests	6 (43%)	8 (57%)
All tests	49 (67%)	24 (33%)

effect will be found. Reaction-time tests are typically recorded in milliseconds, and the other timed tests are recorded in whole seconds. Intelligence tests usually have portions which are timed, although the timing may not be weighted as heavily as whether or not the responses are correct. The last group of tests in the table refers to those which are untimed and unpaced, such as "power" tests of problem solving.

From a review of Table 4, it is clear that to find small drug effects one would use the more highly timed measures. This is where computer-assisted testing may make its greatest contribution. Two comments about computerized testing are in order at this point. First, most tests utilizing a computer have a strong element of motor speed. Thus, even though investigators have labeled their tests as tests of "memory," "decision-making," "attention," etc., if the primary outcome measure in each case is in seconds or milliseconds, the major element may be one of motor speed, not the element which is postulated as being measured. Drugs (such as phenytoin) which are associated with slightly decreased motor speed (91) will therefore tend to generally look bad. However, there is now evidence that when the motor aspects are partialled out, the so-called "cognitive" effects of this agent tend to disappear as well (92).

A second comment about computerized testing is that there are technical facets of enormous importance in terms of outcome. For example, different response boxes may render dramatically different results. The data presented in Fig. 1 graphically illustrate this point. A simple decision-making task was set up in which colored pictures appeared on a

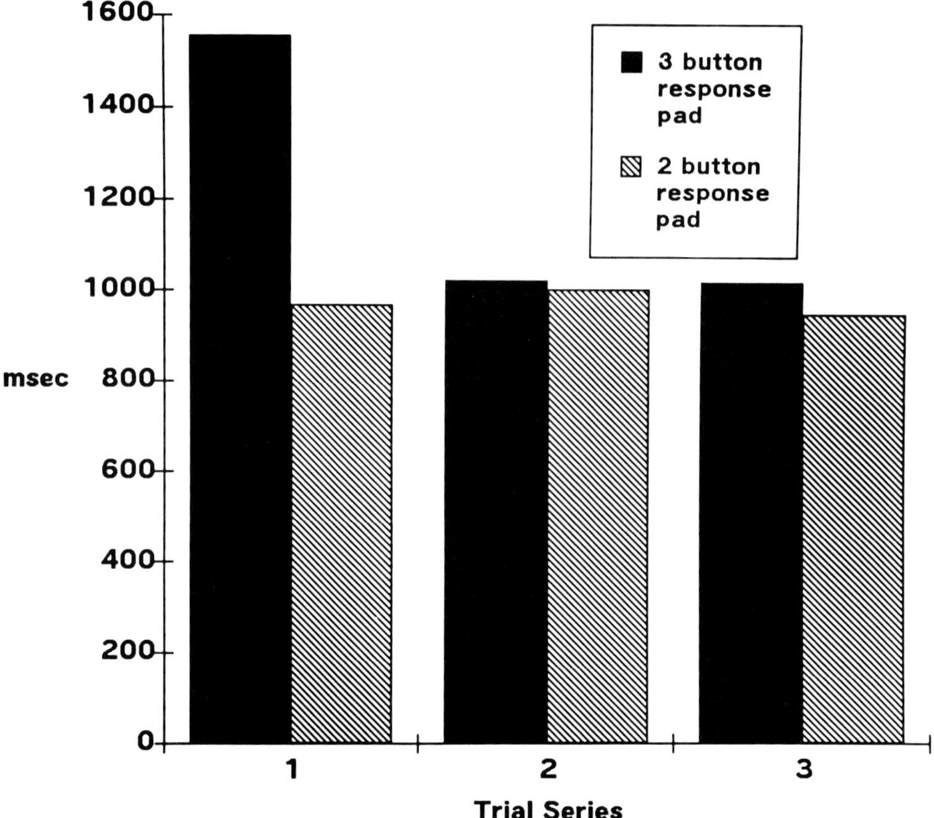

FIG. 1. Average response times (in milliseconds) across three series of 20 trials, each with two different response pads (three-button and two-button types) used by two different series of subjects.

screen, and the task was to hit as quickly as possible the "Yes" button if people were present in the picture and the "No" button if no one was there. People in the pictures either were obviously and conspicuously present or were not present at all. There were 60 trials, which were divided into three groups (labeled 1, 2, and 3) of 20 trials each. Twenty adults completed the task utilizing a three-button response pad modeled after a method used previously by other investigators (43). This response box consisted of "Yes" and "No" buttons which were about 15 cm apart, and each button was about 12 cm from the starting mark; the patient was required to return to this mark each time he or she gave a response. A gross movement of the entire hand was required in order to respond, and patients soon quired in order to respond, and patients soon

learned how to move their hands more quickly. The result was a major practice effect. This is illustrated by the solid bars in Fig. 1. There was an approximately 500-msec practice effect from the first group of 20 trials to the second group. However, 15 other adults were administered the same test with a two-button response pad which did not require a hand movement but which merely required the depressing of the "Yes" or "No" button by the index and middle fingers, respectively, of the preferred hand. The buttons were only 3 cm apart. There was no practice effect with this response pad at all. Thus, the two response pads produced markedly different results, and this is especially significant when it is noted that the typical drug effect in these studies is on the order of 50–100 msec.

Co-medication

The administration of co-medication at the same time that a study drug is being evaluated is common, and it occurred in about 60% of all studies using patients with epilepsy (Table 1). It is well known that these medications interact with one another, and it is reasonable to assume that these interactions might have some effects upon behavior and upon mental abilities. This is in agreement with the fact that co-medication was routinely found in the more poorly controlled studies (I.A.2 and I.B.1.b in Table 1) and that, as shown above, these studies did render results which were somewhat different from better controlled studies. This does not prove that co-medication per se was the critical factor, but it is reasonable to assume that the addition of medications to the drug regimens probably complicated the results. This problem also exists for studies of the effects of antiepileptic drugs upon mental abilities; an illustration of this follows.

Wilensky et al. (31) compared clorazepate and phenobarbital while co-administering phenytoin in 42 adults with uncontrolled partial seizures. Detailed neuropsychological testing was accomplished at the end of the baseline period, as well as at the end of each drug study period, in this double-blind, counterbalanced, crossover study. Seizure control was equivalent for clorazepate and phenobarbital, but there was a definite tendency for the patients to prefer clorazepate because it caused fewer side effects. However, no statistically significant differences were noted on the neuropsychological tests, apparently because the phenytoin levels were higher with clorazepate than with phenobarbital despite the doses remaining constant. Thus, the adverse effects of phenobarbital appear to have been counterbalanced by the reduced phenytoin levels, whereas the higher phenytoin levels with clorazepate offset the less toxic effects of clorazepate. The result was a complete washout in the test data.

The methodological problems summarized above require a more conservative statement of the adverse effects of these drugs upon behavioral and mental abilities than is usually given. The problems typically cause investigators to attribute certain effects to drugs when they should probably be attributed to other factors, but occasionally the opposite is true.

CONCLUSIONS

This chapter has had the primary purpose of reviewing the behavioral effects of medications used to control seizures. A review of 90 studies in the area revealed that the most positive findings were associated with carbamazepine and probably valproic acid, whereas the most negative findings were noted in connection with the barbiturates. Phenytoin is consistently neither positive nor negative in its effects. Although the benzodiazepines tended to be positive in their effects upon behavior, they are now less frequently used as chronic antiepileptic drugs.

Significant problems were uncovered by this review. There is a great lack of agreement as to how behavior is to be measured. There were approximately as many different tests or procedures to measure behavior as there were studies, and it is apparent that progress in the area will be dependent upon a much better consensus about what is to be measured and how measurement is to take place. Attention to this point appears to be a first-line requirement in future research. In addition, it was noted that the outcome of the various studies was dependent upon a series of factors which also require attention. These include the following: (a) characteristics of subjects used, (b) basic study design, including the degree of experimental control, (c) type of psychological test used, (d) type of statistics which are applied, (e) presence of co-medication, and (f) intrinsic subject-related differences which exist between groups despite efforts to eliminate them. Attention to such factors should do much to bring order to this difficult but important area.

ACKNOWLEDGMENTS

The preparation of this chapter and a portion of the research reported therein was supported by grants NS 24823 and NS 17111 awarded by the National Institute of Neurological and Communicative Disorders and Stroke, PHS/DHHS.

REFERENCES

1. Evans RW, Gualtieri CT. Carbamazepine: a neuropsychological and psychiatric profile. *Clin Neuropharmacol* 1985;8:221–241.
2. Parnas J, Flachs H, Gram L. Psychotropic effect of antiepileptic drugs. *Acta Neurol Scand* 1979;60:329–343.
3. Rivinus TM. Psychiatric effects of the anticonvulsant regimens. *J Clin Psychopharmacol* 1982; 2:165–192.
4. Trimble MR. Anticonvulsant drugs and psychosocial development: phenobarbitone, sodium valproate, and benzodiazepines. In: Morselli PL, Pippenger CE, Penry JK, eds. *Antiepileptic drug therapy in pediatrics.* New York: Raven Press, 1983;201–217.
5. Trimble MR, Cull CA. Antiepileptic drugs, cognitive function, and behavior in children. *Cleve Clinic J Med* 1989;56:S140–S149.
6. Andrewes DG, Bullen JG, Tomlinson L, Elwes RDC, Reynolds EH. A comparative study of the cognitive effects of phenytoin and carbamazepine in new referrals with epilepsy. *Epilepsia* 1986;27:128–134.
7. Andrewes DG, Tomlinson L, Elwes RDC, Reynolds E. The influence of carbamazepine and phenytoin on memory and other aspects of cognitive function in new referrals with epilepsy. *Acta Neurol Scand* 1984;69(Suppl 99):23–30.
8. Brown SW, McGowan MEL, Reynolds EH. The influence of seizure type and medication on psychiatric symptoms in epileptic patients. *Br J Psychiatry* 1986;148:300–304.
9. Byrne JM, Camfield PR. Effects of phenobarbital on early intellectual and behavioral development: a concordant twin case study. *J Clin Exp Neuropsychol* 1987;9:393–398.
10. Gillham RA, Williams N, Brodie MJ, Butler E, Larkin JG. Relationship between carbamazepine concentration and cognitive function in patients with epilepsy. In: *Book of abstracts: Seventeenth Epilepsy International Congress,* Jerusalem, September 1987;48.
11. Hassan MN, Laljee HCK, Parsonage MJ. Sodium valproate in the treatment of resistant epilepsy. *Acta Neurol Scand* 1976;54:209–218.
12. Corbett JA, Trimble MR, Nichol TC. Behavioral and cognitive impairments in children with epilepsy: the long-term effects of anticonvulsant therapy. *J Am Acad Child Psychiatry* 1985; 24:17–23.
13. Hoare P. The development of psychiatric disorder among school children with epilepsy. *Dev Med Child Neurol* 1984;26:3–13.
14. Loveland N, Smith B, Forster FM. Mental and emotional changes in epileptic patients on continuous anticonvulsant medication: a preliminary report. *Neurology* 1957;7:856–865.
15. Robertson MM, Trimble MR. Anticonvulsants and mood: the relationship. In: *Book of abstracts: Seventeenth Epilepsy International Congress,* Jerusalem, September 1987;101.
16. Cereghino JJ, Brock JT, Van Meter JC, Penry JK, Smith LD, White BG. Carbamazepine for epilepsy: a controlled prospective evaluation. *Neurology* 1974;24:401–410.
17. Dodrill CB. Effects of sulthiame upon intellectual, neuropsychological, and social functioning abilities among adult epileptics: comparison with diphenylhydantoin. *Epilepsia* 1975;16:617–625.
18. Dodrill CB, Troupin AS. Psychotropic effects of carbamazepine in epilepsy: a double-blind comparison with phenytoin. *Neurology* 1977;27: 1023–1028.
19. Meador KJM, Loring DW, King DW, Huh K, Gallagher BB. Comparative cognitive effects of anticonvulsants. *Neurology* 1989;39:149.
20. Rajotte P, Jilek W, Jilek L, et al. Antiepileptic and psychotropic properties of carbamazepine (Tegretol). *Union Med Can* 1967;96:1200–1206.
21. Wilensky AJ, Ojemann LM, Friel PN, Almes MJ, Levy RH, Dodrill CB. Cinromide in epilepsy: a pilot study. *Epilepsia* 1983;24:401–409.
22. Wilensky AJ, Friel PN, Ojemann LM, Dodrill CB, McCormick KB, Levy RH. Zonisamide in epilepsy: a pilot study. *Epilepsia* 1985;26:212–220.
23. Loiseau P, Strube E, Tor J, Levy RH, Dodrill C. Évaluation neuropsychologique et thérapeutique du stiripentol dans l'épilepsie: résultats préliminaires. *Rev Neurol (Paris)* 1988;3:165–172.
24. Macphee GJA, McPhail EM, Butler E, Brodie MJ. Controlled evaluation of a supplementary dose of carbamazepine on psychomotor function in epileptic patients. *Eur J Clin Pharmacol* 1986;31:195–199.
25. Marjerrison G, Jedlicki SM, Keogh RET, Hrychuck W, Poulakakis GM. Carbamazepine: behavioral, anticonvulsant and EEG effects in chronically-hospitalized epileptics. *Dis Nerv Sys* 1968;29:133–136.
26. Pryse-Phillips WEM, Jeavons PM. Effect of carbamazepine (Tegretol) on the electroencephalograph and ward behaviour of patients with chronic epilepsy. *Epilepsia* 1970;11:263–273.
27. Rennick P, Keiser T, Rodin E, Rim C. The psychotropic effects of carbamazepine in patients with psychomotor epilepsy: results of a double-blind study. In: *Book of abstracts: American Epilepsy Society,* New York, December 1974;18.
28. Rodin EA, Rim CS, Kitano H, Lewis R, Rennick PM. A comparison of the effectiveness of primidone versus carbamazepine in epileptic outpatients. *J Nerv Ment Dis* 1976;163:41–46.
29. Stores G, Williams P. A controlled study of the behavioural effects of carbamazepine and valproate used as single treatment in children with epilepsy. In: *Book of abstracts: Seventeenth Epilepsy International Congress,* Jerusalem, September 1987;116.
30. Troupin AS, Ojemann LM, Dodrill CB. Mephenytoin: a reappraisal. *Epilepsia* 1976;17:403–414.
31. Wilensky AJ, Ojemann LM, Temkin NR, Troupin AS, Dodrill CB. Clorazepate and phenobarbital as antiepileptic drugs: a double-blind study. *Neurology* 1981;31:1271–1276.

32. Wulfsohn M. Carbamazepine (Tegretol) in the long-term treatment of grand mal epilepsy. *S Afr Med J* 1972;46:1091–1092.

33. Hamster W, Petruch F. Psychometric studies before and under carbamazepine treatment. In: Meinardi H, Rowan AJ. *Advances in epileptology: 1977.* Amsterdam: Swets & Zeitlinger, 1978;104–108.

34. Hellström B, Barlach-Christoffersen M. Influence of phenobarbital on the psychomotor development and behaviour in preschool children with convulsions. *Neuropädiatrie* 1980;11:151–160.

35. Herranz JL, Arteaga R, Armijo JA. Side effects of sodium valproate in monotherapy controlled by plasma levels: a study of 88 pediatric patients. *Epilepsia* 1982;23:203–314.

36. Holcombe V, Summit NJ, Brandt J, et al. Effects of Tegretol or phenytoin on cognitive function and behavior in epileptic children younger than six years. *Neurology* 1987;37(Suppl 1):92.

37. Mitchell WG, Chavez JM. Phenobarbital versus carbamazepine for partial seizures in children. *Epilepsia* 1986;27:640.

38. Özdirim E, Renda Y, Epir S. Effects of phenobarbital and phenytoin on the behaviour of epileptic children. In: Meinardi H, Rowan AJ. *Advances in epileptology: 1977.* Amsterdam: Swets & Zeitlinger, 1978;120–123.

39. Schain RJ. Carbamazepine and cognitive functioning. In: *Book of abstracts: Thirteenth Epilepsy International Congress,* Kyoto, Japan, September 1981;250.

40. Smith DB, Craft BR, Collins J, Mattson RH, Cramer JA, and the VA Cooperative Study Group 118. Behavioral characteristics of epilepsy patients compared with normal control. *Epilepsia* 1986;27:760–768.

41. Vining EPG, Mellits ED, Dorsen MM, et al. Psychologic and behavioral effects of antiepileptic drugs in children: a double-blind comparison between phenobarbital and valproic acid. *Pediatrics* 1987;80:165–174.

42. Al-Kaisi AH, McGuire RJ. The effect of sulthiame on disturbed behaviour in mentally subnormal patients. *Br J Psychiatry* 1974;124:45–49.

43. Cull CA, Trimble MR. Behavioural effects of changes in antiepileptic drug regimen in children with epilepsy. In: *Book of abstracts: Seventeenth Epilepsy International Congress,* Jerusalem, September 1987;27.

44. Fischbacher E. Effect of reduction of anticonvulsants on well-being. *Br Med J* 1982;285:423–424.

45. Lehmann HE, Ban TA. Studies with new drugs in the treatment of convulsive disorders. *Int J Clin Pharmacol* 1968;3:231–234.

46. Miles MV, Tennison MB, Greenwood RS. Assessment of antiepileptic drug effects on child behavior using the Child Behavior Checklist. *J Epilepsy* 1988;1:209–213.

47. Pellock JM, Culbert JP, Garnett WR, et al. Assessment of cognitive and behavioral effects of carbamazepine, phenytoin, and phenobarbital in school-aged children. *Epilepsia* 1987;28:597.

48. Rett A. The so-called psychotropic effect of Tegretol in the treatment of convulsions of cerebral origin in children. In: Birkmayer W, ed. *Epileptic seizures—behavior, pain.* Stuttgart: Hans Huber, 1976;194–204.

49. Schain RJ, Ward JW, Guthrie D. Carbamazepine as an anticonvulsant in children. *Neurology* 1977;27:476–480.

50. Singh AN, Saxena BM, Germain M. Anticonvulsive and psychotropic effects of carbamazepine in hospitalized epileptic patients: a long-term study. In: Penry JK, ed. *Epilepsy, the Eighth International Symposium,* 1977;47–56.

51. Bird CAK, Griffin BP, Miklaszewska JM, Galbraith AW. Tegretol (carbamazepine): a controlled trial of a new anti-convulsant. *Br J Psychiatry* 1966;112:737–742.

52. Jacobides GM. Alertness and scholastic achievement in young epileptics treated with carbamazepine (Tegretol). In: Meinardi H, Rowan AJ, eds. *Advances in epileptology: 1977.* Amsterdam: Swets & Zeitlinger, 1978;114–119.

53. Jeavons PM, Clark JE. Sodium valproate in treatment of epilepsy. *Br Med J* 1974;2:584–586.

54. Thompson PJ, Trimble MR. Anticonvulsant serum levels: relationship to impairments of cognitive functioning. *J Neurol Neurosurg Psychiatry* 1983;46:227–233.

55. Trimble MR, Thompson PJ. Anticonvulsant drugs and behaviour. In: Akimoto H, Kazamatsuri H, Seino M, Ward A, eds. *Advances in epileptology: Thirteenth Epilepsy International Symposium.* New York: Raven Press, 1982;205–209.

56. Clyde CA. The influence of personality on response to low doses of benzodiazepines. In: Hindmarch I, Stonier PD, eds. *Clobazam.* London: Royal Society of Medicine, 1981;75–86.

57. Doongaji DR, Sheth A, Apte JS, Lakdawala PD, Khare CB, Thatte SS. Clobazam versus diazepam—a double-blind study in anxiety neurosis. *J Clin Pharmacol* 1978;18:358–364.

58. Harder F, Elsass P, Hendel J, Hvidberg EF, Hjörting-Hansen E. Clinical and psychological effects of intravenous diazepam related to plasma levels. *Int J Oral Surg* 1976;5:226–239.

59. Hendel J, Elsass P, Andreasen PB, Gymoese E, Hvidberg EF. Neuropsychologic effects of diazepam related to single dose kinetics and liver function. *Psychopharmacology* 1976;48:11–17.

60. Saario I, Linnoila M, Mattila MJ. Modification by diazepam or thioridazine of the psychomotor skills related to driving: a subacute trial in neurotic out-patients. *Br J Clin Pharmacol* 1976;3:843–848.

61. Salkind MR, Hanks GW, Silverstone JT. Evaluation of the effects of clobazam, a 1,5 benzodiazepine, on mood and psychomotor performance in clinically anxious patients in general practice. *Br J Clin Pharmacol* 1979;7:113S–118S.

62. Saxena B, Singh AN, Porter WR. Clinical and

experimental comparison of intramuscular lorazepam, diazepam, and placebo: psychometric tests and psychiatric rating scales in the assessment of benzodiazepines. *Curr Ther Res* 1980; 28:260–276.

63. Schwarz E, Kielholz P, Hobi V, Goldberg L, Hofstetter M, Ladewig D. Changes in EEG, blood levels, mood scales and performance scores during long term treatment with diazepam, phenobarbital or placebo in patients. *Prog Neuropsychopharmacol Biol Psychiatry* 1982; 6:249–263.

64. Silverstone JT. Lorazepam in phobic disorders: a pilot study. *Curr Med Res Opin* 1973;1:272–275.

65. Steiner-Chaskel N, Lader MH. Effects of single doses of clobazam and diazepam on psychological functions in normal subjects. In: Hindmarch I, Stonier PD, eds. *Clobazam*. London: Royal Society of Medicine, 1981;23–32.

66. Tansella CZ, Tansella M, Lader M. A comparison of the clinical and psychological effects of diazepam and amylobarbitone in anxious patients. *Br J Clin Pharmacol* 1979;7:605–611.

67. Thompson PJ, Trimble MR. Clobazam and cognitive functions. In: Akimoto H, Kazamatsuri H, Seino M, Ward A, eds. *Advances in epileptology: Thirteenth Epilepsy International Symposium*. New York: Raven Press, 1982;229–231.

68. Uhlenhuth EH, Turner DA, Purchatzke G, Gift T, Chassan J. Intensive design in evaluating anxiolytic agents. *Psychopharmacology* 1977; 52:79–85.

69. Goldberg JB, Kurland AA. Dilantin treatment of hospitalized cultural–familial retardates. *J Nerv Ment Dis* 1970;150:133–137.

70. Idestrom CM, Schalling D, Carlquist U, Sjöqvist F. Acute effects of diphenylhydantoin in relation to plasma levels: behavioral and psychophysiological studies. *Psychol Med* 1972;2:111–120.

71. Lefkowitz MM. Effects of diphenylhydantoin on disruptive behavior: study of male delinquents. *Arch Gen Psychiatry* 1969;20:643–651.

72. Looker A, Conner CK. Diphenylhydantoin in children with severe temper tantrums. *Arch Gen Psychiatry* 1970;23:80–89.

73. Malitz S, Kanzler M. Are antidepressants better than placebo? *Am J Psychiatry* 1971;127:1605–1611.

74. Stephens JH, Shaffer JW. A controlled study of the effects of diphenylhydantoin on anxiety, irritability, and anger in neurotic outpatients. *Psychopharmacologia* 1970;17:169–181.

75. Stephens JH, Shaffer JW, Brown CC. A controlled comparison of the effects of diphenylhydantoin and placebo on mood and psychomotor functioning in normal volunteers. *J Clin Pharmacol* 1974;14:543–551.

76. Trimble MR, Thompson P, Corbett J. Anticonvulsant drugs, cognitive function, and behaviour. In: Sander M, ed. *Psychopharmacology of anticonvulsants*. Oxford: Oxford University Press, 1982;106–121.

77. Camfield CS, Chaplin S, Doyle A-B, Shapir SH, Cummings C, Camfield PR. Side effects of phenobarbital in toddlers; behavioral and cognitive aspects. *J Pediatr* 1979;95:361–365.

78. Gardner DL, Cowdry RW. Positive effects of carbamazepine on behavioral dyscontrol in borderline personality disorder. *Am J Psychiatry* 1986;143:519–522.

79. Groh C. The psychotropic effect of Tegretol in non-epileptic children, with particular reference to the drug's indications. In: Birksmayer W, ed. *Epileptic seizures—behavior, pain*. Stuttgart: Hans Huber, 1976;259–263.

80. Janke W, Ehrhardt J, Munch U. Behavioral effects of carbamazepine after single and repeated administration in emotionally labile subjects. *Neuropsychobiology* 1983;10:217–227.

81. Betts TA, Crowe A, Alford C. Psychotropic effects of sodium valproate. *Br J Clin Pract [Symp Suppl]* 1982;18:145–146.

82. Dureman I, Malmgren H, Norrman B. Comparison studies of chlorazepate administered as a divided daily dose and as a single dose at night. *Psychopharmacology* 1978;57:123–126.

83. Moffatt WR, Siddiqui AR, MacKay DN. The use of sulthiame with disturbed mentally subnormal patients. *Br J Psychiatry* 1970;117:673–678.

84. Smith WL, Philippus MJ, Guard HL. Psychometric study of children with learning problems and 14–6 positive spike EEG patterns, treated with ethosuximide (Zarontin) and placebo. *Arch Dis Child* 1968;43:616.

85. Dikmen S, Temkin N, Weiler M, Wyler AR. Behavioral effects of anticonvulsant prophylaxis: no effect or artifact? *Epilepsia* 1984;25:741–746.

86. Klein DF, Greenberg IM. Behavioral effects of diphenylhydantoin in severe psychiatric disorders. *Am J Psychiatry* 1967;124:847–848.

87. Lindsley DB, Henry CE. The effect of drugs on behavior and the electroencephalograms of children with behavior disorders. *Psychosom Med* 1942;4:140–149.

88. Luchins DJ. Carbamazepine for the violent psychiatric patient. *Lancet* 1983;1:766.

89. Uhlenhuth EH, Stephens JH, Dim BH, Covi L. Diphenylhydantoin and phenobarbital in the relief of psychoneurotic symptoms: a controlled comparison. *Psychopharmacologia* 1972;27:67–84.

90. Dodrill CB. Effects of antiepileptic drugs on abilities. *J Clin Psychiatry* 1988;49:31–34.

91. Dodrill CB. Diphenylhydantoin serum levels, toxicity, and neuropsychological performance in patients with epilepsy. *Epilepsia* 1975;16:593–600.

92. Dodrill CB, Temkin NR. Motor speed is a contaminating variable in the measurement of the "cognitive" effects of phenytoin. *Epilepsia* 1987; 28:587.

Advances in Neurology, Vol. 55, edited by
D. Smith, D. Treiman, and M. Trimble,
Raven Press, Ltd., New York © 1991.

15

Effects of Antiepileptic Drugs on the Developing Central Nervous System

Bruce R. Ransom* and Joann G. Elmore†

*Departments of *Neurology and †Internal Medicine, Yale University School of Medicine,
New Haven, Connecticut 06510*

Clinicians must be concerned about the possibility that anticonvulsants have adverse effects on the developing central nervous system (CNS) for two important reasons: (i) It is frequently necessary to use anticonvulsants to treat epilepsy in pregnant women and infants, and (ii) the CNS is particularly vulnerable to injury during development when neurons and glial cells are proliferating, migrating, and differentiating (1). Unfortunately, very little data from human studies are directly relevant to this question, and what data do exist are difficult to interpret. Animal and *in vitro* studies clearly indicate that, under certain conditions, anticonvulsant drug therapy may injure the developing CNS. Much more analysis will be necessary, however, before the difficult and more far-reaching question of how to best treat epilepsy in pregnant women and infants is answered. The importance of avoiding the tragedy of damage to the developing CNS, as well as avoiding the consequent risk of intellectual impairment or behavioral alteration, should motivate further evaluation of this issue.

Because a great variety of toxic effects have been ascribed to the human use of anticonvulsants, it is necessary to define the type of toxicity that is the focus of this review. Unfortunately, inadequacies in our current understanding of anticonvulsant drug toxicity severely limit the precision of such statements. Of interest here are drug-induced changes in the biochemistry or structure of the developing CNS, occurring either pre- or postnatally, which are not anticipated based on our knowledge of the drug's mechanism(s) of anticonvulsant action. Such effects (e.g., loss of neurons) might be expected to deleteriously influence behavior or aspects of cognitive function and would likely be slowly reversible or irreversible in nature. Excluded from consideration are (a) acute and fully reversible drug effects (such as drowsiness or mild cognitive dysfunction) that can be accounted for by the known pharmacological actions of the drug and (b) drug-induced birth defects that presumably represent derangements of embryogenesis.

The primary goal of this review is to critically assess the information available on the adverse effects of anticonvulsants on the developing CNS. Three kinds of studies will be considered in evaluating this complex issue: (i) human studies on the effects of prenatal anticonvulsant exposure, (ii) animal studies, and (iii) *in vitro* studies using cultured mammalian neurons. We comment on some of the factors which influence the relevance of nonhuman experimental studies to the clinical situation. Finally, we identify some of the remaining questions which future research in this area should seek to answer.

HUMAN STUDIES

Human studies have variably measured neuropsychological function and the potentially related feature of infant head size in attempting to determine if anticonvulsants deleteriously affect brain development. Thus far, none of these studies have satisfactorily determined if anticonvulsant drug exposure during the prenatal period can cause lasting effects on behavior or intellectual function. The effect of anticonvulsants on the objective parameter head circumference has been most frequently studied (see below). Several investigators have shown that the mean head circumference of infants born to mothers with epilepsy receiving anticonvulsant therapy is smaller than that of infants born to mothers without epilepsy (2–7). Long-term follow-up studies of such infants will be necessary to determine if smaller head size has behavioral or cognitive consequences.

Before discussing the issue of drug effects on head circumference, it is pertinent to inquire as to the relationship between head size and intelligence. Head size is "determined by the growth of the brain except in cases of hydrocephalus, craniosynostosis, or other cranial pathology" (8). Small head circumference has been linked with mental retardation (9). Among microcephalic children, I.Q. correlates directly with head size (8); larger than average head size at 1 year of age, on the other hand, correlates with superior intelligence at age 7 (10). Early studies on the relationship between head size and intelligence often evaluated preselected populations which were potentially biased toward mental subnormality. Nelson and Deutschberger (11) attempted to eliminate this bias when they evaluated the relationship between head circumference at 50–54 weeks and I.Q. at 4 years in 9379 children registered in the Collaborative Project on Cerebral Palsy. They found that I.Q. at 4 years varied directly with head circumference at 1 year; children with head sizes in the smallest 0.67% of the population at 1 year of age had a 50% risk of having an I.Q. below 80 at 4 years of age. There is reason to believe, therefore, that any factor which systematically promotes smaller infant head size may also be associated with reduced I.Q.

Hiilesma et al. (2) showed that administration of either carbamazepine alone or combination therapy containing phenobarbital (PB) to pregnant patients with epilepsy is associated with fetal head growth retardation of their offspring. One hundred thirty-three women with epilepsy on low-dose anticonvulsant therapy, along with their 143 babies, were studied (some mothers were twice pregnant during the study). The analysis was restricted to singleton live births after at least 32 weeks of gestation. A control pair (mother and child) was selected for each pair in the epilepsy group and was carefully matched for maternal age, parity, social class, and fetal sex. There were no significant differences between the epilepsy patients and the controls, or between the mothers on different antiepileptic regimens, with regard to maternal stature, head circumference, weight, weight gain during pregnancy, smoking, drinking, consumption of drugs other than anticonvulsants, pregnancy complications, cesarean section, and duration of labor. The mean head circumference (standardized for gestational age and sex) of babies born to mothers on carbamazepine monotherapy was 7 mm less than that of controls ($p < 0.01$), and the mean head circumference of babies born to mothers on drug regimens which included PB or primidone was 6 mm less than that of controls ($p < 0.05$). These differences persisted when head circumferences were further standardized for weight and length, factors which, importantly, were not influenced by anticonvulsant drug exposure. Head size did not correlate with maternal serum drug levels, duration of the mothers' epilepsy, seizure type, number and temporal distribution of seizures during pregnancy, or complications during pregnancy and delivery. No catch-up growth in head circumference occurred by the age of 18 months. Phenytoin by itself had no apparent effect on infant head size, but the average serum level of this drug was quite low (5.2 µg/ml in the third trimester of pregnancy) (2). It should be noted that although the mean head circumference of the infants of treated mothers with epilepsy was smaller than that of the controls, most of the individual values were still within the normal range. Future assessment of the brain function of these children, or of that of a similar population, is required in order to judge the true significance of this finding.

Koch et al. (3) prospectively studied 70 children whose mothers had epilepsy and were on anticonvulsant medication during pregnancy. These children had generally smaller builds, lower body weights, and smaller heads than did the control children ($p < 0.05$). Children exposed to two or more anticonvulsants showed greater reductions in these measurements than did those children exposed to a single drug; no differences were noted among the various anticonvulsants in terms of their tendency to reduce weight, length, and head size. The reduction in head circumference remained demonstrable up to the fourth year of life ($p < 0.01$), although the weight and length returned to normal. Longitudinal assessment of these children's cognitive and linguistic abilities is apparently underway.

Hanson and Smith (12) drew attention to a pattern of fetal abnormalities that appeared to result from exposure to hydantoin anticonvulsants. The affected infants exhibited a multisystem pattern of abnormalities, including craniofacial anomalies, nail and digital hypoplasia, prenatal-onset growth deficiency, and mental deficiency; this clinical pattern was termed the "fetal hydantoin syndrome" (12). The fetal hydantoin syndrome, per se, probably represents a derangement of embryogenesis, but some of the alterations attributed to this syndrome, such as changes in growth or behavior, may be due to nonspecific CNS toxicity as defined above. It has been estimated, using data from the Collaborative Perinatal Project, that the frequency of hydantoin therapy during pregnancy is about two per 1000 pregnancies and that approximately 6000 babies are exposed to this drug yearly in the United States (4).

The effect of hydantoin anticonvulsants on fetal outcome was further evaluated by Hanson et al. (4) in a prospective study of 35 children born to 23 women with epilepsy who were on a hydantoin anticonvulsant during pregnancy; during 20 of these pregnancies the mothers received one or more additional anticonvulsants. Among the offspring, four (11%) met the criteria for the fetal hydantoin syndrome, but 11 other children (31%) showed abnormalities (such as microcephaly and mental deficiency) when evaluated at age 4. Hanson et al. (4) also reported a case–control evaluation of 104 children whose mothers had a convulsive disorder and were treated with hydantoins; 80 also received barbiturates continuously throughout pregnancy. Control subjects, who did not have a seizure disorder and who received no anticonvulsants during pregnancy, were chosen for 100 of the hydantoin cases; these controls were matched for maternal socioeconomic status, maternal age, and race. Anticonvulsant-exposed infants had a significantly smaller head circumference at birth than did the controls ($p < 0.05$), but this difference was not detected when reassessed at age 7. The mean full-scale Wechsler Intelligence Scale for Children (WISC) mental performance score at 7 years of age was lower in drug-exposed children than in the controls ($p < 0.05$). Stratification of these data by maternal hydantoin dosage level, by exposure to hydantoins alone versus hydantoins plus barbiturates, and by racial and sex-specific categories revealed no significant differences (4). The sample size in this study was not adequate to fully exclude such possibilities as a dose–response relationship or the possible contributions of various drug combinations. Furthermore, no clear separation of the role of hydantoins from that of the seizure disorder could be made.

Deblay et al. (5) studied 115 children born to mothers with epilepsy treated with anticonvulsants during pregnancy; 101 mothers received PB and 40 received a hydantoin. There was a high incidence (31%) of small head circumference (≤ 2 S.D. below the mean) at birth, and this was frequently associated later with impaired somatic and psychomotor development.

Because of serious concerns about the effects of some anticonvulsants on the fetus, it has been suggested that carbamazepine is the drug of choice for pregnant women who require anticonvulsant therapy (7). Both Niebyl et al. (13) and Nakane et al. (14) found no relationship between prenatal exposure to carbamazepine and major malformations. However, studies by Hiilesma et al. (2; see above) and Bertollini et al. (15) demonstrated an association between prenatal exposure to carbamazepine and reduced head circumference. Jones et al. (7) reported a specific pattern of malformations in 35 live-born children of women treated prenatally with carbamazepine monotherapy. The observed malformation pattern included minor craniofacial defects (11%), fingernail hyperplasia (21%), and microcephaly (11%). The microcephaly developed postnatally in some of the children in whom it was noted. Twenty-five children who were exposed prenatally to carbamazepine alone had formal neurobehavioral assessment, and five (20%) were found to be developmentally delayed (7).

Similarity in the patterns of malformation was noted between the carbamazepine-exposed children and those with the fetal hydantoin syndrome. Both phenytoin and carbamazepine are metabolized through the arene oxide pathway to an epoxide intermediate (16). Buehler (17) noted that children with more severe clinical signs of the fetal hydantoin syndrome have a lower level of activity of epoxide hydrolase, an enzyme involved in epoxide detoxification. It has been hypothesized that this epoxide intermediate, rather than the specific drug itself, might be the teratogenic agent (7). It should be emphasized again that, although these adverse effects of carbamazepine may represent true teratogenicity (i.e., altered embryogenesis), some of the effects may be the result of nonspecific toxicity on developing neurons.

Nelson and Ellenberg (6) evaluated extensive data from the Collaborative Perinatal Project of the National Institute of Neurological and Communicative Disorders and Stroke on the relationship between maternal seizure disorders and neurological outcome in offspring. Their findings address the critical issue of the influence of maternal epilepsy on fetal outcome, independent of drug treatment. This study followed 54,000 pregnant women prospectively from the first prenatal visit until the children born of those pregnancies reached the age of 7 years. The offspring of women with a "current seizure disorder" ($N = 410$; see definition below), the subset of this "current seizure disorder" group who had seizures during pregnancy ($N = 204$), and controls ($N = 43,926$) were compared. The term "current seizure disorder" indicated that "at least one seizure occurred within 5 years of the birth of the child" (6); eclamptic seizures and convulsions accompanying insulin overdosage in diabetic women were excluded. Among other things, this study provides important epidemiological data on the manner in which pregnant women with epilepsy are managed. Of the treated women with a current seizure disorder, 20% took PB only, 30% took phenytoin only, and 50% took both;

other medications were prescribed in a small number of cases. Seventy percent of the women who had seizures during pregnancy received anticonvulsant treatment during pregnancy. Thirty-five percent of women with a current seizure disorder but with no seizures noted during pregnancy were treated during pregnancy. A small percentage of the control seizure-free gravid women received anticonvulsant medications (mainly PB); treatment was probably instituted in most of these women because of toxemia.

Control patients who received anticonvulsants, as compared to nontreated control patients, were noted to have more stillbirths ($p < 0.001$), smaller head size of the child (defined as ≤ 2 S.D., $p < 0.02$), and more "bad outcomes," including death ($p < 0.001$). When women with toxemia were excluded from this analysis, only the excess of stillbirths remained significant. The investigators concluded that in control women who do not have seizures, the apparent excess risk associated with anticonvulsant treatment was actually related to the maternal condition for which the drug was given. Neither low birth weight (below 2501 g) nor neonatal seizures were more frequent in the infants of women with current seizure disorders (6). At 1 year of age, there was a twofold excess of children with small head circumferences (≤ 2 S.D. below the mean for birth weight, gestational age, sex, and race) among the progeny of women with current seizure disorders ($p < 0.005$). Low I.Q., which was defined as an I.Q. below 70 on the WISC administered when the children were 7 years old, was observed more frequently in the progeny of women with current seizures than in the progeny of the control population. These differences in I.Q. were statistically significant only among blacks. In mothers with a current seizure disorder, fetal characteristics (including head circumference) were not found to be significantly affected by anticonvulsant therapy.

In a thoughtful discussion, Nelson and Ellenberg (6) point out that, despite this study being a very large prospective controlled evaluation, many factors could have confounded their data. For example, drug levels and compliance were not monitored. They conclude that "this report does not provide evidence of a role for antiepileptic medications in determining the less favorable outcomes of pregnancy in women with current seizure disorders, but we could not rule out such a role" (6). However, this study clearly shows that fetal head size and intelligence, features which are regularly assessed in looking for prenatal drug effects, are also affected by the maternal seizure disorder itself. Without carefully controlling for this latter variable, it will not be possible to determine the role which drugs play in unfavorable fetal outcomes.

Studies revealing a possible association between anticonvulsant medications during pregnancy and small head circumference of exposed offspring have prompted investigations on possible mechanisms for this effect. Anticonvulsant drugs may influence growth and thyroid hormones in nonpregnant women with epilepsy (18–21). Kaneko et al. (22) measured growth hormone, thyrotropin, and thyroid hormone levels in the sera of pregnant women and correlated these data with fetal head circumference. Blood levels of thyrotropin, thyroxine, and growth hormone were all lower in mothers with epilepsy, but the decrease in thyroxine level correlated best with smaller fetal head circumference.

ANIMAL STUDIES

Rodents have been used in most studies looking for toxic effects of anticonvulsants on the developing nervous system. The majority of this work has focused on PB, perhaps because the greater aqueous solubility of this drug compared to that of other anticonvulsants makes it easier to work with experimentally. The first animal studies examined the effects of prenatal or postnatal anticonvulsant therapy on brain weight; subsequent studies have extended this analysis to a cellular level. It is obviously of great importance to know if drug-induced changes in the CNS are associated with behavioral or cognitive alterations. Unfortunately, relatively little work has been done on this critical issue.

In one of the earliest reports, neonatal rats treated from postnatal day 3 to 20 with 60 mg/kg/day of PB had reduced body, whole-brain, and cerebellar weights, compared to those of control animals, when evaluated at 21 days of age (23). Because undernutrition had been known to be associated with decreased brain weight (1), subsequent studies controlled for this variable. Schain and Watanabe (24) compared body, whole-brain, and cerebellar weights in neonatal animals treated with PB (same protocol as above) and in undernourished control animals. Although the mean body weight of PB-treated animals was 10% greater than that of undernourished animals, the mean whole-brain and cerebellar weights of the PB-treated animals were still significantly less than those in the undernourished animals. Diaz and Schain (25) also concluded that neonatal rats exposed to PB (60 mg/kg/day; from day 4 to 18) have diminished brain weight in excess of that expected to occur as a result of a reduction in body weight. In this study, PB-treated neonatal rats were force-fed so that their average weight remained similar to that of controls. In spite of this forced normalization of body weight, the drug-treated rats had a significant (12%) reduction in brain weight. The neonates receiving 60 mg/kg/day of PB exhibited normal gross motor activity but were slightly less active when stimulated in an open-field enclosure (25). Neonatal animals receiving only 15 mg/kg/day of PB showed no reduction in brain growth. Rats exposed to PB (60 mg/kg/day) at a later stage of development (from day 25 to 39) also showed reduced brain weight (26).

Similar effects of PB on brain weight have been obtained using mice (27). After exposure to PB from gestation day 6 to parturition, the brains of male offspring were evaluated at 50 days of age and were found to be 8% smaller with respect to body weight. Importantly, no differences in body weight or physical development were noted. PB was administered by incorporating it into the food supply of the pregnant mice, and blood levels ranged between 40 and 200 μg/ml. Treated animals "often showed slight signs of intoxication but were able to eat and groom normally" (27). Mice of both sexes exposed to PB postnatally (from day 2 to 21) also evidenced reduced brain weight, as compared to that of an untreated control group, at 50 days of age. Male mice exposed to PB, but not females, had a significantly (16%) lower body weight than did the controls.

Histological evaluation of the brains of mice exposed to PB during development reveals approximately a 33% reduction in the number of Purkinje cells in the cerebellum and a 15–33% reduction in hippocampal pyramidal cells. Neonatal, but not prenatal, PB exposure causes a significant reduction in cerebellar and hippocampal granule cells and less extensive neuronal loss in the cerebral cortex. The investigators pointed out that in contrast to other insults (including x-irradiation and undernutrition), neonatal exposure to PB destroys already formed neurons (e.g., Purkinje cells and hippocampal pyramidal neurons) as well as the more susceptible populations of cells, such as cerebellar granule cells, which proliferate and differentiate during the period of drug administration (28).

Neonatal, but not prenatal, exposure to PB causes a long-lasting reduction in the number of Purkinje cell dendritic spines in mice for as long as 4 weeks after the end of drug exposure, as determined by analysis of Golgi-stained cells (29). No drug effects were noted in terms of overall dendritic size or the number of dendritic branches. Rats exposed to PB during the late prenatal period and postnatally until day 21 do exhibit a subtle rearrangement of their cerebellar Purkinje cell dendrites (30). It is noteworthy that these rats were treated with a relatively low dose of PB (10 mg/kg/day), which resulted in a 20% reduction in the number of Purkinje cells but which had no effect on overall cerebellar weight, and that these effects were apparent even as long as 4 months after drug treatment (30).

Ultrastructural degenerative changes have been described in mouse cerebellar neurons and myelin after prenatal and neonatal exposure to PB (31). Prenatal exposure was achieved by giving pregnant mice PB in their food from gestation day 9 through 18 as previously discussed (see above); neonates were exposed to PB (50 mg/kg/day) from day 2 to 21. Electron microscopy was carried out at day 50, and a significant increase in degenerative changes in the cerebellar cortex was noted in treated animals in comparison to controls. These changes included (a) mitochondrial degeneration and intracellular lamellar bodies in neurons, especially in neuronal processes in the molecular and granular cell layers, and (b) myelin degeneration. Similar changes have been noted after perinatal treatment with phenytoin (32).

The long-term behavioral consequences of perinatal exposure to anticonvulsants have not been well studied. Early studies suggested mild, long-lasting deficits in certain types of learning behavior in rodents exposed to PB during development (see ref. 33). In a more recent study, rats were exposed to PB (60 mg/kg/day) from postnatal day 6 to 36 and tested in a cold-water T maze 10–20 days after the drug was stopped. Treated animals ran the maze faster than did controls and made fewer errors (34); no significant differences in maze performance were seen when animals were tested 3 months after PB had been discontinued. The treated animals exhibited increased excitability, and it was suggested that the improved performance of these animals may have reflected greater motivation.

Mice treated neonatally with PB exhibit long-term deficits in a delayed spontaneous alternation task and the radial eight-arm maze, behaviors which are believed to be mediated, in part, by cholinergic mechanisms and to depend upon the hippocampus (35,36). As previously mentioned, the hippocampus suffers cell loss after early exposure to PB (see above) and also shows a transient change in a cholinergic enzyme (36). It is as yet unknown if these structural and neurochemical changes underlie the noted behavioral alterations.

Rodents exposed prenatally to PB exhibit greater open-field activity than do controls, and this effect persists into adulthood (37). Reduced levels of whole-brain dopamine and norepinephrine were noted at 21 days of age, but these neurochemical changes were not detected in adult animals and therefore are probably not responsible for the behavioral alterations; this study did not eliminate the more subtle possibility of persistent regional differences in neurotransmitters, however (37). The abnormal open-field activity of treated animals was believed to be partially related to slower habituation to novel environmental stimuli (37).

Male rats exposed prenatally to PB exhibit permanent changes in reproductive behavior and have permanent decreases in plasma and brain testosterone levels (38). PB might be acting indirectly on gonadotropin, or it might be exerting its action by a direct effect on synthetic enyzmes. Androgenic receptors are widespread throughout the CNS and may be critical for establishing the form of the adult CNS by influencing sexually dimorphic brain regions (see, e.g., ref. 39). To our knowledge, no human studies have followed up on this important experimental observation.

The metabolism of anticonvulsants, as well as the concentration dependency of their actions and toxic effects, may vary between different animal species and humans and may also vary in relationship to developmental stage. These important issues have not been systematically analyzed, and therefore they impose one of the potential limitations in our ability to extrapolate the findings from animal studies to humans. This difficulty is illustrated by discussing the variability of PB serum and brain levels in neonatal rodents.

It is important to relate PB's retarding effects on brain development to the serum or brain levels of this drug which were achieved by the various dosage regimens. Trough levels of PB in neonatal rats given 60 mg/kg/day of this drug averaged 2 μg/ml in one study (21-day old rats) (24) and ranged between 7 and 13 μg/ml in another (18-day-old rats) (25). The plasma half-life of PB in 21-day-old rats was estimated to be about 5 hr (24); the rapid metabolism of PB by rats of this age may explain their ability to receive large barbiturate dosages with relatively minor behavioral effects (see, e.g., ref. 23). In two-day-old mice receiving 40 or 50 mg/kg/day of PB, the brain levels remained between 30 and 50 μg/g for a 24-hr period following drug administration; in 20-day-old animals receiving the same dosage of PB, maximum brain concentrations were less than 15 μg/g and fell to near zero by 4 hr after injection (28). In mice, therefore, the metabolism of PB increases rapidly during the first 20 days of life. It is not clear whether this is simply due to induction of degradative enzymes by PB or whether it represents a true developmental difference. In absolute terms, these rodent blood levels of PB are roughly similar to therapeutic levels in human infants, although the speed of PB metabolism is more rapid in rodents (40).

Are the dosages of PB used in these animal studies relevant to the dosages used in humans? This question has no simple answer. The issue is not just whether the blood and brain levels of drug are comparable, but also whether the effects of similar drug levels are physiologically, metabolically, and pharmacologically equivalent. Incomplete evidence indicates that similar brain levels of PB, as an example, have similar actions on brain function in humans and rodents (see ref. 41); it is less clear whether this is the case during brain development, mainly as a result of minimal investigative effort thus far. Tentatively then, it appears that the dosage range of PB used in animal studies is roughly equivalent to that used in humans, and thus the results of animal experimentation may be providing clues which are highly relevant to the effects of anticonvulsants on the immature human nervous system.

The animal studies reviewed here strongly suggest that at least one anticonvulsant, PB, adversely affects the developing CNS. Perinatal exposure to this drug may be particularly harmful to certain brain regions, especially the cerebellum and the hippocampus. These structures are believed to have primary roles in learning and memory (see, e.g., ref. 42). Behavioral studies have demonstrated some changes in the performance of previously drug-exposed animals on certain tasks, but results to date have not been impressive (see above); further studies on learning and memory in drug-exposed animals seem advisable. One can be justifiably concerned that the vastly more complex behavioral repertoire of humans, compared to rodents, would be more susceptible to alteration if pre- or postnatal exposure to an anticonvulsant produced major changes in the anatomic substrates of these behaviors.

IN VITRO STUDIES

In vitro preparations offer several advantages in attempting to identify toxic effects of chronic drug exposure. Drugs can be applied directly to cultured CNS neurons at known concentrations that can be easily verified at later times by directly assaying the compound in the culture medium (ref. 43). The possibility that observed effects on the target tissue might be mediated indirectly by effects of the drug on other organ systems or by biotransformation of the administered drug is largely eliminated. Finally, characteristics of the cultured cells, including their density and individual morphology, can be directly assayed after various periods of chronic drug exposure. A number of anticonvulsants have been examined using this powerful approach.

Bergey et al. (44) found that PB (30–120 μg/ml), in a concentration-dependent fashion, reduces the survival of large spinal cord neurons derived from embryonic mice and exposed to PB from day 14 to 28 in culture. PB also decreases the activity of the acetylcholine-synthesizing enzyme, choline acetyltransferase, in these cultures. Both of these effects are partially reversed when the cultures are switched from PB-containing medium to normal medium for 2 weeks. These investigators found that the parent molecule of PB, barbituric acid, has no effects on neuronal density or enzyme activity at concentrations up to 930 μM.

The above results were confirmed and extended by Serrano et al. (43). They found that PB (20–90 μg/ml) causes a concentration-dependent reduction in all classes of neurons in mouse spinal cord cultures exposed to the drug for 4–6 weeks beginning on day 14 (Fig. 1). Neuronal density was also decreased by chronic exposure to barbituric acid (172 mM), a result which conflicts with that reported by Bergey et al. (44). Thus, the issue of whether or not non-anticonvulsant barbiturates (such as barbituric acid) produce neuronal toxicity after chronic exposure remains undecided.

By quantitatively evaluating the morphology of individual neurons injected with Lucifer yellow, it was found that PB exposure also produces a concentration-dependent reduction in the length and branching frequency of dendrites (Fig. 2). The dendritic processes of cultured spinal cord neurons are densely crusted with synaptic terminals, as is the case *in vivo* (45,46). The loss of dendritic surface area caused by PB would reduce the number

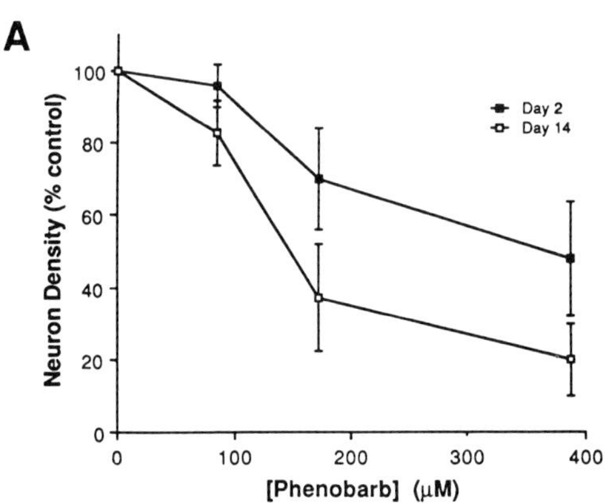

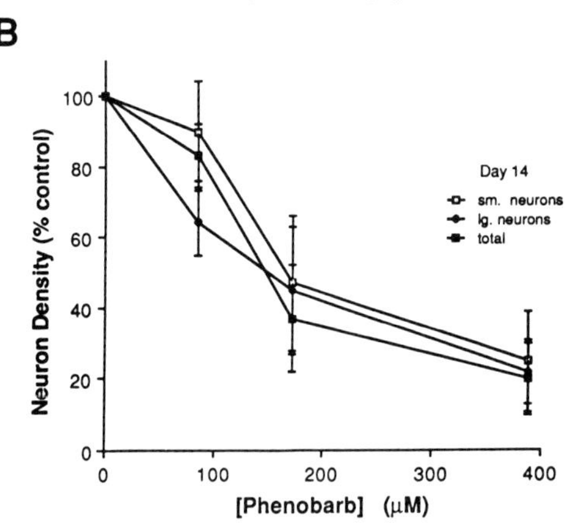

FIG. 1. Effect of chronic exposure to different concentrations of PB on neuronal density in cell cultures of mouse spinal cord. Cultures were exposed to PB from day 2 or day 14 after plating and were evaluated after a total of 8 weeks in culture. The percent neuron density, relative to control cultures, is displayed as a function of chronic exposure to different PB concentrations. Each point represents the average neuron density in nine separate culture dishes. **A:** There was a concentration-dependent decline in neuron density that was greater in cultures exposed to PB from day 14 than in those exposed from day 2. The difference between the day 2 and day 14 exposure conditions at PB concentrations of 172 and 388 μM was significant at the $p < 0.01$ level. **B:** Reduction in the density of the main neuronal subcategories in cultures exposed from day 14 was comparable to the reduction in the density of total cells. Small neurons were defined as phase bright cells with distinct processes whose greatest somal diameter was ≤20 μm, and large neurons were similar cells whose greatest somal diameter was >20 μm. Total neurons represents the combination of small and large neurons as defined above, in addition to "other" neurons (phase bright cells gathered in tight aggregates whose processes were not easily seen with phase optics). Thus all cells, regardless of size, were equally affected by PB. (From ref. 43, with permission.)

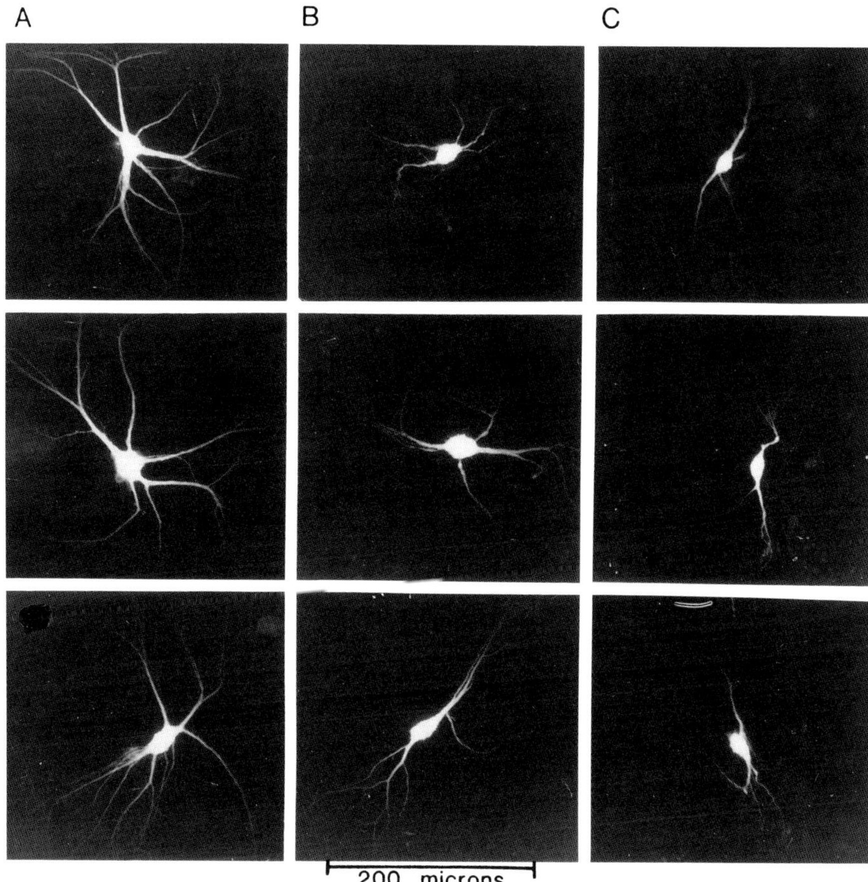

FIG. 2. Chronic exposure to PB alters neuronal morphology. Spinal cord neurons, exposed from day 14 to PB at various concentrations [86 μM (**B**) and 388 μM (**C**)], were injected with the stain Lucifer yellow at 6 weeks of age (i.e., 4 weeks of PB exposure); unexposed neurons of the same age were also stained [control (**A**)]. PB-treated neurons, in general, showed a concentration-dependent reduction in the extent of dendritic branching. (From ref. 43, with permission.)

of synaptic contacts received by an individual cell and thereby potentially impair neuronal information transfer (46). Curiously, Serrano et al. (43) found that the negative effects of PB were much more dramatic if cultures were exposed to the drug from day 14 as opposed to instituting exposure from day 2 in culture (e.g., Fig. 1). This counterintuitive result remains unexplained but raises the interesting possibility that deleterious drug effects on the CNS may be critically dependent upon the developmental stage.

Other anticonvulsants also have adverse effects on cultured neurons. Phenytoin exposure (culture day 10 to 17), in a concentration-dependent manner (15–50 μg/ml), reduced the number of neurons in mouse cerebral cortex cultures; neurons containing gamma-aminobutyric acid (GABA) were reduced to the same extent as was the total neuronal population (47). A number of specific biochemical functions were assayed after mouse cerebral cortical cultures were chronically exposed (culture day 9 to 20) to phenytoin (30 μg/ml), carbamazepine (24 μg/ml), valproic acid (162 μg/ml), ethosuximide (196 μg/ml), and diazepam (3.6 μg/ml) (48,49). At these concentrations, phenytoin and valproic acid strongly decreased (a) high-affinity uptake of GABA and β-alanine, (b) choline acetyltransferase activity, and (c) benzodiazepine binding. Ethosuximide and diazepam were less toxic, and carbamazepine had no significant toxicity in relationship to these parameters. All of these drugs caused a significant loss of neurons, however, except for ethosuximide (48,49). The total drug concentrations in these studies were about 1.5 to 2 times the high therapeutic concentrations in human serum, but the free concentrations were relatively higher than would have been expected in human serum because of less protein binding *in vitro* (48). The *in vitro* effects of these drugs over a range of free concentrations more comparable to those used in humans should be studied. It would also be important to study how the duration and timing of drug exposure influences outcome (see ref. 43).

The mechanisms by which anticonvulsants decrease neuronal survival and which in other ways adversely affect the developing nervous system remain unclear. Perhaps these drugs block the action of a trophic substance which is critical for neuronal survival; a number of such trophic molecules or factors have been described (50–52). Such molecules will be present *in vitro* as well as *in vivo*, especially when cultures are supplemented with animal serum or grown with background cells. Alternatively, these drugs might block certain forms of electrical activity which could impact on neuronal survival (53).

The effects of PB on neuronal morphology (see, e.g., ref. 43) are intriguing. PB, as well as other anticonvulsants, have been shown to inhibit depolarization-dependent calcium uptake by synaptosomes (41). Because growth-cone elongation in growing neurons may be dependent upon an influx of calcium (54), process simplification following chronic anticonvulsant exposure could represent the outcome of a long-term reduction in growth-terminal calcium influx.

Anticonvulsants could act indirectly to influence the survival or morphology of developing neurons. Late prenatal and early neonatal exposure to PB causes a permanent reduction in plasma and brain testosterone levels in rats (38). A subclass of spinal neurons is very sensitive to alterations in testosterone levels; reduced levels cause a marked reduction in dendritic branching (55). The altered sexual behavior in rats which may fol-

low from diminished levels of testosterone during development could be partly due to changes in neuronal interactions mediated by the altered dendritic morphology of the spinal neurons. Other hormones, such as those of the thyroid, influence the survival of neurons in the developing brain and may be affected by anticonvulsants (22,31,56). That anticonvulsant-induced changes in hormone levels may secondarily account for the changes in the developing brain is made increasingly attractive by the recent discovery that adrenal hormones exert a powerful influence on neuronal survival in the hippocampus (57).

DISCUSSION AND CONCLUSIONS

Animal and *in vitro* studies indicate that at some concentrations and for certain periods of exposure, a variety of anticonvulsant medications adversely affect the developing CNS. The ill effects include loss of neurons or alteration in their form, decreased transmitter-related enzyme activity or high-affinity uptake, and less well documented changes in behavior. Interpretation of these data vis-à-vis human anticonvulsant usage must be done with great caution, however. Concentrations of anticonvulsants used in nonhuman studies may not be functionally comparable to drug levels which are clinically efficacious in humans; this could be the result of either (a) intrinsic differences in CNS structure and function or (b) differences in pharmacokinetics and drug distribution. Nevertheless, to the extent that neuronal development in animals and *in vitro* can be compared to the situation in humans, these accumulated results raise serious concerns about long-term exposure of the developing human nervous system to anticonvulsants.

Although there have been some excellent human investigations into the issue regarding the effect of anticonvulsants on the developing fetus and child, these studies all suffer from certain methodological shortcomings or the lack of long-term evaluation, which have prevented us from obtaining a clear answer. In many of the studies reviewed, the use of two or more drugs simultaneously makes it difficult to draw conclusions about individual agents. Because drug effects on fetal outcome may be concentration-dependent, regular monitoring of anticonvulsant drug levels is essential but has rarely been systematically employed. As noted by Nelson and Ellenberg (6), the effects of anticonvulsant medications must be disentangled from the effects of maternal epilepsy itself on fetal outcome. In some studies, the two groups of pregnant women with epilepsy (i.e., treated and untreated) were not randomly chosen and often differed in terms of (a) severity and type of epilepsy and (b) frequency of seizures. Pregnant women with epilepsy who require treatment cannot be readily compared to pregnant women with epilepsy who do not require treatment; these patient groups probably differ in a variety of ways which, independent of anticonvulsant treatment, may influence fetal outcome.

The ideal human study to determine whether prenatal anticonvulsant exposure adversely affects CNS development, and whether it has consequent adverse effects on cognition and behavior, would be prospective and would randomly and blindly assign carefully matched groups of pregnant women with epilepsy to single anticonvulsant drugs (i.e., monotherapy) or placebo. The study would require long-term follow-up of the exposed infants so that subtle changes in behavior or intellectual ability could be assessed and correlated with any other measures of difference such as head circumference, growth, etc. In reality, ethical considerations, including the need to provide optimum care for the epilepsy populations under study, preclude undertaking such an investigation in its purest form. A more practical version of the ideal study, however, could be carried out. We believe that a rigorously planned, large, multicenter study is warranted by virtue of the large number of unborn fetuses at risk for drug-induced CNS injury and the available human, animal, and *in vitro* studies which raise serious concerns that anticonvulsants may damage the developing CNS.

ACKNOWLEDGMENTS

This work was supported by NIH grant NS 15589 (BRR) from the National Institute of Neurological and Communicative Disorders and Stroke.

REFERENCES

1. Dobbing J. The later development of the brain and its vulnerability. In: Davis JA, Dobbing J, eds. *Scientific foundations of pediatrics*. Philadelphia: WB Saunders, 1974;568.
2. Hiilesma VK, Teramo K, Granstrom ML, Bardy AH. Fetal head growth retardation associated with maternal antiepileptic drugs. *Lancet* 1981; 165–167.
3. Koch S, et al. Antiepileptika wahrend der Schwangerschaft. *Dtsch Med Wochenschr* 1983; 108:250–257.
4. Hanson JW, Myrianthopoulos NC, Sedgwick HMA, et al. Risks to the offspring of women treated with hydantoin anticonvulsants, with emphasis on the fetal hydantoin syndrome. *J Pediatr* 1976;89:662–668.
5. Deblay MF, Vert P, Andre M. L'enfant de mère epileptique. *Nouv Presse Med* 1982;11:173–176.
6. Nelson KB, Ellenberg JH. Maternal seizure disorder, outcome of pregnancy, and neurologic abnormalities in the children. *Neurology* 1982; 32:1247–1254.
7. Jones KL, Lacro RV, Johnson KA, Adams J. Patterns of malformation in the children of women treated with carbamazepine during pregnancy. *N Engl J Med* 1989;320:1661–1666.
8. Pryor HB, Thelander H. Abnormally small head size and intellect in children. *J Pediatr* 1968; 73:593–598.
9. O'Connell EJ, Feldt RH, Stickler GB. Head circumference, mental retardation and growth failure. *Pediatrics* 1965;36:62–65.
10. Fisch RO, Bilek MK, Horrobin JM, Chang PN. Children with superior intelligence at seven years of age. *Am J Dis Child* 1976;130:481–487.
11. Nelson KB, Deutschberger J. Head size at one year as a prediction of four year IQ. *Neurology* 1970;12:487–495.
12. Hanson JW, Smith DW. The fetal hydantoin syndrome. *J Pediatr* 1975;87:285.
13. Niebyl JR, Black DA, Freeman JM, Luff RD. Carbamazepine levels in pregnancy and location. *Obstet Gynecol* 1979;53:139–140.
14. Nakane Y, Okuma T, Takahashi R, et al. Multi-institutional study on the teratogenicity and fetal toxicity of antiepileptic drugs: a report of a collaborative study group in Japan. *Epilepsia* 1980;21:663–680.
15. Bertollini R, Kallon B, Mastroiacooo P, Robert E. Anticonvulsant drugs in monotherapy: effect on the fetus. *Eur J Epidemiol* 1987;3:164–171.
16. Lindhout D, Hoppener RJ, Meinardi H. Teratogenicity of antiepileptic drug combinations with special emphasis on epoxidation (of carbamazepine). *Epilepsia* 1984;25:77–83.
17. Buehler BA. Epoxide hydrolase activity in fibroblasts: correlation with clinical features of the fetal hydantoin syndrome. *Proc Greenwood Govt Cent* 1987;6:117.
18. Fichsel H, Knopfle G. Effects of anticonvulsant drugs on thyroid hormone in epileptic children. *Epilepsia* 1978;19:323–336.

19. Liewendahl K, Majuri H, Helenius T. Thyroid function tests in patients on long-term treatment with various anticonvulsant drugs. *Clin Endocrinol* 1978;8:185–191.

20. Luoma PV, Myllula VV, Hokkanen E. Elevated serum growth hormone levels in patients treated with anticonvulsants. In: Canger R, Angeleri F, Penry JK, eds. *Advances in epileptology: XIth Epilepsy International Symposium.* New York: Raven Press, 1980;431–433.

21. Yeo PPB, Bates D, Howe JG, Ratcliffe WA, Schardt CW, Heath A, Evered DC. Anticonvulsants and thyroid function. *Br Med J* 1978;1:1581–1583.

22. Kaneko S, et al. Foetal head growth retardation due to antiepileptic drugs: with reference to GH, TSH, T4, T3 and reverse T3 concentrations. *Folia Psychiatr Neurol Jpn* 1983;37(1):25–32.

23. Schain RJ, Watanabe K. Effect of chronic phenobarbital administration upon brain growth of the infant rat. *Exp Neurol* 1975;47:509–515.

24. Schain RJ, Watanabe K. Origin of brain growth retardation in young rats treated with phenobarbital. *Exp Neurol* 1976;50:806–809.

25. Diaz J, Schain RJ. Phenobarbital: effects of long term administration on behavior and brain of artificially reared rats. *Science* 1978;199:90–91.

26. Diaz J. Disruption of the brain growth spurt in adolescent rats by chronic phenobarbital administration. *Exp Neurol* 1983;79:559–563.

27. Yanai J, Rosselli-Austin L, Tabakoff B. Neuronal deficits in mice following prenatal exposure to phenobarbital. *Exp Neurol* 1979;64:237–244.

28. Yanai J, Bergman A. Neuronal deficits after neonatal exposure to phenobarbital. *Exp Neurol* 1981;73:199–208.

29. Yanai J, Iser C. Stereologic study of Purkinje cells in mice after early exposure to phenobarbital. *Exp Neurol* 1981;74:707–716.

30. Hannah RS, Roth SH, Spira AW. Effect of phenobarbital on Purkinje cell growth patterns in the rat cerebellum. *Exp Neurol* 1988;100:354–364.

31. Fishman RHB, Gaathon A, Yanai J. Early barbiturate treatment eliminates peak serum thyroxide levels in neonatal mice and produces ultrastructural damage in the brains of adults. *Dev Brain Res* 1982;5:202–205.

32. Delcerro MP, Snider MS. Cerebellar alterations resulting from Dilantin intoxication: an ultrastructural study. In: Fields WS, Willis WD, eds. *The cerebellum in health and disease.* St. Louis: WH Green, 1970;380–411.

33. McBride MC, Rosman NP. Absence of behavioral effects of intrauterine phenobarbital exposure in rats. *Exp Neurol* 1984;86:53–65.

34. McBride MC, Rosman NP, Davidson SJ, Oppenheimer EY. Long-term behavioral effects of phenobarbital in suckling rats. *Exp Neurol* 1985;89:59–70.

35. Pick CG, Yanai J. Long term reduction in spontaneous alterations after early exposure to phenobarbital. *Int J Dev Neurosci* 1984;2:223–228.

36. Kleinberger N, Yanai J. Early phenobarbital-induced alterations in hippocampal acetylcholinesterase activity and behavior. *Dev Brain Res* 1985;22:113–123.

37. Middaugh LD, Simpson LW, Thomas TN, Zemp JW. Prenatal maternal phenobarbital increases reactivity and retards habituation of mature offspring to environmental stimuli. *Psychopharmacology* 1981;74:349–352.

38. Gupta C, Yaffe SJ, Shapiro BH. Prenatal exposure to phenobarbital permanently decreases testosterone and causes reproductive dysfunction. *Science* 1982;216:640–642.

39. Nordeen EJ, Nordeen KW, Sengelaub DR, Arnold AP. Androgens prevent normally occurring cell death in a sexually dimorphic spinal nucleus. *Science* 1985;229:671–673.

40. Painter MJ, Pippenger C, MacDonald H, Pitlick W. Phenobarbital and diphenylhydantoin levels in neonates with seizures. *J Pediatr* 1978;92(2):315–319.

41. Prichard JW, Ransom BR. Phenobarbital: mechanisms of action. In: Levy R, Mattson R, Meldrum B, Penry JK, Dreifuss FE, eds. *Antiepileptic drugs.* New York: Raven Press, 1989;267–282.

42. McCormick DA, Thompson RF. Cerebellum: essential involvement in the classically conditioned eyeblink response. *Science* 1983;223:296–299.

43. Serrano EE, Kunis DM, Ransom BR. Effects of chronic phenobarbital exposure on cultured mouse spinal cord neurons. *Ann Neurol* 1988;24:429–438.

44. Bergey GK, Swaiman KF, Schrier BK, et al. Adverse effects of phenobarbital on morphological and biochemical development of fetal mouse spinal cord neurons in culture. *Ann Neurol* 1981;9:584–589.

45. Ransom BR, Neale E, Henkart M, et al. Mouse spinal cord in cell culture: I. Morphology and intrinsic neuronal electrophysiologic properties. *J Neurophysiol* 1977;40:1132–1150.

46. Gelfan S, Kao G, Ruchkin DS. The dendritic tree of spinal neurons. *J Comp Neurol* 1973;139:385–412.

47. Swaiman KF, Neale EA, Schrier BK, Nelson PG. Toxic effect of phenytoin on developing cortical neurons in culture. *Ann Neurol* 1983;13:48–52.

48. Neale EA, Sher PK, Graubard BI, et al. Differential toxicity of chronic exposure to phenytoin, phenobarbital, or carbamazepine in cerebral cortical cell cultures. *Pediatr Neurol* 1985;1:143–150.

49. Sher PK, Neale EA, Graubard BI, et al. Differential neurochemical effects of chronic exposure of cerebral cortical cell culture to valproic acid, diazepam, or ethosuximide. *Pediatr Neurol* 1985;1:232–237.

50. Gurney ME, Heinrich SP, Mark RL, Yin H. Molecular cloning and expression of neuroleukin, a neurotrophic factor for spinal and sensory neurons. *Science* 1986;234:566–574.

51. Thoenen H, Edgar D. Neurotrophic factors. *Science* 1985;229:238–242.

52. Brenneman DE, Neale EA, Foster GA, et al. Non-neuronal cells mediate neurotrophic action

of vasoactive intestinal peptide. *J Cell Biol* 1987;104:1603–1610.

53. Bergey GK, Fitzgerald SC, Schrier BK, Nelson PG. Neuronal maturation in mammalian cell culture is dependent on spontaneous electrical activity. *Brain Res* 1981;207:49–58.

54. Bolsover SR, Spector I. Measurements of calcium transients in the soma, neurite, and growth cone of single cultured neurons. *J Neurosci* 1986;6:1934–1940.

55. Kurz EM, Sengelaub DR, Arnold AP. Andro-
gens regulate the dendritic length of mammalian motoneurons in adulthood. *Science* 1986;232:395–398.

56. DeVoogd TJ. Androgens can affect the morphology of mammalian CNS neurons in adulthood. *Trends Neurosci* 1987;10:341.

57. Sloviter RS, Valiquette G, Abrams GM, et al. Selective loss of hippocampal granule cells in the mature rat brain after adrenalectomy. *Science* 1989;243:535–538.

Advances in Neurology, Vol. 55, edited by
D. Smith, D. Treiman, and M. Trimble,
Raven Press, Ltd., New York 1991.

16

Antiepileptic Drugs in Affective Illness

Clinical and Theoretical Implications

Robert M. Post, Lori L. Altshuler, Terence A. Ketter, Kirk Denicoff,
and Susan R. B. Weiss

Biological Psychiatry Branch, National Institute of Mental Health, Bethesda, Maryland 20892

In seeking treatments other than lithium for patients with refractory bipolar affective illness, we chose to first study an anticonvulsant for a variety of empirical and theoretical reasons. Structures within the limbic system have long been implicated in modulation of normal and pathological emotional repertoires (1–13). Whereas previous theory-driven pharmacological approaches to the affective disorders had centered around neurotransmitter specificity, we shifted the focus to a drug that might target anatomical rather than neurotransmitter effects. Of the anticonvulsants, carbamazepine was chosen because it had one of the best profiles of efficacy in complex partial seizures and in preclinical models of seizures arising from limbic areas of brain as compared with other areas (14,15). Subsumed within the concept that carbamazepine was an effective limbic anticonvulsant was the fact that carbamazepine inhibited at least some stages of limbic kindling (14,16–22). This model has been used as a conceptual bridge to understand the unfolding of symptoms in manic–depressive illness (23–25), although there is little evidence for a literal kindling-like physiological phenomenon occurring in patients with primary affective disorders.

We were further bolstered in this reasoning by the extensive, although largely uncontrolled, reports of the potential psychotropic effect of carbamazepine. For example, Dalby (26), in his series in 1971, reported 11 of 18 patients who had periodic depressions resembling those seen in primary endogenous depression and who responded to carbamazepine. He cited a number of instances in which this occurred in spite of inadequate seizure control, suggesting that improvement in mood and behavior might be occurring independently of the anticonvulsant efficacy of carbamazepine. In addition, in his review in 1975, approximately 50% of some 2500 patients with epilepsy treated with carbamazepine were reported to show positive psychotropic effects (27). At the time, it was highly controversial as to whether these putative psychotropic effects of carbamazepine were due to a primary effect of the drug or merely were secondary to substitution of this agent for more behaviorally toxic anticonvulsants and/or better seizure control achieved (28,29). The clear demonstration of positive psychotropic effects of carbamazepine in non-epilepsy patients with primary affective disorders obviates the controversy and strongly implicates a direct psychotropic effect of carbamazepine independent of the other factors noted above. After we decided to initiate the protocol for studying the anticonvulsant carbamazepine in primary affective disorders, we became aware of Okuma et al.'s work (30) which had suggested that the drug had positive effects in uncontrolled clinical trials of patients with manic–depressive illness. Earlier work, by Takezaki and Hanaoka (31), had reported the acute antimanic and prophylactic efficacy of carbamazepine.

In this chapter we briefly review the evidence for the efficacy of a variety of anticonvulsant modalities in the acute and prophylactic treatment of manic–depressive illness. We start with a consideration of electroconvulsive therapy as the best documented and most efficacious treatment of acute depressive episodes and include it under the rubric of an anticonvulsant, since recent data suggest that it is, in fact, a potent anticonvulsant modality in both humans and experimental animals (32,33).

The question is raised and discussed as to whether the anticonvulsant properties of these agents are, in fact, related to their psychotropic effects in manic–depressive patients. This issue obviously becomes crucial when considering mechanisms of action of the anticonvulsants, both in seizure disorders and in affective disorders. Some evidence suggests that temporal factors such as the time course of onset of efficacy may be different in seizure and affective disorders, suggesting that different mechanisms are involved (34). Evidence is addressed on the issue of whether limbic sites of action of the anticonvulsants are, in fact, related to their positive effects in manic–depressive illness. Finally, the kindling analogy for the evolution of symptoms in the course of affective illness is discussed in the context of its potential derivative theoretical implications for a differential pharmacotherapy as a function of illness, since this analogy may help in elucidation of the phenomenon of conditioned tolerance.

ANTICONVULSANTS IN AFFECTIVE DISORDERS

Electroconvulsive Therapy

Electroconvulsive therapy (ECT) is highly effective in the acute treatment of manic and depressive episodes (35–38), although it is impractical and virtually unstudied for long-term or prophylactic treatment. Not only have a wealth of studies documented the efficacy of ECT as being superior to that of most traditional (38) or novel agents such as carbamazepine (Fig. 1), but a series of recent double-blind investigations of active ECT against sham ECT have further convincingly documented its effectiveness (39).

The induction of electroconvulsive seizures (ECS) in animals is a potent anticonvulsant (32,33). ECS prevent both the development (Fig. 2 and Table 1) and the expression of completed amygdala-kindled seizures (Fig. 3 and Table 2) and may thus be regarded as having both antiepileptogenic (i.e., prevents development of seizures) and anticonvulsant (i.e., prevents expression of completed seizures) effects. In this regard, ECS are more potent than carbamazepine, which, in the rat, is ineffective in preventing the development of amygdala kindling (22,40). Similarly, ECT is a potent anticonvulsant in humans, as evidenced by (a) the increase in seizure thresholds as a function of treatment duration and (b) its occasional effective use as a primary anticonvulsant in patients with refractory seizure disorders (41).

The mechanisms by which ECS and ECT exert their anticonvulsant principles have not been adequately delineated, although several factors have been postulated. Chronic ECS up-regulates adenosine receptors and alters a variety of peptides implicated in the regulation of convulsive excitability, including thyrotropin-releasing hormone (TRH), endogenous opiates, somatostatin, etc. (42). Best documented is a role for opiates; the cerebrospinal fluid (CSF) of animals receiving chronic ECS confers a naloxone-reversible anticonvulsant principle when transferred to the CSF of other animals (43,44). Whether these effects are related to the efficacy of ECS in manic–depressive illness remains to be further delineated.

Carbamazepine, the Keto-derivative of Carbamazepine (Oxcarbazepine), and Carbamazepine-10,11-epoxide

Acute Mania

Carbamazepine and its congeners appear to exert acute antimanic effects in the treatment of patients with primary affective disorders (45). A series of 13 studies which were double-blind and placebo-controlled documented a rapid onset of action in the first week of treatment; time course and incidence of im-

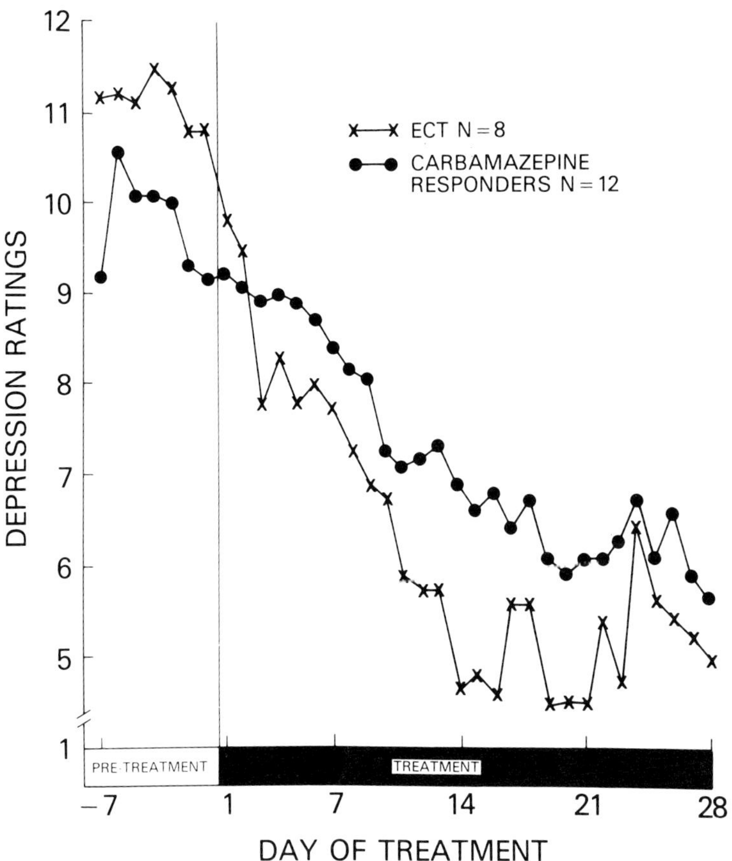

FIG. 1. Time course of antidepressant effects in electroconvulsive therapy (ECT) responders and in carbamazepine responders. Note that even when carbamazepine-responsive patients (12/35) are selected to compare with unselected ECT-treated patients (all were pharmacologically refractory) on our Unit, the time course of response is more rapid with ECT.

provement were parallel to those achieved with the antipsychotic neuroleptics (see Table 3). This antimanic efficacy is particularly notable in light of the fact that carbamazepine, unlike the neuroleptic agents, does not block either (a) stimulant-induced hyperactivity in animals or (b) dopamine receptors *in vitro* (46–48). Thus, carbamazepine is exerting its antimanic efficacy through a mechanism other than dopamine receptor blockade. This confers several potential advantages, including the virtual lack of acute extrapyramidal side effects and the absence of longer-term tardive dyskinesia (49). It also makes the drug more acceptable to many patients because of a lack of extrapyramidal side effects; furthermore, it

provides a theoretical rationale for the combined use of carbamazepine with neuroleptics in the refractory patient, since these two drugs are apparently acting through different pharmacological mechanisms.

As illustrated in Fig. 4, the keto-derivative of carbamazepine, oxcarbazepine has also been reported to have antimanic effects parallel to that of the neuroleptics (50) The 10,11-epoxide metabolite of carbamazepine has active anticonvulsant effects in animals (22) and in humans, and it is also active in the treatment of trigeminal neuralgia (51). Clinical trials are currently in progress to assess whether the epoxide also has acute antimanic efficacy; such evidence will be helpful in as-

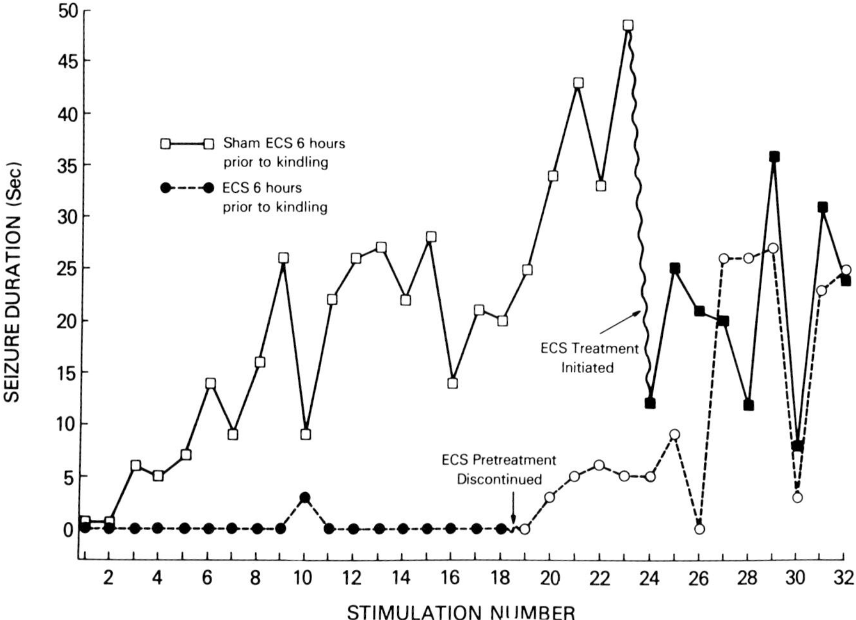

FIG. 2. Electroconvulsive seizures (ECS) inhibit the development of amygdala kindling and suppress completed kindled seizures. ECS administered 6 hr prior to each amygdala stimulation blocks the development of kindling. However, when electroconvulsive therapy (ECT) treatment was discontinued on day 19, the remaining animals showed a relatively normal rate of kindling development. When active ECT was given to the previously sham-treated group on day 24, acute anticonvulsant effects of ECS were again evident.

TABLE 1. *Effects of electroconvulsive seizures (ECS) on development of amygdala kindling*

Investigators	Interval between ECS and kindling	Effect on after discharge duration	Effect on seizures
Babington and Wedeking (173)	0.5 hr	NA[a]	↓ ↓ ↓
	20 hr	NA	↓ ↓ ↓
	24 hr	NA	↓ ↓
Post et al. (174)	6 hr	—	↓ ↓ ↓
Post et al. (32)	24 hr [(A) 1 min later]	—	—
Tsuru et al. (175)	24 hr (5 min later)	—	↓ ↓
	ECS alone (20 days)	—	—
Urca and Frenk (176)	5 min	↓	↓ ↓ ↓
	0.3 sec later	—	↓
	24 hr	—	—
	ECS alone (18 days)	—	—
Handforth (177)	22 hr	—	↓ ↓
	24 hr (immediately afterward)	—	↓ ↓

[a]NA, data not available.

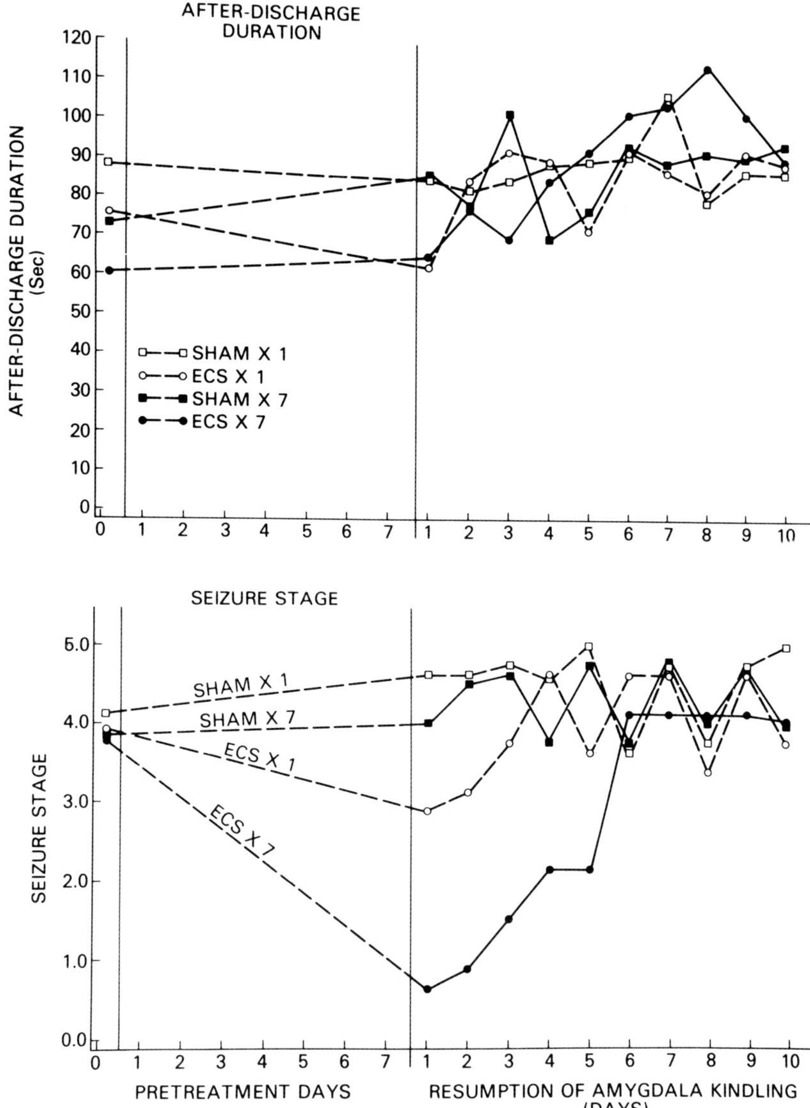

FIG. 3. Electroconvulsive seizures (ECS) inhibit amygdala-kindled seizures without affecting after-discharges. Animals were amygdala-kindled until the first stage 3 or 4 seizure was observed. During the next 7 days, rats received only real or sham ECS. Compared with sham electroconvulsive therapy (ECT) controls, seven daily ECS, but not a single ECS followed by a 6-day delay, markedly suppressed kindled seizures when amygdala stimulation was resumed ($p < 0.0001$; $F = 3.59$; df = 19.92). Afterdischarge duration was not significantly affected. The suppressive effects of repeated ECS persisted for 5 days. On day 5, kindled seizure stage was significantly reduced ($p < 0.04$, $t = -2.40$; df = 9) as was seizure duration ($p < 0.005$; $t = -3.65$).

TABLE 2. *Effects of electroconvulsive seizures (ECS) on completed amygdala-kindled seizures*

Investigators	Interval	Type	Seizures	Duration
Babington and Wedeking	15 min	Single	↓ ↓ ↓	
(173)	30 min	Single	↓ ↓ ↓	
	60 min	Single	↓ ↓	
	120 min	Single	↓ ↓	
	180 min	Single	↓	
	240 min	Single	↓	
Urca and Frenk (176)[a]	—		—	
Handforth (177)[a]	12–24 hr	Multiple	↓ ↓ ↓	24–48 hr
Post et al. (32)	24 hr	Single (6-day delay)	—	
		Multiple (×7)	↓ ↓ ↓	1–5 days

[a] Eighteen or 20 days of prior ECS had no effect on development of kindling.

certaining mechanisms of action shared by the psychoaffective compounds in this series (52,53).

Preliminary data suggest that carbamazepine may be effective in a subgroup of patients inadequately responsive to the traditional antimanic agent lithium carbonate (45). For example, inadequate responses to lithium have been reported in (a) patients with more severe mania, more psychotic mania, or more dysphoric mania, (b) patients with more rapid cycling, and (c) patients without a family history of manic–depressive illness in first-degree relatives. In one or more studies, these very same variables associated with relatively inadequate response to lithium have been associated with greater degrees of response to carbamazepine (45). These data suggest the possibility that in addition to severity, pattern, and course of illness, pharmacoresponsivity may differ in manic–depressive illness of the inherited versus the acquired form. It is also of interest that the documentation of the acute antimanic efficacy of carbamazepine in double-blind studies (Table 3) is considerably more robust than that available for lithium carbonate at the time of its Food and Drug Administration (FDA) approval in 1973.

Acute Depression

The incidence and degree of acute antidepressant efficacy of carbamazepine has been much less well delineated as compared to its antimanic effectiveness. Post et al. (54; and *unpublished observations*, 1990) reported moderate-to-marked antidepressant effects in 17 of 54 acutely depressed patients studied in a double-blind fashion using a B–A–B design. Neumann et al. (55) compared five patients on carbamazepine with five patients on trimipramine and found equivalent effects. A variety of uncontrolled observations also supports a possible antidepressant effect of carbamazepine, although clinical trials of this agent compared with others (and compared with placebo) in our randomized, controlled design remain to be conducted.

Preliminary evidence suggests that patients with more severe depression at the outset, more discrete episodes in the past, and less chronicity may be among those who respond best to the agent (54). Although the cohort consisted largely of those with bipolar depression (i.e., those with a prior history of mania or hypomania), several unipolar depressed patients were among the responders. Whether the drug is less effective in unipolar patients than in bipolar patients remains to be further clarified. There was no evidence that the presence or absence of even mild electroencephalographic (EEG) abnormalities, psychosensory symptoms (Figs. 5 and 6), or a positive family history was associated with degree of acute antidepressant carbamazepine response. In fact, preliminary evidence suggested that those who responded better to lithium had greater numbers of psychosensory symptoms than those who did not respond (Fig. 7) (56). It is noteworthy, however, that the degree of decrease in thyroid indices (T_4) and free T_4 was associated with the degree of antidepressant response ($r = -0.56$, $p < 0.001$) (57). That is, paradoxically, those with greatest degree of thyroid suppression were among those who responded best to the drug (58). These data parallel those of Baumgartner et al. (59), who reported that degree of thyroid decreases were also associated with degree of antidepressant responses to maprotiline and cloripramine.

Cowdry and Gardner's reports (60,61) on carbamazepine in the treatment of patients with borderline personality disorders are of particular interest to this discussion of the psychotropic effects of carbamazepine in the affective disorders, even though these patients with borderline personality disorder represent an unusual diagnostic subgroup with markedly unstable levels of depression. These investigators reported that carbamazepine was particularly effective in decreasing episodes of dyscontrol whereas the anticonvulsant alprazolam actually increased them, which led to the discontinuation of the alprazolam trial. Based on this important clinical effect of carbamazepine, therapists reported that patients were much improved during double-blind administration of carbamazepine when compared to those receiving placebo. However, patients' subjective ratings of mood were not significantly altered by carbamazepine [and several experienced extended depressions (62)], whereas patients reported greater degrees of mood improvement on the monoamine oxidase inhibitor (MAOI) tranylcypromine. These data highlight the possible differential effects of carbamazepine on aggression and impulsivity as opposed to primary effects on mood in patients with borderline personality disorder, and they also highlight the differential efficacy among the anticonvulsants as revealed by an exacerbation of dyscontrol episodes by alprazolam.

Prophylaxis

A number of controlled and quasi-controlled clinical trials, as well as a large series of open clinical studies, demonstrate the prophylactic efficacy of carbamazepine in the prevention of both manic and depressive episodes (see Table 4). Moderate-to-marked prophylactic responses have been observed in approximately 65% of lithium-refractory manic–depressive patients, although a number of

recent studies also suggest that carbamazepine shows approximately equal efficacy when compared to that of lithium carbonate in patients entered into randomized clinical trials (63–66).

Preliminary data again suggest possible differences in clinical predictors of response to these two agents, with lithium being less effective in rapid or continuously cycling patients (67–71) and possibly in those with an age of onset before age 20 (72). In contrast, carbamazepine has been reported to be highly effective in rapid-cycling patients (see Table 4), and one study suggests that it is more effective in those with early onset (73). Joffe (74) has reported that lithium is less effective in rapid cyclers, that carbamazepine is particularly effective in this subgroup, and that the combination is required for those with continuous cycling patterns. Clearly, further work is required to delineate possible clinical and biological predictors of response to these agents.

Differential Response Among Anticonvulsants and Combination Therapy

Response to one anticonvulsant is not necessarily associated with positive response to another drug of this class. For example, as illustrated in Fig. 8, one patient showed an excellent response during a series of double-blind clinical trials of carbamazepine compared with placebo, showed no response to the anticonvulsant valproic acid, and may have further deteriorated during clinical treatment on a double-blind basis with phenytoin (75). Conversely, we have observed differential response in the opposite direction—that is, lack of response to carbamazepine and positive response to valproate, as illustrated in Fig. 9. These data are of considerable importance from the clinical perspective, suggesting the utility of sequential clinical trials of the anticonvulsant agents in lithium-nonresponders. They also suggest the possibility that differential mechanisms of action of the anticonvulsants may confer differential clinical responsivity in the affective disorders as well as in the seizure disorders.

The role of combined treatment of carbamazepine or valproate with lithium carbonate remains to be further documented. Although

TABLE 3. *Controlled studies of carbamazepine in acute mania*[a]

Investigators	N	Diagnosis	Design	Dose of CBZ (mg/day) [blood level]	Other drugs	Duration	Results
Ballenger and Post (136) Post et al. (45,178)	19	M–D psychosis	Double-blind (B–A–B–A)	600–2000 [7–15.5 µg/ml]	None	11–56 days	12/19 improved; time course similar to that of neuroleptics; frequent relapses on placebo substitution
Okuma et al. (179)	32 CBZ 28 CPZ	M–D psychosis ICD-9	Blind vs. CPZ 150–450 mg	300–900 [2.7–11.7 µg/ml] [mean $= 7.2 \pm 3.4$]	Bedtime hypnotics	3–5 weeks	21/32 improved on CBZ (marked to moderate) 15/28 improved on CPZ
Klein et al. (180)	11 3	Manic Excited SA	Blind vs. placebo (addition to Hal)	600–1600 [6–18 µg/ml]	Hal (15–45 mg/ day), all patients	5 weeks	10/14 improved on CBZ + Hal (7/13 improved on placebo + Hal)
Muller and Stoll (50) Muller and Stoll (50)	6 OXCB2 10 Hal	M–D M–D	Blind vs. placebo Blind vs. Hal (15–20 mg)	600–1200 mg 900–1200 mg OXCBZ	Hal & hypnotics	3 weeks 2 weeks	?/6 $p < 0.01$ better than placebo ?/10 OXCBZ = Hal
Grossi et al. (181)	18 CBZ 19 CPZ	M–D	Blind vs. CPZ (randomized) 200–500 mg CPZ	200–1200 mg	?	21 days	10/15 improved on CBZ 13/17 improved on CPZ CBZ had fewer side effects than CPZ
Emrich et al. (182)	7	Manic psychoses	Double blind (B–A–B)	1800–2100 Oxcarbazepine	None	Variable	6/7 (> 25% improvement on IMPS)
Lerer et al. (183)	14 CBZ 14 Li	M–D	Blind vs. Li (randomized)	600–2600 mg (3.3–14 µg/ml)	Chloral hydrate Barbiturates HS	28 days	4/14 improved on carbamazepine 11/14 improved on lithium

Study	N	Diagnosis	Design	Dose	Concomitant medication	Duration	Results
Brown et al. (184) Cookson (185)	9 CBZ 9 Hal	Manic	Blind vs. Hal (20–80 mg/ day)	400–1600 mg	CPZ to 3 CBZ pts. CPZ to 5 Hal pts.	42 days	CGI = $p < 0.05$ (Li) BPRS = NS 6/8 marked improvement CBZ 3/9 marked improvement Hal; 2 Hal patients switched into depression; CBZ better efficacy & acceptance
Lenzi et al. (186)	11 CBZ 11 Li	M–D & SA	Blind vs. Li (900 mg) (0.6–1.2 mEq/ liter)	400–1600 mg (7–12 µg/ml)	CPZ, all patients	19 days	Equal efficacy in CBZ & Li groups; less CPZ required in CBZ group acutely; CBZ better on paranoia; fewer EPS
Desa et al. (187)	5	Manic	Blind vs. placebo (addition to Li)	400 mg (fixed dose)	?	4 weeks	CBZ + Li ($p < 0.05$) better on BRMS scores than Li alone by 2nd week
Okuma et al. (188)	50 CBZ 51 Li	M–D	Blind vs. Li	400–1200 mg	Neuroleptics	4 weeks	31/50 improved on carbamazepine 30/51 improved on lithium; onset earlier on CBZ
Okuma et al. (188)	103 CBZ 98 placebo	SA S Atypical P	Blind vs. placebo		Neuroleptics		50% improved on CBZ 30% improved on placebo 100/159 (63%) improved on CBZ

13 studies in 297 patients.

[a]CBZ, carbamazepine; CPZ, chlorpromazine; Li, lithium; IMPS, Inpatient Multidimension Rating Scale; BRMS, Bech–Raefelson Mania Scale; CGI, Clinical Global Impressions; BPRS, Brief Psychiatric Rating Scale; EPS, Extrapyramidal side effects; Hal, haloperidol; M–D, manic–depressive; SA, schizoaffective; S, schizophrenic; P, paranoid; OXCBZ, oxcarbazepine; NS, not significant; HS, nighttime; ICD-9, International Classification of Diseases-9.

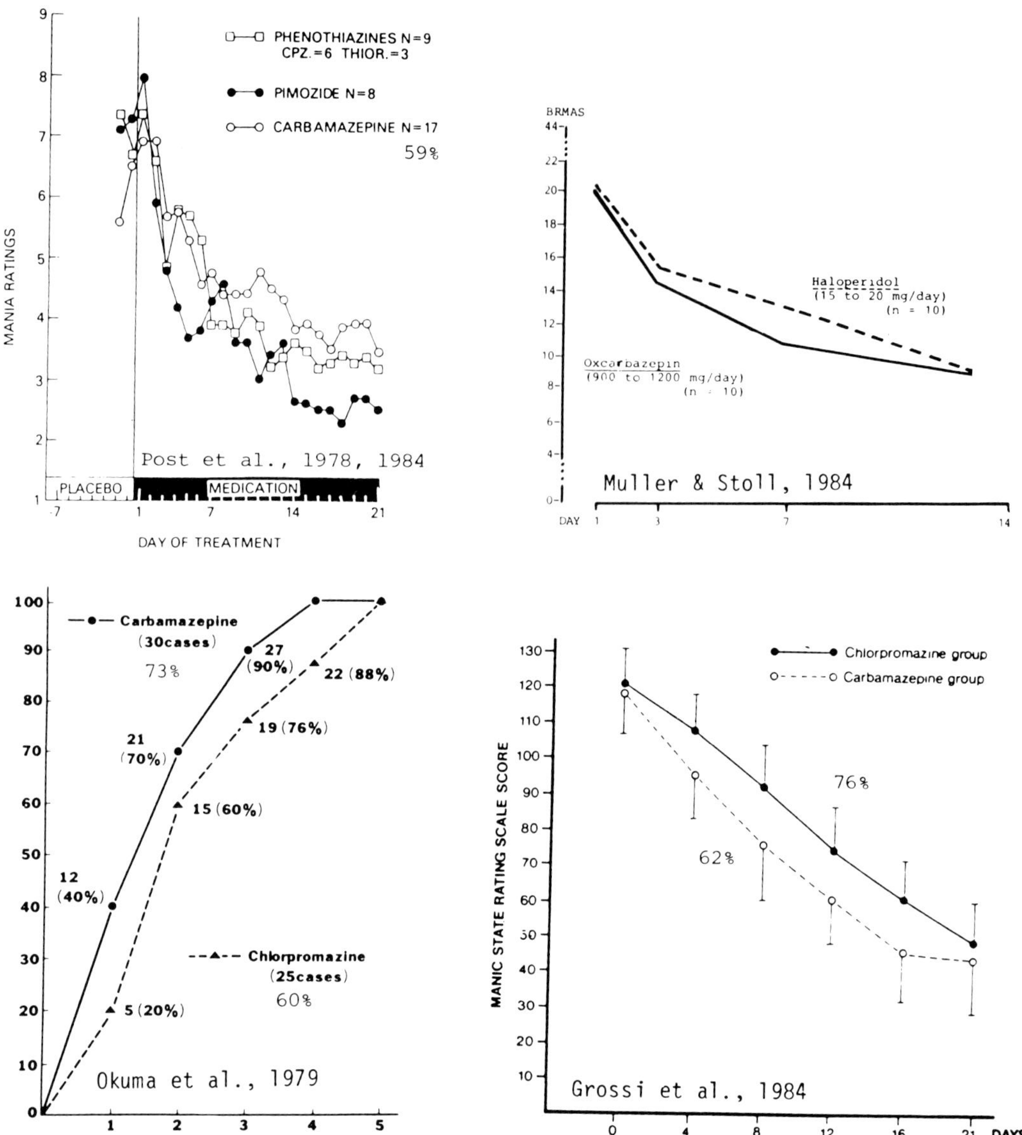

FIG. 4. Controlled comparisons of carbamazepine and neuroleptics in mania. These studies are typical of those in the literature (*N* = 6; see ref. 205 for review), and they indicate an approximate equal time course, magnitude, and incidence of antimanic response to carbamazepine (or its keto-congener) compared with various neuroleptics. CPZ, chlorpromazine; THIOR, thioridazine hydrochloride; BRMAS, Bech–Raefelsen on Mania Scale. (Adapted from refs 50, 135, 178, 179, 181).

one subgroup of patients is clearly responsive to acute or long-term treatment with carbamazepine alone, a different subgroup appears to require treatment with the combination (see Fig. 10, where most patients were treated with the combination of lithium and carbamazepine). Parallel data seem to be emerging for the lithium–valproate combination. Many of the open studies of carbamazepine and valproate prophylaxis have included these drugs as additions to previously ineffective treatment modalities, usually including lithium carbonate. In a proportion of patients, relapses have been observed upon lithium dis-

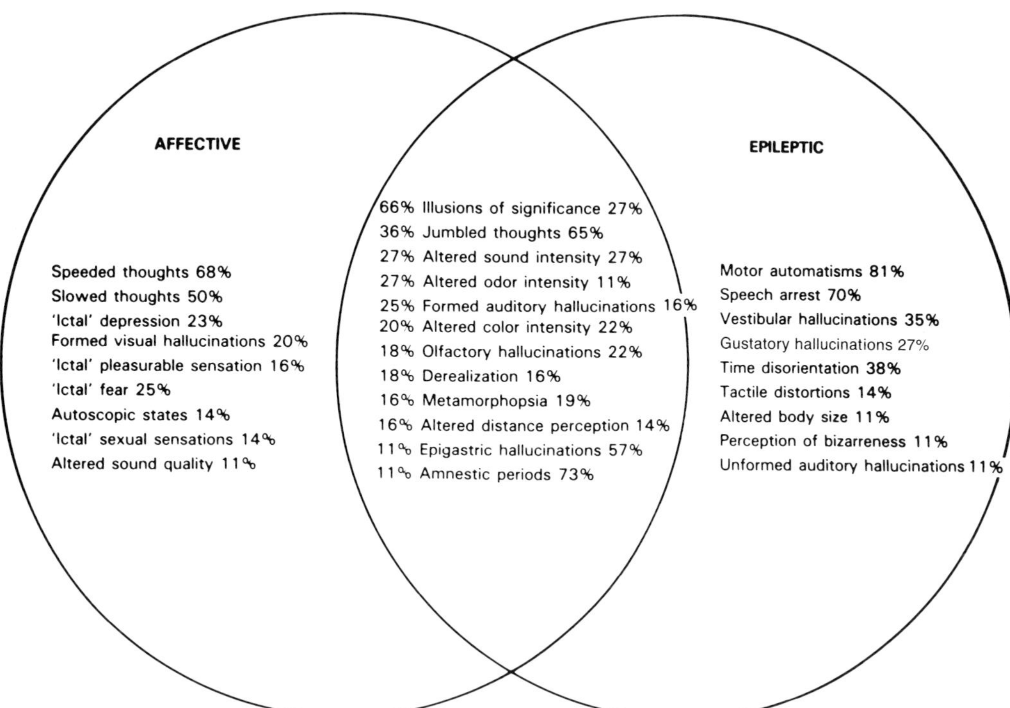

FIG. 5. Distribution of psychosensory symptoms reported by patients with affective illness compared with those reported by patients with epilepsy. Note high incidence of overlapping psychosensory symptoms in the middle of the Venn diagram. These symptoms represent those reported by both affective patients (percentages on left of middle column) and epileptic patients (percentages on right of middle column) at a rate significantly greater than that of controls. Symptoms in left circle were significant with respect to controls for affectives only; those in right circle, for epileptics only. Note that all symptoms were reported by less than 10% of controls.

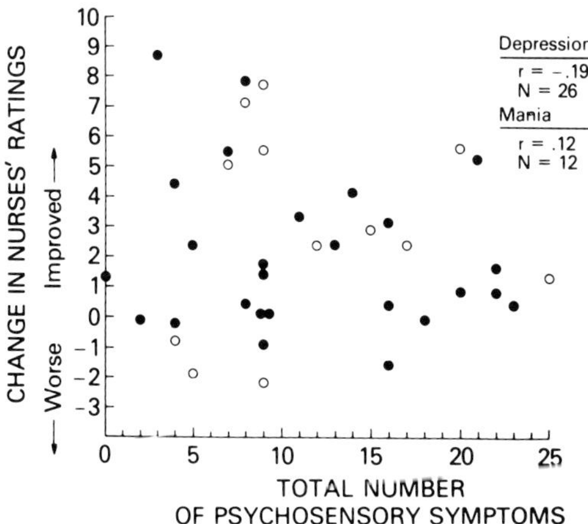

FIG. 6. Psychosensory symptoms do not predict antidepressant (●) or antimanic (○) response to carbamazepine. Note that there was no hint of a positive relationship between lifetime history of psychosensory symptoms rated on the Silberman–Post Psychosensory Rating Scale (SPPRS) based on detailed clinical interviews (56) and degree of antimanic or antidepressant response to carbamazepine. Individual subscales of the SPPRS also are not associated with marked or moderate response (Ketter, Bierer, and Post, *unpublished observations,* 1990).

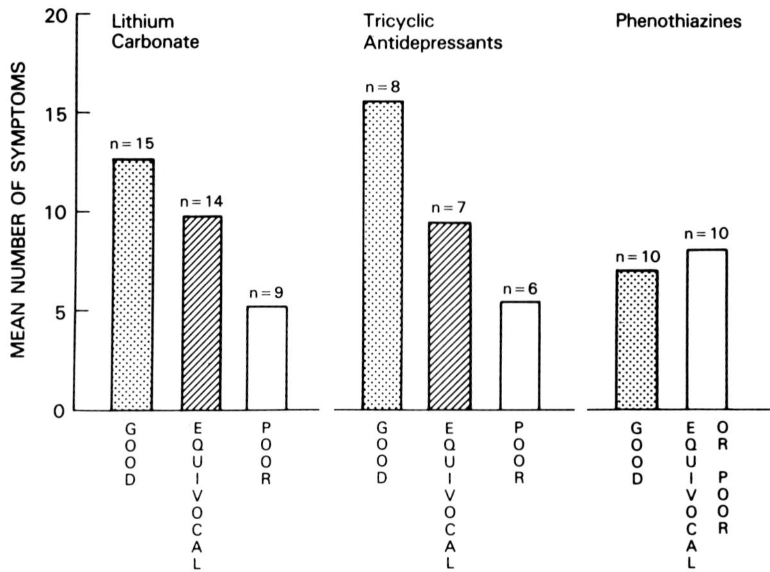

FIG. 7. Relationship of drug response in affective illness to history of occurrence of epileptic-like psychosensory symptoms. Paradoxically, greater numbers of psychosensory symptoms were associated with good responses to lithium (the classical treatment for affective illness) but not to the anticonvulsant carbamazepine (see Fig. 6).

continuation. From the clinical standpoint, the physician should be aware of this necessity for combination treatment in a subgroup of refractory patients (76–80) and should engage in lithium discontinuation only under carefully controlled circumstances, particularly in light of recent data indicating that lithium discontinuation can be associated with withdrawal-emergent episodes that are often of considerable severity (69,81–85).

Valproate

Although valproate is less well studied than carbamazepine, preliminary data suggest that valproate possesses acute and prophylactic antimanic properties (see Table 5). However, only two studies of its antimanic efficacy have been conducted on a double-blind basis, and no studies have been done with regard to its prophylaxis. Nonetheless, a series of clinical observations support the long-term prophylactic effects of valproate—particularly when used in combination with lithium, which had previously been ineffective alone. Puzynski and Klosiewicz (86) suggest only a moderate

effect of valproate when used in rapid cyclers, with a lesser degree of effectiveness on depressed (as compared with manic) episodes. McElroy et al. (87) have reported six cases (five of which had previously been unresponsive to the anticonvulsant carbamazepine) in which valproate produced rather dramatic improvement in rapid- and continuous-cycling patients.

Again, it would appear that there is an urgent need for both (a) the systematic assessment of the long-term effects of the alternative anticonvulsant agents in the treatment of the affective disorders and (b) the determination of clinical and biological markers of response. The effects of valproate in epilepsy are thought to be based on gamma-aminobutyric acid (GABA) potentiation, whereas those of carbamazepine are thought to involve other mechanisms (34,53). This profile of different mechanisms of action, along with the different profile of clinical antiepileptic efficacy, lays the groundwork for both (a) differential clinical responsivity, which appears to be pertinent with regard to affective illness, and (b) the possible utility of combination treatment. This has not been systematically

TABLE 4. *Controlled and quasi-controlled[a] studies of carbamazepine prophylaxis in manic–depressive illness[b]*

Investigators	N	Diagnosis	Design	Dose of CBZ (mg/day) [blood level]	Other drugs	Duration	Results
Post et al. (135, 189)	7	6 M–D 1 confusional psychosis	4 Blind 3 Open	800–2000 mg [11.3 µg/ml] [7.5–15.5 µg/ml]	None for 3 patients Li in 3 Neuroleptics in 1	6–51 mos.	6/7 improved, especially Li nonresponsive cyclers
Okuma et al. (190)	12 CBZ 10 Placebo	M–D	CBZ vs. placebo (blind, randomized)	400–600 mg [5.6 ± 2.0 µg/ml]	Acute treatments added during episode breakthroughs	12 mos. either Rx	6/10 improved on CBZ 2/9 improved on placebo ($p < 0.10$ diff.)
Placidi et al. (63)	CBZ 20 Li 27	M–D SA M–D + SA	CBZ vs. Li (blind, randomized)	400–1600 mg [7–12 µg/ml]	Acute treatments added during episode breakthroughs	36 mos.	21/29 marked-to-moderate improvement on CBZ 20/27 on Li improved by relapse criteria
Kishimoto and Okuma (73)	18	BP I & II	Open crossover A–B or B–A vs. Li (400–800 mg)	200–600 mg		> 1 yr each $\overline{X}$ = 52.4 mos. CBZ $\overline{X}$ = 42.2 mos. Li	Significantly fewer hospitalizations on CBZ; CBZ effective in Li nonresponders
Watkins et al. (64)	19 CBZ Li	7 UP 12 BP	CBZ vs. Li (double blind, randomized)	[5–12 µg/ml]	Antidepressants as needed		16/19 improved on CBZ 15/18 improved on Li $p < 0.001$ increases in mos. of remission both drugs; Li > CBZ
Bellaire et al. (65)	50 CBZ	18 UP 24 BP 8 SA	CBZ vs. Li (open, randomized)	600–800 mg [0.2–12.5 µg/ml]		24 mos.	Global efficacy and tolerance NS; favor CBZ
Lusznat et al. (66)	20 CBZ 20 Li	M–D	CBZ vs. Li (blind, randomized)	[6–12 µg/ml]	Neuroleptics; antidepressants as needed	12 mos.	9/16 satisfactory on CBZ 5/17 satisfactory on Li; CBZ NS, better than Li on readmission, depression side effects

Controlled studies: 58/81 (72%) response to CBZ
Uncontrolled studies: 286/445 (64%) response to CBZ
Total: 344/526 (65%) response

[a]Blinded, crossover, or randomized.
[b]CBZ, carbamazepine; Li, lithium; M–D, manic–depressive; SA, schizoaffective; UP, unipolar; BP, bipolar; NS, not significant; Rx, treatment.

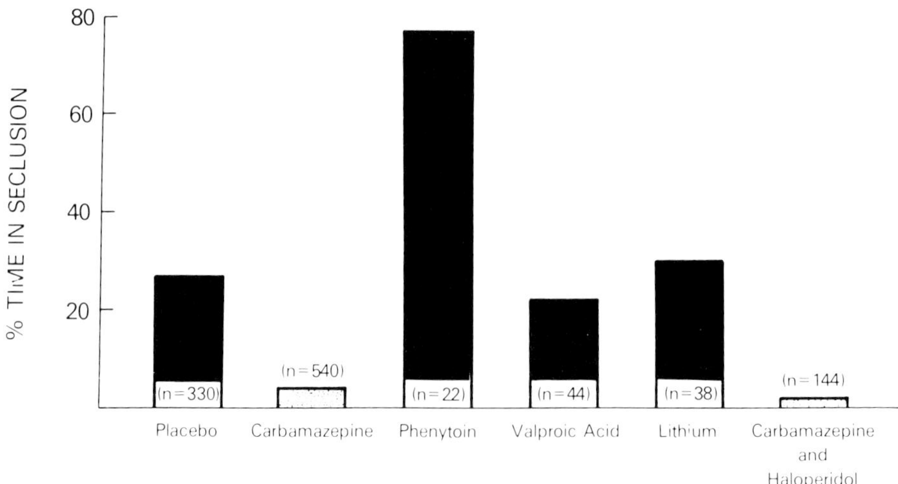

FIG. 8. Selective response to carbamazepine, but not to placebo, lithium, or other anticonvulsants (valproate and phenytoin), in a psychotically manic patient (75). Carbamazepine alone or in combination with haloperidol dramatically decreased percentage of time in seclusion (based on number of hours in each 24-hr day) over extended double-blind clinical trials; *n* indicates the number of days on each treatment. Placebo days were not consecutive; instead, they were interspersed before and in between active trials, confirming selective response to carbamazepine in an "off–on–off–on" design.

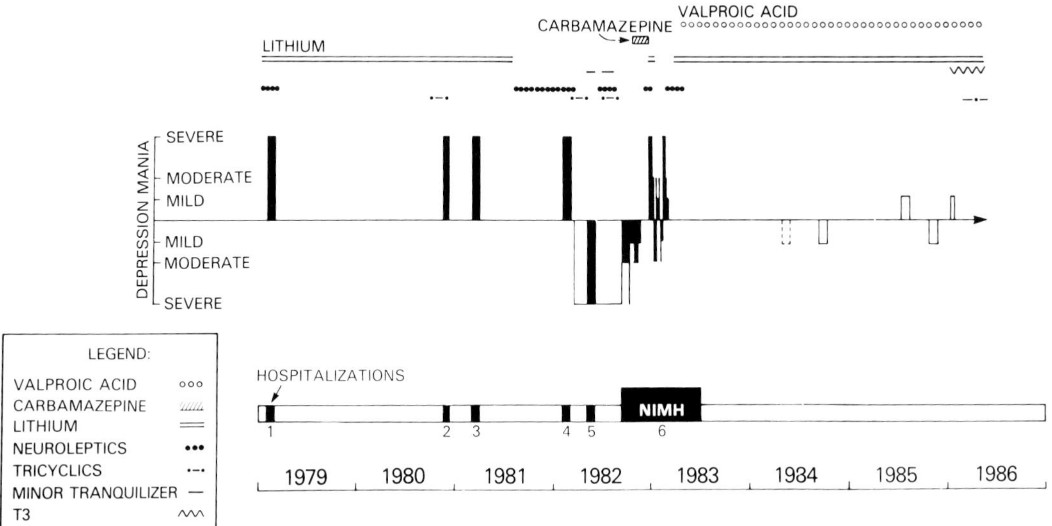

FIG. 9. Prophylactic response to valproate in a carbamazepine nonresponder. Manic episodes are plotted above the mood line, and depressive episodes are plotted below it. Shaded episodes indicate hospitalizations; dotted lines indicate a mild depression, the timing of which is not precise. This male with bipolar disorder, in his early 50s, experienced repeated episodes of dysphoric, psychotic mania that required hospitalization in spite of adequate lithium treatment (1979–81). At NIMH, he experienced a breakthrough manic episode during carbamazepine treatment. The addition of valproate to lithium resulted in an excellent response where lithium alone had been unsuccessful. The patient did not experience a manic breakthrough requiring hospitalization until 1989. This case and others observed in our studies suggest that loss of efficacy can develop for valproate as well as for carbamazepine (see Figs. 17 and 18) and lithium.

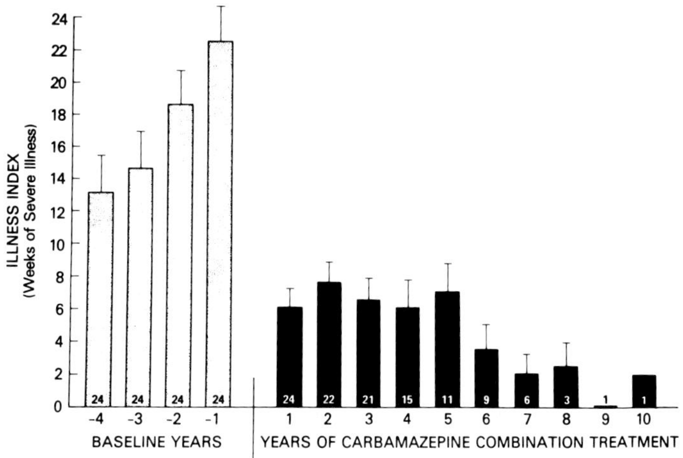

FIG. 10. Carbamazepine prophylaxis in primary affective illness. The illness index represents the number of weeks ill per year multiplied by the severity of the illness based on life-chart criteria (mild = 0.25; moderate = 0.5; severe or incapacitating = 1.0). Carbamazepine, usually in conjunction with lithium, decreased the number, severity, and duration of manic and depressive episodes in a group of lithium-refractory patients. Response was sustained in approximately 50%, but the other half showed some loss of efficacy in the second, third, or fourth year of treatment. The numbers in columns equal the number of patients followed for up to 10 years of open-label follow-up (see Fig. 17 and ref. 206 for details).

explored in affectively ill patients, although preclinical evidence (88) and preliminary clinical evidence from several groups suggests that the carbamazepine–valproate combination may be effective in the refractory seizure patients (89–91).

Benzodiazepine-Active Anticonvulsants

Although diazepam administered orally in humans is not an effective anticonvulsant, the administration of clonazepam and alprazolam (as well as lorazepam, chlorazepate, and clobazam) by this route does appear to be sufficient to exert anticonvulsant effects. In a double-blind evaluation, Chouinard et al. (92) have reported that clonazepam is as effective as lithium carbonate in the treatment of acute mania. However, neuroleptics were used conjointly, and clonazepam appeared to be associated with a significant degree of sedation. Further clinical trials are required in order to delineate the degree and incidence of acute antimanic responses to this agent and to separate sedative and nonspecific effects from important primary therapeutic effects.

Nonetheless, at the present time there would appear to be a role for clonazepam as an adjunctive and nighttime supplement to existing antimanic therapies for the patient showing breakthrough manic symptoms. Because a substantial proportion of well-maintained patients with epilepsy will show the emergence of tolerance to the anticonvulsant effects of benzodiazepines (89,93,94), one would further wonder about the long-term efficacy of clonazepam and related agents in mania or prophylaxis. Preliminary observations of Kishimoto, Okuma, and associates (*personal communication*, 1988) suggest that clonazepam may be a useful adjunctive treatment in the prevention of some patients' recurrent episodes, but as many as one-third of patients may show tolerance to this effect. Aronson et al. (95) reported that all five lithium-refractory patients who had their neuroleptic therapy tapered during the addition of clonazepam for prophylaxis had suffered relapses (three became manic and two became delusionally depressed). These data speak for only a limited role for clonazepam as an adjunct to acute treatments; antidepressant effectiveness has not been systematically

assessed, although reports suggest either improvement (207) or exacerbation of depression in some patients.

The antipanic drug alprazolam has been reported to possess antidepressant properties for those with mild-to-moderate depression, but it appears to be less effective in patients with more severe endogenous or psychotic depressions (96). Moreover, it should be used cautiously in the bipolar patient as there are a series of reports of the induction of mania with this anticonvulsant agent (97–99), apparently in parallel with similar reports with traditional tricyclic, heterocyclic, and MAOI antidepressants.

Whereas clonazepam acts exclusively at the central-type benzodiazepine receptor (which modulates chloride channels), carbamazepine does not appear to exert its anticonvulsant effects through this site; instead, carbamazepine acts through the so-called "peripheral-type" benzodiazepine receptor (100,101). Alprazolam has major effects at the central-type receptor site, although preliminary evidence suggests that it may also have some effects at the peripheral-type site (102).

Other Anticonvulsants in Affective Disorders

Phenytoin

Although phenytoin was originally suggested to be an acute antimanic agent (103, 104), a study reported lack of effect on five or six patients (105); systematic controlled clinical studies remain to be conducted. Similarly, the utility of phenytoin in long-term prophylaxis has not been adequately studied. Knowledge of the overall clinical efficacy of this anticonvulsant is of considerable clinical and theoretical importance, particularly in light of evidence that it shares with carbamazepine an ability to stabilize sodium channels (106,107). Should the two drugs emerge with equal efficacy in the primary affective disorders, this might help suggest a role for sodium-channel stabilization in the therapeutic efficacy. To the extent that carbamazepine is more effective (as preliminary data would suggest), this would indicate (a) a less likely role for the common effect on sodium channels and (b) a role for some other effect of carbamazepine not shared by phenytoin (34,53). To date, we have not observed a positive response to phenytoin in any of the first five patients treated with phenytoin on a double-blind basis.

GABA Agonists

Progabide and its congeners, which appear to exert their efficacy as indirect potentiators of GABA and have been reported to be effective anticonvulsant agents, have received preliminary clinical trials in acute depression (108–110). Both open studies and one controlled study (in comparison with those on imipramine) suggest acute antidepressant efficacy for these compounds. Further studies of these drugs, as well as studies of other GABA-active agents (including gamma-vinyl GABA), would appear warranted in light of these promising initial findings and also in light of the clinical importance of such a demonstration for the implication of a GABAminergic mechanism in effective treatment of the affective disorders (111–113). The non-anticonvulsant $GABA_B$ agonist L-baclofen is discussed below (see also Fig. 12).

Acetazolamide

A single study by Inoue et al. (114) reported that the anticonvulsant acetazolamide (Diamox) was effective in the treatment of patients with atypical confusional psychoses, particularly those which were associated with dreamy states and which were temporally related to puerperal and premenstrual episodes. Whether this drug would be effective in more traditional manic patients and in prophylaxis remains to be determined. However, the patients in Inoue et al.'s study were sometimes responsive to this agent when they were not responsive to either lithium or carbamazepine, again suggesting possible differential responsivity among the anticonvulsants. Since acetazolamide has been associated with the development of tolerance to its anticonvulsant effects in animal models and in humans, there would be concern about the maintenance of its long-term effectiveness in patients with psychiatric disorders as well.

Ethosuximide

Although open studies of ethosuximide suggest possible efficacy in the treatment of patients with borderline personality disorders (115), systematic clinical trials have not been reported in patients with primary affective disorder. Again, knowledge of the clinical efficacy of this compound would be of considerable theoretical importance in ascertaining whether agents with selective effects on petit mal or absence epilepsy may also be effective in the treatment of patients with the affective disorders.

MECHANISMS OF PSYCHOTROPIC EFFICACY OF THE ANTICONVULSANTS

Given the evidence of efficacy of carbamazepine in bipolar affective disorder and its widespread use for that indication, as well as the emerging evidence for that of valproate and possibly other of the anticonvulsants, a critical issue is whether the mechanisms conferring anticonvulsant effects are the same as those related to the therapeutic benefits seen in the affective disorders. The differential efficacy of different anticonvulsants in individual patients with affective disorders suggests that there is not a unitary anticonvulsant principle that cuts across efficacy in all patients with affective disorders. However, if we take carbamazepine as an example, evidence of the time course of onset of efficacy in different disorders suggests the possibility that the mechanisms mediating the anticonvulsant effects of carbamazepine may be different from those involved in affective illness.

As illustrated in Fig. 11, there is considerable evidence that the anticonvulsant and antinociceptive effects of carbamazepine usually occur rapidly, possibly emerging within 24–48 hr in the treatment of trigeminal neuralgia (116). Moreover, it is clear that in many animal models, the single injection of carbamazepine may be acutely effective as an anticonvulsant (14,22). Positive effects of carbamazepine on sleep in manic–depressive patients also occur acutely and are clearly evident within the first week of treatment (45). In contrast, the antimanic effects of carbamazepine emerge over a longer period of time

and appear to require 2–3 weeks to become maximal. Furthermore, the lag in onset of efficacy of carbamazepine is clearly most evident in terms of acute antidepressant effects. In this instance, it is rare to see significant effects within the first week of treatment, and maximal effects often require 2–5 weeks of treatment (54).

These data suggest that a considerable lag in onset in the antidepressant effects is associated with the mechanisms of action of carbamazepine, which require considerable periods of time and/or chronic drug administration in order to become manifest. In this fashion, we can provisionally allocate different mechanisms of action of carbamazepine on the basis of their time course of biochemical and pharmacological effects. For example, the acute anticonvulsant effects of carbamazepine have been most closely associated with the ability of carbamazepine to bind acutely to peripheral-type benzodiazepine receptor sites and function as a peripheral-type benzodiazepine receptor antagonist such as PK-11195. The peripheral-type benzodiazepine effects of carbamazepine are documented by the fact that the ligand RO5-4864 reverses the anticonvulsant effects of carbamazepine, but not those of diazepam, on amygdala-kindled seizures (100,101). In contrast, the central-type antagonist, RO-15-1788, reverses the anticonvulsant effects of diazepam but does not reverse those of carbamazepine. Alpha-2-adrenergic mechanisms are also implicated in carbamazepine's acute anticonvulsant effects on amygdala-kindled seizures, since the alpha-2 antagonist yohimbine reverses the anticonvulsant effects of carbamazepine [although the alpha-2 agonist clonidine itself is not sufficient as an anticonvulsant agent (Weiss et al., *unpublished observations*, 1988)].

Carbamazepine also binds to type 2 sodium channels and stabilizes sodium influx (107, 117). This mechanism, in conjunction with that of phenytoin, has been suggested as a prime candidate for the acute anticonvulsant effects of carbamazepine in some seizure models. Carbamazepine's ability to decrease the release of the excitatory amino acid aspartate acutely may also be important to its anticonvulsant effects in some systems (118).

Terrence et al. (119) have suggested that

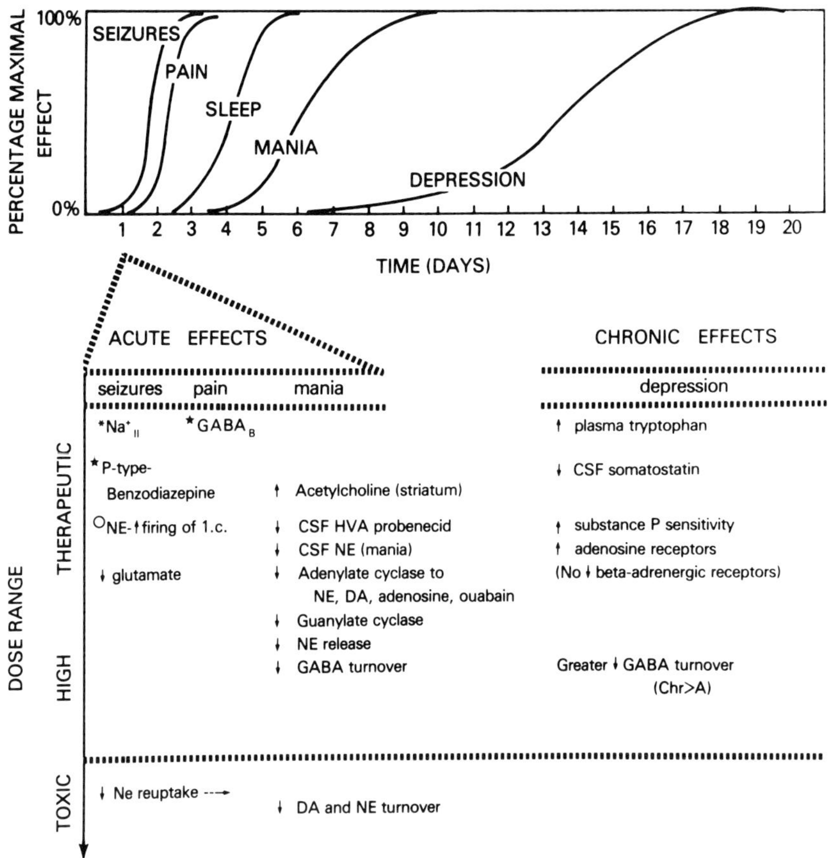

FIG. 11. Time course of clinical and biochemical effects of carbamazepine. Seizure and paroxysmal pain syndromes respond rapidly to carbamazepine, whereas maximal effects in mania and depression are delayed 2–3 weeks or more, respectively. Thus, acute effects observed in animals and humans are likely to be related to anticonvulsant and antinociceptive efficacy, whereas chronic effects are more likely to be related to antidepressant mechanisms. GABA, gamma-aminobutyric acid; NE, norepinephrine; CSF, cerebrospinal fluid; DA, dopamine; Chr, chronic; A, acute; HVA, homovanillic acid.

$GABA_B$ mechanisms of carbamazepine are related to carbamazepine's antinociceptive effects, because (a) the putative $GABA_B$ agonist L-baclofen is effective in the treatment of trigeminal neuralgia clinically and (b) the inactive isomer D-baclofen reverses the antinociceptive effects of both carbamazepine and L-baclofen in appropriate preclinical models of trigeminal neuralgia. In contrast, baclofen is not an effective anticonvulsant during amygdala-kindled seizures, and D-baclofen is ineffective in reversing the anticonvulsant effects of carbamazepine during these seizures (Weiss et al., *unpublished data*, 1988). These data suggest that the $GABA_B$ effects of carbamazepine are not important to carbamazepine's anticonvulsant effects but that they are important to its antinociceptive effects.

These data leave open the possibility that $GABA_B$ effects may or may not be critical to carbamazepine's psychotropic effects in manic–depressive illness. Preliminary data collected by these investigators in collaboration with R. Joffe and K. Kramlinger suggest that L-baclofen [at doses that are effective in trigeminal neuralgia (120)] was ineffective as an antidepressant in four patients (Fig. 12), including one patient (#361) who subsequent-

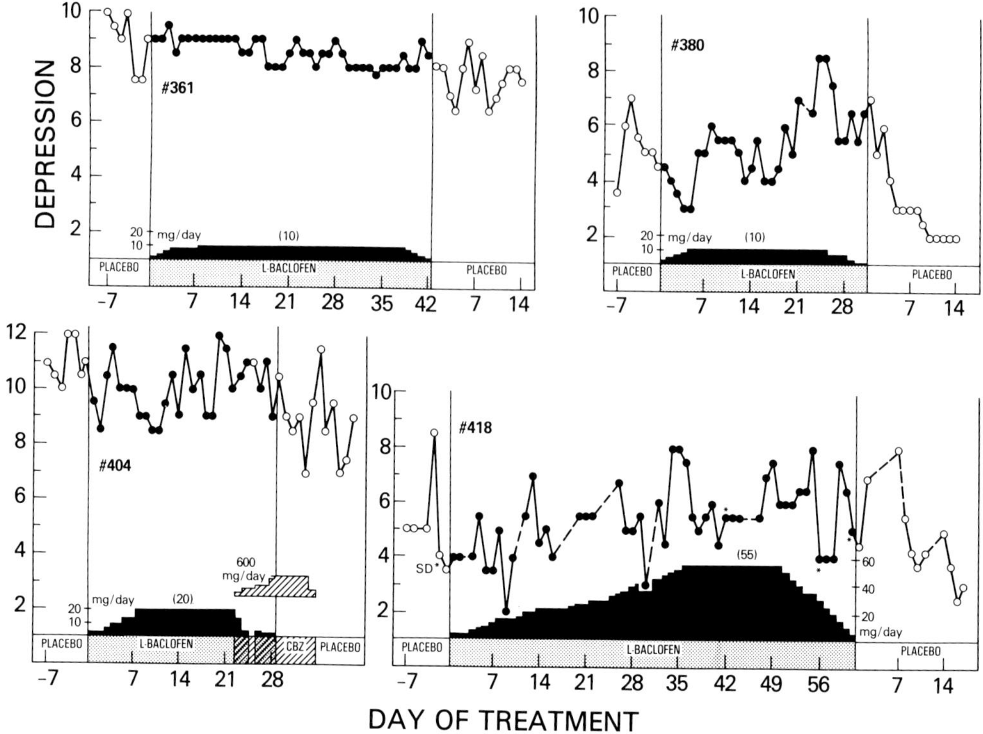

FIG. 12. Lack of antidepressant response to L-baclofen in four depressed patients. Ordinate equals blind nurses' ratings on the Bunney–Hamburg global depression scale during placebo (○) and L-baclofen treatment (●). Dose of L-baclofen is also indicated in shaded bars (based on mg/day). Abscissa indicates days of treatment. Patients #380 and #418 showed exacerbations of depression during treatment with L-baclofen, but they showed improvement upon its withdrawal with placebo substitution. CBZ, carbamazepine.

ly responded to carbamazepine. In patient #418, doses as high as 50 mg/day were utilized, suggesting that even high doses are ineffective as antidepressants. However, these high doses remain to be administered to a patient who is carbamazepine-responsive in order to definitively document that adequately high doses are ineffective in this type of patient. Nonetheless, these preliminary data suggest the likelihood that the efficacy of carbamazepine in affective disorders is not mediated through a GABA$_B$ mechanism, in contrast to what has been postulated for carbamazepine's antinociceptive effects. These data are of considerable interest in light of the suggestion of Lloyd et al. (113) that all of the antidepressant modalities up-regulate GABA$_B$ receptors in the frontal cortex of rats after chronic, but not acute, treatment. Since our

patients remained stable or deteriorated on L-baclofen and several improved upon drug withdrawal (#380 and #418), it is possible that decreases (rather than increases) in GABA$_B$ tone are important to antidepressant effects and are related to the up-regulation observed by Lloyd et al. (113).

Carbamazepine exerts a variety of effects on systems that have been putatively associated with the induction of mania or its treatment. Carbamazepine, for example, decreases norepinephrine, dopamine, and GABA turnover and blocks adenylate cyclase activity stimulated by norepinephrine, dopamine, and adenosine (34,53). Thus, effects on any of these systems (or several others) remain active candidates for carbamazepine's antimanic activity. In addition, carbamazepine exerts a variety of biochemical effects that appear to require chronic drug administration; these may be more closely associated with the antidepressant effects of carbamazepine than with those only requiring acute administration. As illustrated in Fig. 11, chronic administration of carbamazepine is associated with increases in adenosine receptors (121–123) [as is ECT but not lithium (124)], substance P levels (125), and sensitivity (126) in rat striatum (effects paralleled by lithium carbonate). In addition, the effects of carbamazepine on GABA turnover are greater during chronic administration than during acute administration (118). In humans, chronic administration of carbamazepine is associated with increases in plasma free total tryptophan (127) and decreases in somatostatin in CSF (128,129). Chronic drug treatment is also associated with decreases in peripheral indices of thyroid function (58) and increased secretion of urinary free cortisol and a high incidence of escape from dexamethasone suppression (130).

So far, none of these mechanisms has been closely linked to the psychotropic effects of carbamazepine, with the possible exception of greater decreases in thyroid function being associated with greater degrees of antidepressant efficacy (57,58). Reliable and valid animal models of affective disorders are not readily available at this time. Thus, the search for the critical mechanism of carbamazepine responsible for its positive effects in the affective disorders depends on other methods of study, either in the clinical situation or in indirect preclinical models.

One strategy recently elucidated has been to use a seizure model which requires chronic administration of carbamazepine in order to demonstrate efficacy. In this fashion, one might be able to use a seizure model in order to dissect possible mechanisms of anticonvulsant action that might be more closely associated with psychotropic effects.

As illustrated in Fig. 13, we have found that chronic administration of carbamazepine will block the development of local-anesthetic-kindled seizures (131). Carbamazepine blocks the development and lethality of cocaine-kindled seizures as well as the development of lidocaine-kindled seizures. It is remarkable that this effect is only achieved with chronic oral administration and not achieved by intermittent pretreatments with carbamazepine

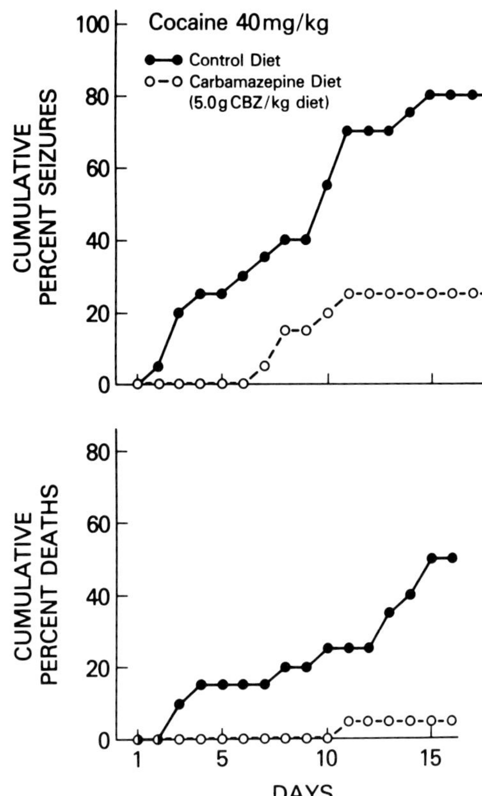

FIG. 13. Chronic carbamazepine (CBZ) prevents the development of cocaine-kindled seizures and mortality. The percentage of rats experiencing cocaine-induced seizures and deaths is shown on a daily basis with or without carbamazepine co-treatment (N = 20 per group). Rats treated with carbamazepine were fed a diet containing the drug beginning 4 days before the first cocaine injection and were continued on this diet throughout the experiment. Chronic carbamazepine in the diet markedly suppressed the development of the cocaine-induced seizures and deaths; repeated intermittent dosing either is ineffective (see Fig. 14) or, at high doses (50 mg/kg i.p.), exacerbates cocaine kindling.

by the intraperitoneal route (a method that is highly effective in preventing amygdala-kindled seizures) (Fig. 14).

These data suggest that chronic administration (but not repeated, intermittent administration) of carbamazepine is sufficient to block the development of local-anesthetic-kindled seizures and their associated lethality.

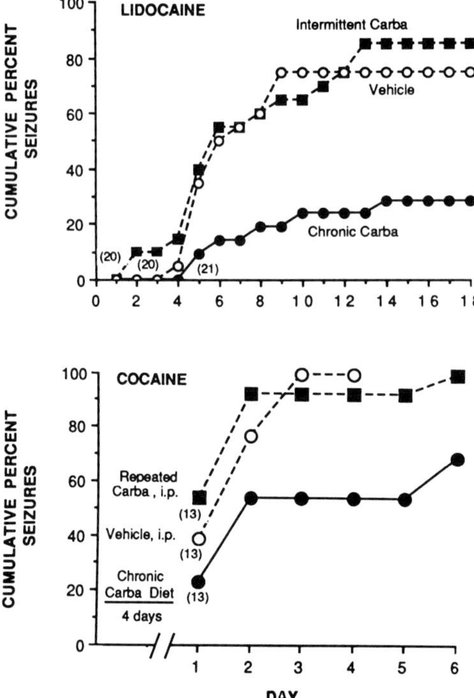

FIG. 14. Pretreatment with chronic carbamazepine (Carba) in diet (not repeated injection) is required to block both lidocaine- (**top**) and cocaine-kindled (**bottom**) seizures. Rats were treated with chronic Carba (diet), i.p.-injected Carba (15 mg/kg), or vehicle for four days prior to either lidocaine (65 mg/kg i.p.) or cocaine (65 mg/kg i.p.) injections and were continued on this regimen throughout the study. The repeated i.p. Carba had no effect on the development of either lidocaine- or cocaine-kindled seizures, whereas chronic Carba was highly effective (see ref. 131 for details).

Moreover, they suggest that a different profile of effects may be induced by chronic drug administration as opposed to repeated, intermittent drug administration. Finally, to the extent that chronic administration of carbamazepine is required for the initiation of its psychotropic effects in patients with manic–depressive illness, the effects of carbamazepine on local-anesthetic-kindled seizures, which also require chronic administration, may provide an important model system not directly employing an animal model of depression. For example, preliminary data suggest

that intrathecal administration of corticotropin-releasing factor (CRF) will reverse the anticonvulsant effects of carbamazepine on local-anesthetic-kindled seizures; however, the specificity of this effect remains to be determined, since CRF alone will also exacerbate cocaine-kindled seizures (Weiss et al., *unpublished observations*, 1988). In addition to providing a possible model for examining biochemical effects implicated in carbamazepine's psychotropic action, the current findings also underscore the possibility that carbamazepine may be clinically useful in the treatment of cocaine addiction and its associated toxicities (131–133). Preliminary evidence in support of this contention is already available from Halikas et al. (134), who found that chronic carbamazepine treatment of cocaine abusers (as well as treatment of mixed cocaine and heroin abusers) reduced cocaine craving and appeared to change the threshold for cocaine-induced paranoia and seizures in one patient who was repeatedly experiencing these phenomena.

ARE LIMBIC SUBSTRATES INVOLVED IN THE PSYCHOTROPIC EFFECTS OF CARBAMAZEPINE?

Although the limbic concept was importantly involved in our initial decisions to study carbamazepine (135,136), little direct data are available to support a specific limbic site of action of carbamazepine in affective illness (15). Drugs with greater relative effects on limbic system seizures (complex partial; see Table 6) than on seizures manifested in other areas of the brain (such as absence; see Table 7) should be more effective in the treatment of manic–depressive illness if this hypothesis were correct. In this regard, carbamazepine, one of the most promising psychotropic agents for the treatment of manic–depressive illness, does have the best ratio in inhibiting amygdala-kindled compared with cortical-kindled foci (see Table 8) (14,137). However, phenytoin is equally effective in treating clinical seizures of the psychomotor–complex-partial category, even though it is notably less effective in the initial phases (development and completed) of amygdala-kindled seizures. In Albright and Burnham's scheme, valproate

TABLE 6. *Results of clinical trials: complex partial seizures*[a]

Drug	Number of clinical trials		
	Unchanged	Moderate	Excellent
Carbamazepine	—	1	8
Clonazepam	3	6	5
Valproate	2	5	3
Phenytoin	—	—	1
Primidone	—	1	1
Phenacemide	1	1	1
Methsuximide	2	4	—
Mephenytoin	—	2	—
Trimethadione	—	1	—
Paramethadione	1	—	—
Ethotoin	1	—	—
Metharbital	1	—	—
Phenobarbital	(No clinical trials)		

[a]From ref. 204, with permission.

has the second best limbic/cortical ratio compared with carbamazepine, and it is of interest that it appears also to be effective in the acute and prophylactic treatment of some refractory bipolar patients. Clinical studies of the efficacy of a drug such as ethosuximide in bipolar illness would be of great use in the assessment of whether limbic nonselective agents [i.e., those with relatively selective antiabsence effects (138)] were also equally effective in the affective disorders.

Another possible approach implicating limbic substrates in the mechanism of action of carbamazepine would be to see an association between evidence of limbic system dysfunction and degree of clinical response. In a variety of areas where preliminary data exist, there is little evidence to support this contention. For example, most studies, including our own, are demonstrating responses in patients with normal EEGs (in many instances, studied with nasopharyngeal electrodes and sleep deprivation). Although several studies have reported the efficacy of carbamazepine in patients with abnormal EEGs, there appears to be an equal degree of clinical improvement in patients without this phenomenon; recently, Luchins (139,140) has described equal

TABLE 7. *Results of clinical trials: absence seizures*[a]

Drug	Number of clinical trials		
	Unchanged	Moderate	Excellent
Clonazepam	—	2	9
Valproate	—	2	8
Ethosuximide	—	3	5
Phensuximide	—	1	4
Trimethadione	—	4	3
Methsuximide	2	3	2
Paramethadione	—	1	1
Phenytoin	—	—	1
Phenobarbital	—	2	—
Mephenytoin	2	1	—
Metharbital	—	1	—
Primidone	3	—	—
Phenacemide	2	—	—
Ethotoin	1	—	—
Carbamazepine	(No clinical trials)		

[a]From ref. 204, with permission.

TABLE 8. *Relative potency of anticonvulsants in suppressing amygdala-kindled local seizures*[a]

Anticonvulsant	Amygdala to cortical after discharge suppression (%)
Carbamazepine	55
Sodium valproate	37
Phenobarbital	33
Phenytoin	30
Methsuximide	25
Clonazepam	22
Ethosuximide	14
Diazepam	0

[a]From ref. 14, with permission.

degrees of anti-aggressive effects of carbamazepine in patients with and without EEG abnormalities. The same can be said for psychosensory phenomena.

If one assumes that a history of psychosensory distortion similar to that reported with temporal lobe epilepsy is a marker for limbic system dysfunction (8,56,141,142), then patients with affective illness who report prominent psychosensory symptoms should show a better clinical response to carbamazepine than those without. Again, preliminary clinical data suggest that this is not the case, as illustrated in Fig. 6. Contrary to predictions, the evidence suggests that those with greater degrees of psychosensory symptoms actually show greater (rather than lesser) degrees of response to lithium carbonate (56) (Fig. 7).

If one employs the limbic-active probe procaine as a challenge strategy for limbic system dysfunction, then degree of procaine-induced activation of clinical EEG or endocrine parameters should provide an index of carbamazepine response (143). Although the numbers of affectively ill patients studied to date have been insufficient to reach definitive conclusions in this regard, the preliminary evidence from patients with borderline personality disorder suggests no close relationship between degree of procaine-induced change and degree of response to carbamazepine. The lack of supporting clinical evidence taken in conjunction with the findings that carbamazepine is highly effective in a variety of types of seizures, many of which do not in-

volve limbic system dysfunction, leaves the issue of the "limbic" basis of carbamazepine's effects in affective illness very much unresolved.

THE KINDLING ANALOGY IN AFFECTIVE ILLNESS: IMPLICATIONS FOR CARBAMAZEPINE

While kindling continues to be a highly useful and heuristically valuable analogy for helping to conceptualize the unfolding and evolving course of manic–depressive illness, there is little evidence to support a direct kindling effect in patients with manic–depressive illness. On the most obvious level, it is apparent that patients with manic–depressive illness do not show convulsive disturbances. Moreover, the vast majority of patients also present without any evidence of EEG abnormalities. Although it might be argued that covert evidence of local spiking and seizure discharges may not be apparent in surface electrodes, the burden of proof remains on the investigator who claims that such discharges exist (144). Even though depth EEG studies in patients with manic–depressive illness do not appear ethically feasible at the present time, other techniques may provide a partial resolution to this difficult problem. Recent studies of magnetoencephalography yield the promise of being able to localize foci deep within the brain (145). Systematic series of studies have yet to be completed in patients with the affective disorders using this technique, however.

Studies are available of deep structures visualized by techniques of positron emission tomography (PET). Many structures in the brain appear to be relatively hypometabolic during phases of bipolar depression, with values returning to or above normal following the switch into euthymia or hypomania (146). In our study, there was no evidence of a discrete area of increased uptake in the temporal lobe or other areas of the brain, and, in fact, temporal lobe structures were relatively hypometabolic in the small series of depressed patients compared with controls (147). Thus, preliminary evidence from PET would suggest a closer approximation to the PET findings of patients with epilepsy in the interictal state rather than any focal area of increase as might

TABLE 9. *Carbamazepine in paroxysmal and dysrhythmic syndromes[a]*

Seizures	**Motor and verbal tics**
Temporal lobe epilepsy (TLE) (complex partial seizures)	Gilles de la Tourette's syndrome
Grand mal seizures	Hemifacial spasm
Alcohol withdrawal seizures	Paroxysmal dysarthria
Amygdala-kindled seizures	**Muscle irritability**
	Myokymia
	Muscle hypertonicity
Paroxysmal pain syndromes	**Myoclonic tinnitus[c]**
Trigeminal neuralgia	**Autonomic dysregulation**
Tabes (lightning pain)	Autonomic epilepsy (with flushing and hypertension)
Phantom limb pain	Autonomic epilepsy (with heaches and abdominal pain)
Post-herpetic neuralgia[b]	**Affective dysregulation**
Glossopharyngeal neuralgia	Manic–depressive illness
Recurrent episodes of headache	Affective dysregulation of TLE
Cardiac arrhythmia	
Digitalis-induced ventricular arrhythmias	
Multiple sclerosis	

[a]From ref. 15, with permission. See ref. 15 for further references.

[b]Effective only on lancinating component of pain.

[c]In three studies of tinnitus, acute response to lidocaine was predictive of longer-term response to carbamazepine.

be expected to occur with an ictal process (148,149).

A final caveat is clearly in order. Given the fact that some types of kindled seizures and some stages of kindling but not others are differentially sensitive to the anticonvulsant effects of carbamazepine (Fig. 14), one should be particularly cautious in making any inference that a kindling process might exist on the basis of the efficacy of carbamazepine in a given syndrome. The logical fallacy in this assumption is clearest in the case of trigeminal neuralgia or in the case of the efficacy of carbamazepine in the treatment of various cardiac arrhythmias where an epileptic process is not implicated and the kindling phenomenon may be irrelevant. Shaikh et al. (150) have also reported that carbamazepine suppresses feline affective defensive aggression (but not quiet biting attack) elicited by midbrain periaqueductal gray stimulation in the absence of convulsive activity.

Nonetheless, it is possible that the mechanisms of action of carbamazepine that stabilize various types of dysrhythmic processes not only in the epilepsics but also in the paroxysmal pain syndromes and other phenomena, including cardiac arrhythmias and myokymias, could also be implicated in the psychotropic effects of carbamazepine (Table 9). That is, even in the absence of seizure focus in patients with manic–depressive illness or a kindling process, one could change set points, thresholds, or other types of neural processes involved in the regulation of neural excitability that could be important to carbamazepine's psychotropic effects. Carbamazepine appears to be particularly effective in blocking syndromes with paroxysmal, as opposed to chronic, symptomatology (Table 10). With this series of caveats in mind, we do wish to preliminarily explore the kindling model, since it might bear on two phenomena important in the treatment of manic–depressive patients—i.e., the possibility that pharmacotherapy may occur differentially as a function of course of illness, and that the phe-

TABLE 10. *Paroxysmal syndromes treated with carbamazepine*

Paroxysmal component (positive effect)	Chronic component (no effect)
+ + + Seizures	− − Status epilepticus
+ + + Trigeminal neuralgia	− − Chronic pain syndromes
+ PTSD (posttraumatic stress disorder) —flashback and terrors	− − Numbness depression
+ Episodic dyscontrol	
+ Dyscontrol acts	− − Mood in borderlines
+ (Panic)	− ? Generalized anxiety
+ Acute depression	− − Chronic depression
+ + + Mania	

nomenon of conditioned tolerance may occur in a small proportion of patients as an explanatory mechanism for observed loss of efficacy.

Differential Pharmacotherapy as a Function of Course of Illness

The kindling phemonenon provides clear-cut evidence for the differential efficacy of pharmacological interventions as a function of stage of kindling evolution. If we divide kindling into three stages (development, completed, spontaneous), it is readily apparent that drugs are effective in some stages of kindling but not in others. In the developing stage of kindling, electrical or pharmacological stimulation that was initially inadequate to produce a seizure eventually becomes sufficient to produce a seizure (151,152). The second stage of kindling involves repeated seizure induction with the same stimulation, and we have called this the "completed" phase. However, after sufficient numbers of repetitions of kindled seizures, animals evolve into the stage of spontaneity where seizures occur in the absence of exogenous stimulation, either electrically or pharmacologically (153–156). Preliminary evidence also exists for spontaneity during lidocaine-kindled seizures. That is, animals subjected to many dozens of lidocaine-kindled seizures have been observed to show similar patterns of seizures spontaneously without drug administration (Contel and Post, *unpublished observations*).

Although carbamazepine is effective in blocking the development of electrically kindled seizures in cats (18) and nonhuman primates (19), it is ineffective at any dose and method of administration in blocking the development of amygdala-kindled seizures in the rat (19,20,22,40). This is particularly remarkable because carbamazepine is the most effective agent in blocking the completed amygdala-kindled seizure (Table 8). Conversely, the glutamate antagonist MK801 is effective in inhibiting the development phase of amygdala kindling in the rat, but similar doses are unable to inhibit the completed kindled seizure (157).

Pinel (158) has demonstrated an even more remarkable double dissociation with diazepam and phenytoin. Diazepam is highly effec-

tive in the developing and completed stages of kindling but is without effect on spontaneous seizures, whereas phenytoin shows (a) the opposite pattern of inefficacy in the early and intermediate phases of kindling and (b) a highly effective profile on spontaneous seizures. Thus, as summarized in Fig. 15, there is clear-cut evidence for a differential pharmacotherapy as a function of stage of kindling evolution. This pharmacological dysjunction implies that different biochemical and/or physiological mechanisms are incorporated in different stages of the kindling process. Some evidence exists to support the contention that the neural substrates of kindling do change in different stages of its evolution. For example, following repeated kindled seizures there appears to be sprouting in some mossy fiber nerve terminals in the hippocampus (159). Pinel (155) has also demonstrated the remarkable finding that with the evolution from completed kindled seizure stage to that of spontaneity, the afterdischarge focus evoked at the electrode in the kindled focus actually disappears. Thus the spontaneous seizure is not associated with spiking at the original kindled focus, and whether a spike focus occurs elsewhere in the brain during the spontaneous seizure remains to be documented.

Moreover, there is also evidence for differential pharmacological response in different phases as a function of seizure type. As we have already mentioned, carbamazepine is highly effective in blocking local anesthetic-induced kindling development, whereas it is ineffective at this same stage on amygdala kindling development in the rat. Thus, the hazards of inferring a kindling mechanism on the basis of the efficacy of a given drug are indeed apparent. The evidence of a differential pharmacotherapy also indicates that different stages of the kindling process are subserved by different biophysiological mechanisms or anatomical substrates.

This would also appear to be the case in a model of learning and memory, such as long-term potentiation (LTP); in this situation the development of LTP is inhibited by glutamate antagonists such as AP5, but its expression is not affected by these drugs (160). Similar pharmacological dysjunctions and dissociations are evident in the phenomenon of behavioral sensitization. For example, neuroleptics

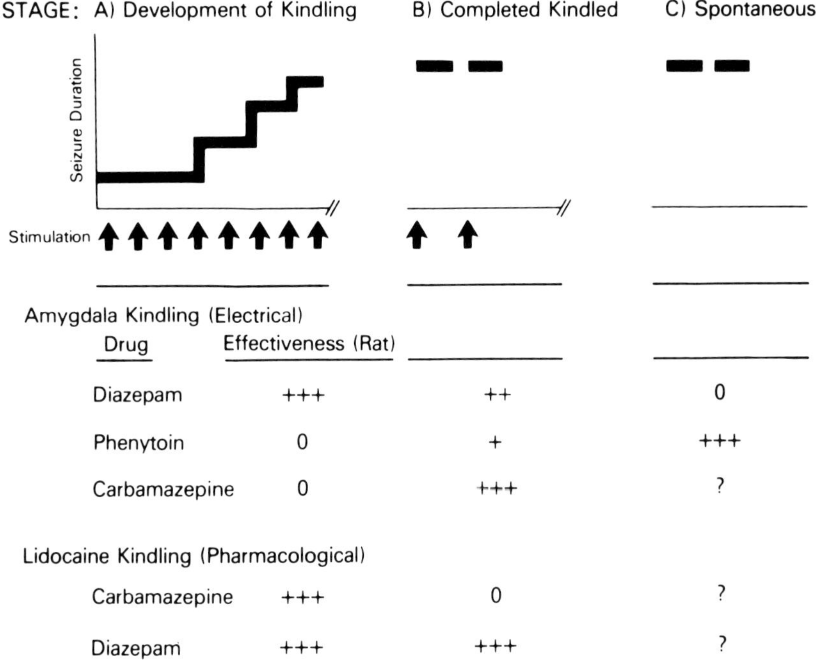

	Amygdala Kindling (Electrical) Effectiveness (Rat)		
Drug			
Diazepam	+++	++	0
Phenytoin	0	+	+++
Carbamazepine	0	+++	?

Lidocaine Kindling (Pharmacological)

Carbamazepine	+++	0	?
Diazepam	+++	+++	?

FIG. 15. Pharmacology of kindling as a function of stimulus type and stage of development. Anticonvulsants are effective in some stages of amygdala kindling but not in others. Moreover, the same anticonvulsant, carbamazepine, is differentially effective in different stages of amygdala-kindling as compared with lidocaine-kindling—that is, a double-dissociation. Pinel (158) reported another remarkable double-dissociation where diazepam is effective in amygdala-kindling early (**A** and **B**) but not late (**C**) in kindling, whereas phenytoin shows the opposite profile.

will block the development of behavioral sensitization to cocaine, but they are not effective in terms of the expression of this phenomenon (48).

Thus, we can ask whether similar dysjunctions also occur in the pharmacology of the affective disorders as a function of stage in their evolution. As reviewed earlier, there is some evidence that patients with rapid cycling are less responsive to lithium carbonate when compared to those without the pattern (74). While rapid cycling can, in rare instances, emerge at the outset of bipolar illness, it is more likely to occur as a function of the later stages of the illness. As such, it is possible that carbamazepine and valproic acid and related anticonvulsants may be effective in later rapid-cycling stages of the illness when lithium alone is ineffective or only partially effective. Similarly, tricyclic antidepressants and MAOIs appear to be among the treatments of choice for severe depressive recurrences;

however, these agents may be relatively contraindicated in the later stages of bipolar illness, where they might be associated with the induction of manic episodes, rapid-cycling phenomena, or continuous-cycling phenomena (161–166).

These are just several examples of how the pharmacotherapy of the affective disorders may change as a function of stage of evolution of the illness. The schema shown in Fig. 16 is highly provisional and is presented for its heuristic value to stimulate further systematic studies of this variable in pharmacotherapy, rather than as evidence that is well documented. Thus, it may be useful for the clinician and the theoretician to consider the possibility that in addition to illness- and patient-related subtypes with differential pharmacoresponsivity, this may also occur as a function of stage in evolution of the illness. In addition to being relevant in the preclinical kindling models, this principle is also ob-

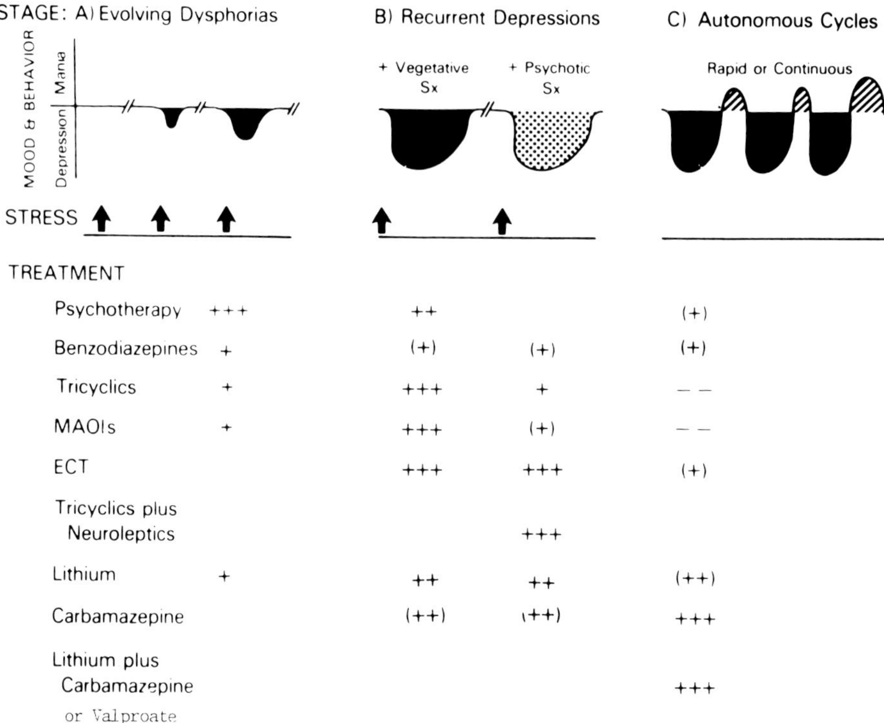

FIG. 16. Psychopharmacotherapy of affective illness as a function of type and stage of development: a hypothetical schema. MAOIs, monoamine oxidase inhibitors; ECT, electroconvulsive therapy. Just as different stages of kindling are differentially responsive to pharmacological interventions (see Fig. 15), we postulate that a differential effectiveness of therapeutic agents may also exist as a function of the longitudinal course of affective illness (see ref. 24 for details). Although some of the existing literature is convergent with this idea, this schema remains to be directly tested.

viously highly relevant in the area of cancer chemotherapies, where treatments may be radically different for primary and metastatic phases of the same illness. Independent of the adequacy of the responsivity to the anticonvulsants in the early phases of manic–depressive illness, which also appears promising (63–66), it would appear that the anticonvulsants, particularly carbamazepine and valproate, do offer important clinical options for the lithium-refractory manic–depressive patient, who perhaps has a more "malignant" course of illness than do many other patients with lithium-responsive disease.

Conditioned Tolerance to Carbamazepine

A fundamental way that we might use the kindling seizure analogy to elucidate a possi-

ble principle of relevance to the pharmacotherapy of affective illness centers around the phenomenon of conditioned tolerance. Repeated administration of carbamazepine prior to amygdala-kindled seizures eventually results in loss of anticonvulsant efficacy to the drug (167). This cannot be attributable to pharmacokinetic changes, since it will be reversed by a period of administering carbamazepine immediately after a kindled seizure occurs. Thus, animals with identical histories of drug administration can be made responsive or unresponsive to carbamazepine based on the temporal contingencies. Following the development of tolerance to carbamazepine, this effect will be reversed by a period of inducing seizures without any drug at all, but it will not be reversed by an extended period of time without either seizures or drug. Also, the administration of carbamazepine alone without seizure induction is ineffective in reversing contingent tolerance.

Conditioned tolerance appears to be selective with respect to the inducing drug, since animals that are tolerant to carbamazepine are responsive to the benzodiazepine diazepam. However, there does appear to be a cross-tolerance between anticonvulsants acting at the "peripheral-type" benzodiazepine receptor site, such that animals that are demonstrating conditioned tolerance to the anticonvulsant effects of carbamazepine are also tolerant to the anticonvulsant effects of PK-11195, the selective antagonist for the benzodiazepine receptor.

In this preclinical model, we have attempted to discern methods for slowing the development of conditioned tolerance (167). Remarkably, we have found that using a higher dose of carbamazepine (25 mg/kg instead of 15 mg/kg) is ineffective in slowing the development of conditioned tolerance. Moreover, alternating injections of carbamazepine and diazepam in an attempt to prevent once-daily amygala-kindled seizures is ineffective in slowing the development of kindled conditioned tolerance to the anticonvulsant effects of carbamazepine. Chronic oral administration of carbamazepine, which would (hypothetically) help break the associations between acute drug treatment and seizure induction (i.e., the drug would be in the animal continuously and not just prior to a seizure), was sufficient to decrease the rate of tolerance development. This latter demonstration may also explain why tolerance is not typically observed clinically in chronic treatment of epilepsy patients where, in fact, blood levels are maintained steadily and seizures occur intermittently, thereby minimizing the possible pairing of drug and seizure state.

Nonetheless, we feel that the phenomenon of contingent tolerance may be relevant to some patients with refractory seizure disorders, particularly where initially responsive patients show deterioration in their clinical course (89). The preclinical models suggest the possibility that a period of time off medication may be helpful in reinstituting pharmacological efficacy even if this is only transient. Preliminary data in support of this hypothesis are evident in two cases in the study of Pakalnis et al. (168). Similarly, a period of time off medication may be helpful in reversing tolerance phenomena that develop in a subgroup of patients chronically treated with carbamazepine for trigeminal neuralgia and other related paroxysmal pain syndromes (119,120,169).

Finally, we would wonder whether this phenomenon might also be relevant for the subgroup of patients with emerging refractoriness to carbamazepine following initial successful prophylaxis of affective episodes with the drug (Fig. 17). Frankenburg et al. (170) implied that a loss of efficacy occurred in a number of their patients followed over several years. In addition, Fawcett and Kravits (*personal communication*) have observed a similar phenomenon which is not always responsive to increasing the dose of carbamazepine. While there are many possible reasons for the loss of efficacy to a given psychotropic agent in the pharmacoprophylaxis of the affective disorders (171), we suggest that the phenomenon of conditioned tolerance may be relevant. As illustrated in Fig. 18, a patient who was showing repeated acute responses to carbamazepine for two severe depressions appeared to have an initially successful response to carbamazepine. However, with continued administration, minor depressive episodes continued to break through with increasing severity and duration until full-blown and incapacitating episodes (although not requiring rehospitalization as previously occurred during the medication-free state) occurred repeatedly.

This progressive emergence of affective episodes is parallel to the progressive emergence of amygdala-kindled seizures in spite of carbamazepine pretreatment (i.e., contingent tolerance) and suggests the possible utility of a period of time off carbamazepine in an attempt to renew medication responsivity. Donaldson (172) and Fawcett (*personal communication*, 1988) have suggested that tolerance to the antidepressant effects of the MAOIs might also develop, and Fawcett noted that periods of time off drug might renew effectiveness. These data are consistent with our formulation of contingent tolerance.

Thus, it is possible that the phenomenon of contingent tolerance may be relevant to a subgroup of patients who might show loss of efficacy to agents such as (a) carbamazepine,

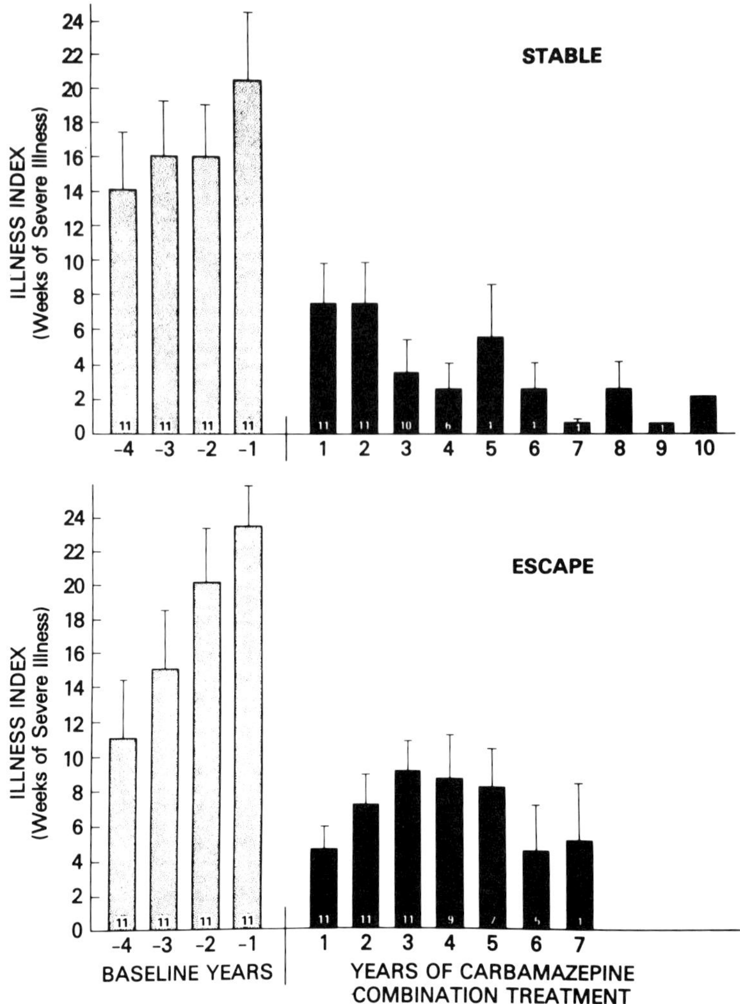

FIG. 17. Persistence of carbamazepine prophylaxis as assessed by the illness index (i.e., duration of illness multiplied by severity; see legend to Fig. 10). Some patients show stable long-term responsiveness to carbamazepine **(top)**, whereas another group (with a faster rate of clinical deterioration in the 4 years prior to starting carbamazepine) shows a pattern of escape or loss of prophylactic efficacy **(bottom)** after the first year of treatment (black bars).

tricyclic antidepressants, and MAOI antidepressants (which are not traditionally associated with tolerance development in most animal models) and (b) benzodiazepines, acetazolamide, alcohol, and other anticonvulsants which display tolerance phenomena readily. Nonetheless, it is possible that patients who develop refractoriness during treatment of their seizure disorder, trigeminal neuralgia, or affective disorder may be displaying this phenomenon on the basis of con-

tingent tolerance and would benefit from either (a) a period of medication-free evaluation or (b) the switch to another drug of a different category which might not be associated with cross-tolerance phenomena.

CONCLUSIONS

From the clinical perspective, the anticonvulsant drugs, particularly carbamazepine

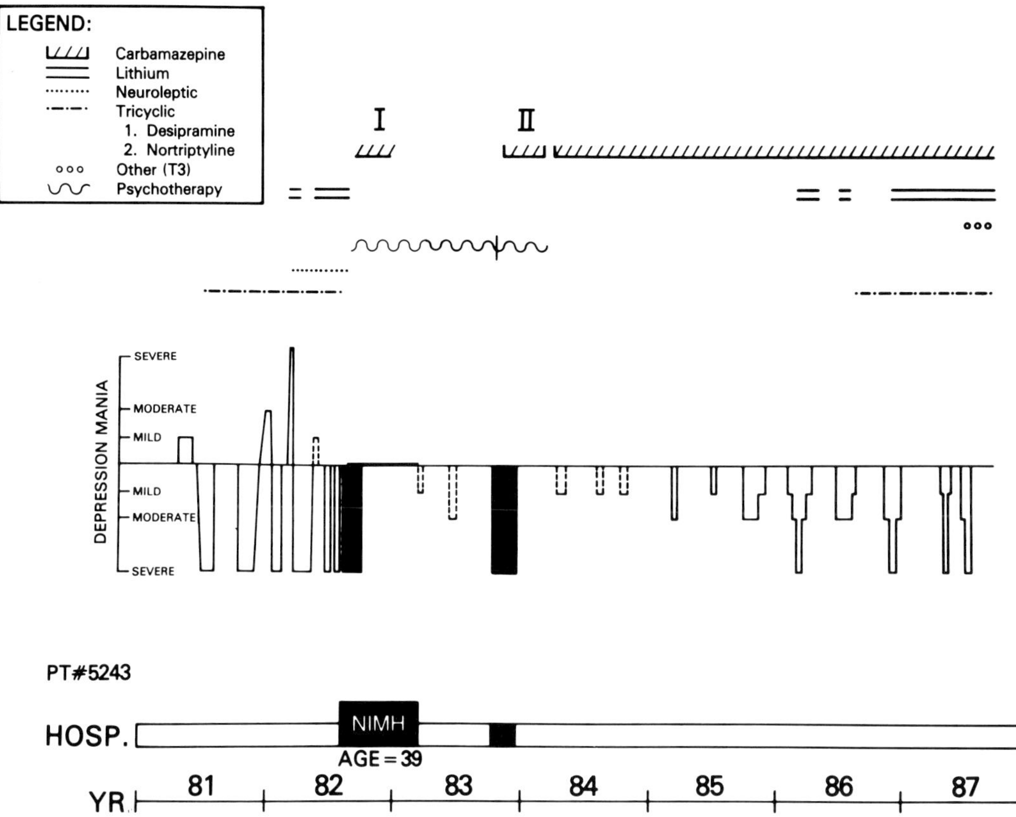

FIG. 18. Good acute response to carbamazepine (I, II) but progressive emergence of episodes. This rapid-cycling bipolar female showed a pattern of rapid cycling on tricyclic antidepressants with or without lithium treatment prior to NIMH admission. A severe depression responded to treatment with carbamazepine, but the drug was discontinued because of minor liver enzyme elevations. After a brief interval of wellness, the patient became severely depressed and required rehospitalization elsewhere in 1983. She did not respond to various treatments (not illustrated) until carbamazepine was reinstituted. The patient did well, experiencing only mild-to-moderate depressions in 1984 and 1985 on carbamazepine prophylaxis, but her depression became progressively more severe in 1986 in spite of adjunctive therapy with lithium and antidepressants. This gradual reemergence of severe depression during carbamazepine prophylaxis appears to represent the development of tolerance to its psychotropic effects. The patient again responded when an MAOI (tranylcypromine) was added to her carbamazepine prophylaxis (not shown).

and valproate, now provide alternative or adjunctive treatments to lithium carbonate for the refractory bipolar patient. The considerable data on carbamazepine and lesser data on other drugs strongly supports the idea that carbamazepine may possess psychotropic properties in patients with epilepsy independent of its improvement in seizure control or substitution for more behaviorally toxic agents. While preliminary evidence suggests that many of the factors that are associated with a relatively poorer response to lithium (i.e., manic severity, dysphoria, rapid cycling, and nonfamilial occurrence) may be associated with better response to carbamazepine and other anticonvulsants, these observations need further confirmation in more systematic clinical trials. Moreover, it is increasingly clear from individual case studies (Figs. 8 and 9), as well as from small series, that response to one anticonvulsant may not predict response to another, suggesting important differences in patient subgroups, different mechanisms of action of the anticonvulsants, and even the possibility that response to pharmacotherapeutic agents could differ as a function of stage of evolution of the syndrome.

Because of carbamazepine's unique clinical profile as an anticonvulsant, antinociceptive, antimanic, and antidepressant agent, comparing the time course of clinical effects with the time course of carbamazepine's biological actions may help dissect mechanisms of action of this drug that are unique or common to different clinical syndromes. Comparative analyses of lithium, carbamazepine, and valproate—each of which appears to have better antimanic than antidepressant efficacy (at least acutely), as well as some efficacy in long-term prophylaxis—should also prove valuable. This clinical profile contrasts with that of ECT, where effects appear to be as good (or better) in depression as in mania. Moreover, comparing the mechanisms of action of these bimodal agents (lithium, carbamazepine, and ECT) with those of the unimodal antidepressants of the tricyclic, heterocyclic, and MAOI class should also reveal mechanisms that underlie common mood-stabilizing properties, as opposed to unimodal antidepressant activity and the concomitant vulnerability for inducing manic episodes, rapid cycling, or continuous cycling.

Similarly, the anticonvulsant drugs provide unique agents for further systematic study of the possible role of limbic and related structures in the pathophysiology of the affective disorders and their response to treatment. Sensitization to the psychomotor stimulants and kindling may provide interesting analogies for syndromes which show progressive evolution in behavioral and physiological concomitants such as those observed in affective illness. The kindling model may help to identify those structures and principles that may underlie progression of symptoms over time, and it may also help to determine the differential pharmacotherapy as a function of stage of illness. Pharmacologically kindled seizures with lidocaine and cocaine may also uniquely provide a seizure model that requires chronic administration (as opposed to repeated, intermittent administration) of carbamazepine for effective prevention. As such, these seizure models may be more directly pertinent to

mechanisms involving chronic carbamazepine which are important to its psychotropic properties in patients with affective disorders. Lastly, we have utilized the kindling model to dissect the phenomena of conditioned tolerance, which may be of value in elucidating a possible mechanism for loss of efficacy of anticonvulsant, antinociceptive, and psychotropic agents.

Thus, it is clear that there is a rich interplay between seizures and anticonvulsant agents in the treatment of the affective disorders. ECT was originally developed as a therapeutic tool based on the observations of the inverse relationship between seizures and psychosis. It is now apparent that ECT also exerts potent anticonvulsant effects in animals and humans, providing a further leverage point in understanding the mechanism of action of this treatment as well as those of the more routinely used pharmacological anticonvulsant agents. In the past decade there has been a revolution in the treatment of bipolar affective disorder, with the introduction of a new series of treatments for the bipolar patient. We look forward to the further treatment advances that the next decade may yield, and we anxiously await further insights relating to the mechanism of action of the anticonvulsants in both the seizure and the affective disorders.

REFERENCES

1. Papez JW. A proposed mechanism of emotion. *Arch Neurol Psychiatry* 1937;38:725–743.
2. MacLean PD. The limbic system and its hippocampal formation: studies in animals and their possible application to man. *J Neurosurg* 1954;11:29–44.
3. MacLean PD. The limbic brain in relation to the psychoses. In: Black P, ed. *Physiological correlates of emotion.* New York: Academic Press, 1970;129–146.
4. MacLean PD. A triune concept of the brain and behavior. In: Boag TJ, Campbell D, eds. *The Clarence M. Hicks memorial lectures, 1969.* Toronto: University of Toronto Press, 1973;2–66.
5. Gellhorn E. *Biological foundations of emotion.* Glenview, IL: Scott, Foresman & Co., 1968.
6. Monroe R. *Episodic behavioral disorders.* Cambridge, MA: Harvard University Press, 1970.
7. Isaacson RL. *The limbic system.* New York: Plenum Press, 1974.
8. Gloor P, Olivier A, Quesney LF, Andermann F, Horowitz S. The role of the limbic system in experiential phenomena of temporal lobe epilepsy. *Ann Neurol* 1982;12:129–144.

9. Stevens JR, Mark VH, Erwin F, Pachico P, Suematsu K. Deep temporal stimulation in man. *Arch Neurol* 1969;21:157–167.

10. Stevens JR. Psychomotor epilepsy and schizophrenia: a common anatomy? In: Brazier MAB, ed. *Epilepsy: its phenomena in man.* New York: Academic Press, 1973;190–214.

11. Stevens JR. Interictal clinical manifestations of complex partial seizures. In: Penry JK, Daly DD, eds. *Complex partial seizures and their treatment. Advances in neurology,* vol 11. New York: Raven Press, 1975;85–112.

12. Heath RG. Correlation of brain function with emotional behavior. *Biol Psychiatry* 1976;11:463–480.

13. Trimble MR. Interictal psychoses of epilepsy. *Acta Psychiatr Scand* 1984;69:9–20.

14. Albright PS, Burnham WM. Development of a new pharmacological seizure model: effects of anticonvulsants on cortical- and amygdala-kindled seizures in the rat. *Epilepsia* 1980;21:681–689.

15. Post RM, Uhde TW. Are the psychotropic effects of carbamazepine in manic–depressive illness mediated through the limbic system? *Psychiatr J Univ Ottawa* 1985;10:205–219.

16. Babington RG, Horovitz ZP. Neuropharmacology of SQ 10,996, a compound with several therapeutic indications. *Arch Int Pharmacodyn Ther* 1973;202:106–118.

17. Babington RG. The pharmacology of kindling. In: Hanin I, Usdin E, eds. *Animal models of psychiatry and neurology.* Oxford: Pergamon Press, 1977;141–149.

18. Wada JA, Sato M, Wake A, Green JR, Troupin AS. Prophylactic effects of phenytoin, phenobarbital, and carbamazepine examined in kindled cat preparations. *Arch Neurol* 1976;33:426–434.

19. Wada JA. Pharmacological prophylaxis in the kindling model of epilepsy. *Arch Neurol* 1977;34:389–395.

20. Albertson TE, Joy RM, Stark LG. Carbamazepine: a pharmacological study in the kindling model of epilepsy. *Neuropharmacology* 1984;23:1117–1123.

21. Ashton D, Wauquier A. Behavioral analysis of the aspects of 15 anticonvulsants in the amygdaloid kindled rat. *Psychopharmacology* 1979;65:7–13.

22. Weiss SRB, Post RM. Carbamazepine and carbamazepine-10,11-epoxide inhibit amygdala kindled seizures in the rat but do not block their development. *Clin Neuropharmacol* 1987;10:272–279.

23. Post RM, Rubinow DR, Ballenger JC. Conditioning, sensitization, and kindling: implications for the course of affective illness. In: Post RM, Ballenger JC, eds. *Neurobiology of mood disorders.* Baltimore: Williams & Wilkins, 1984;432–466.

24. Post RM, Rubinow DR, Ballenger JC. Conditioning and sensitization in the longitudinal course of affective illness. *Br J Psychiatry* 1986;149:191–201.

25. Post RM, Weiss SRB. Kindling and manic–depressive illness. In: Trimble MR, Bolwig TG, eds. *The clinical relevance of kindling.* Chichester, England: John Wiley & Sons, 1989; 209–230.

26. Dalby MA. Antiepileptic and psychotropic effect of carbamazepine (Tegretol) in the treatment of psychomotor epilepsy. *Epilepsia* 1971; 12:325–334.

27. Dalby MA. Behavioral effects of carbamazepine. In: Penry JK, Daly DD, eds. *Complex partial seizures and their treatment. Advances in neurology,* vol 11. New York: Raven Press, 1975;331–343.

28. Rivinus TM. Psychiatric effects of the anticonvulsant regimens. *J Clin Psychopharmacol* 1982;2:165–192.

29. Parnas J, Flachs H, Gram L. Psychotropic effect of antiepileptic drugs. *Acta Neurol Scand* 1979;60:329–343.

30. Okuma T, Kishimoto A, Inoue K, et al. Antimanic and prophylactic effects of carbamazepine on manic–depressive psychosis. *Folia Psychiatr Neurol Jpn* 1973;27:283–297.

31. Takezaki H, Hanaoka M. The use of carbamazepine (Tegretol) in the control of manic–depressive psychosis and other manic, depressive states. *Clin Psychiatry* 1971;13:173–182.

32. Post RM, Putnam F, Contel NR, Goldman B. Electroconvulsive seizures inhibit amygdala kindling: implications for mechanisms of action in affective illness. *Epilepsia* 1984;25:234–239.

33. Post RM, Putnam F, Uhde TW, Weiss SRB. ECT as an anticonvulsant: implications for its mechanism of action in affective illness. In: Malitz S, Sackeim HA, eds. *Electroconvulsive therapy: clinical and basic research issues. Annals of the New York Academy of Sciences,* vol 462. New York: New York Academy of Sciences, 1986;376–388.

34. Post RM. Time course of clinical effects of carbamazepine: implications for mechanisms of action. *J Clin Psychiatry* 1988;49:35–46.

35. Milstein V, Small JG, Klapper MH, Small IF, Miller MJ, Kellams JJ. Uni- versus bilateral ECT in the treatment of mania. *Convulsive Ther* 1987;3:1–9.

36. Mukherjee S, Sackeim HA, Lee C. Unilateral ECT in the treatment of manic episodes. *Convulsive Ther* 1988;4:74–80.

37. Fink M. *Convulsive therapy: theory and practice.* New York: Raven Press, 1979.

38. Fink M. Theories of the antidepressant efficacy of convulsive therapy (ECT) In: Post RM, Ballenger JC, eds. *Neurobiology of mood disorders.* Baltimore: Williams & Wilkins, 1984; 721–730.

39. Brandon S, Cowley P, McDonald C, Neville P, Palmer R, Wellstood-Eason S. Electroconvulsive therapy: results in depressive illness from the Leicestershire trial. *Br Med J* 1984;288:22–25.

40. Baltzer V, Klebs K, Schmutz M. Effects of oxcarbazepine, a compound related to carbamazepine, and of GP 47 779, its main metabolite in

man, on the evolution of amygdaloid-kindled seizures in the rat. Paper presented at the Epilepsy International Congress, Kyoto, Japan, 1981.

41. Sackeim, HA, Decina P, Malitz S, Resor SR, Prohovnik I. Anticonvulsant and antidepressant properties of electroconvulsive therapy: a proposed mechanism of action. *Biol Psychiatry* 1983;18:1301–1310.

42. Nakajima T, Post RM, Pert A, Ketter T, Weiss SRB. Perspectives on the mechanism of action of electroconvulsive therapy: anticonvulsant, dopaminergic, and C-fos oncogene effects. *Convulsive Ther* 1989;5:274–295.

43. Holaday JW, Tortella FC, Long JB, Belenky GL, Hitzeman RJ. Endogenous opioids and their receptors: evidence for involvement in the postictal effects of electroconvulsive shock. *Ann NJ Acad Sci* 1986;462:124–139.

44. Tortella FC, Long JB. Characterization of opioid peptide-like anticonvulsant activity in rat cerebrospinal fluid. *Brain Res* 1988;426:139–146.

45. Post RM, Uhde TW, Roy-Byrne PP, Joffe RT. Correlates of antimanic response to carbamazepine. *Psychiatry Res* 1987;21:71–83.

46. Koella WP, Levin P, Baltzer V. The pharmacology of carbamazepine and some other antiepileptic drugs. In: Birkmayer W, ed. *Epileptic seizures—behavior—pain.* Bern: Hans Huber, 1976;32–50.

47. Post RM, Jimerson DC, Bunney WE Jr, Goodwin FK. Dopamine and mania: behavioral and biochemical effects of the dopamine receptor blocker pimozide. *Psychopharmacology* 1980;67:297–305.

48. Weiss SRB, Post RM, Pert A, Woodward R, Murman D. Context-dependent cocaine sensitization: Differential effect of haloperidol on development versus expression. *Pharmacol Biochem & Behav* 1989;34:655–661.

49. Post RM, Rubinow DR, Uhde TW, Ballenger JC, Linnoila M. Relationship of the efficacy of carbamazepine to dopaminergic mechanisms. *Arch Gen Psychiatry* 1986;43:392–396.

50. Muller AA, Stoll K-D. Carbamazepine and oxcarbazepine in the treatment of manic syndromes: studies in Germany. In: Emrich HM, Okuma T, Muller AA, eds. *Anticonvulsants in affective disorders.* Amsterdam: Excerpta Medica, 1984;139–147.

51. Tomson T, Bertilsson L. Potent therapeutic effect of carbamazepine-10,11-epoxide in trigeminal neuralgia. *Arch Neurol* 1984;41:598–601.

52. Marangos PJ, Post RM, Patel J, Zander K, Parma A, Weiss S. Specific and potent interactions of carbamazepine with brain adenosine receptors. *Eur J Pharmacol* 1983;93:175–182.

53. Post RM. Mechanisms of action of carbamazepine and related anticonvulsants in affective illness. In: Meltzer H, Bunney WE Jr, eds. *Psychopharmacology: a generation of progress.* New York: Raven Press, 1987;567–576.

54. Post RM, Uhde TW, Roy-Byrne PP, Joffe RT. Antidepressant effects of carbamazepine. *Am J Psychiatry* 1986;143:29–34.

55. Neumann J, Seidel K, Wunderlich H-P. Comparative studies of the effect of carbamazepine and trimipramine in depression. In: Emrich HM, Okuma T, Muller AA, eds. *Anticonvulsants in affective disorders.* Amsterdam: Excerpta Medica, 1984;160–166.

56. Silberman EK, Post RM, Nurnberger J, Theodore W, Boulenger J-P. Transient sensory, cognitive, and affective phenomena in affective illness: a comparison with complex partial epilepsy. *Br J Psychiatry* 1985;146:81–89.

57. Post RM, Kramlinger KG, Joffe RT, Gold PW, Uhde TW. Effects of carbamazepine on thyroid function. In: *Abstracts of the 140th annual meeting of the American Psychiatric Association,* Chicago, Illinois, May 1987, Symposium 104-D, p. 142.

58. Roy-Byrne PP, Joffe RT, Uhde TW, et al. Carbamazepine and thyroid function in affectively ill patients: clinical and theoretical implications. *Arch Gen Psychiatry* 1984;41:1150–1153.

59. Baumgartner A, Graf K-J, Kurten I, Meinhold H. The hypothalamic–pituitary–thyroid axis in psychiatric patients and healthy subjects, Part 3: the TRH test and thyroid hormone determinations as predictors of therapeutic response and long-term outcome in major depression and schizophrenia. *Psychiatr Res* 1988;24:306–315 & 324–332.

60. Cowdry RW, Gardner DL. Pharmacotherapy of borderline personality disorder. *Arch Gen Psychiatry* 1988;45:111–119.

61. Gardner DL, Cowdry RW. Anticonvulsants and personality disorders. In: McElroy SL, Poper HS Jr, ed. *Use of anticonvulsants in psychiatry: recent advances.* Clifton, NJ: Oxford Health Care, 1988;127–140.

62. Gardner DL, Cowdry RW. Development of melancholia during carbamazepine treatment in borderline personality disorder. *J Clin Psychopharmacol* 1986;6:236–239.

63. Placidi GF, Lenzi A, Lazzerini F, et al. The comparative efficacy and safety of carbamazepine versus lithium: a randomized, double-blind 3-year trial in 83 patients. *J Clin Psychiatry* 1986;47:490–494.

64. Watkins SE, Callender K, Thomas DR, Tidmarsh SF, Shaw DM. The effect of carbamazepine and lithium on remission from affective illness. *Br J Psychiatry* 1987;150:180–182.

65. Bellaire W, Demish K, Stoll K-D. Carbamazepine versus lithium in prophylaxis of recurrent affective disorders. *Psychopharmacol [Suppl] Abstr XVI CINP Congr* 1988;96:287 [Abstract 31.03.03].

66. Lusznat RM, Murphy DP, Nunn CMH. Carbamazepine vs. lithium in the treatment and prophylaxis of mania. *Br J Psychiatry* 1988;153:198–204.

67. Abou-Saleh MT, Coppen A. Who responds to prophylactic lithium? *J Affective Disord* 1986;10:115–125.

68. Goodnick PJ, Fieve RR, Schlegel A, Baxter N. Predictors of interepisode symptoms and relapse in affective disorder patients treated with lithium carbonate. *Am J Psychiatry* 1987; 144:367–369.

69. Bouman TK, Niemantsverdriet-van Kampen JG, Ormel J, Slooff CJ. The effectiveness of lithium prophylaxis in bipolar and unipolar depressions and schizo-affective disorders. *J Affective Disord* 1986;11:275–280.

70. Hanus H, Zapletalek M. The prophylactic lithium treatment in affective disorders and the possibilities of the outcome prediction. *Sbornik Ved Pr Lek Fak Univ Karlovy* 1984;27:5–75.

71. Prien RF, Kupfer DJ, Mansky PA, Small JG, Tuason VB, Voss CB, Johnson WE. Drug therapy in the prevention of the recurrences in unipolar and bipolar affective disorders. Report of the NIMH collaborative study group comparing lithium carbonate, imipramine, and a lithium carbonate–imipramine combination. *Arch Gen Psychiatry* 1984;41:1096–1104.

72. Strober M. Juvenile onset of bipolar affective illness. In: *Abstracts of the annual meeting of the American College of Neuropsychopharmacology*, Puerto Rico, December 1988, p. 19.

73. Kishimoto A, Okuma T. Antimanic and prophylactic effects of carbamazepine in affective disorders. In: *Abstracts of 4th world congress of biological psychiatry*, Philadelphia, September 8–13, 1985.

74. Joffe RT. Carbamazepine lithium and life course of bipolar affective disorder: a clinical evaluation. *Acta Psychiatrica Scandinavica*, 1990, in press.

75. Post RM, Berrettini W, Uhde TW, et al. Selective response to the anticonvulsant carbamazepine in manic–depressive illness: a case study. *J Clin Psychopharmacol* 1984;4:178–185.

76. Kishimoto A, Omura F, Umezawa Y, Fukuma E. Combined therapy with lithium and carbamazepine. In: *New research abstracts, 137th annual meeting of the American Psychiatric Association*, Los Angeles, California, May 1984, Abstract NR22.

77. Lipinski JF, Pope HG Jr. Possible synergistic action between carbamazepine and lithium carbonate in the treatment of three acutely manic patients. *Am J Psychiatry* 1982;139:948–949.

78. Keisling R. Carbamazepine and lithium carbonate in the treatment of refractory affective disorders. *Arch Gen Psychiatry* 1983;40:223.

79. Kramlinger KG, Post RM. The addition of lithium to carbamazepine: antidepressant efficacy in treatment-resistant depression. *Arch Gen Psychiatry* 1989;46:794–800.

80. Kramlinger KG, Post RM. Adding lithium carbonate to carbamazepine: antimanic efficacy in treatment-resistant mania. *Acta Psychiatr Scand* 1989;79:378–385.

81. Mander AJ. Clinical prediction of outcome and lithium response in bipolar affective disorder. *J Affective Disord* 1986;11:35–41.

82. Mander AJ, Loudon JB. Rapid recurrence of mania following abrupt discontinuation of lithium. *Lancet* 1988;2:15–17.

83. Lenz G, Lovrek A, Thau K, et al. Lithium-withdrawal study in schizoaffective patients. In: Birch NJ, ed. *Lithium: inorganic pharmacology and psychiatric use*. Oxford: IRL Press, 1988;161–162.

84. Tondo L, Floris GF, Burrai C, Pani PP. Lithium withdrawal: an outcome. In: Birch NJ, ed. *Lithium: inorganic pharmacology and psychiatric use*. Oxford: IRL Press, 1988;155–156.

85. Greil W, Schmidt ST. Terminating lithium long-term treatment. In: Birch NJ, ed. *Lithium: inorganic pharmacology and psychiatric use*. Oxford: IRL Press, 1988;149–153.

86. Puzynski S, Klosiewicz L. Valproic acid amide as a prophylactic agent in affective and schizoaffective disorders. In: Emrich HM, Okuma T, Muller AA, eds. *Anticonvulsants in affective disorders*. Amsterdam: Excerpta Medica, 1984; 68–75.

87. McElroy SL, Keck PE Jr, Pope HG Jr, et al. Valproate in the treatment of rapid-cycling disorder. *J Clin Psychopharmacol* 1988;8:275–279.

88. Bourgeois BFD. Anticonvulsant potency and neurotoxicity of valproate alone and in combination with carbamazepine or phenobarbital. *Clin Neuropharmacol* 1988;11:348–359.

89. Callaghan N, Goggin T. Adjunctive therapy in resistant epilepsy. *Epilepsia* 1988;29:S29–S35.

90. Walker JE, Koon R. Carbamazepine versus valproate versus combined therapy for refractory partial complex seizures with secondary generalization. *Epilepsia* 1988;29:693.

91. Dean JC, Penry JK. Carbamazepine/valproate therapy in 100 patients with partial seizures failing carbamazepine monotherapy: long term follow-up. *Epilepsia* 1988;29:687.

92. Chouinard G, Young SN, Annable L. Antimanic effect of clonazepam. *Biol Psychiatry* 1983;18:451–466.

93. Allen J, Jawad S, Oxley J, Trimble M. Development of tolerance to anticonvulsant effect of clobazam. *J Neurol Neurosurg Psychiatry* 1985;48:284–285.

94. Schmutz M, David J, Grewal RS, Bernasconi R, Baltzer V. Pharmacological and neurochemical aspects of tolerance. In: Koella WP, ed. *Tolerance to beneficial and adverse effects of antiepileptic drugs*. Raven Press: New York, 1986; 25–36.

95. Aronson TA, Shukla S, Hirschowitz J. Clonazapam treatment of five lithium-refractory patients with bipolar disorder. *Am J Psychiatry* 1989;146:77–80.

96. Lydiard RB, Laraia MT, Ballenger JC, Howell EF. Emergence of depressive symptoms in patients receiving alprazolam for panic disorder. *Am J Psychiatry* 1987;144:664–665.

97. Arana GW, Pearlman C, Shader RI. Alprazolam-induced mania: two clinical cases. *Am J Psychiatry* 1985;142:368–369.

98. Goodman WK, Charney DS. A case of alprazolam, but not lorazepam, inducing manic symptoms. *J Clin Psychiatry* 1987;48:117–118.

99. Strahan A, Rosenthal J, Kaswan M, Winston A. Three case reports of acute paroxysmal excitement associated with alprazolam treatment. *Am J Psychiatry* 1985;142:859–861.

100. Weiss SRB, Post RM, Patel J, Marangos PS. Differential mediation of the anticonvulsant effects of carbamazepine and diazepam. *Life Sci* 1985;36:2413–2419.

101. Weiss SRB, Post RM, Marangos PJ, Patel J. "Peripheral-type" benzodiazepines: behavioral effects and relationship to the anticonvulsant effects of carbamazepine. In: Wada J, ed. *Kindling III.* New York: Raven Press, 1986; 375–392.

102. Costa E, Manev H, Alho H, Favaron M, Szekely AM, Guidotti A. Neuronal death elicited by glutamate: mechanism of action of its pharmacological inhibition: In: *Abstracts, XVIth CINP annual meeting,* Munich, August 15–19, 1988, p. 116, Abstract FR01.05.

103. Kalinowsky L, Putnam T. Attempts at treatment of schizophrenia and other nonepileptic psychosis with Dilantin. *Arch Neurol Psychiatry* 1943;49:414–423.

104. Kubanek JL, Rowell RC. The use of Dilantin in the treatment of psychotic patients unresponsive to other treatment. *Dis Nerv Syst* 1946; 7:47–50.

105. Freyhan FA. Effectiveness of diphenylhydantoin in management of nonepileptic psychomotor excitement states. *Arch Neurol Psychiatry* 1945;53:370–374.

106. Willow M, Catterall WA. Inhibition of binding of [³H]batrachotoxinin A 20-alpha-benzoate to sodium channels by the anticonvulsant drugs diphenylhydantoin and carbamazepine. *Mol Pharmacol* 1982;22:627–635.

107. McLean MJ, Macdonald RL. Carbamazepine and 10,11-epoxycarbamazepine produce use- and voltage-dependent limitation of rapidly firing action potentials of mouse central neurons in cell culture. *J Pharmacol Exp Ther* 1986; 238:727–738.

108. Morselli PL, Fournier V, Macher JP, et al. Therapeutic action of progabide in depressive illness: a controlled clinical trial. In: Bartholini G, Lloyd KG, Morselli PL, eds. *GABA and mood disorders: experimental and clinical research. (LERS) monograph series,* vol 4. New York: Raven Press, 1986;119–126.

109. Perris C, Tjallden G, Bossi L, Perris H. Progabide versus nortriptyline in depression: a controlled trial. In: Bartholini G, Lloyd KG, Morselli PL, eds. *GABA and mood disorders: experimental and clinical research. LERS monograph series,* vol 4. New York: Raven Press, 1986;135–138.

110. Weiss E, Brunner H, Clere G, et al. Multicenter double-blind study of progabide in depressed patients. In: Bartholini G, Lloyd KG, Morselli PL, eds. *GABA and mood disorders: experimental and clinical research. LERS monograph series,* vol 4. New York: Raven Press, 1986;127–133.

111. Emrich HM, Altmann H, Dose M, von Zerssen D. Therapeutic effects of GABA-ergic drugs in affective disorders. A preliminary report. *Pharmacol Biochem Behav* 1983;19:369–372.

112. Berrettini W, Post RM. GABA and affective illness. In: Post RM, Ballenger JC, eds. *Neurobiology of mood disorders.* Baltimore: Williams & Wilkins, 1984;673–685.

113. Lloyd KG, Thuret EW, Pilc A. GABA and the mechanism of action of antidepressant drugs. In: Bartholini G, Lloyd KG, Morselli PL, eds. *GABA and mood disorders: experimental and clinical research. LERS monograph series,* vol 4. New York: Raven Press, 1986;33–42.

114. Inoue H, Hazama H, Hamazoe K, et al. Antipsychotic and prophylactic effets of acetazolamide (Diamox) on atypical psychosis. *Folia Psychiatr Neurol Jpn* 1984;38:425–436.

115. Andrulonis PA, Donnelly J, Glueck BC. Preliminary data on ethosuximide and the episodic dyscontrol syndromes. *Am J Psychiatry* 1980; 137:1455–1456.

116. Swerdlow M. Anticonvulsant drugs and chronic pain. *Clin Neuropharmacol* 1984;7:51–82.

117. Willow M, Gonoi T, Catterall WA. Voltage clamp analyses of the inhibitory actions of diphenylhydantoin and carbamazepine on voltage-sensitive sodium channels in neuroblastoma cells. *Mol Pharmacol* 1985;27:549–558.

118. Bernasconi R, Martin P. Effects of antileptic drugs on the GABA turnover rate. *Arch Pharmacol* 1979;307:R63.

119. Terrence CF, Sax M, Fromm GH, Chang C-H, Yoo CS. Effect of baclofen enantiomorphs on the spinal trigeminal nucleus and steric similarities of carbamazepine. *Pharmacology* 1983;27: 85–94.

120. Fromm GH, Terrence CF. Comparison of L-baclofen and racemic baclofen in trigeminal neuralgia. *Neurology* 1987;37:1725–1728.

121. Marangos PJ, Weiss SRB, Montgomery P, et al. Chronic carbamazepine treatment increases brain adenosine receptors. *Epilepsia* 1985;26: 493–498.

122. Marangos PJ, Montgomery P, Weiss SRB, Patel J, Post RM. Persistent upregulation of brain adenosine receptors in response to chronic carbamazepine treatment. *Clin Neuropharmacol* 1987;10:443–448.

123. Marangos PJ, Weiss SRB, Post RM. Carbamazepine and brain adenosine receptors. In: Wasterlain, CG, Vert P, eds. Neonatal Seizures, New York: Raven Press, 1990;203–209.

124. Newman M, Zohar J, Kalian M, Belmaker RH. The effects of chronic lithium and ECT on A_1 and A_2 adenosine receptor systems in rat brain. *Brain Res* 1984;291:188–192.

125. Mitsushio H, Takashima M, Mataga N, Toru M. Effects of chronic treatment with trihexy-

phenidyl and carbamazepine alone or in combination with haloperidol on Substance P content in rat brain: a possible implication of Substance P in affective disorders. *J Pharmacol Exp Ther* 1988;245:982–989.

126. Jones RS, Mondadori C, Olpe HR. Neuronal sensitivity to substance P is increased after repeated treatment with tranylcypromine, carbamazepine or oxaprotaline, but decreased after repeated electroconvulsive shock. *Neuropharmacology* 1985;24:627–633.

127. Pratt J, Jenner P, Johnson AL, Showon SD, Reynolds EH. Anticonvulsant drugs alter plasma tryptophan concentrations in epileptic patients: implications for antiepileptic action and mental function. *J Neurol Neurosurg Psychiatry* 1984;47:1131–1133.

128. Rubinow DR, Post RM, Gold PW, Ballenger JC, Reichlin S. Effects of carbamazepine on cerebrospinal fluid somatostatin. *Psychopharmacology* 1985;85:210–213.

129. Steardo L, Barone P, Hunnicutt E. Carbamazepine lowering effect on CSF somatostatin-like immunoreactivity in temporal lobe epilepsy. *Acta Neurol Scand* 1986;74:140–144.

130. Rubinow DR, Post RM, Gold PW, Uhde TW. Effect of carbamazepine on mean urinary free cortisol excretion in patients with major affective illness. *Psychopharmacology* 1986;88:115–118.

131. Weiss SRB, Post RM, Szele F, Woodward R, Nierenberg J. Chronic carbamazepine inhibits the development of local anesthetic seizures kindled by cocaine and lidocaine. *Brain Res* 1989;497:72–79.

132. Weiss SRB, Post RM, Costello M, Woodward R, Tandeciarz S, Nutt D. Carbamazepine retards the development of cocaine-kindled seizures but not sensitization to cocaine's effects on hyperactivity and stereotypy. *Neuropsychopharmacol* 1990;3:273–281.

133. Post RM, Weiss SRB, Pert A. Cocaine-induced behavioral sensitization and kindling: implications for the emergence of psychopathology and seizures. In: Kalivas PW, Nemeroff CB, eds. *Mesocorticolimbic dopamine system.* New York: New York Academy of Sciences, 1988;292–308.

134. Halikas JA, Kemp KD, Kuhn KL, Carlson GA, Crea F. Carbamazepine for cocaine addiction? [letter] *Lancet* 1989;1:623–624.

135. Post RM, Ballenger JC, Reus VI, Lake CR, Lerner P, Bunney WE Jr. Effects of carbamazepine in mania and depression. In: *New research abstracts. 131st annual meeting of the American Psychiatric Association,* Atlanta, Georgia, May 1978. Abstract 7.

136. Ballenger JC, Post RM. Therapeutic effects of carbamazepine in affective illness: a preliminary report. *Commun Psychopharmacol* 1978;2:159–178.

137. Albright PS. Effects of carbamazepine, clonazepam, and phenytoin on seizure threshold in amygdala and cortex. *Exp Neurol* 1983;79:11–17.

138. Shouse MN, Stoh PJ, Vreeken T. Anticonvulsant drug selectively affects kindling and penicillin V epilepsy, especially during seizure-prone sleep or awakening states in cats. *Epilepsia* 1989;30:7–16.

139. Luchins DJ. Carbamazepine in normal EEG violent psychotics. In: *Proceedings of the 137th annual meeting of the American Psychiatric Association,* Los Angeles, California, May 1984.

140. Luchins DJ. Carbamazepine in violent non-epileptic schizophrenia. *Psychopharmacol Bull* 1984;20:569–571.

141. Halgren E. The amygdala contribution to emotion and memory: current studies in humans. In: Ben-Ari Y, ed. *The amygdaloid complex. INSERM Symposium,* no. 20. Amsterdam: Elsevier/No. Holland Biomedical Press, 1981;395–408.

142. Maldonado HM, Delgado-Escuetta AV, Walsh GO, Swartz BE, Rand RW. Complex partial seizures of hippocampal and amygdalar origin. *Epilepsia* 1988;29:420–433.

143. Kellner CH, Post RM, Putnam FK, et al. Intravenous procaine as a probe of limbic system activity in psychiatric patients and normal controls. *Biol Psychiatry* 1987;22:1107–1126.

144. Lennox WG. *Epilepsy and related disorders.* Boston: Little, Brown, 1960.

145. Rose DF, Smith PD, Sato S. Magnetoencephalography and epilepsy research. *Science* 1987;238:329–335.

146. Baxter LR, Phelps ME, Mazziotta JC, Gruzi BH, Schwartz JM. Differentiation of depressive disorders with positron emission tomography. In: *Abstracts of the 140th annual meeting of the American Psychiatric Association,* Chicago, Illinois, May 1987, p. 45, Abstract 11A.

147. Post RM, DeLisi LE, Holcomb HH, Uhde TW, Cohen R, Buchsbaum MS. Glucose utilization in the temporal cortex of affectively ill patients: positron emission tomography. *Biol Psychiatry* 1987;22:46–54.

148. Engel J Jr, Kuhl DE, Phelps ME. Patterns of human local cerebral glucose metabolism during epileptic seizures. *Science* 1982;218:64–66.

149. Theodore WH, Fishbein D, Deitz M, Baldwin P. Complex partial seizures: cerebral metabolism. *Epilepsia* 1987;28:319–323.

150. Shaikh MB, Edinger HM, Seigel A. Carbamazepine regulates feline aggression elicited from the midbrain periaqueductal gray. *Pharmacol Biochem Behav* 1988;30:409–415.

151. Goddard GV, McIntire DC, Leech CK. A permanent change in brain function resulting from daily electrical stimulation. *Exp Neurol* 1969;25:295.

152. Racine R. Kindling: the first decade. *Neurosurgery* 1978;3:234–252. Rivinus TM. Psychiatric effects of the anticonvulsant regimens. *J Clin Psychopharmacol* 1982;2:165–192.

153. Pinel JPJ, Rovner LI. Electrode placement and kindling-induced experimental epilepsy. *Exp Neurol* 1978;58:335–346.

154. Pinel JPJ, Rovner LI. Experimental epileptogenesis: kindling-induced epilepsy in rats. *Exp Neurol* 1978;58:190–202.

155. Pinel JPJ. Kindling-induced experimental epilepsy in rats: cortical stimulation. *Exp Neurol* 1981;72:559–569.

156. Wada JA, Sato M, Corcoran ME. Persistent seizure susceptibility and recurrent spontaneous seizures in kindled cats. *Epilepsia* 1974;15:465–478.

157. McNamara JO, Russell RD, Rigsbee L, Bonhaus DW. Anticonvulsant and antiepileptic actions of MK-801 in the kindling and electroshock models. *Neuropharmacology* 1988;27:563–568.

158. Pinel JPJ. Effects of diazepam and diphenylhydantoin on elicited and spontaneous seizures in kindled rats: a double dissociation. *Pharmacol Biochem Behav* 1983;18:61–63.

159. Sutula T, Xiao-Xian H, Cavazos J, Scott G. Synaptic reorganization in the hippocampus induced by abnormal functional activity. *Science* 1988;239:1147–1150.

160. Collingridge GL, Bliss TVP. NMDA receptors—their role in long-term potentiation. *Trends Neurosci* 1987;10:288–293.

161. Wehr TA, Goodwin FK. Rapid cycling in manic–depressives by tricyclic antidepressants. *Arch Gen Psychiatry* 1979;36:555–559.

162. Wehr TA, Goodwin FK. Can antidepressants cause mania and worsen the course of affective illness? *Am J Psychiatry* 1987;144:1403–1411.

163. Kukopulos A, Reginaldi D, Laddomada P, Floris G, Serra G, Tondo L. Course of the manic–depressive cycle and changes caused by treatment. *Pharmakopsychiatria* 1980;13:156–167.

164. Kukopulos A, Caliari B, Tundo A, et al. Rapid cyclers, temperament, and antidepressants. *Compr Psychiatry* 1983;24:249–258.

165. Wehr TA, Sack DA, Rosenthal NE, Cowdry RW. Rapid cycling affective disorder: contributing factors and treatment response. *Am J Psychiatry* 1988;145:179–184.

166. Kupfer DJ, Carpenter LL, Frank E. Possible role of antidepressants in precipitating mania and hypomania in recurrent depression. *Am J Psychiatry* 1988;145:804–808.

167. Weiss SRB, Post RM. Development and reversal of conditioned inefficacy and tolerance to the anticonvulsant effects of carbamazepine. *Epilepsia* 1990;in press.

168. Pakalnis A, Drake MD Jr, John K, Kellum JB. Forced normalization: acute psychosis after seizure control in seven patients. *Arch Neurol* 1987;44:289–292.

169. Killian JM, Fromm GH. Carbamazepine (Tegretol) in the treatment of neuralgia: use and side effects. *Arch Neurol* 1968;19:129–136.

170. Frankenburg FR, Tohen M, Cohen BM, et al. Long-term response to carbamazepine: a retrospective study. *J Clin Psychopharmacol* 1988;8:130–132.

171. Leverich GS, Post RM, Rosoff AS. Factors associated with relapse during maintenance treatment of affective disorders. *International Clin Psychopharm*, 1990;5:135–156.

172. Donaldson SR. Tolerance to phenelzine and subsequent refractory depression: three cases. *J Clin Psychiatry* 1989;50:33–35.

173. Babington RG, Wedeking PW. Blockade of tardive seizures in rats by electroconvulsive shock. *Brain Res* 1975;88:141–144.

174. Post RM, Putnam FW, Contel NR. Electroconvulsive shock inhibits amygdala kindling. In: *Proceedings of the 11th annual meeting of the Society for Neuroscience.* Los Angeles, California, 1981, p. 587, Abstract 187.13.

175. Tsuru N, Ninomiya H, Fukuoka H, Nakahara D. Alterations of amygdaloid kindling phenomenon following repeated electroconvulsive shocks in rats. *Folia Psychiatr Neurol Jpn* 1981;35:167–174.

176. Urca G, Frenk H. Electroconvulsive shock disrupts amygdaloid kindling: dissociation between behavioral and electrographic events. *Exp Neurol* 1982;78:492–502.

177. Handforth A. Postseizure inhibition of kindled seizures by electroconvulsive shock. *Exp Neurol* 1982;78:483–491.

178. Post RM, Ballenger JC, Uhde TW, Bunney WE Jr. Efficacy of carbamazepine in manic–depressive illness: implications for underlying mechanisms. In: Post RM, Ballenger JC, eds. *Neurobiology of mood disorders.* Baltimore: Williams & Wilkins, 1984;777–816.

179. Okuma T, Inanaga K, Otsuki S, et al. Comparison of the antimanic efficacy of carbamazepine and chlorpromazine: a double-blind controlled study. *Psychopharmacology* 1979;66:211–217.

180. Klein E, Bental E, Lerer B, et al. Carbamazepine and haloperidol in excited psychoses. *Arch Gen Psychiatry* 1984;41:165–170.

181. Grossi E, Sacchetti E, Vita A, et al. Carbamazepine vs. chlorpromazine in mania: a double-blind trial. In: Emrich HM, Okuma T, Muller AA, eds. *Anticonvulsants in affective disorders.* Amsterdam: Excerpta Medica, 1984;177–187.

182. Emrich HM, Dose M, von Zerssen D. The use of sodium valproate, carbamazepine and oxcarbazepine in patients with affective disorders. *J Affective Disord* 1985;8:243–250.

183. Lerer B, Moor N, Meyendorff E, et al. Carbamazepine versus lithium in mania: a double-blind study. *J Clin Psychiatry* 1987;48:89–93.

184. Brown D, Silverstone T, Cookson J. Carbamazepine compared to haloperidol in acute mania. *Int Clin Psychopharmacol* 1989;4:229–238.

185. Cookson JC. Carbamazepine in acute mania: a practical review. *Int Clin Psychopharmacol* 1987;2:11–22.

186. Lenzi A, Lazzerini F, Grossi E, et al. Use of carbamazepine in acute psychosis: a controlled study. *J Int Med Res* 1986;14:78–84.
187. Desai NG, Gangadhar BN, Channabasavanna SM, et al. Carbamazepine hastens therapeutic action of lithium in mania. In: *Proceedings of the international conference on new directions in affective disorders*, Jerusalem, 1987.
188. Okuma T, Yamashita I, Takahashi R, et al. Double blind controlled studies on the therapeutic efficacy of carbamazepine in affective and schizophrenic patients. *Psychopharmacol* [*Suppl*] *Abstr XVI CINP Congr* 1988;96:102 [Abstract TH 18.5].
189. Post RM, Uhde TW, Ballenger JC, Squillace KM. Prophylactic efficacy of carbamazepine in manic–depressive illness. *Am J Psychiatry* 1983;140:1602–1604.
190. Okuma T, Inanaga K, Otsuki S, et al. A preliminary double-blind study of the efficacy of carbamazepine in prophylaxis of manic depressive illness. *Psychopharmacology* 1981;73:95–96.
191. Lambert PA, Carraz G, Borselli S, et al. Le dipropylacetamide dans le traitement de la psychose maniaco–depressive. *Encephale* 1975;1:25–31.
192. Lambert PA. Acute and prophylactic therapies of patients with affective disorders using valpromide (dipropylacetamide). In: Emrich HM, Okuma T, Muller AA, eds. *Anticonvulsants in affective disorders*. Amsterdam: Excerpta Medica, 1984;33–44.
193. Semadeni GW. Clinical study of the normothymic effects of dipropylacetamide. *Acta Psychiatr Belg* 1976;76:458–466.
194. Emrich HM, von Zerssen D, Kissling W, Moller H-J, Windorfer A. Effect of sodium valproate in mania. The GABA-hypothesis of affective disorders. *Arch Psychiatr Nervenkr* 1980;229:1–16.
195. Emrich HM, Dose M, von Zerssen D. Action of sodium-valproate and of oxcarbazepine in patients with affective disorders. In: Emrich HM, Okuma T, Muller AA, eds. *Anticonvulsants in affective disorders*. Amsterdam: Excerpta Medica, 1984;45–55.
196. Vencovsky E, Soucek K, Kabes J. Prophylactic effect of dipropylacetamide in patients with bipolar affective disorder—short communication. In: Emrich HM, Okuma T, Muller AA, eds. *Anticonvulsants in affective disorders*. Amsterdam: Excerpta Medica, 1984;pp. 66–67.
197. Brennan MJW, Sandyk R, Borseek D. Use of sodium-valproate in the management of affective disorders: basic and clinical aspects. In: Emrich HM, Okuma T, Muller AA, eds. *Anticonvulsants in affective disorders*. Amsterdam: Excerpta Medica, 1984;56–65.
198. Prasad AJ. The role of sodium valproate as an anti-manic agent. *Pharmatherapeutica* 1984;4:6–8.
199. McElroy SL, Keck PE Jr, Pope HG Jr. Sodium valproate: its use in primary psychiatric disorders. *J Clin Psychopharmacol* 1987;7:16–24.
200. Brown R. U.S. experience with valproate in manic depressive illness: a multicenter trial. *J Clin Psychopharmacol* 1989;50:13–16.
201. Hayes SG. Long-term use of valproate in primary psychiatric disorders. *J Clin Psychopharmacol* 1989;50(suppl):35–39.
202. Calabrese JR and Delucchi GA. Spectrum of efficacy of valproate in 55 patients with rapid-cycling bipolar disorder. *Am J Psychi* 1990;147:431–434.
203. Sovner R. The use of valproate in the treatment of mentally retarded persons with typical and atypical bipolar disorders. *J Clin Psychopharmacol* 1989;50(suppl):40–43.
204. Porter RJ, Penry JK. Efficacy and choice of antiepileptic drugs. In: Meinardi H, Rowan AJ, eds. *Psychology, pharmacology, and new diagnostic approaches. Advances in epileptology, 1977*. Amsterdam: Swets & Zeitlinger, 1978;220–230.
205. Post RM. Alternatives to lithium for bipolar affective illness. In: Tasman A, Goldfinger SM, Kaufmann CA, eds. *Review of Psychiatry*, Vol. 9, Washington, DC: American Psychiatric Press, 1990:170–202.
206. Post RM, Leverich G, Rosoff AS and Altshuler LL. Carbamazepine prophylaxis in refractory affective disorders: A focus on long-term followup. *J of Clin Psychopharmacol* 1990;in press.
207. Kishimoto A, Kamata K, Sugihara T, Ishiguro S, Hazama H, Mizukawa R, Kunimoto N. Treatment of depression with clonazepam. *Acta Psychiatr Scand* 1988;77:81–86.

Advances in Neurology, Vol. 55, edited by
D. Smith, D. Treiman, and M. Trimble,
Raven Press, Ltd., New York © 1991.

17

Effects of Temporal Lobe Surgery on Behavior

Rebecca Rausch

*Reed Neurological Research Center, Department of Psychiatry and Biobehavioral Sciences and
Department of Neurology, University of California, Los Angeles,
Los Angeles, California 90024*

BEHAVIOR STUDIES IN TEMPORAL LOBE SURGERY FOR EPILEPSY

An acceptable treatment for medically intractable seizures documented to originate from a temporal lobe is unilateral temporal lobe surgery. In carefully selected cases, the surgery has proven highly effective in controlling seizure activity (1,2). The most direct behavior consequence of surgery is a selective decrease in memory functioning. On the other hand, successful surgical treatment has also been shown to relate to improvement in selective cognitive functions, emotional status, and psychosocial functioning.

The specific pattern and extent of postoperative memory change are dependent upon (a) the anatomical boundaries of the resection and (b) the functional significance of the removed tissue. The locus and extent of temporal lobe tissue excised may vary among the several surgical centers as well as within a given center. The surgical parameters are dependent upon the following factors:

1. seizure onset characteristics;
2. interictal epileptiform activity (determined by surface, depth, and/or intraoperative monitoring);
3. identifiable underlying pathology;
4. functional localization determined, in part, by the intracarotid sodium amylobarbital procedure and/or speech/cognitive mapping; and
5. surgical philosophy of the surgical center.

Standardized Resections

The various surgical approaches for intractable temporal lobe epilepsy have been eloquently described by Crandall (3). In selective surgical centers, if the primary epileptic focus is documented to originate from within the mesial temporal lobe, standardized temporal lobe resections are performed. The standard resection, first described by Falconer (4,5), removes the mesial component of the involved temporal lobe, including 2.5 cm of hippocampus, hippocampal gyrus, uncus, two-thirds of the amygdala, and the lateral temporal neocortex. To avoid primary language cortex, the left language-dominant temporal lobe neocortical resection is slightly smaller than the right temporal lobe resection. The left resection extends 5.0–5.5 cm from the anterior tip as measured along the middle temporal gyrus; the right nondominant temporal lobe resection extends 6.0–6.5 cm from the anterior tip. The magnetic resonance imaging (MRI) scan is frequently used to confirm the parameters of the surgery (3).

Behavior studies utilizing patients who are candidates for or who have undergone a standardized temporal lobe resection have provided systematic data addressing the functional significance of the resected temporal lobe area. Such studies have utilized within-group comparisons; that is, the same patients were studied both prior to and following surgery. This approach enabled identification of the direct effects of left and right temporal lobe surgery on the epileptic brain.

In addition, between-subjects designs have been incorporated; groups of patients who have undergone either a standardized left versus right temporal lobectomy were compared. The strengths of these latter studies lay in their lateralization of hemispheric functions. Patients' performances in both types of studies have been compared to either matched nonsurgical epilepsy patients, patients with surgery outside the temporal lobe, or normal controls, with groups matched for age, education, and/or socioeconomic status. Lastly, the standardized resection typically involved an "en bloc" removal of the tissue. Neuropathological analyses of the resected tissue provide potential quantitative data that document preoperative selective lesions within the temporal lobe. Correlation of this information with preoperative selective cognitive deficits have provided evidence for functional specificity of temporal lobe substructures (see, e.g., ref. 6).

Variation in Surgical Boundaries

In contrast to surgical programs that utilize a standardized approach, centers that vary the boundaries of surgery according to the extent of involved tissue provide potentially rich material to compare the effects of lesion parameters. Brenda Milner and her colleagues at the Montreal Neurological Institute (MNI) have studied a large series of such patients. These endeavors have addressed the memory effects of both (a) large versus small mesial temporal lobe lesions and (b) mesial versus lateral temporal lobe lesions.

However, as pointed out by Awad et al. (7), studies correlating extent of resection with memory deficits have relied mostly upon intraoperative linear measurements. Recent data indicate that there have been limitations to the accuracy of such measures. As with the standardized approach, MRI has been reported as an important surgical adjunct to provide additional measures of the anatomical boundaries of the resection (8). The correlation between extent of removal of temporal lobe subregions (as documented by postoperative MRI scans) and postoperative cognitive deficits appears to be a promising brain–behavior research tool.

Cross-Center Behavior Comparisons

Factors limiting comparison of the effects of temporal lobe surgery among surgical centers include patient selection, temporal factors, medication, seizure activity, and variations in surgical approach (9). For example, cognitive changes associated with a large temporal lobe resection at a center that utilizes a standardized resection for localized temporal lobe seizures are likely to differ from those associated with a similar large resection but at a center that tailors the surgery to the extent of cortical involvement. Patients from the latter center, when compared to those from the former one, are more likely to have greater preexisting brain pathology. Also, since our present technology is less than optimal in identifying underlying pathology (10), patients from the latter center are also more likely to have damaged tissue (albeit non-epileptic) outside the resection boundary. The most obvious temporal factor affecting the extent of cognitive changes associated with surgery is the time interval between surgery and assessment. The extent or presence of memory deficits associated with similar surgeries will differ significantly if one assessment is performed 1 month after surgery and the other one is performed 1 year after surgery. During the early postoperative period, enhanced cognitive deficits may be observed as a result of transient effects of surgery on nonresected brain tissue (e.g., edema; see refs. 11 and 12).

COGNITIVE EFFECTS OF SURGERY

As mentioned above, the cognitive consequences of temporal lobe surgery are dependent not only upon the anatomical parameters of the surgery but also upon the functional significance of the involved tissue. In regard to the latter, it should be emphasized that the majority of such seizure patients have had long-standing intractable epilepsy. Major hemispheric reorganization of brain function may have occurred prior to surgery. In testing with intracarotid sodium amylobarbital (see below), shifting of language dominance from the left to the right hemisphere has been demonstrated to occur in a significant number of patients with left temporal lobe epilepsy

(13,14). The shift in hemispheric language dominance is frequently present even though the patient remains right-handed (14,15). In addition, intrahemispheric functional changes may occur (16). For example, functions normally dependent upon anterior neocortical areas may shift more posteriorly. Intraoperative functional mapping has been useful in the localization of selective language behavior sites in the temporal neocortex (17). Thus, even in centers that perform standardized temporal lobe surgery, prediction of the specific profile of cognitive deficits subsequent to temporal lobe surgery is limited. Nevertheless, as will be discussed below, two general cognitive changes potentially associated with temporal lobe surgery include (i) a risk for global amnesia and (ii) modality-specific cognitive deficits.

Risk for Global Amnesia

If unilateral resection of mesial temporal lobe structures is undertaken in a patient whose contralateral temporal lobe cannot maintain global memory functioning, a severe amnesic syndrome will occur. Strong evidence for this conclusion is provided by the classic case of H.M., a patient with intractable epilepsy who became severely amnesic following an experimental surgery to control his epilepsy. The surgery included bilateral removal of the hippocampal gyrus, hippocampal pes, amygdala, and uncus, leaving intact the lateral neocortex. Since surgery, this patient has exhibited severe and persistent impairment in the conscious learning of new information (18,19).

Direct evidence that unilateral resections may result in an amnesic syndrome if the contralateral temporal lobe is dysfunctional is available from detailed case reports by Penfield and Milner (20) and by Penfield and Mathieson (21). The patient in the latter study underwent two surgeries of the left temporal lobe, with an amnesic syndrome occurring after the second surgery (see Fig. 1). The first surgery involved excision of only the anterior 4 cm of the lateral temporal lobe but left intact the mesial structures, including amygdala, hippocampus, hippocampal gyrus, and uncus. The second surgery leading to the amnesic syndrome removed the latter structures. Au-

topsy was performed on the patient years later and revealed marked neuronal loss within the hippocampus of the unresected right temporal lobe. Taken together, these two cases (20,21) strongly indicate that, following a unilateral mesial temporal lobe resection, new declarative learning requires the presence of functional contralateral mesial temporal lobe structures.

To avoid amnesic syndromes in patients undergoing unilateral temporal lobe surgery, Milner et al. (22) of the MNI introduced the use of the carotid sodium amylobarbital procedure. The procedure has been adopted by most epilepsy-surgery programs, although there have been numerous modifications of the original protocol (15,23,24). Generally, the intracarotid sodium amylobarbital procedure (IAP) involves injection of sodium amylobarbital directly into the internal carotid artery of the proposed surgical hemisphere. This results in a temporary, 2- to 3-minute pharmacological ablation of the proposed surgical hemisphere. During this time, a brief assessment of language and memory competence of the contralateral hemisphere is made.

Ever since the introduction of the IAP for memory testing at the MNI, there have been no reports from that center of severe amnesia following unilateral temporal lobe surgery (25). Data from the University of California— Los Angeles (UCLA) also indicate good outcome with this procedure. Rausch et al. (26) recently reported that impaired memory performance during drug perfusion of a hemisphere correlated significantly with a seizure focus in the noninjected hemisphere. Furthermore, severe hippocampal damage in the noninjected hemisphere was found to be systematically detected by poor memory performance; one exception was a patient whose posterior cerebral artery ipsilateral to the drug injection did not perfuse. Thus, the perfusion pattern of the drug must be considered in estimating the validity of the procedure. It should be noted that one case of a postoperative amnesic syndrome has been identified by the IAP (27).

Whereas several centers highly regard the diagnostic value of the IAP, others have reported difficulties with the procedure (28). The marked variations in protocols performed among the various surgical centers must be

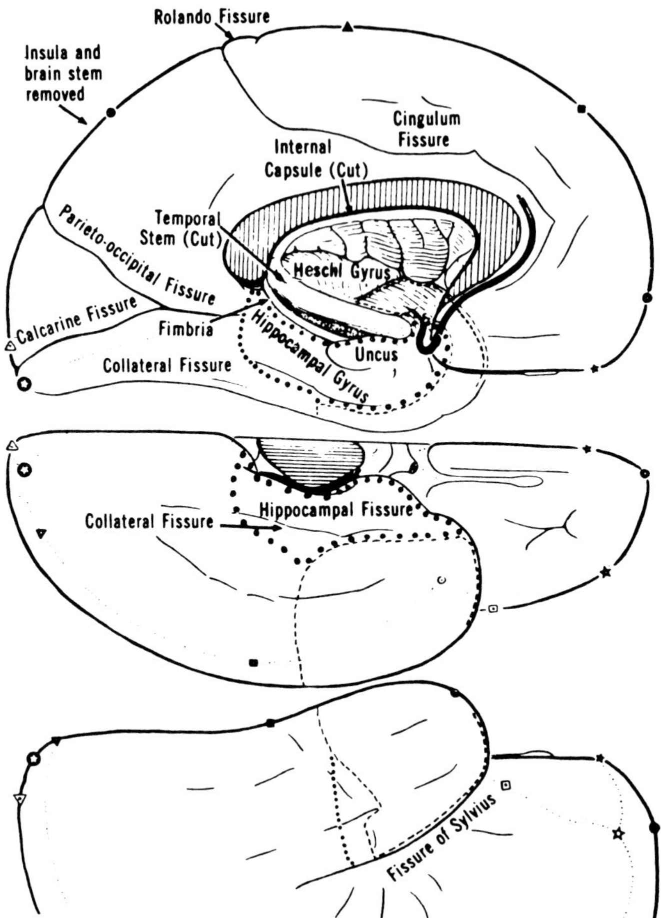

FIG. 1. Surgeon's postoperative drawing. Cortical excision indicated by the fine broken line did not produce amnesia. Excision indicated by the dotted line resulted in amnesia. Autopsy showed that at least 1 cm more of hippocampus proper and hippocampal gyrus was spared. (From ref. 21, with permission.)

considered. Patient selection, speed and dosage of injection, and behavioral assessment techniques have all been reported as variants (25). Such differences in patient selection and protocols are most likely to be important in the conflicting results reported. For example, one center reporting unreliable results with the IAP has found a 20% memory failure rate in the areas of brain ipsilateral to the proposed temporal lobe surgery. This is in marked contrast to several other centers, whose failure rates in the areas of brain ipsilateral to the site of surgery were 1% or less (25).

Selective Cognitive/Memory Changes

Unlike bilateral temporal lobe surgery, unilateral temporal lobe surgery typically results in selective memory losses. The most prominent deficiency is not in primary memory (e.g., as indicated by the patient's immediate digit span) or in long-term memory but, instead, in the conscious learning and retention of selective *new* memories. Studies of patients who have undergone unilateral temporal lobe surgeries support material-specific memory deficits associated with the side of temporal lobe removal. Resection of the speech-dominant (left) temporal lobe has been found to impair verbal memory (29,30), whereas resection of the nondominant (right) temporal lobe depresses nonverbal memory (31–34). In spite of the selective memory loss, other cognitive functions such as gross language, visual–perceptual, and intellectual skills are generally spared (11,12,31).

The postoperative cognitive changes are related, in part, to the extent of seizure control following surgery. Rausch and Crandall (35) reported that, following left (language-dominant) temporal lobe surgery, patients whose seizures were controlled by surgery (as well as those whose seizures were not controlled by surgery) showed a reduction in verbal memory functioning. However, those patients with seizures controlled by surgery exhibited less deterioration in scores than did those whose seizures continued postoperatively. A minor deficiency in the verbal learning of those patients successfully treated has a lesser impact in light of the associated cognitive increments. Temporal lobe epilepsy patients successfully treated with surgery improve in intellectual scores, frontal lobe function, and selective memory functions associated with the nonsurgical hemisphere (35–37).

Left (Language-Dominant) Temporal Lobe Changes

As a result of the continued integrity of general language and cognitive status among temporal lobectomy patients, studies delineating the nature of their verbal memory deficits have been possible. Studies of patients who have undergone left (language-dominant) temporal lobe resections have identified deficits in multiple verbal memory processes. These can be classified as deficiencies in (a) rote-verbal learning, (b) semantic organization/ learning, and (c) confrontational naming. The first two deficiencies reflect the previously described weakness in conscious new verbal learning. The third deficiency—difficulty in confrontational naming—differs from the others: A selective weakness exists in the ability to retrieve from old memories (e.g., that of re-

calling names). The three affected domains will be described below, with speculations as to underlying anatomical substrates.

Rote-Verbal Learning

Deficits in rote-verbal learning are a well-documented consequence of left temporal lobe dysfunction. For example, several reports demonstrate that patients who have undergone a left temporal lobectomy are markedly impaired in the ability to learn unrelated word-pairs from the Wechsler Memory Scale (WMS) (38; also see refs. 31, 35, and 39). The memory deficit is enhanced if an interrupted delay intervenes between learning and recall. The deficiency in learning is not as marked if the words are semantically related. Thus, unlike unrelated word-pairs, learning of related word-pairs from the WMS has not been consistently depressed in this patient group (40). Also, while a rote-verbal learning deficiency has been reported in both auditory and visual modalities (41), the deficit has been most consistently observed in the auditory domain (42). It is possible that visual presentation of word-pairs encourages multiple encoding strategies.

A rote-verbal learning deficit in left temporal lobectomy patients is easily demonstrated by word-list learning tasks (43,44).[1] For example, using the Bushke Selective Reminding Task (45), a specific type of word-list learning, left temporal lobectomy patients have been shown to have difficulties in several verbal learning processes (43). On first presentation trials of the word-list, left temporal lobectomy patients entered fewer words into long-term storage [as defined by Bushke (45)] than did either patients with right temporal lobectomy or normal controls. In addition, once the words were learned or entered into long-term storage on later trials, left temporal lobectomy patients were impaired in their ability to consistently recall the words. The processing deficits in initial learning and in recall were parallel and appeared to reflect similar underlying deficiencies. It should be

---

[1]Several tasks described as rote learning incorporate other learning strategies. They are discussed here because the primary learning strategy is rote.

noted that the left temporal lobectomy patients performed significantly better on the list-learning task if the words were semantically related than if they were unrelated (43). Thus, the left temporal lobectomy patients were aided in learning by the semantic characteristics of the words.

Semantic/Organizational Learning

Left temporal lobectomy patients have also been shown to have subtle deficits in *semantic/organizational* memory. Left temporal lobectomy patients do not organize or cluster in the free recall of a list of words to the same extent as do controls (44). They demonstrate a deficiency, as measured by reaction speed, in semantically classifying drawings or words (46), and they overgeneralize in their recall of semantically related material (47). In addition, there is a tendency (although not as extreme as for frontal-lobe-damaged patients) for left temporal lobectomy patients to make more intrusion errors in word-list learning when compared to normal controls (43). Although left temporal lobectomy patients have been noted to perform worse than normal controls on several semantic measures, it should be emphasized that such deficiencies are mild and less evident than rote-verbal learning impairments. Also, as mentioned above, left temporal lobectomy patients are able to utilize semantic characteristics of words to aid their deficient rote-learning skills.

Recalling the details and gist of a recent story reflects both rote-learning and complex semantic and grammatical processing. Left temporal lobectomy patients have been shown to be deficient in such behavior as assessed by the Logical Prose Subtest of the WMS. However, depressed performance on this measure has not been as reliably observed as that on the more rote-verbal learning tasks (47,48). Indeed, it is not unusual to find left temporal lobectomy patients with significantly impaired rote-learning skills and intact recall of prose (40).

Confrontational Naming

A mild depression in confrontational naming is a sequela of left temporal lobectomy. The naming weakness is frequently not obvious to the casual observer but can be demonstrated by formal testing [e.g., by the Boston Naming Test (49)]. In many instances, the deficiency can be quite frustrating to the patient. Figure 2 shows proposed boundaries of language areas of the cortex; a standardized left temporal lobe resection is superimposed. To avoid potential naming problems with left temporal lobe resections, functional mapping has been used to localize primary language areas (17).

Proposed Anatomical Substrates

Several deficiencies in processing of verbal material associated with left temporal lobe surgery appear to be related to different temporal lobe subregions. There has been a tendency in the literature to attribute all temporal lobe memory functions to mesial structures. The interpretation is due, in part, to reports of global memory deficits associated with bilateral temporal lobe damage. Left mesial temporal lobe structures are generally regarded to be responsible for all verbal memory functions, and right mesial temporal lobe structures are hypothesized to be responsible for all nonverbal memory functions. However, new evidence from studies indicates that different types of memory-processing deficits

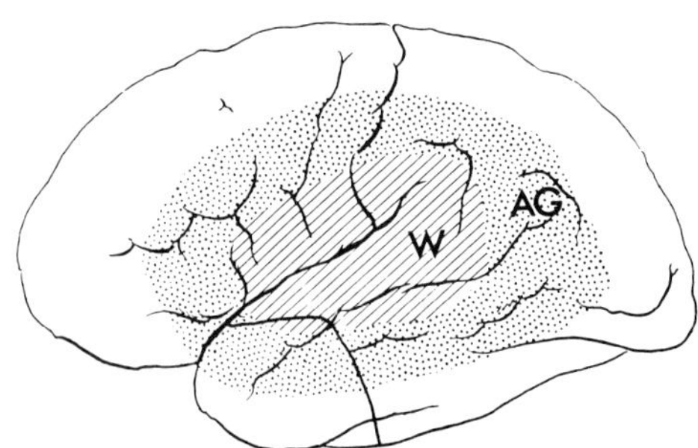

FIG. 2. Outline of left hemisphere cortex indicating areas where pathology produces aphasia. Pathology in areas marked by diagonal lines almost invariably produces aphasia. Pathology in areas marked by stippling frequently results in aphasia. Solid line represents excision line of a standardized left temporal lobe surgery. W: Wernicke's area, AG: Angular area. (Modified from ref. 51, with permission.)

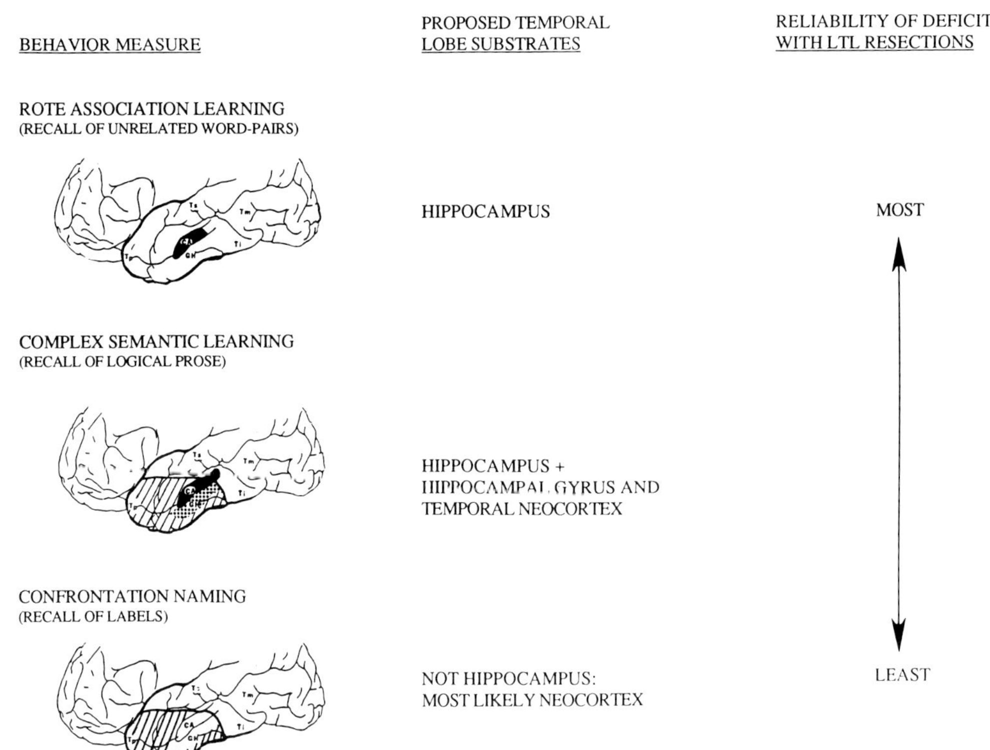

FIG. 3. Behavior measures sensitive to left (language-dominant) temporal lobe (LTL) surgery.

occur with verbal and nonverbal modalities in patients with lesions of various temporal lobe subregions.

Figure 3 shows three measures frequently impaired following left (language-dominant) temporal lobe surgery. The measures are listed in order of the predictability or reliability of being depressed following standardized temporal lobe surgery. Anatomical subregions of the temporal lobe that may potentially be involved in the mediation of such behaviors are also listed.

Rote-verbal (association) learning (i.e., the learning of unrelated word-pairs), as mentioned earlier, is a highly predictable deficit following left temporal lobe surgery. Data from our laboratory indicate that this measure is dependent upon the extent of damage within the hippocampus proper (6). In such studies, damage to the various subregions of the temporal lobe is determined by quantitative pathological analyses on resected temporal lobe tissue. We find that preoperative performance on learning and retaining unrelated word-pairs significantly correlates with the volumetric density of primary neurons in Ammon's horn subfields of the left hippocampus. The correlated behavioral measure is not related to the integrity of the left hippocampal gyrus or lateral neocortex, nor is it related to the integrity of right temporal lobe structures. The behavior function appears to be dependent solely upon the integrity of the left hippocampus proper.

Deficiencies in processing logical prose are less reliably observed in left temporal lobectomy patients. Our research suggests that this measure may be more dependent upon more recently evolved cortex (such as hippocampal gyrus) than upon the archicortex of the hippocampus. Consistent with this view, Ojemann and Dodrill (50) have presented data indicating that lateral left temporal lobe neocortex may be important for maintaining such behavior.

Confrontational naming or word-finding deficiencies following left (language-dominant) temporal lobe resections are difficult to predict. Some patients may show a moderate impairment after surgery, whereas others may show no significant decrease in this ability. Our experience with patients with varying preoperative lesion sites indicates that naming is more dependent upon lateral neocortical structures than upon hippocampus or hippocampal gyrus. Similarly, there have been numerous reports of naming problems associated with neocortical lesions of the dominant temporal lobe (51).

Collectively, these findings indicate that, following a dominant standardized temporal lobe resection, memory deficits closely tied to damage to hippocampus proper are more reliably found than those memory problems more related to neocortical dysfunction. We suggest that the relative sparing of functions associated with extrahippocampal regions reflect the type of cortex involved. This interpretation is supported by the observations of Butters et al. (52) in 1974. They noted, in studies with lower primates, that phylogenetically older neuroanatomical structures (such as the hippocampus—an allocortex) have less recovery of function following damage than do phylogenetically newer areas (such as the hippocampal gyrus and temporal neocortex).

Right Temporal Lobe Changes

Researchers from the MNI have suggested that the nonverbal memory changes associated with right temporal lobe surgery may vary as a function of extent of mesial versus lateral temporal lobe resections. Their studies indicate that extensive mesial temporal lobe resections elicit deficits in learning unfamiliar sequences [i.e., series of turns in a maze (53)], as well as in recalling complex designs with little or no inherent organization (34). The extent of lateral right temporal lobe resections has been implicated in the recall of abstract complex designs with intrinsic structures (54,55).

From our experience at UCLA, deficiencies associated with right-sided (nondominant) standardized temporal lobe lesions have not been as consistently observed as have those associated with standardized dominant temporal lobe lesions (40). Our research shows that right temporal lobectomy patients frequently perform worse on tests of recall of nonverbal material than do left temporal lobe patients and normal controls. However, in the various studies, differences among the several subject groups do not consistently reach significance (9,48). Measures found to be depressed in selective studies in patients who have undergone standardized right temporal lobe resections were the delayed recall of WMS Visual Reproduction Subtest, the Rey Osterrieth Delayed Recall (56), and a modified version of Kimura's Nonsense Figure Test (57). These measures are identical or similar to those reported by MNI to be sensitive to right temporal lobe dysfunction. The differences in surgical results reported from the various surgical centers may reflect a number of variables, including patient selection, surgical approach, and temporal factors (9). It is hoped that future collaborative efforts will be developed to address such issues.

Inconsistent findings of nonverbal deficiencies in patients with standardized right temporal lobe resections are in marked contrast to those verbal deficits strongly correlated with standardized left temporal lobe surgery. It should be noted that a standardized right temporal lobe resection is larger (e.g., it removes approximately 1 cm additional neocortex) than a standardized left temporal lobe resection. There are several explanations for the failure to find consistent deficits with standardized right temporal lobe surgery. First, precise behavior correlates of right anterior temporal lobe may not have been identified. Second, functional correlates of the right hemisphere may not be as tightly associated with its anatomical substrates as those of the left hemisphere. This would result in greater functional plasticity of the right temporal lobe. Third, the right temporal lobe patient groups are not as well-defined as the left (language-dominant) temporal lobe group. The IAP is routinely used to identify hemispheric language dominance in this population. The technique, however, does not allow detection of shifting of nondominant hemispheric (i.e., nonverbal) functions. Thus, there may be a significant population of right temporal lobe patients in whom basal right hemispheric non-dominant functions have shifted to coexist with left hemispheric language functions.

Summary of Cognitive/Memory Changes

Unilateral temporal lobe resection in a patient with an intact contralateral hemisphere memory system is likely to result in selective memory deficits. The extent of memory deficiencies and selective associated cognitive improvements are related to the success of the surgery to relieve seizures. Verbal memory deficiencies associated with left temporal lobe resections have been more consistently reported than have nonverbal memory deficits purported to occur with right temporal lobe resections. Different types of verbal memory deficits appear to be dependent, in part, upon different left temporal lobe substructures. Surgical outcome studies must consider not only the parameters of the surgeries but also the different types of memory processes.

PERSONALITY EFFECTS OF SURGERY

The relationship of temporal lobe surgery and personality factors is extensively reviewed in Chapters 5 and 12 of this volume and will only be briefly discussed here. To date, there has been no strong evidence to indicate that temporal lobectomy for epilepsy produces any consistent psychiatric effect that "is independent of the relief of epilepsy and of the previous personality" (58). Emotional changes that have been most frequently observed are found in patients whose seizures have been controlled. Ferguson and Rayport (59) have described the emotional adjustments that may occur following cessation of a long-standing seizure disorder. For the most part, however, reports have stressed emotional improvements in patients following successful seizure control. Hermann et al. (60) recently documented short-term improvements in multiple indices of psychological distress and psychological well-being following successful surgery. They reported that improvements continued up to 3 months postoperatively and remained constant at 6 months follow-up. It should be noted that

psychosis has not been reported to be aided by successful surgery, except in those rare individuals with a transient psychosis related to the ictal or postictal period.

PSYCHOSOCIAL EFFECTS OF SURGERY

A major drawback of intractable epilepsy is its adverse effect on psychosocial functioning, a significant consideration when evaluating the indication for surgical intervention. It is generally assumed that successful surgical control of seizures will result in psychosocial improvement. Published clinical studies document improved psychosocial functioning in most individuals following surgery for temporal lobe seizures (35,58,61). Psychosocial improvement is strongly influenced by the extent of seizure control. Indeed, when seizure control is taken into account, enhanced psychosocial functioning is not documented unless seizures are completely controlled by surgery (35,60).

In 1982, Rausch and Crandall (35) reported on the changes that occur postoperatively on four measures of psychosocial function: degree of dependency, work performance, family relationships and non-family relationships. These measures, previously used by Horowitz and Cohen (62) and Taylor and Falconer (63) in their studies of temporal lobe epilepsy patients, are shown in Table 1. Three groups of patients were studied before and after surgery. Group A consisted of temporal lobectomy patients whose seizures were controlled by surgery; Group B consisted of patients who showed a significant reduction in seizure frequency ($\geq 75\%$) but who continued to have seizures; and Group C received little or no benefit from surgical treatment. Another group of patients, designated IO, were individuals who underwent diagnostic depth electrodes to localize seizure onset but without success; thus, definitive surgery was not performed. For the present study, these latter patients served as a control group. Patients and family members were interviewed extensively prior to and following temporal lobe surgery.

Figure 4 shows that postoperative improvement in psychosocial functioning is directly related to relief from seizures. Patients whose

TABLE 1. *Psychosocial measures used by Rausch and Crandall (35)*

Degree of dependency:	A rating of 1–6. The lowest score is "1," which represents "self-sufficiency, ability to care for others where necessary"; the highest score is "6," which indicates "personal needs only or unable to care for self."
Work, housework, or school performance:	A rating of 1–5, with "1" representing "works steadily and efficiently with no limitations or able to run home efficiently" and "5," indicating "unable to work, dependent at home on others."
Family relationships:	A rating of 1–5, with "1" representing "social adjustment normal" and "5" representing "unable to live with family as a direct consequence of epilepsy or personality difficulties."
Non-family relationships:	A rating of 1–5, with "1" representing "relations normal" and "5" indicating "unable to make relationships outside of the family."

seizures were completely controlled by surgery, Group A, were the only patients to show improvement in the psychosocial measures. The psychosocial levels of patients in Group B (patients whose seizures showed a worthwhile reduction), Group C, or Group IO did not change significantly. Group A patients improved in three of the four measures: degree of dependency, work performance, and non-family relations. Family relationships did not change in any of the patient groups. This re-

flects the difficulty frequently encountered in attempts to modify family dynamics. It is noteworthy that changes in psychosocial functioning are independent of the language-dominant hemisphere as a surgical site. Hence, verbal deficits associated with left-sided surgery are apparently not a major determinant of postoperative functioning.

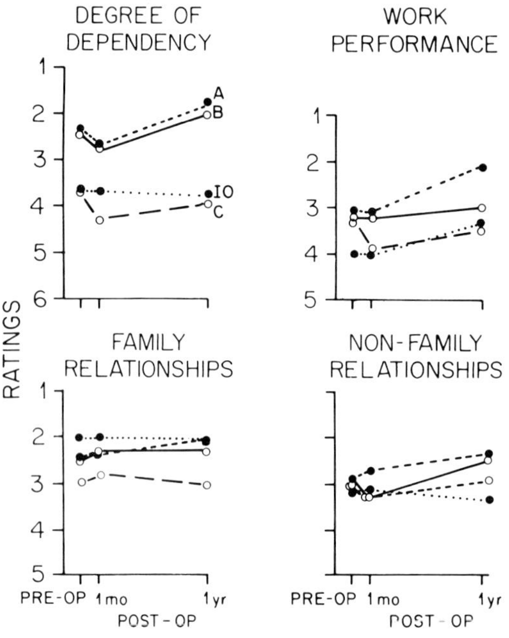

Data from these studies have also provided prognostic information. Patients whose seizures were controlled by surgery and who improved psychosocially after surgery (Group A) functioned at a higher level before surgery than did the other groups. Preoperatively, they exhibited higher levels of psychosocial functioning, higher intellectual scores, and fewer seizures. Thus, it appears that patients who were least affected by their seizure disorder reaped the most benefit from surgical treatment.

PREDICTION OF OPTIMAL OUTCOME

The above study indicates that patients who become seizure-free following surgery will also benefit psychosocially from surgery. With new advances, patients who undergo temporal lobe surgery now are more likely to have their seizures completely controlled (1). The question thus becomes, which of those patients who undergo "successful" surgery will benefit the most psychosocially? In 1986, a study was undertaken to identify *before* surgery those patients who would most likely benefit the most psychosocially from successful seizure control (64). The dependent variable was a psychosocial measure composed of those four measures used in the Rausch and

FIG. 4. Psychosocial functioning prior to and at 1 month and at 1 year following temporal lobe surgery. The patient groups are described in the text. (From ref. 64, with permission.)

Crandall (35) study (i.e., degree of dependency, work performance, family relationships, non-family relations) plus a fifth measure, personal satisfaction. Scores in personal satisfaction, a scale originally described by Horowitz and Cohen (62), ranged from a high of "1" (i.e., satisfied or reasonably contented) to a low of "5" (i.e., suicidal discontented).

The choice of the dichotomized predictive variables was based on preliminary studies (64) and included:

1. *Age at surgery:* < 30 years versus ⩾ 30 years.

2. *Preoperative good family support* (Yes versus No): Appropriate relative [e.g., spouse (if patient is married) or parents and siblings (if patient is single)] provides the patient with emotional security, is supportive in stressful/critical situations, and helps the patient follow medical instructions, including the taking of medicines and getting to appointments if the patient requires this assistance. The relative does not deprecate the patient's self-esteem but rather provides positive reassurance.

3. *Degree of psychopathology:* < 3 versus > 3 MMPI clinical scales ⩾ 2 standard deviations above mean (i.e., *t*-scores ⩾ 70).

4. *MacAndrew scale* (< 24 versus > 24): A subscale of the MMPI useful as a measure of an addictive personality. This measure has been shown to relate to personality characteristics of alcoholics. We interpret the scale as a measure of taking psychological responsibility for one's own behavior.

In addition to the four predictor variables identified above, the following two direct consequences of surgery were included in the analyses:

5. *Extent of seizure control:* While all patients received significant reduction of seizure frequency, patients could be further categorized in a finer scale as to extent of control (as reported in results of surgery). Seizure control scores were dichotomized as 1 versus 2 or 3.

6. *Cognitive decrease:* For the present study, a significant cognitive decrease is defined as "one in which scores on the appropriate memory tests dropped considerably (greater than 1 standard deviation) and in which the patient or family reported associated difficulty in this area."

The probability of improvement was determined by the number of patients with positive signs on a particular measure who improved psychosocially after surgery divided by the number of patients with positive signs:

Probability of improvement

$$= \frac{\text{Number of patients with positive signs who improve}}{\text{Number of patients with positive signs}}$$

Table 2 shows the conditional probabilities of improvement in psychosocial status after surgery. Note the third column. Given the fact that a given seizure patient has met our center's diagnostic criteria for surgery (65), there

TABLE 2. *Predictors of positive psychosocial outcome*[a]

		Estimate of probability + 1 SD	
Predictor	N	Improved/same	Highest level
If surgery	41	0.83 ± 0.06	0.37 ± 0.08
No or mild cognitive decrease	25	0.96 ± 0.04	0.36 ± 0.10
Excellent seizure control	27	0.89 ± 0.06	0.44 ± 0.10
No or mild psychopathology[b]	17	0.94 ± 0.06	0.59 ± 0.12
Good family support[b]	26	0.92 ± 0.05	0.58 ± 0.10
Nonaddictive personality[b]	22	0.91 ± 0.06	0.45 ± 0.11
Young age at surgery[b]	32	0.84 ± 0.07	0.41 ± 0.09
All preoperative variables[b]	8	1.00	1.00
All variables	3	1.00	1.00

[a]From ref. 64, with permission.
[b]Preoperative variables.

was an estimated 83% chance of improvement in overall psychosocial functioning postoperatively. Thirty-four of the 41 patients operated upon improved postoperatively. Three of these patients' postsurgical scores were essentially the same as those preoperatively. However, since the raters felt that improvement occurred in all areas (but not to a degree to change the rating scale), these patients were rated as improved. The percentage of patients who had good indicators and who improved is shown separately for each measure. Of the preoperative measures, only young age at surgery ($<$ 30 years) did not increase our predictive power. There were eight patients in our study who had all preoperative factors in the positive direction, and all of these patients improved after surgery. Interestingly, the combination of any two of the three contributing preoperative predictors (no or mild psychopathology, good family support, and non-addictive personality) was 100% in predicting improvement after surgery.

The fourth column does not represent a change in psychosocial functioning but represents, instead, the attainment of the highest levels of psychosocial functioning (i.e., working with no limitations; self-sufficient; good social adjustment; and high self-satisfaction). It is more difficult to predict who will achieve the highest levels of functioning as opposed to who will improve. If all positive variables are present preoperatively, our predictive power appears high. The highest predictive power derived from the combination of any two combined variables included good family support in conjunction with either of the personality factors.

Prediction of a decline in psychosocial functioning is difficult; see the third column in Table 3. For any given negative predictor, the highest estimate for an individual is still less than 50%. When considering the combination of any two predictors of poor outcome, it was the combination of poor family support with significant cognitive decrease or the combination of poor family support with addictive personality that increased the predictive value of decreased psychosocial functioning after surgery.

The power in predicting failure to attain the highest psychosocial levels is displayed in the fourth column of Table 3. Family support again played a predominant role. The best predictor of less-than-optimal outcome was poor family support. Not one of the 15 patients with poor family support realized high levels of psychosocial functioning, despite the presence of many positive indices.

CONCLUSIONS

Several variables have been identified that enhanced our ability to predict psychosocial change and functioning levels after surgery for temporal lobe seizures. These include good family support, no or mild psychopathology, and responsibility for one's own behavior and personality. Of the several variables, good family support appears to be most cru-

TABLE 3. *Predictors of negative psychosocial outcome[a]*

Predictor	N	Estimate of probability + 1 SD	
		Worse	Less than highest level
If surgery	41	0.17 ± 0.06	0.63 ± 0.08
Cognitive decrease	16	0.38 ± 0.12	0.63 ± 0.12
Occasional seizures	14	0.29 ± 0.12	0.79 ± 0.11
Psychopathology[b]	17	0.29 ± 0.12	0.82 ± 0.09
Poor family support[b]	15	0.33 ± 0.12	1.00
Addictive personality[b]	12	0.33 ± 0.12	0.75 ± 0.13
Older age at surgery[b]	9	0.22 ± 0.14	0.78 ± 0.14
All preoperative variables[b]	2	1.50 ± 0.35	1.00
All variables	1	1.00	1.00

[a]From ref. 64, with permission.
[b]Preoperative variables.

cial. Thus, in addition to medical factors, environmental and psychological influences are also highly significant in determining the overall success of temporal lobe surgery.

ACKNOWLEDGMENTS

The author wishes to thank Catherine Ary and Maria Melendez for assistance during various phases of preparation of this chapter. The research described was supported, in part, by PHS grant NS 02808.

REFERENCES

1. Engel J Jr. *Surgical treatment of the epilepsies.* New York: Raven Press, 1987.
2. Spencer SS, Spencer DD, Williamson PD, Mattson RH. The localizing value of depth electroencephalography in 32 refractory epileptic patients. *Ann Neurol* 1982;12:248–253.
3. Crandall PH. Cortical resections. In: Engel J Jr, ed. *Surgical treatment of the epilepsies.* New York: Raven Press, 1987;377–404.
4. Falconer MA. Surgical treatment of temporal lobe epilepsy. *NZ Med J* 1967;66:539–544.
5. Falconer MA. Anterior temporal lobectomy for epilepsy. In: Rob C, Smith R, eds. *Operative surgery.* London: Butterworths, 1971;142–149.
6. Rausch R, Babb TL. Evidence for memory specialization within the mesial temporal lobe in man. In: Engel J Jr, Ojemann GA, Luders HO, Williamson PD, eds. *Fundamental mechanisms of human brain function.* New York: Raven Press, 1987;103–109.
7. Awad IA, Katz A, Hahn JF, Kong AK, Ahl J, Luders H. Extent of resection in temporal lobectomy for epilepsy. I. Interobserver analysis and correlation with seizure outcome. *Epilepsia* 1989;30:756–762.
8. Katz A, Awad IA, Kong AK, et al. Extent of resection in temporal lobectomy for epilepsy. II. Memory changes and neurologic complications. *Epilepsia* 1989;30:763–776.
9. Rausch R, Ary CM. Supraspan learning in patients with unilateral anterior temporal lobe resections. *Neuropsychologia* 1990;in press.
10. Engel J Jr, Driver MV, Falconer MA. Electrophysiological correlates of pathology and surgical results in temporal lobe epilepsy. *Brain* 1975;98:129–156.
11. Milner B. Psychological aspects of focal epilepsy and its neurosurgical management. In: Purpura DP, Penry JK, Walter RD, eds. *Advances in neurology,* vol 8. New York: Raven Press, 1975;299–321.
12. Rausch R. Differences in cognitive function with left and right temporal lobe dysfunction. In: Benson DF, Zaidel E, eds. *The dual brain.* New York: Guilford Press, 1985;247–261.
13. Rasmussen T, Milner B. Clinical and surgical studies of the cerebral speech areas in man. In: Zulch KJ, Creutzfeldt O, Galbraith GC, eds. *Cerebral localization.* New York: Springer-Verlag, 1975;238–257.
14. Rausch R, Walsh GO. Right hemisphere language dominance in right handed epileptic patients. *Arch Neurol* 1984;41:1077–1080.
15. Rausch R, Risinger M. Intracarotid sodium amobarbital technique. In: Boulton AA, Baker G, eds. *Neuromethods.* Clifton: Humana Press, 1990;in press.
16. Satz P, Strauss E, Wada J, Orsini DL. Some correlates of intra- and interhemispheric speech organization after left focal brain injury. *Neuropsychologia* 1988;26:345–350.
17. Lesser RP, Luders H, Klem G, et al. Extraoperative cortical functional localization in patients with epilepsy. *J Clin Neurophysiol* 1987;4:27–53.
18. Scoville WB. The limbic lobe and memory in man. *J Neurosurg* 1954;11:64–66.
19. Scoville WB, Milner B. Loss of recent memory after bilateral hippocampal lesions. *J Neurol Neurosurg Psychiatry* 1957;20:11–21.
20. Penfield W, Milner B. Memory deficit produced by bilateral lesions in the hippocampal zone. *Arch Neurol Psychiatry* 1958;79:475–497.
21. Penfield W, Mathieson G. Memory: autopsy findings and comments on the role of hippocampus in experiential recall. *Arch Neurol* 1974;31:145–154.
22. Milner B, Branch C, Rasmussen T. Study of short-term memory after intracarotid injection of sodium amytal. *Trans Am Neurol Assoc* 1962;87:224–226.
23. Klove HJ, Trites RL, Grabow JD. Intracarotid sodium amytal for evaluating memory function. *Electroencephalogr Clin Neurophysiol* 1970;28:418–419.
24. Blume W, Grabow J, Darley F, Aronson A. Intracarotid amobarbital test of language and memory before temporal lobe lobectomy for seizure control. *Neurology* 1973;23:812–819.
25. Rausch R. Psychological evaluation. In: Engel J Jr, ed. *Surgical treatment of epilepsies.* New York: Raven Press, 1987;181–195.
26. Rausch R, Babb TL, Engel J Jr, Crandall PH. Memory following intracarotid amobarbital injection contralateral to hippocampal damage. *Arch Neurol* 1989;46:783–788.
27. Rausch R, Babb TL, Brown WJ. A case of amnestic syndrome following selective amygdalohippocampectomy. *J Clin Exp Neuropsychol* 1985;7:643.
28. Loring DW, Lee GP, Meador KJ, et al. The intracarotid amobarbital procedure as a predictor of memory failure following unilateral temporal lobectomy. *Neurology* 1990;in press.
29. Meyer V, Yates AJ. Intellectual changes following temporal lobectomy for psychomotor epilepsy: preliminary communication. *J Neurol Neurosurg Psychiatry* 1955;103:44–52.
30. Milner B. Psychological defects produced by temporal-lobe excision. *Res Publ Assoc Res Nerv Ment Dis* 1958;36:244–257.

31. Milner B. Visual recognition and recall after right temporal-lobe excision in man. *Neuropsychologia* 1968;6:191–209.

32. Rausch R, Serafetinides EA, Crandall PH. Olfactory memory in patients with anterior temporal lobectomy. *Cortex* 1977;13:445–452.

33. Smith ML, Milner B. The role of the right hippocampus in the recall of spatial location. *Neuropsychologia* 1988;19:781–793.

34. Jones-Gotman M. Memory for designs: the hippocampal contribution. *Neuropsychologia* 1986;24:193–203.

35. Rausch R, Crandall PH. Psychological status related to surgical control of temporal lobe seizures. *Epilepsia* 1982;23:191–202.

36. Hermann BP, Wyler AR, Richey ET. Wisconsin Card Sorting Test performance in patients with complex partial seizures of temporal-lobe origin. *J Clin Exp Neuropsychol* 1988;10:467–476.

37. Novelly RA, Augustine EA, Mattson RH, et al. Selective memory improvement and impairment in temporal lobectomy for epilepsy. *Ann Neurol* 1984;15:64–67.

38. Wechsler D, Stone CP. *Wechsler memory scale.* New York: Psychological Corporation, 1945.

39. Blakemore CP, Falconer MA. The long term effects of anterior temporal lobectomy on certain cognitive functions. *J Neurol Neurosurg Psychiatry* 1967;30:364–367.

40. Rausch R. Anatomical substrates of interictal memory deficits in temporal lobe epileptics. *Int J Neurol* 1990;in press.

41. Milner B. Brain mechanisms suggested by studies of the temporal lobes. In: Millikan CH, Darley FL, eds. *Brain mechanisms underlying speech and language.* New York: Grune & Stratton, 1967;122–132.

42. Meyer V. Cognitive changes following temporal lobectomy for relief of temporal lobe epilepsy. *Arch Neurol Psychiatry* 1959;81:299–309.

43. Ribbler A, Rausch R. Performance of patients with unilateral temporal lobectomy on selective reminding procedures using either related or unrelated words. *Cortex* 1990;in press.

44. Weingartner J. Verbal learning in patients with temporal lobe lesions. *J Verb Learn Verb Behav* 1968;7:520–526.

45. Bushke H. Selective reminding for analysis of memory and learning. *J Verb Learn Verb Behav* 1973;12:543–550.

46. Wilkins A, Moscovitch M. Selective impairment in semantic memory after temporal lobectomy. *Neuropsychologia* 1978;16:73–79.

47. Rausch R. Lateralization of temporal lobe dysfunction and verbal encoding. *Brain Lang* 1981;12:92–100.

48. Rausch R, Boone K, Ary CM. Right hemisphere language dominance in temporal lobe epilepsy: clinical and neuropsychological correlates. *J Clin Exp Neuropsychol* 1990;in press.

49. Kaplan E, Goodglass H, Weintraub S. *The Boston naming test.* Philadelphia: Lea & Febiger, 1983.

50. Ojemann GA, Dodrill CB. Verbal memory deficits after left temporal lobectomy for epilepsy. *J Neurosurg* 1985;62:101–107.

51. Benson DF. Aphasia. In: Heilman KM, Valenstein E, eds. *Clinical neuropsychology.* New York: Oxford University Press, 1985;17–47.

52. Butters N, Rosen JJ, Stein DG. Recovery of behavioral functions after sequential ablation of the frontal lobes of monkeys. In: Stein DG, Rosen JJ, Butters N, eds. *Plasticity and recovery of function in the central nervous system.* New York: Academic Press, 1974;429–466.

53. Corkin S. Tactually-guided maze learning in man: effects of unilateral cortical excisions and bilateral hippocampal lesions. *Neuropsychologia* 1965;3:339–351.

54. Jones-Gotman M. Right hippocampal excision impairs learning and recall of a list of abstract designs. *Neuropsychologia* 1986;24:659–670.

55. Taylor LB. Localization of cerebral lesions by psychological testing. *Clin Neurosurg* 1969;16:269–287.

56. Osterrieth P. Le test de copie d'une figure complexe. *Arch Psychol* 1944;30:206–356.

57. Kimura D. Right temporal lobe damage. *Arch Neurol* 1963;8:264–271.

58. Taylor DC. Mental state and temporal lobe epilepsy. *Epilepsia* 1972;13:727–765.

59. Ferguson SM, Rayport M. The adjustment to living without epilepsy. *J Nerv Ment Dis* 1965;140:26–37.

60. Hermann BP, Wyler AR, Ackerman B, Rosenthal T. Short-term psychological outcome of anterior temporal lobectomy. *J Neurosurg* 1989;71:327–334.

61. Augustine EA, Novelly RA, Mattson RH, et al. Occupational adjustment following neurosurgical treatment of epilepsy. *Ann Neurol* 1984;15:68–72.

62. Horowitz MJ, Cohen FM. Temporal lobe epilepsy: effect of lobectomy on psychosocial functioning. *Epilepsia* 1968;9:23–41.

63. Taylor DC, Falconer MA. Clinical, socio-economic, and psychological adjustment after temporal lobectomy. *Br J Psychiatry* 1968;114:1247–1261.

64. Crandall PH, Rausch R, Engel J Jr. Preoperative indications for optimal surgical outcome for temporal lobe epilepsy. In: Wieser HG, Elger CE, eds. *Presurgical evaluation of epileptics.* Berlin-Heidelberg: Springer-Verlag, 1987;325–334.

65. Engel J Jr, Rausch R, Lieb JP, Kuhl DE, Crandall PH. Correlation of criteria used for localizing epileptic foci in patients considered for surgical therapy for epilepsy. *Ann Neurol* 1981;9:215–244.

Advances in Neurology, Vol. 55, edited by
D. Smith, D. Treiman, and M. Trimble,
Raven Press, Ltd., New York © 1991.

18

Behavioral Changes Following Corpus Callosotomy

Alexander G. Reeves

Section of Neurology, Dartmouth Medical School, Hanover, New Hampshire 03756

HISTORICAL BACKGROUND

During a 6-month period between 1939 and 1940, Van Wagenen and Herren (1) transected the corpus callosum in a small series of patients with intractable generalized epilepsy. It was reported that seizure control improved. Subsequent series have amply supported the benefits of corpus callosotomy for some patients with generalized seizures and partial seizures with secondary generalization which are refractory to medical and more traditional epilepsy surgeries (2–20).

Akelaitis (21,22) reported on the neuropsychological changes in 10 of Van Wagenen's patients after callosotomy. Although he noted a difficulty with bimanual cooperation between the right and left hands, he was loath to attribute the change to section of the callosum. Instead, he postulated it to be the result of lateralized operative or preoperative brain damage.

Traditional neuropsychological testing revealed no significant deficits; this was in accord with Dandy (23), who made this observation on the removal of pineal tumors in 1936:

The corpus callosum is split longitudinally from its posterior extremity to a point anteriorly where the third and lateral ventricle comes into view; this incision is bloodless. Usually this incision takes most and sometimes all of this structure to its downward bend. No symptoms follow its division. This simple experiment at once disposes of the extravagant claims to function of the corpus callosum.

Van Wagenen and Herren (1) had justified transecting the callosum by also attributing neurological deficits attributed to callosal lesions in the past to extracallosal pathologies. Nevertheless, Trescher and Ford (24) in 1937 reported on alexia in the left visual field of a patient who had had section of the posterior callosum by Dandy and opined that "special methods of examination are required to demonstrate the essential symptoms." In spite of this caveat, until Sperry and his colleagues (25,26) had undertaken their studies on the split-brain monkey, the right questions were not asked.

Callosotomy as a treatment for intractable generalized seizures lay fallow from 1940 when Van Wagenen's series was interrupted by World War II, until Joseph Bogen and co-workers (27,28) rekindled the procedure in the early 1960s. One of Sperry's young colleagues, Michael Gazzaniga, was assigned to this new project (29). A series of studies of the bisected human callosum ensued; this series continues today and has so far elucidated a great wealth of information and speculation on the functions of the forebrain commissures and the right and left cerebral hemispheres (30–32).

The neuropsychological consequences of transection of the corpus callosum—and, by necessity, the underlying hippocampal commissure—have now been well described and are uniform enough to allow some predictability. Even so, the brains of patients with intractable seizures are generally and variably defective, which must be kept in mind when attempting to extrapolate findings to normal brain functions.

NEUROLOGICAL OBSERVATIONS

Standard neuropsychological and psychosocial assessments have shown little or no negative effects when compared with premorbid levels of activity (18,21,22,33–35). Most patients show improvements, at least in part, on the basis of decreased seizures and anticonvulsant loads (18,33,34). Some negative effects have been recorded in a small number of patients and will be elaborated below. These have rarely outweighed the benefits of improved seizure control (36). In this chapter, I will discuss the neuropsychological effects of anterior section (anterior half to two-thirds), posterior section (posterior half plus the hippocampal commissure), and complete section of the callosum, plus hippocampal commissure. Unless otherwise stated, the model subject will be left hemisphere-dominant for verbal language and right-handed.

Anterior Section

An acute and easily observable syndrome is characteristic in the hours and days following anterior callosal section (37). In our experience, this syndrome occurs (at least in part) in most patients. The major finding is a decrease in the spontaneity of speech; it may be so severe that the patient is completely mute, or it may be as mild as a slowness in initiating speech (37,38). Typically, once begun, speech, although it may continue to be slow, is not dysphasic (37). Other components of the syndrome can include variable degrees of paresis of the nondominant leg, a disinhibited forced grasping reflex in the nondominant hand, and urgency incontinence (37). Although the syndrome usually lasts from days to weeks, a small number of patients have been disabled for months or longer (37,39, 40).

It has been suggested that either operative traction on the nondominant frontal parasagittal region or acute parasagittal disconnec-

tion, or both, are responsible for the syndrome (37). In support of traction injury are (a) the presence of contralateral paresis of the leg, presumably the result of compression of the parasagittal portion of motor strip which represents the leg, and (b) the contralateral forced grasp response, a finding which has been related to premotor, supplementary motor, and adjacent cingulate cortex lesions (41).

Speech arrest follows unilateral stimulation of the nondominant supplementary motor area which lies anterior to the primary motor cortex (42). A role in the generation of speech and movement in general has been postulated for the supplementary motor area of the dominant and nondominant hemispheres (43–48). Whether traction on the supplementary motor area alone or a combination of traction plus diaschisis from disconnecting the two callosally interconnected supplementary motor areas (49) is the cause of the mutism (37,50) is a moot point at present. Most important is the observation that the disability is usually temporary.

One center has reported several patients who developed dysphasic difficulties following anterior, posterior, and complete callosotomy, and these deficits have been attributed to preoperative bilateral or mixed cerebral dominance for verbal language (51) and an implied callosally mediated hemispheric interdependence for these functions. This will be discussed further below.

Posterior Section

Interhemispheric sensory disconnection occurs following section of the posterior half of the callosum (30,31). The dominant and nondominant hemispheres are no longer able to internally transmit somesthetic or visual information to each other. Visual and tactile scanning of both halves of the environment nevertheless allows both sides of the brain to have equal access to both sides of the world. The potential disability from posterior callosal section is therefore greatly diminished.

Although there is no obvious behavioral indication of disconnection, the effects of posterior half section are readily evident at the bedside. Rapid presentation of visual stimuli (tachistoscopic) in the nondominant visual field is not reported by the patient, whose language-dominant hemisphere has no access to the information and no verbal capacity in the nondominant hemisphere to report what has been seen.

The splenium is the major route for interhemispheric visual transfer (49). If the section is carried rostrally to the callosal midpoint, encompassing parietal interconnections, tactile separation occurs. Objects placed in the nondominant hand of the blindfolded subject cannot be identified by the dominant hemisphere. The dominant hemisphere reports that it has not seen or felt anything, but it can be demonstrated that there are no nondominant hemisphere elementary visual or tactile deficits. Objects presented tachystoscopically to the nondominant visual field can be correctly identified behind a screen by the nondominant hand. Similarly, objects palpated by the hand can be re-identified from a group of objects by the same hand. What is missing is the ability to say what has been seen and felt on the left.

Auditory stimuli reach both ears almost equally from both sides of the environment. Internally, the pathways to the auditory cortex are bilateral from both cochlear systems, so each ear has access to both hemispheres. Nevertheless, with dichotic listening tasks, auditory disconnection can be demonstrated when the posterior temporal lobes are separated by posterior callosal sectioning (52). When a verbal command is given to perform a task with the nondominant hand, no problem is encountered. The dominant hemisphere, which is alone capable of understanding the command, presumably controls the nondominant motor cortex through the non-severed anterior callosum which interconnects the two frontal motor systems. If the anterior callosum is then split, completing hemispheric disconnection (with the exception of the anterior commissure), the patient (his dominant hemisphere) no longer correctly performs a command to carry out a task with the nondominant hand. He may respond in some fashion with the nondominant hand, possibly either by (a) a perseveration of a response by the dominant hand which has been observed by the nondominant hemisphere or (b) a mimicking of a movement made by the examiner. It is presumed that the nondominant hemisphere is able to recognize the prosody (music) of a command and therefore attempts to accommodate the examiner by using nonverbal cues.

Complete Section

Most split-brain procedures are now carried out in two stages to decrease the acute postoperative morbidity of a prolonged surgical procedure (53) and to avoid the complete split-brain syndrome if possible. One-stage complete callosotomy is not, to our knowledge, practiced today. If inadequate seizure control is achieved by anterior section [the usual preliminary procedure in most centers (36)], the callosotomy is completed. The most recent multicenter data indicate anterior section to be approximately 50% as effective for control of seizures when compared to complete section (36).

The classic split-brain syndrome follows complete callosotomy (30–32). The sensory disconnection seen with posterior section is present, and now the dominant hemisphere no longer has access to the motor cortex of the nondominant hemisphere for the execution of skilled distal movements (54). Each hemisphere, however, is able to control some proximal movements of the ipsilateral limb through ipsilateral uncrossed motor pathways (54). The nondominant (left) hand no longer will respond correctly to verbal commands for skilled movements. Nevertheless, some incorrect behavior of the nondominant hand will usually be seen because (a) the dominant (left) hemisphere can initiate some proximal movements of the ipsilateral nondominant upper limb and (b) the nondominant hemisphere can perceive these movements of the left arm and can also preceive the prosody of a command. If the examiner inadvertently first asks the subject to carry out a command with the dominant-hemisphere hand and is then asked to use the nondominant-hemisphere hand the same way, more often than not the task is completed correctly. The nondominant hemisphere, perceiving the prosody of a command and the proximal movement of the nondominant arm, copies what it has just seen the dominant arm do, leaving the novice examiner with the impression that the nondominant hemisphere has verbal language capability. If the examiner begins with a command to carry out a task with the nondominant hand or follows the dominant-hand task with a different command for the nondominant hand, the disconnection is revealed.

Thus, the nondominant hand no longer responds appropriately to verbal commands. A number of our patients, when asked what is wrong with their nondominant hand, have responded with considerable insight that the hand will not cooperate, implying that their dominant-hemisphere self is not in control of their nondominant-hemisphere self.

Furthermore, the nondominant hand is frequently noted in the postoperative period to act in an antagonistic manner towards the dominant hand. Basic manual tasks such as eating, opening and closing doors, turning faucets on and off, and washing hands may be difficult because the nondominant hand may terminate an action which the dominant hemisphere has initiated. For example, the dominant hand (as is frequently used when initiating a manual activity) may turn on the hot water. Both hands reach for the water to begin the well-learned bimanual task of washing. The nondominant hand recoils from what appears to be too hot water and then turns off the faucet. The dominant hand turns the faucet on again, appearing to tolerate the heat better. Ultimately, the nondominant hand tolerates the heat or the dominant hand decreases the heat.

Cooperation is established for previously well-learned bimanual tasks, presumably by use of external cues in most patients over a short period of time (weeks to months). New bimanual tasks are learned with difficulty, a problem which may need to be considered with younger patients. A recent report suggests that younger patients are, in fact, more able to accommodate hemispheric separation—at least with somesthetic-directed functions (55). This may be on the basis of greater plasticity of sensory integration allowed by greater use of ispilaterally projecting sensory pathways in the developing brain (55). Furthermore, in time it is apparent that some patients are able to control some hand–finger movements with ipsilateral motor pathways (56).

Interhemispheric antagonism has remained a chronic problem in a small number of patients. Persistent and disabling difficulties with daily hygiene, dressing, and shopping (56), and in one case (Reeves and Roberts, *unpublished observations*) in almost all daily activities, have occurred. The latter patient has such great antagonism between his two hemispheres that his left and right arms abuse each other, potentially causing physical injury. The dominant (left) hemisphere has verbally expressed great hostility towards the left arm and leg, considering them another hostile person. This antagonistic behavior has created a paralyzing disability which far outweighs the benefits of the excellent seizure control afforded by callosotomy in this patient. No retrospective clues are available to allow prediction of a predisposition towards such a disabling behavioral result in other patients. Fortunately, it is most unusual, and developing cooperation between hemispheres is the rule.

One of our patients (Reeves and Roberts, *unpublished observations*) developed excellent cooperation within days of complete callosal section. When asked to carry out a task with her nondominant-hemisphere-controlled left hand (e.g., show me three fingers with your left hand), she quickly learned to place the left hand into her right hand, which would then arrange the fingers appropriately. The nondominant hemisphere in this patient willingly followed the lead of the dominant hemisphere using external cues just as it had done before surgery using internal callosally transmitted cues.

In other tasks (such as picture completions and Kohs block pattern reproduction), the dominant hemisphere, frequently less capable with visuospatial problems, has allowed the more capable nondominant hemisphere to take charge and complete the task.

One left-handed patient with left-hemisphere dominance for verbal language is no longer able to write more than random letters or digits with his left hand following callosotomy. He has subsequently learned to write fluently with his right hand (57). Similarly, a patient in our series, preoperatively right-handed but with right-hemisphere verbal language dominance, became left-handed for writing following callosotomy (Reeves and Roberts, *unpublished observations*). In both of these instances, it is presumed that the dominant hemisphere was exercising callosally mediated contralateral control of the motor system for writing. Although they had writing difficulties, neither of these two patients had other evident dysphasic difficulties. In both, one 20 and the other 11 years old, compensation was ultimately successful and writing was learned with the contralateral hand. Right-hemisphere dominance with right-handedness is rare, but it should be expected that some left-handed patients will need to transfer writing skills to their right hand after complete callosotomy.

A number of other, more benign behavioral examples of hemispheric independence have been observed.

A 14-year-old right-handed boy who lives by the seashore had many of the usual food aversions seen in youngsters. In particular, he had a strong aversion for white bait, a favorite of his family, which is a finger food dish of small fish, fried and eaten uneviscerated. His aversion was visual and imaginative. He had never tasted the dish. Following complete callosotomy, he was seen to be taking the fish with his left hand, putting them in his mouth and eating them. His hamburger was untouched, and when his mother exclaimed over the new acceptance, he responded (with his dominant left hemisphere) that he was puzzled too, but that the fish were in fact good. Thereafter, he also ate the fish with his right hand. Presumably his right hemisphere was naive to the aversion and was simply copying the rest of the family, who were evidently enjoying the dish.

Another right-handed, left-hemisphere-dominant patient, while discussing her newly controlled seizures with her physician on the phone, exclaimed that she could not continue to talk because her mother was coming into the room, and her left hand apparently did not want her to continue the conversation. It was trying to hang up the phone. When asked if this was a problem, she said no and that she would call back later, and then her left hand hung up the phone.

MEMORY DEFICITS

Memory dysfunction has been noted in a minority of patients following partial and complete callosotomy (56,58,59). A deficit in learning new material has been noted which may result from disconnecting two damaged and interdependent hippocampal formations by severing the callosum and hippocampal commissure (56,60). Zaidel and Sperry (59) and later Dimond (61) noted deficits in attentional capacity following complete callosotomy which could account for the observed memory difficulties. The conclusions drawn from the series of 10 patients studied by Zaidel and Sperry (59) were criticized by LeDoux et al. (58) for not having preoperative data in patients with multiple preoperative reasons for memory and attentional difficulties. These included brain damage, seizures, and high-dose anticonvulsant medications. A patient studied pre- and postoperatively by LeDoux et al. (58) showed no postoperative defects but, in fact, showed improved memory functions. This controversy notwithstanding, it is apparent that memory difficulties do occur in some patients (56), but as a rule are not of great enough significance to outweigh the psychological benefits of improved seizure control and a decreased anticonvulsant load (32,33).

LATERALIZED CEREBRAL DEFICITS

A small number of patients have emerged from surgery with persistent lateralized hemispheric deficits not seen prior to callosotomy. The centers reporting these findings have postulated the severance of successful, callosally mediated compensation for ancient lateralized cortical lesions (60,62). Although the sample from which conclusions can be drawn is small, it is suggested that the presence of mixed bilateral hemispheric dominance for verbal language functions may sometimes lead to dysphasic deficits following callosotomy. In particular, it was suggested that difficulties may be more likely to arise if the hemisphere controlling handedness is not the language-dominant hemisphere (51). Although transfer of writing capacity occurred following callosotomy in the two patients reported above who had crossed hemisphere control of writing, no dysphasic difficulties were noted (39) (Reeves and Roberts, *unpublished observations*).

Preoperative carotid amytal testing (The WADA test) (63) is, for the time being, recommended (when feasible) for patients undergoing callosotomy to determine the presence of unusual combinations of language dominance, which might predict postoperative difficulties (36).

CONCLUSIONS

Dandy (23) and Akelaitis (21,22) were not prepared to ask the right questions. If they had simply flashed cards manually at the bedside, tested graphesthesia and stereognosis, and asked their patients to carry out tasks with their nondominant hand, they would have discovered the significance of the corpus callosum for communication in the human brain. Their observation that little overt negative behavioral change occurs following calosotomy has been largely corroborated and continues to justify callosotomy as a therapy for patients with intractable epilepsy. The positive effects on behavior which follow decreased seizures, along with the decreased need for anticonvulsants, outweigh (with few exceptions) the observable, but inconsistent, chronic negative effects. The split-brain syndrome is easily demonstrated and well accommodated by most patients. It continues to be an extraordinary resource for studies of the highest functions of the brain.

REFERENCES

1. Van Wagenen WP, Herren RY. Surgical division of commissural pathways in the corpus callosum: relation to spread of an epileptic attack. *Arch Neurol Psychiatry* 1940;44:740–759.
2. Bogen JE, Vogel PJ. Neurologic status in the long term following complete cerebral commissurotomy. In: Michel F, Schott B, eds. *Les syndromes de disconnextion calleuse chez l'homme.* Lyon: Hôpital Neurologique, 1975; 227–251.
3. Luessenhop AJ. Interhemispheric commissurotomy: the split brain operation as an alternate to hemispherectomy for control of intractable seizures. *Am Surg* 1970;36:265–268.
4. Wilson DH, Reeves AG, Gazzaniga MS. "Central" commissurotomy for intractable generalized epilepsy: series two. *Neurology,* 1982; 32:687–697.
5. Amacher AL. Midline commissurotomy for the treatment of some cases of intractable epilepsy. *Childs Brain,* 1976;2:54–58.
6. Avila JO, Radvany J, Huck FR, Pires de Camargo CH, Marino R, Ragazzo PC, Riva D. Anterior callosotomy as a substitute for hemispherectomy. *Acta Neurochir [Suppl]* 1980;30:137–143.
7. Saint-Hilaire JM, Giard N, Bouvier G, Labrecque R. Anterior callosotomy in frontal lobe epilepsies. In: Reeves AG, ed. *Epilepsy and the corpus callosum.* New York: Plenum Press, 1985;303–314.
8. Rayport M, Ferguson SM, Corrie WS. Outcomes and indications of corpus callosum section for intractable seizure control. *Appl Neurophysiol* 1983;46:47–51.
9. Geoffroy G, Lassonde M, Delisle F, Decarie M. Corpus callosotomy for control of intractable epilepsy in children. *Neurology (Cleve)* 1983; 33:891–897.
10. Gates J, Rosenfeld W, Maxwell RE, Lyons R. Response of multiple seizure types to callosotomy. *Epilepsia* 1985;26:543.
11. Wada JA, Moyes P. Anterior callosal bisection in medically refractory generalized seizure patients. *Epilepsia* 1982;24:262.
12. Waterman K, Purves SJ, Kosaka B, Straauss E, Wada JA. An epileptic syndrome caused by mesial frontal lobe seizure foci. *Neurology* 1987; 37:577–588.
13. Rappaport ZH, Lerman P. Corpus callosotomy in the treatment of secondary generalizing intractable epilepsy. *Acta Neurochir (Wien)* 1988; 94:10–14.
14. Garcia-Flores E. Corpus callosum section in patients with intractable epilepsy. *Acta Neurophysiol* 1987;50:390–397.
15. Makari GS, Holmes GL, Murro AM, Smith JR, Flanigin HF, Cohen MJ, Huh K, Gallagher BS, Ackell AB, Campbell R, King DW. Corpus callosotomy for the treatment of intractable epilepsy in children. *J Epilepsy* 1989;2:1–7.
16. Reeves AG, O'Leary PM. Total corpus callosotomy for control of medically intractable epilepsy. In: Reeves AG, ed. *Epilepsy and the corpus callosum.* New York: Plenum Press, 1985; 269–280.
17. Spencer SS, Gates JR, Reeves AG, Spencer DD, Maxwell RE, Roberts DW. Corpus callosum section. In: Engel J Jr, ed. *Surgical treatment of the epilepsies.* New York: Raven Press, 1987: 425–444.
18. Goodman RN, Williamson PD, Reeves AG, Spencer SS, Spencer DD, Mattson RH, Roberts DW. Interhemispheric commissurotomy for congenital hemiplegia with intractable epilepsy. *Neurology* 1985;35:1351–1354.
19. Nordgren RE, Reeves AG, Roberts DW. Corpus callosotomy for intractable seizures in children. *Ann Neurol* 1988;24:316.
20. Roberts DW, Reeves AG. Effect of commissurotomy on complex partial epilepsy in patients without a resectable seizure focus. *Appl Neurophysiol* 1987;50:398–400.

21. Akelaitis AJE. Studies on corpus callosum: higher visual function in each hemisphere's field following complete section of the corpus callosum. *Arch Neurol Psychiatry* 1941;45:786–796.

22. Akelaitis AJE. A study of gnosis, praxis and language following section of the corpus callosum and anterior commissure. *J Neurosurg* 1944;1:94–102.

23. Dandy WE. Operative experiences in cases of pineal tumors. *Arch Surg* 1936;33:19–46.

24. Trescher JH, Ford FR. Colloid cyst of the third ventricle. Report of a case: operative removal with section of posterior half of the corpus callosum. *Arch Neurol Psychiatry* 1937;37:959–973.

25. Myers RE, Sperry RW. Intraocular transfer of a visual form discrimination habit in cats after section of the optic chiasm and corpus callosum. *Anat Rec* 1953;115:351–352.

26. Sperry RW. Cerebral organization and behavior. *Science* 1961;133:1749–1757.

27. Bogen JE, Vogel PJ. Treatment of generalized seizures by cerebral commissurotomy. *Surg Forum* 1963;14:431–433.

28. Bogen JE, Fisher ED, Vogel PJ. Cerebral commissurotomy: a second case report. *JAMA* 1965;194:1328–1329.

29. Bogen JE, Gazzaniga MS. Cerebral commissurotomy in man: minor hemisphere dominance for certain visuospatial functions. *J Neurosurg* 1965;23:394–399.

30. Gazzaniga MS. *The bisected brain*. New York: Appleton–Century–Crofts, 1970.

31. Gazzaniga MS, LeDoux JE. *The integrated mind*. New York: Plenum Press, 1978.

32. Gazzaniga MS. Some contributions of split-brain studies to the study of human cognition. In: Reeves AG, ed. *Epilepsy and the corpus callosum*. New York: Plenum Press, 1985;341–348.

33. Ferrell RB, Culver CM, Tucker GJ. Psychosocial and cognitive function after commissurotomy for intractable seizures. *J Neurosurg* 1984;58:374–380.

34. Ritter FJ, Gates JR, Maxwell RE, Jacobs MP, Skare SS. Behavioral changes in children following corpus callosotomy (Abstract).

35. Oepen G, Schultz-Weiling R, Zimmermann P, Straesser S, Gilsbach J. Long-term effects of partial callosal lesions. *Acta Neurochir* 1985;77:22–28.

36. Spencer S, Gates JR, Reeves AG, Spencer DD, Maxwell RE, Roberts D. Corpus callosum section. In: Engel J Jr, ed. *Surgical treatment of the epilepsies*. New York: Raven Press, 1987;425–444.

37. Ross MK, Reeves AG, Roberts DW. Post-commissurotomy mutism. *Ann Neurol* 1984;16:114.

38. Bogen JE. Linguistic performance on the short term following cerebral commissurotomy. In: Whitaker HA, Whitaker HA, eds. *Studies in neurolinguistics*, vol 2. New York: Academic Press, 1976;193–224.

39. Rayport M, Ferguson SM, Corrie WS. Mutism after corpus callosum section for intractable seizure control. *Epilepsia* 1984;25:663.

40. Sussman NM, Gur RC, Gur RE, O'Connor MJ. Mutism as a consequence of callosotomy. *J Neurosurg* 1983;59:514–519.

41. Twitchell TE. The automatic grasping responses of infants. *Neuropsychologia* 1965;3:247–259.

42. Penfield W, Roberts L. *Speech and brain mechanisms*. New York: Atheneum, 1966;119–137.

43. Ross M, Damasio H, Eslinger P. The role of the supplementary motor area (SMA) and anterior cingulate (AC) in the generation of movement. *Neurology* 1986;36(Suppl 1):346.

44. Gelmers HJ. Non-paralytic motor disturbances and speech disorders: the role of the supplementary motor area. *J Neurol Neurosurg Psychiatry* 1983;46:1052–1054.

45. Damasio AR, Geschwind N. The neural basis of language. *Annu Rev Neurosci* 1984;7:127–147.

46. Brust JCM, Plank C, Burke A, Guobadia MMI, Healton EB. Language disorder in a right-hander after occlusion of the right anterior cerebral artery. *Neurology* 1982;32:492–497.

47. Caplan LR, Zervas NT. Speech arrest in a dextral with right mesial frontal astrocytoma. *Arch Neurol* 1978;35:252–253.

48. Alexander MP, Schmitt MA. The aphasia syndrome of stroke in the left anterior cerebral artery territory. *Arch Neurol* 1980;37:97–100.

49. Pandya DN, Rosene DL. Some observations on trajectories and topography of commissural fibers. In: Reeves AG, ed. *Epilepsy and the corpus callosum*. 1985;329–337.

50. Macfarlene V, Ross MK, Reeves AG, Roberts DW, Bouvier G, Rouleau I. Anterior callosotomy and the parasagital frontal lobe syndrome: Submitted for publication.

51. Spencer DD, Spencer SS, Sass KJ, Novelly RA, Williamson PD, Mattson RH. Corpus callosum section for epilepsy. III. Neurologic and neuropsychological effects. *Neurology* 1988;38:25.

52. Musiek FE, Reeves AG, Baron JA. Release from central auditory competition in the split-brain patient. *Neurology* 1985;35:983–987.

53. Wilson DH, Reeves AG, Gazzaniga MS. "Central" commissurotomy for intractable generalized epilepsy: series two. *Neurology* 1982;32:687–697.

54. Volpe BT. Observation of motor control in patients with partial and complete callosal section: implications for current theories of apraxia. In: Reeves AG, ed. *Epilepsy and the corpus callosum*. New York: Plenum Press, 1985;381–391.

55. Lassonde M, Sauerwain H, Geoffrey G, Decarie M. Effects of early and late transection of the corpus callosum in children. *Brain* 1986;109:953–967.

56. Ferguson SM, Rayport M, Corrie WS. Neuropsychiatric observations on behavioral consequences of corpus callosum section for seizure control. In: Reeves AG, ed. *Epilepsy and the corpus callosum*. New York: Plenum Press, 1985;501–514.

57. Gur RE, Gur RC, Sussman NM, O'Connor MJ,

Vey MM. Hemispheric control of the writing hand: the effect of callosotomy in a left-hander. *Neurology* 1984;34:904–908.

58. LeDoux JE, Risse GL, Springer SP, Wilson DW, Gazzaniga MS. Cognition and commissurotomy. *Brain* 1974;100:87–104.

59. Zaidel E, Sperry RW. Memory impairment after commissurotomy in man. *Brain* 1974;97:263–272.

60. Novelly RA, Lifrak MD. Forebrain commissurotomy reinstates effects of preexisting hemisphere lesions: an examination of the hypothesis. In: Reeves AG, ed. *Epilepsy and the corpus callosum*. New York: Plenum Press 1985;467–500.

61. Dimond SJ. Depletion of attentional capacity after total commissurotomy in man. *Brain* 1976; 99:347–356.

62. Campbell AL Jr, Bogen JE, Smith A. Disorganization and reorganization of cognitive and sensorimotor functions in cerebral commissurotomy: compensatory roles of the forebrain commissures and cerebral hemispheres in man. *Brain* 1981;104:493–551.

63. Wada J, Rasmussen T. Intracarotid injection of sodium amytal for the lateralization of speech dominance: experimental and clinical observations. *J Neurosurg* 1960;17:266–282.

Advances in Neurology, Vol. 55, edited by
D. Smith, D. Treiman, and M. Trimble,
Raven Press, Ltd., New York © 1991.

19

Ictal Manifestations of Temporal Lobe Seizures

Heinz-Gregor Wieser

*Department of Neurology, University Hospital Zurich,
CH-8031 Zurich, Switzerland*

Temporal lobe epilepsy (TLE) is frequent and unfortunately often drug-resistant. This implies that epileptologists, and especially those engaged in the surgical treatment of TLE, spend quite a lot of their time studying psychomotor seizures (the term "complex partial seizures" (CPS) is used synonymously) by analyzing carefully the accompanying subjective experiences as well as objective descriptions given by relatives and other observers. In addition, with the advent of prolonged video–EEG monitoring facilities, the habitual seizures of many patients can now be videotaped, so that detailed studies of the ictal semiology of temporal lobe (TL) seizures are much easier to conduct. Despite these fortunate circumstances, CPS of TL origin often remain puzzling and still are an attractive field warranting further research. A characteristic of this seizure type is the rich variety of ictal clinical manifestations encompassing (a) changes in higher cognitive functions ("psychical phenomena"), (b) changes in the emotional–affective sphere in conjunction with vegetative, motor, and distinct sensory symptoms, and (c) automatisms. To attribute a specific anatomic origin to different symptoms and signs of CPS carries the risk of losing the many intimate relations between them and the characteristic overall gestalt.

It is problematic to describe this seizure type in terms of symptom catalogues: too varied and intimate are the interrelationships between observed clinical signs and symptoms, as exemplified by the variable relationship between different degrees of perturbed consciousness and several forms of automatic behavior. The evolution of a seizure—that is, its

"march of symptoms," the time and duration of each of them, the contextual background of a new symptom within a setting of already existing other symptoms, factors triggering the seizure, and environmental influences, as well as distinct traits of the "interictal personality" of the affected person—should be considered too when describing the clinical symptom complex of any single CPS or even the constellation of symptoms in any individual patient.

The difficulties of a meaningful analysis further increase with the attempt to correlate ictal behavior with the underlying ictal epileptic discharge, especially if spatiotemporal aspects, possible "distant" effects, and spread are to be considered (1). Although some distinct electroclinical correlations have been derived, we are far away from understanding all conditions that lead to the appearance of a specific ictal behavior. Most of the correlations are "conditional"; that is, they have a multifactorial aspect. For example, amygdala discharges might well correlate with oroalimentary automatisms in a given patient; this, however, does not imply that the electrical stimulation of this nuclear mass must reproduce this type of automatic behavior in all patients, or even in this same patient. In fact, it is more likely that the patient, following stimulation of his/her amygdala, does not have a clouding of consciousness with chewing; instead, he/she experiences either a distinct "strange feeling" (probably associated with an ascending epigastric aura), "some kind of memory flashback," or an unexplainable sudden feeling of fear (2,3), etc.

However, seen as whole, the seizures of a

given patient may be remarkably stereotyped and typical. I remember one patient whose 6-year-old son, who often had witnessed the attacks of his father, was able to distinguish easily between two slightly different habitual seizure types, which later on turned out to correlate with differently lateralized seizure onset in mediobasal limbic TL structures; however, from the medical descriptions that listed the various ictal symptoms and signs, this did not become apparent.

In this chapter we want to briefly summarize some of our earlier studies dealing with the "electroclinical features of the psychomotor seizure" (4). These data are based on 213 spontaneous psychomotor seizures from 29 candidates for TL surgery. The seizures have been carefully selected according to rigorous criteria. They were recorded with simultaneous 32-channel stereotactic depth and surface electroencephalography (EEG); behavior was synchronously split-screen videotaped, and direct interactive observation by trained personnel was required. After encoding these seizures into computer-readable matrices (time-dependent appearances of symptoms; spatiotemporal EEG discharges differentiating between five degrees of EEG patterns per location), chronotopographical electroclinical correlation analyses (cluster analysis; principal component analysis, multidimensional scaling) were conducted. In the second part of this chapter we refer to another additional 272 CPS recorded in 68 patients during radiotelemetric long-term video monitoring of both surface and four-contact foramen ovale electrode EEG with simultaneous split-screen recording of behavior. This part of the chapter centers around the issue of the bilaterality of mediobasal limbic seizures.

In the third part we present a few of our electrocerebral stimulation data. This study (5) is based on a total of 2223 stimulations performed in 116 patients who have been evaluated for possible surgical therapy of their drug-resistant seizures. Electrical stimulations were performed at the end of the stereoelectroencephalographic evaluation with the aim of obtaining additional confirmatory evidence for the assumed localization of the primary epileptogenic area, but also to study the functions of the accessible brain structures.

RESULTS OBTAINED FROM AN ELECTROCLINICAL CORRELATION STUDY OF STEREOELECTROENCEPHALO-GRAPHICALLY RECORDED SPONTANEOUS PSYCHOMOTOR SEIZURES

Frequency of Observed Ictal Symptoms and Location of Seizure Discharges

Figure 1 is a graph of observed clinical symptoms and signs, and Fig. 2 shows the location of those depth electrodes from which high-frequency discharges (>10 Hz, mostly 20–30 Hz) and/or clonic discharges (bursts of high-frequency discharges) were recorded during the analyzed seizures.

As can be seen from Fig. 1, the following symptoms were frequently observed: *visceromotor symptoms* such as changes in heart rate, respiration, and pupil diameter, as well as "flush" or pallor; *digestive symptoms* such as salivation, flatulence, and sometimes borborygmi; *viscerosensitive symptoms* such as epigastric ascending constriction, nausea, and "cephalic" aura; and *behavioral symptoms* such as change of posture and/or position, altered facial expression, change of affectivity, etc. Consciousness was usually retained initially, but it gradually appeared to be clouded to a degree that the patients became unresponsive. Some patients did not even react to painful stimuli. Some patients suddenly became arrested and were unresponsive from the very beginning of an attack or after having experienced their aura (see also Fig. 6). Automatisms with oroalimentary, exploratory, and verbal manifestations also have a high rank order in this graph, whereas "psychic phenomena" constituted only 10% of the 1448 symptoms recorded. In the symptom catalogue that we used, 13 symptoms might be included in the category of "psychic phenomena": visual, auditory, vestibular, and somatosensory (somesthetic) hallucinations; visual illusions; recollections such as déjà vu experiences; forced thinking; strange feeling and "souvenir"; and emotions such as anxiety (fear), sadness, and a general "malaise." Most illusions and hallucinations were complex ones (as opposed to elementary) and were either unimodal (with a predominance of

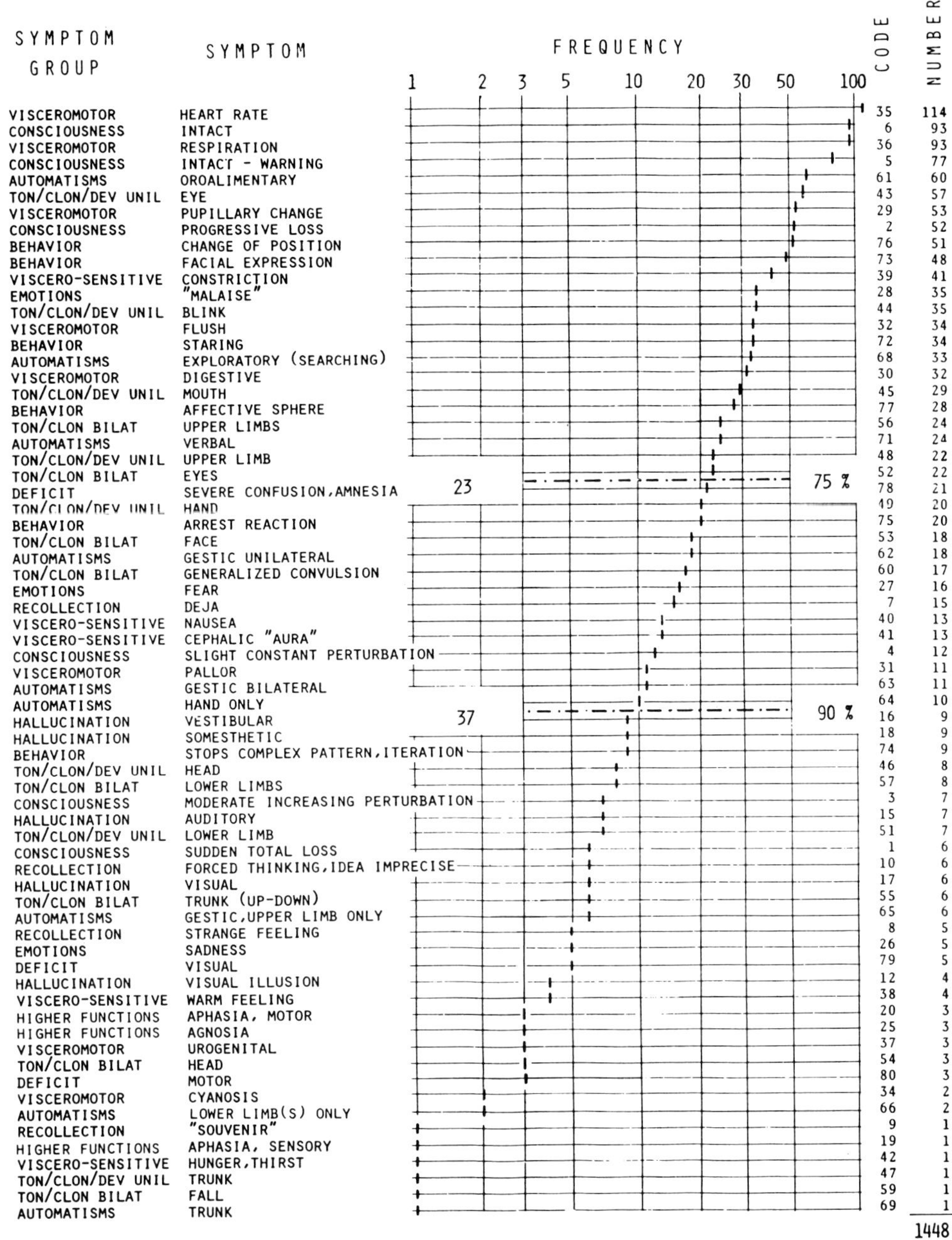

FIG. 1. Graph of ictal symptoms arranged in descending order of how often each was observed. A total of 1448 observations in 213 seizures indicate an average of seven encoded symptom observations per seizure. Sixty-eight of the 80 coded symptoms actually occurred in this population of 29 selected patients. Twenty-three symptoms constituted 75% of all symptom observations, and 37 accounted for 90%. (From ref. 4, with permission.)

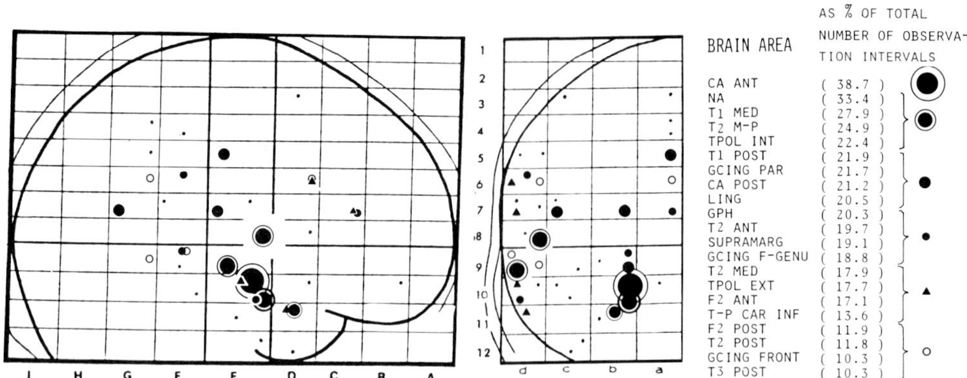

FIG. 2. Number of 10-sec seizure intervals with high-frequency tonic or clonic seizure activity ("activity 3 + 4") as percent of total number of observations per location. (From a total of 563 10-sec seizure intervals and a total of 7409 electrical activity encodings, it can be determined that, on average, 13.2 different brain structures were simultaneously monitored in a patient). In this graph, both hemispheres are combined; moreover, only brain locations with more than 100 observations are considered. In essence, this graph illustrates the key role of mediobasal limbic structures in the origin and/or sustenance of the ictal discharge in psychomotor seizures. (From ref. 4, with permission.)

the visual sense) or polymodal. Very often the polymodal experiences had the character of an "evoked memory" with clear-cut relations to specific personality traits of the affected individual. Therefore they are rightly called "dreamy states," "déjà vu," or "déjà vecu" experiences.

March of Ictal Symptoms and Spread of Ictal Discharges

With the temporal sequence of symptoms encoded, it was easy to look for the most frequently observed initial symptoms (see Fig. 3) and "primictal symptom constellations" and then to calculate for each symptom the probability of pairwise symptom transitions. These results could then be displayed as a kind of symptom group chain, and graphically visualized by connecting symptom groups with arrows, starting with the most frequent initial constellations and proceeding according to their transition probability. Figure 4 shows a three-dimensional display of metric multidimensional scaling of the 19 symptom groups with the most frequent symptom group transitions, which are illustrated by superimposed arrows on the scaled symptom cloud.

Correlation of Ictal Symptoms with the Discharging Brain Sites Over the Entire Seizure

Several computer analyses have been conducted with this electroclinical seizure matrix, including cluster analysis (with different weighting of the discharging brain sites according to the observed EEG patterns), multidimensional scaling of symptoms and brain locations (i.e., anatomical versus "functional" distances), and principal component analysis (PCA).

For the purpose of this chapter we want to refer to some results of the PCA (4), concentrating only on the four strongest factors (principal components) out of a total of 48 (see Fig. 5).

The main findings of this analysis, which combined 80 theoretically possible original intracortical locations and 80 symptoms and condensed them into 48 synthetic variables, might be summarized as follows:

1. The original variables were not independent: 48 factors represent 73% of the total variance.

2. Although the sorted factors did not show any stepwise increase, there appeared to be a

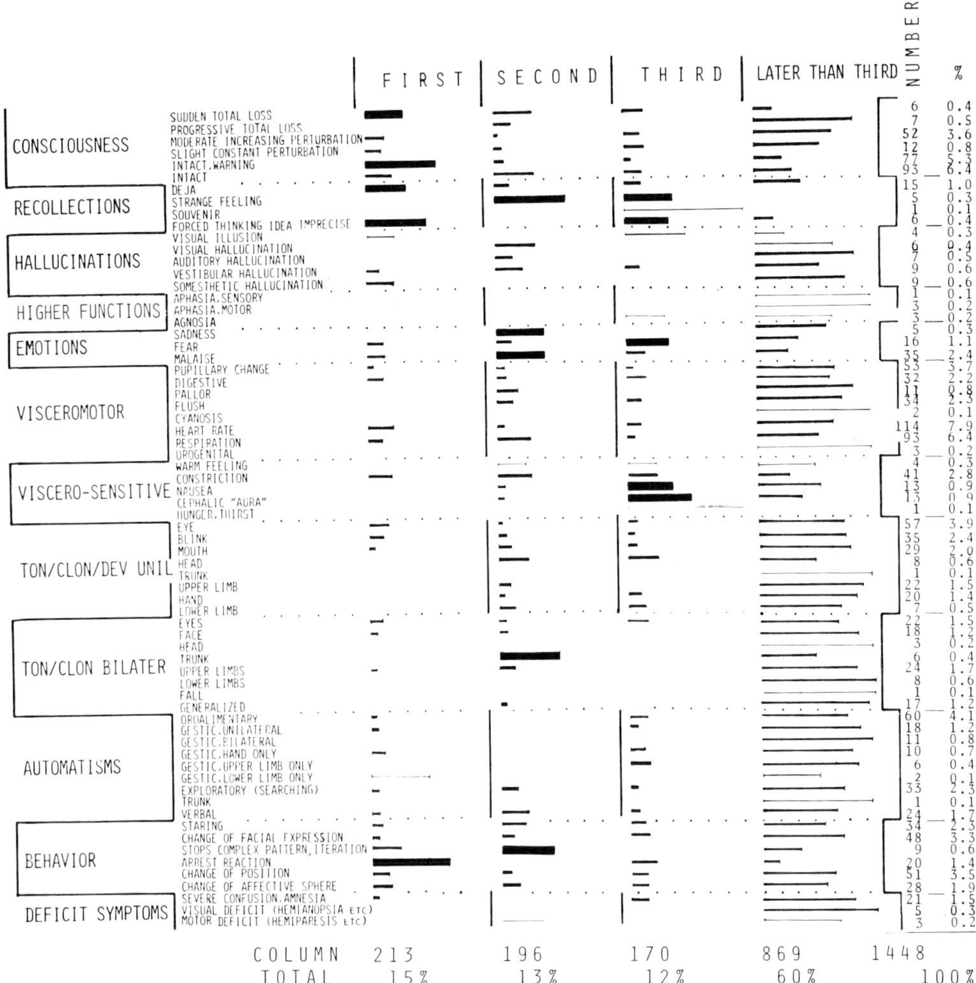

FIG. 3. Sequencing and relative occurrence of seizure symptoms. For every symptom, the sum of bar length totals 100%. The absolute frequency of observation of each symptom is given at the right. Bar thickness represents: symptom observed < 5 times (▬), symptom observed ≥ 5 times (▬). The five most frequently occurring symptoms per vertical column (first, second, etc.) are enhanced (■). (From ref. 4, with permission.)

bend near factor 18. This is where mainly "mixed factors" (consisting of symptoms and ictally discharging locations) give way to factors consisting of clinical symptoms only. These latter factors with their symptoms might therefore be considered as possessing no localizational value.

3. "Mixed factors" made up a much larger part of the total variance than did "pure symptom" factors: The interpretation is that the majority of the observed symptoms did have a "localizational adherence."

4. The strongest factor (factor 1 with an eigenvalue of 7.72; see Fig. 5), however, did not contain symptoms: This might indicate that the totality of the term "psychomotor seizure" is best characterized by the ictal discharge affecting the indicated locations, which in fact are to a great degree the limbic core structures, including mediobasal tem-

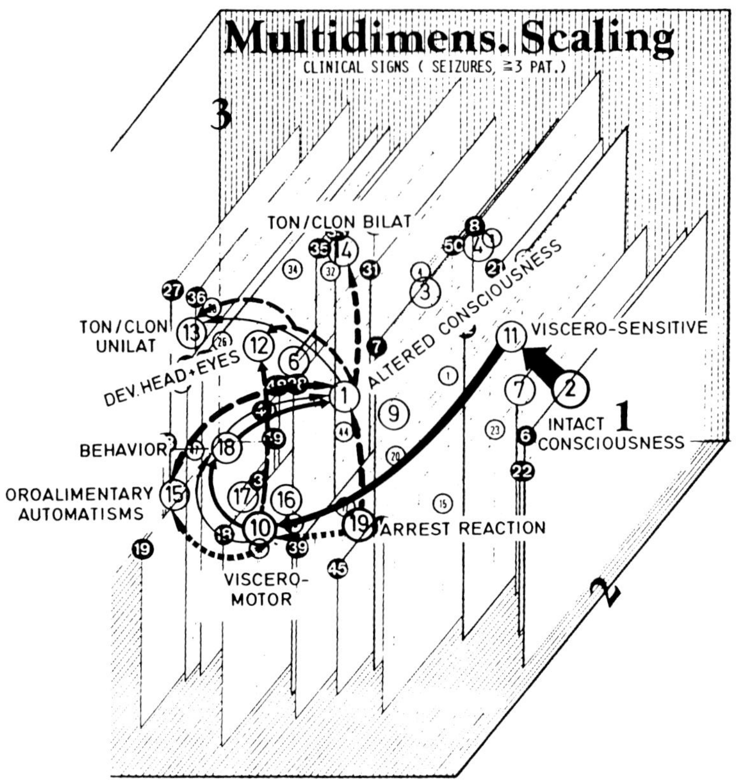

FIG. 4. "March of symptoms": The most important symptom group transitions are marked by arrows using the "pseudospatial" presentation of the multidimensionally scaled ictal symptoms. Larger encircled numbers represent the following symptom groups: 1—altered consciousness; 2—intact consciousness, warning; 3—recollections; 4—visual phenomena; 7—somesthetic hallucinations; 8—aphasia + agnosia; 9—affective–emotional changes; 10—visceromotor; 11—viscerosensitive; 12—deviation eyes + head; 13—motor: tonic–clonic unilateral; 14—motor: tonic–clonic bilateral; 15—oroalimentary automatisms; 16—gesticulatory automatisms; 17—verbal automatisms; 18—behavioral changes; 19—arrest reaction. (From ref. 4, with permission.)

poral structures, the cingulate gyrus, and orbitofrontal cortex.

5. Furthermore, one can also derive from this figure that the strongest factor 1 depicts a unilateral discharge and that only the following factors 2 and 3 show a bilateral discharging constellation. Factor 2 is associated with such symptoms as "confusion–amnesia," "change of affectivity," and "exploratory automatisms." Factor 3 might indicate the often seen suprasylvian spread of neocortical lateral posterior discharges associated with pronounced motor phenomena, whereas factor 4 most probably depicts the rare situation of a relatively well circumscribed insular–opercular discharge associated with the symptoms of "auditory hallucinations" and "constriction," as well as with "sensory aphasia" (if in the dominant hemisphere)?

SEIZURE SPREAD TO THE OPPOSITE HEMISPHERE: HOW BILATERAL ARE LIMBIC SEIZURES?

In the above-mentioned study (4) we have addressed this question and came to the following conclusions:

1. Forty-four percent of the analyzed 213 psychomotor seizures with unilateral onset showed contralateral propagation.

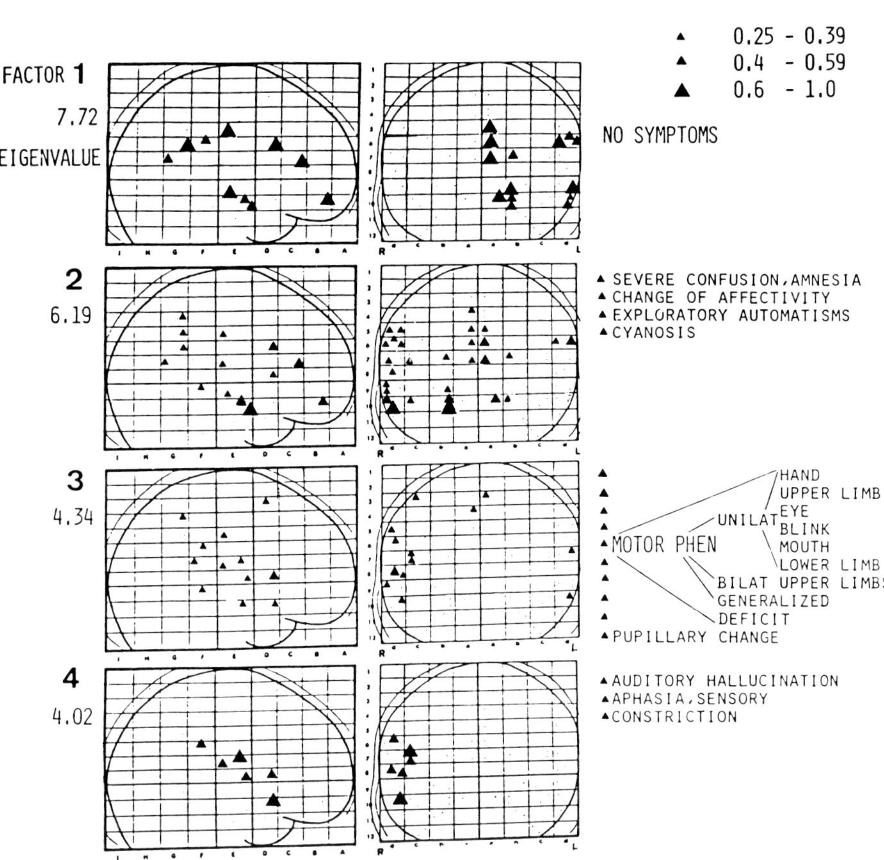

FIG. 5. Principal component analysis of stereoelectroencephalographically recorded brain sites (80 locations) and 80 ictal symptoms in 563 10-sec intervals of 213 psychomotor seizures. Graphical display of the four strongest "factors" (principal components) classified according to their eigenvalue. Only one lateral view is shown which superimposes left and right hemisphere locations. Information concerning lateralization is as follows: Factor 1 has a stronger adherence to the left hemisphere than to the right hemisphere, whereas factor 4 has a stronger adherence to the right hemisphere than to the left hemisphere. Both factors are "unilateral" ones (i.e., either left or right-hemispheric), whereas factors 2 and 3 are "bilateral" (i.e., the ictal discharge involves both hemispheres). (Modified from ref. 4, with permission.)

2. Propagation of the ictal discharge to the contralateral hemisphere was within the first 10 sec in 60%, within the second 10-sec interval in 24%, within the third 10-sec interval in 7.5%, and within the fourth 10-sec interval in 8.5%.

3. Contralateral propagation was more likely to occur when the discharging brain volume in the seizure initiating hemisphere was already relatively large—that is, at a time when ipsilateral seizure spread has reached a certain "critical" value. Before contralateral propagation, the hippocampal formation of the hemisphere showing the seizure onset displayed epileptic discharges in 94%.

4. If contralateral propagation occurred, the contralateral hippocampal formation was the sole recipient of the ictal discharge in 77%, and it was affected together with other contralateral brain sites in 95%.

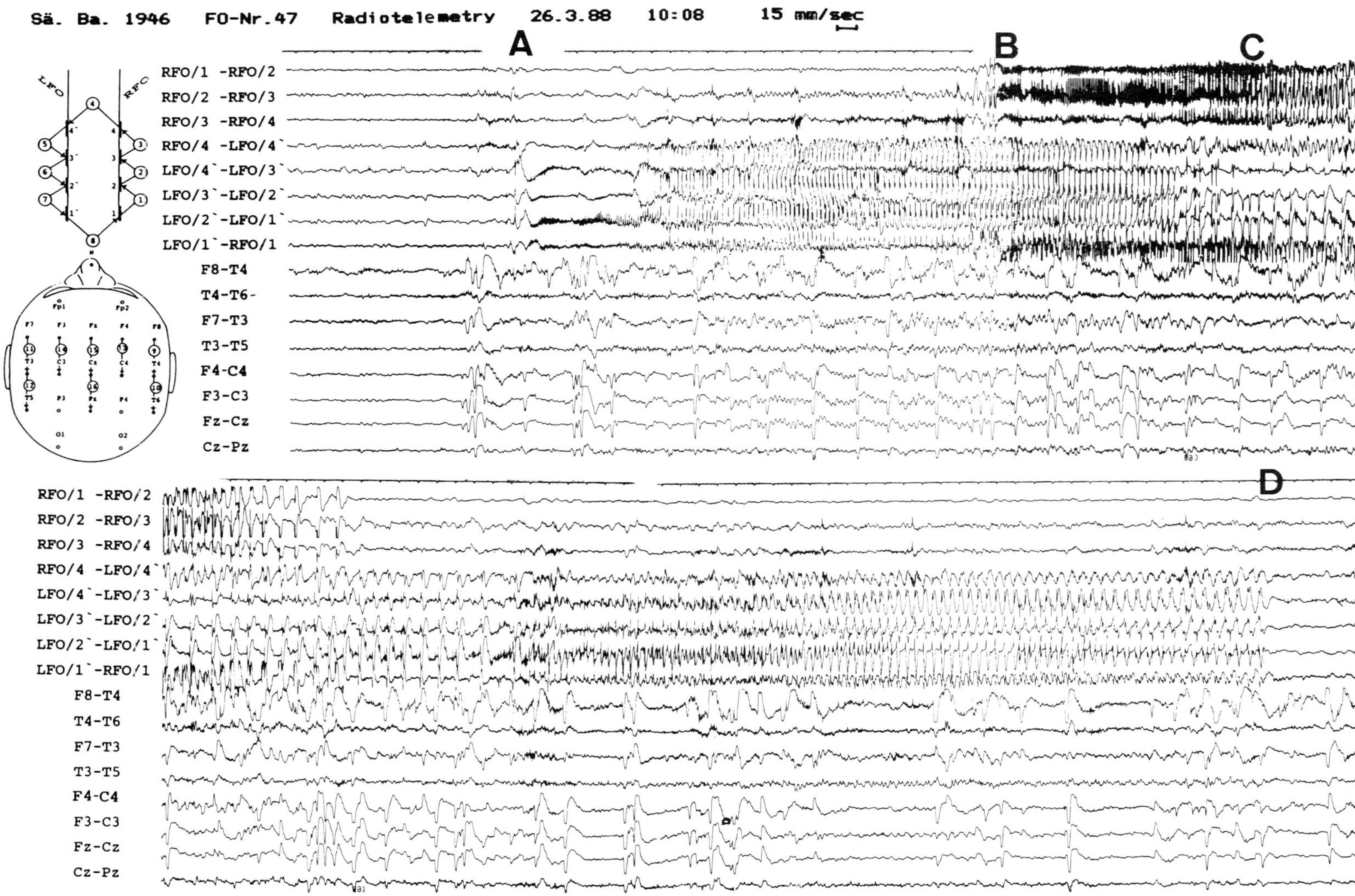

Sä. Ba. 1946 F0-Nr.47 Radiotelemetry 26.3.88 10:08 15 mm/sec
A
B
C
D
RFO/1 -RFO/2
RFO/2 -RFO/3
RFO/3 -RFO/4
RFO/4 -LFO/4'
LFO/4'-LFO/3'
LFO/3'-LFO/2'
LFO/2'-LFO/1'
LFO/1'-RFO/1
F8-T4
T4-T6
F7-T3
T3-T5
F4-C4
F3-C3
Fz-Cz
Cz-Pz
RFO/1 -RFO/2
RFO/2 -RFO/3
RFO/3 -RFO/4
RFO/4 -LFO/4'
LFO/4'-LFO/3'
LFO/3'-LFO/2'
LFO/2'-LFO/1'
LFO/1'-RFO/1
F8-T4
T4-T6
F7-T3
T3-T5
F4-C4
F3-C3
Fz-Cz
Cz-Pz

These findings let us speak of an attractor function of the contralateral hippocampal formation in psychomotor seizures, although the routes mediating this transhemispheric spread were not clear.

Recently we readdressed the issue of contralateral seizure spread by studying our patients who had been evaluated as possible candidates for selective amygdalohippocampectomy (6) with the use of bilaterally implanted four-contact foramen ovale electrodes (7) (see Fig. 6).

The findings from 272 analyzed seizures and 77 auras recorded in 68 patients within an average of 105 hr (range: 5–262) per patient can be summarized as follows:

On average, a patient had 4.0 seizures and 1.1 auras recorded; 201 seizures were classified as CPS, 19 as CPS with secondary generalization (SG), 30 as simple partial seizures (SPS), and 22 as generalized from the outset. During the monitoring period, 49 patients had only CPS without SG; four patients had only CPS with SG; two patients had CPS without, as well as with, SG; one patient had only SPS; four patients had SPS as well as CPS; one patient had CPS with SG and SPS; two patients had CPS as well as CPS with SG and SPS; four patients had generalized seizures from the outset; one patient had no seizures recorded.

Seizure onset (as determined by simultaneous scalp and bilateral foramen ovale electrodes) was always within the same mediobasal TL in 68% of patients; it was unilateral within the mediobasal TL, but with shifting lateralization, in 10%; 3% of patients had always unilateral, but regional, seizure onset, affecting more than mediobasal TL structures; in 19%, seizure onset was outside the mediobasal TL (and affected foramen ovale electrodes only during the course of the seizure).

Seizure duration was calculated for 31 patients who had a total of 130 seizures: Mean seizure duration was 72 ± 43 sec. It was the longest in CPS with SG (104 ± 37 sec), followed by CPS without SG (72 ± 42 sec), followed by SPS (49 ± 28 sec). In 39% of 31 patients, all recorded seizures propagated to the contralateral mediobasal TL; in 19% of patients, all recorded seizures remained unilateral; 23% had unilaterally remaining seizures as well as unilaterally originating seizures with spread to the contralateral hemisphere; 19% had bilateral seizure onset. Of 130 seizures (in 31 patients), 116 (89%) originated unilaterally and 14 (11%) originated bilaterally. Of those with unilateral onset, 74 (64%) spread to the contralateral TL whereas 42 (36%) did not. CPS showed contralateral propagation in 69% of cases, whereas SPS showed this type of propagation in only 26%. Those seizures propagating to the opposite hemisphere displayed contralateral mediobasal TL discharges 22 ± 18 sec (range 1–60 sec) after seizure onset.

Siegel (*unpublished data*) studied the seizures of 17 patients who met the requirement of CPS with unilateral mediobasal TL seizure onset. Using a previous categorization (8), he classified them during the entire length according to their predominant ictal features ("overall clinical gestalt"): (a) absence-like, (b) automatisms, (c) psychosensorial symptoms, (d) psychic symptoms, (e) visceromotor, and (f) viscerosensitive. In most of the seizures, combinations had to be noted in order to characterize the entire gestalt.

FIG. 6. Radiotelemetric foramen ovale (FO) electrode (upper eight channels) and simultaneous scalp EEG recording from a 42-year-old female showing a spontaneous complex partial seizure with the following features: left mediobasal temporal onset; Intermediate propagation to the contralateral right mediobasal TL structures (end of top sequence); and a reprise with shifting back to the seizure-originating structures. Continuous record starts at upper left and ends at lower right. Channels 1–8 are bipolar recordings from the right and left FO electrodes in a closed chain. Channels 9–16 are bipolar scalp derivations (10–20 system; collodion-fixed chlorinated Ag/AgCl cup electrodes). Clinical semiology: Coinciding with the seizure onset (**A**), the patient experiences her habitual aura, which she described as a crescendo-like sensation of increasing fear. At **B** the patient stopped her activity, looked vacant, and arrested. At **C** she started moving, but her activities were purposeless. At the end of the discharge (**D**), she started protocoling her attack.

TABLE 1. *Analysis of the complex partial seizures (CPS) of 17 patients (all CPS with unilateral mediobasal temporal lobe seizure onset): predominant clinical features ("overal clinical gestalt") in relation to whether contralateral propagation occurred or not during foramen ovale electrode evaluation*[a]

	Predominant clinical ictal features					
Type of seizure	Absence-like	Auto-matisms	Psycho-sensorial symptoms	Psychic symptoms	Viscero-motor	Viscero-sensitive
CPS without contralateral propagation (N = 4)	75%	75%	25%	25%	50%	100%
CPS with contralateral propagation (N = 13)	62%	100%	46%	62%	54%	69%

[a]From A. M. Siegel (*unpublished data*), with permission.

TABLE 2. *List of symptoms evoked by electrical brain stimulation*[a]

Observed symptoms and signs	Frequency of observation	Percentage of positive stimulation
Brief movements of extremities and/or head	202	12.1
Arrest	164	9.8
Focal twitches and cloni	142	8.6
Gestural automatisms	142	8.6
Eye movements	139	8.3
Postural changes; reactive movements; acceleration or slowing of movements; restlessness	136	8.2
Unspecific warning	131	7.9
Change of respiration	130	7.8
Opening or closure of eyes or mouth	128	7.7
Gastric and epigastric ascending sensation and oppression	127	7.6
Blinking	123	7.4
Oroalimentary automatisms	115	6.9
Phonation, groaning	101	6.1
Inadequate reaction to commands; "blocked" feeling; increased reaction time	84	5.0
Flush, pallor	83	5.0
Problems with language and/or speech	71	4.3
Dyslexia, dyscalculia	65	3.9
Cardiac symptoms (tachycardia, bradycardia)	57	3.4
Cephalgic sensation	57	3.4
Fear, anxiety	53	3.2
Clouding of consciousness	51	3.1
Visual (positive + negative symptoms)	43	2.6
Unlocalized itching sensation	43	2.6
Amnesia for time of stimulation	35	2.1
Vomiting, nausea	27	1.6
Smiling (?pleasure?)	26	1.6
Alteration of time and space; depersonalization	26	1.6
Funny feeling	23	1.4
Staring	21	1.3
Recollection, déjà experience, dreamy state	17	1.0
Vertigo	10	0.6

[a]Symptoms have been arranged in decreasing frequency of observation and have been expressed in relation to the total of 1665 stimulations which were accompanied by clinical symptoms, regardless of whether an afterdischarge was observed or not (percentage of positive stimulation). Numbers of stimulations per indicated brain region are given in Table 3.

As can be noted in Table 1, seizures with contralateral propagation had automatisms in 100%.

CLINICAL SYMPTOMS PROVOKED BY INTRACEREBRAL ELECTRICAL STIMULATION

In 116 stereoelectroencephalographically examined patients, a total of 2223 stimulations have been performed that produced clinical and/or electrical effects. These stimulations were analyzed with regard to their anatomo-electroclinical characteristics. Fifty-four percent of the stimulations were in the right hemisphere, and 46% were in the left hemisphere; 952 stimulations (43%) were accompanied by one symptom (636 stimulations) or more than one clinical symptom (316 stimulations), but without an afterdischarge. Two hundred thirty-two stimulations (10%) that evoked clinical symptoms were accompanied

by a local afterdischarge at the stimulation site; 481 stimulations (22%) gave rise to a regional afterdischarge with clinical symptoms. The remaining 548 stimulations (25%) produced a local or regional afterdischarge, but no clinical signs or symptoms.

Table 2 lists the observed electrically provoked symptoms and signs according to their frequency. The brain areas from which six particularly interesting symptoms were elicited are depicted in Table 3 and Fig. 7. Figure 8 gives an example of this stimulation data and exemplifies how solid conclusions can be drawn regarding the functional specialization of certain brain structures, despite the sampling problem.

CONCLUDING REMARKS

An overview like this cannot be comprehensive. Many studies on the ictal semiology, particularly the pioneering ones from the

TABLE 3. *Brain areas from which the six indicated symptoms have been evoked by electrical stimulation[a]*

Brain region	Arrest	Gastric and epigastric sensations	Fear and anxiety	Altered time and space, depersonalization	Staring	Recollection déjà vu, dreamy state	Total positive stimulation
Amygdalar and periamygdalar	15	32	14	8	4	7	80/253 (31.6)
Hippocampal	14	34	11	8	3	5	75/148 (50.1)
Parahippocampal gyrus	23	28	12	1	4	3	71/192 (37)
Total	(31.7)[b]	(74.0)[b]	(69.8)[b]	(65.4)[b]	(52.4)[b]	(88.2)[b]	
mediobasal	52	94	37	17	11	15	226/593
limbic	(3.1)	(5.6)	(2.2)	(1.0)	(0.7)	(0.9)	(38.1)
Temporal	22	9	5	4	1	—	41/232
neocortical	(1.3)	(0.5)	(0.3)	(0.2)	(0.06)		(17.7)
Extratemporal	90	24	11	5	9	2	141/840
	(5.4)	(1.4)	(0.7)	(0.3)	(0.5)	(0.1)	(16.8)
Total	164[b]	127[b]	53[b]	26[b]	21[b]	17[b]	408/1665
(% of 1665)	(9.8)	(7.7)	(3.2)	(1.6)	(1.3)	(1.0)	(24.5)

[a]Out of a total of 1665 stimulations (with or without afterdischarges) that were accompanied by clinical symptoms, 408 stimulations evoked the indicated symptoms and signs. For the purpose of this table, the sites of stimulation have been categorized into five brain regions: extratemporal; lateral temporal neocortex (temporal neocortical); parahippocampal gyrus; hippocampus; and amygdala and surrounding structures. When combined, the three latter structures represent the temporal mediobasal limbic structures (total mediobasal limbic). Number in parentheses are percentages referring to the total of 1665 stimulations. The percentages of positive stimulations (with all kinds of symptoms and signs included) per brain area are indicated at the extreme right.

[b]Percentage refers to vertical total.

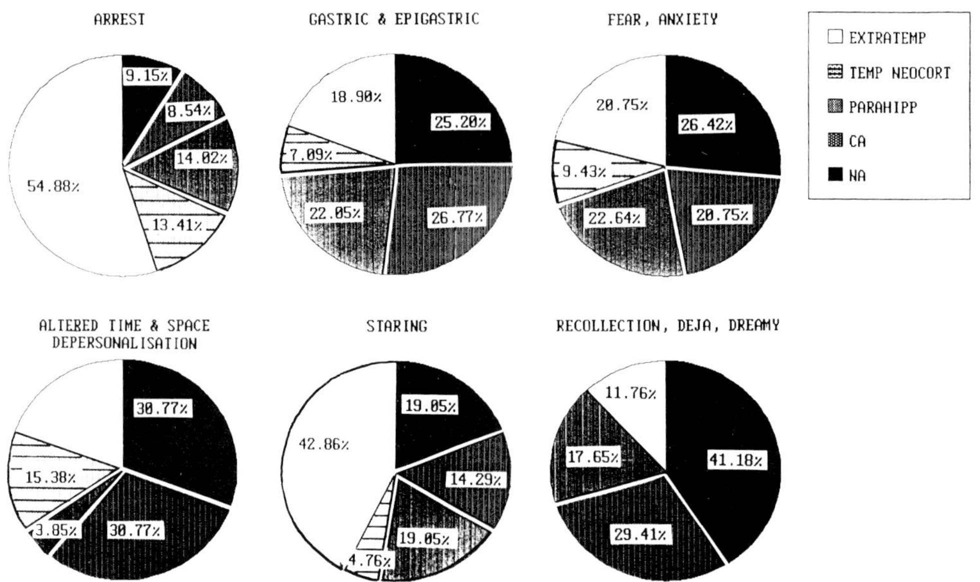

FIG. 7. Relative distribution of brain regions from which the six indicated symptoms have been evoked by electrical stimulation (for absolute numbers refer to Table 3).

schools of Montreal (Montreal Neurological Institute [2,9–14]) and Paris (Hôpital St. Anne [15–17]), as well as from other distinguished workers in this field (18–25), should be discussed in detail.

Reports from the surgical programs of these pioneering surgical centers form the basis of much of our knowledge on the ictal symptomatology of CPS with temporal but also with extratemporal, especially frontal, origin. This is not surprising if one considers that the temporal lobes are the most frequent target for epilepsy surgery and that the careful analysis of the electroclinical accompaniments of habitual attack patterns still remains the most important step in the presurgical evaluation of possible candidates for surgical treatment (9,22).

Although earlier investigations, directed at stimulating the accessible cortex during surgery, were not completely in agreement with results derived from chronically studied patients with depth electrodes (stereoelectroencephalography), during the last decade a rather good agreement of the results from various centers has emerged: Olfactory hallucinations are observed most typically with ictal discharges of the uncus, elementary auditory hallucinations are associated with seizure activity in or near Heschl's gyri, and vertiginous sensations are linked with discharges in the posterior temporal operculum or adjacent parietal region (25). Oroalimentary automatisms might indicate seizure discharges in the amygdala (15), and gustatory sensations might indicate discharges in the insula (10). Although

FIG. 8. Example of topographical mapping of stimulation effects. The three graphs on the left depict sites from which visual symptoms have been elicited (only stimulations without an afterdischarge have been considered here). Because of the uneven distribution of stimulation sites, these left-sided graphs have to be compared with the ones on the right, in which the frequency of stimulations (evoking a symptom but no afterdischarge) is shown. The brain is visualized with three planes: lateral surface (**top**), paramedian (**middle**), and most medial (**bottom**). (From ref. 5, with permission.)

SYMPTOM GROUP VISUAL

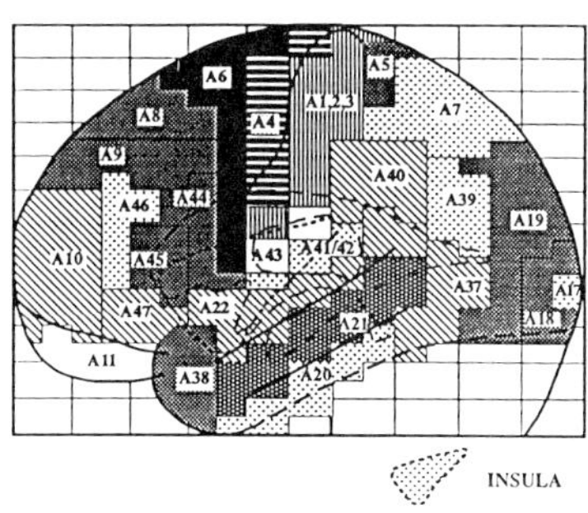

AREAS OF BRODMANN:
LATERAE

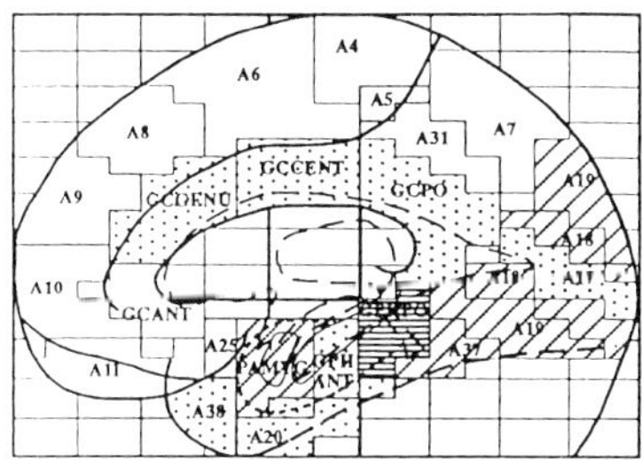

AREAS OF BRODMANN: MEDIAL I
(INTERMEDIATE TL)

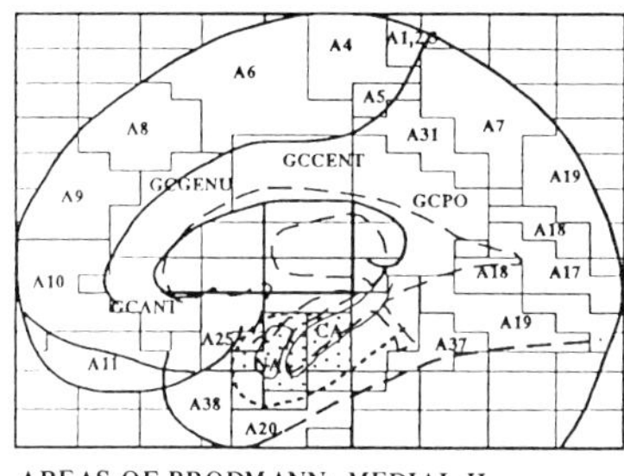

AREAS OF BRODMANN: MEDIAL II
(DEEP TL)

NUMBER OF STIMULATIONS PROVOKING
VISUAL SYMPTOMS

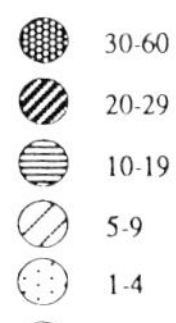

NUMBER OF STIMULATIONS PROVOKING
SYMPTOMS BUT NO AFTERDISCHARGES
PER BRODMANN'S AREA

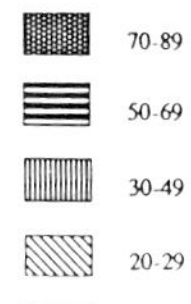

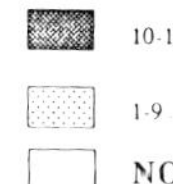

it was initially believed that complex hallucinations, illusions, and memories reflect seizure activity in the lateral temporal or temporoparieto-occipital neocortex, several investigators (2,3,26) have elicited complex psychical phenomena (including complex visual hallucinations) by stimulating medial temporal structures, and without spread of afterdischarges to lateral neocortex. More refined methods of investigating patients during long-lasting focal epileptic discharges of certain temporal lobe structures have revealed autonomic phenomena and subtle cognitive deficits of material-specific memory and language capabilities (27,28). Thus, the hope might not be unfounded that, with the help of refined analysis methods of the EEG in association with simultaneous biochemical measurements (29,30), a further substantial step towards a comprehensive understanding of some of the key symptoms of ictal (but also "interictal") behavior and personality changes (31) can be undertaken.

One major aim of this chapter, therefore, was to show that careful analyses of ictal symptoms not only are an essential prerequisite for correct diagnosis and treatment, but also offer a unique chance to gain fascinating insights into the still mysterious functions of human brain.

REFERENCES

1. Wieser HG. Human limbic seizures: EEG studies, origin, and spread. In: Meldrum BS, Ferrendelli JA, Wieser HG, eds. *Anatomy of epileptogenesis.* London: John Libbey, 1988;127–138.
2. Gloor P, Olivier A, Quesney LF, Andermann F, Horowitz S. The role of the limbic system in experiential phenomena of temporal lobe epilepsy. *Ann Neurol* 1982;12:129–144.
3. Halgren E, Walter RD, Cherlow DG, Crandall PH. Mental phenomena evoked by electrical stimulation of the human hippocampal formation and amygdala. *Brain* 1978;101:83–117.
4. Wieser HG. *Electroclinical features of the psychomotor seizure.* Stuttgart (London): Gustav Fischer (Butterworths), 1983.
5. Schmid M. Analyse klinischer und elektrischer Reizantworten nach zerebralen elektrischen Stimulationen. Thesis, University of Zurich, 1990.
6. Wieser HG, Siegel AM, Yasargil GM. The Zurich amygdalo-hippocampectomy series: a short up-date. *Acta Neurochir* 1990(suppl); Vol. 50 in press.
7. Wieser HG, Moser S. Improved multipolar foramen ovale electrode monitoring. *J Epilepsy* 1988;1:13–22.
8. Wieser HG. The phenomenology of limbic seizures. In: Wieser HG, Speckmann E-J, Engel J Jr, eds. *The epileptic focus.* London: John Libbey, 1987;113–136.
9. Gloor P. Commentary: Approaches to localization of the epileptogenic lesion. In: Engel J Jr, ed. *Surgical treatment of the epilepsies.* New York: Raven Press, 1987;97–100.
10. Penfield W, Jasper HH. *Epilepsy and the functional anatomy of the human brain.* Boston: Little, Brown, 1954.
11. Penfield W, Kristiansen K. *Epileptic seizure patterns.* Springfield, IL: Charles C Thomas, 1951.
12. Quesney LF. Clinical and EEG features of complex partial seizures of temporal lobe origins. *Epilepsia [Suppl]* 1986;27:S27–S45.
13. Rasmussen T. Localizational aspects of epileptic seizure phenomena. In: Thompson RA, Green JR, eds. *New perspectives in cerebral localization.* New York: Raven Press, 1982;177–203.
14. Rasmussen T. Characteristics of a pure culture of frontal lobe epilepsy. *Epilepsia* 1983;24:482–493.
15. Bancaud J. Epileptic attacks of temporal lobe origin in man. *Jpn J EEG–EMG [Suppl]* (Didactic Lectures, Xth ICECN, Kyoto, 1981) 1981;61–71.
16. Bancaud J, Talairach J, Bonis A, Schaub C, Szikla G, Morel P, Bordas-Ferer M. *La stéréoélectroencéphalographie dans l'epilepsie.* Paris: Masson, 1965.
17. Geier S, Bancaud J, Talairach J, Bonis A, Enjelvin M, Hossard-Bouchaud H. Automatisms during frontal lobe epileptic seizures. *Brain* 1976;99:447–458.
18. Ajmone-Marsan C. Clinical-electrographic correlations of partial seizures. In: Wada JA, ed. *Modern perspectives in epilepsy.* Montreal: Eden Press, 1978;76–98.
19. Ajmone-Marsan C. Commentary: Clinical characteristics of partial seizures. In: Engel J Jr, ed. *Surgical treatment of the epilepsies.* New York: Raven Press, 1987;121–127.
20. Delgado-Escueta AV, Bacsal FE, Treiman DM. Complex partial seizures on closed-circuit television and EEG: a study of 691 attacks in 79 patients. *Ann Neurol* 1981;11:292–300.
21. Delgado-Escueta AV, Swartz BE, Maldonado HM, Walsh GO, Rand RW, Halgren E. Complex partial seizures of frontal lobe origin. In: Wieser HG, Elger CE, eds. *Presurgical evaluation of epileptics.* Berlin: Springer, 1987;267–299.
22. Engel J Jr. Approaches to localization of the epileptogenic lesion. In: Engel J Jr, ed. *Surgical treatment of the epilepsies.* New York: Raven Press, 1987;75–95.
23. Spencer SS, Spencer DD, Williamson PD, Mattson RH. Sexual automatisms in partial complex seizures. *Neurology* 1983;33:527–533.
24. Wada JA, Purves SJ. Oral and bimanual–bipedal activity as ictal manifestations of frontal lobe epilepsy [Abstract] *Epilepsia* 1984:25:668.

25. Williamson PD, Wieser HG, Delgado-Escueta AV. Clinical characteristics of partial seizures. In: Engel J Jr, ed. *Surgical treatment of the epilepsies*. New York: Raven Press, 1987;101–120.

26. Wieser HG. Zur Frage der lokalisatorischen Bedeutung epileptischer Halluzinationen. In: Karbowski K, ed. *Halluzinationen bei Epilepsien und ihre Differentialdiagnose*. Berne: Verlag Hans Huber, 1982;67–92.

27. Stodieck SRG, Wieser HG. Autonomic phenomena in temporal lobe epilepsy. *J Autonom Nerv Syst* [Suppl] 1986;611–621.

28. Wieser HG, Hailemariam S, Regard M, Landis T. Unilateral limbic epileptic status activity: stereo-EEG, behavioural, and cognitive data. *Epilepsia* 1985;26:19–29.

29. Buchli R, Meier D, Boesiger P, Isler P, Wieser HG. Phosphorus-31 MR spectroscopy in focal epilepsies [Abstract]. *7th Annual Meeting of the Society for Magnetic Resonance in Medicine*. August 22–26, 1988, San Francisco.

30. Wieser HG, Do K, Perschak H, Cuénod M. Modulation of extracellular aspartate level during epileptiform events in primary epileptogenic area of patients [Abstract]. Satellite Symposium of the XXXI International Congress on the Physiological Sciences, Helsinki, 1989: *Physiology, pharmacology and development of epileptogenic phenomena*, July 4–8, 1989, Frankfurt, p. 68.

31. Wieser HG, Landis T. Is the "interictal behaviour syndrome of temporal lobe epilepsy" really an "interictal" phenomenon? *Neurol Psychiatr* 1983;6:70–78.

Advances in Neurology, Vol. 55, edited by
D. Smith, D. Treiman, and M. Trimble,
Raven Press, Ltd., New York © 1991.

20

Frontal Lobe Seizures and Epilepsies in Neurobehavioral Disorders

Antonio V. Delgado-Escueta*, Barbara E. Swartz*,
Gregory O. Walsh*, Patrick Chauvel†, Jean Bancaud†,
and Dominique Broglin†

*California Comprehensive Epilepsy Program, Southwest Regional Epilepsy Center/
Neurology and Research Services, West Los Angeles VA Medical Center, West Los Angeles,
California 90073; Department of Neurology, University of California, Los Angeles,
Los Angeles, California 90024; and †INSERM Unit 97, Epilepsy Research Unit, and the
Neurosurgical Department, Centre Paul Broca, 75014 Paris, France*

THE CLINICAL CHALLENGE OF FRONTAL LOBE SEIZURES AND EPILEPSIES (FLS/E) IN NEUROBEHAVIORAL DISORDERS

The epilepsies are a common disorder affecting approximately 20–40 million people in the world. Although there are no totally accurate figures on the number of individuals who suffer from epileptic seizures in the United States, conservative estimates of various epidemiologic studies indicate that approximately 0.6% of the population is under treatment for recurrent seizures; the annual incidence rate is 48 per 100,000 population, and the prevalence rate is 650 per 100,000 (1–3).

The National Commission for the Control of Epilepsy and its Consequences (Publication No. NIH 78-311) calculated that there are one to two million epilepsy patients in the United States, of which approximately 600,000 are of frontal lobe origin. About 171,000 of these patients with frontal lobe epilepsies continue to have incapacitating seizures even in the presence of antiepileptic drugs (1–3).

Seizures from frontal lobe epilepsies are more common than previously estimated. Be-

cause the frontal lobe is the largest lobe in the cerebral cortex, both discrete and widespread epileptogenic lesions frequently occur in its vicinity (1–3). Its clinical manifestations are poorly recognized, because many types of seizures come from different frontal regions; furthermore, its large volume presents sampling problems. Frontally originating discharges spread rapidly to other frontal or extratemporal areas, thereby preventing accurate localization and lateralization. Alternatively, the frontal lobe can be invaded by spreading parietal or parieto-occipital discharges. Frontal lobe seizures are also underreported, because they are frequently mistaken for other conditions. In particular, complex partial seizures involving the paralimbic (anterior cingulate, paraolfactory, and caudal orbitofrontal regions) frontal lobe are frequently mistaken for hysterical or psychogenic seizures, impulse dyscontrol, and disinhibited or aggressive behavior of affective and schizophrenic disorders (1–4).

To improve the practitioners awareness and accuracy of diagnosis, we will present algorithms for differentiating frontal and extrafrontal seizures as they relate to history-taking, neurological examination, and diagnosis (2). These algorithms, especially those for seizures of medial frontal and orbital frontal origin, can aid the practitioner in separating frontal lobe epilepsies from pseudoepileptic neurobehavioral disorders.

APPROACHING THE PATIENT WITH SUSPECTED FRONTAL LOBE SEIZURES

The approach to the patient with suspected frontal lobe seizures follows the same principles as the approach to patients with seizures in general (2–4). A multidisciplinary team approach is vital to the successful management of epilepsy and of frontal lobe seizures. The physician in charge should manage and coordinate the efforts of neurologic, psychological, psychiatric, and social-service professionals, and he or she should foster understanding among the patient's family, employers, and school personnel. The team approach should follow six steps: (i) verify that seizures are indeed epileptic in nature, (ii) define the type of frontal lobe seizures and the epilepsy syndrome, (iii) prove the likely cause of epileptic seizures and stop trigger factors, (iv) establish an early treatment plan with antiepileptic drugs, (v) monitor seizure control and recognize adverse effects on the patient's quality of life, and (vi) evaluate for possible surgical treatment if seizures are resistant to antiepileptic drugs (2–4). In this chapter, we will discuss primarily the diagnosis of frontal lobe seizures and epilepsies focusing on the practical issues surrounding steps i, ii, and iii.

Verifying That Neurobehavioral Disorders Are Frontal Lobe Seizures

Frontal lobe seizures are frequently mistaken for pseudoepileptic and nonepileptic behavioral episodes when the patient has episodic fugue states, altered consciousness, or impaired responsiveness, or when episodes of aggression and violence characterize disinhibited states, or when behavior is bizarre, disruptive and antisocial (1–3). Because syncope is commonly associated with pseudoepileptic hysterical seizures, the common faint should be differentiated from frontal lobe drop attacks or what had been incorrectly termed "temporal lobe syncope" (3).

Bimanual, bipedal, or bicycling movements, running in fear, mimics of swimming, and frenetic, bizarre, flailing-arm-and-leg automatisms of frontal lobe seizures are commonly called "hysterical" (2,3). Conversely, impulse dyscontrol with directed aggression and violence are often mistaken for the disinhibited state of frontal lobe seizures. Prolonged postictal psychoses which follow a series of frontal lobe psychomotor seizures can be misdiagnosed as schizophrenia. Although closed-circuit television (CCTV) videotaping, biotelemetry of the electroencephalogram (EEG), and Holter monitoring of the electrocardiogram have shown important clinical differences among these conditions, the history and clinical setting are frequently the most important determinants of the diagnosis (see Table 1).

Syncope: The Hysterical Faint; Psychoses

Syncope (see Table 1) occurs in as many as 25–30% of young, physically healthy adults. In true syncope, postural tone and consciousness are suddenly lost and the patient falls, most frequently because of a temporary decrease in cerebral blood flow. The latter result from either a fall in systemic arterial pressure (vasovagal syncope) or a decrease in cardiac output (cardiac syncope). The clinical picture of pallor, sweats, visual blurring, a sensation of imminent loss of consciousness followed by flaccidity, upward deviation of the eyes, and loss of consciousness (simple syncope) is paralleled by the appearance of 2- to 4-Hz high-amplitude slow waves on the EEG. The persistence of cerebral anoxia for more than 15 sec will be reflected by tonic spasms and one or two generalized jerks (convulsive syncope). The EEG becomes slow and has low voltage, but it promptly returns to normal after consciousness is regained (2).

During the hysterical faint, loss of consciousness is usually feigned, there is neither a fall in systemic arterial pressure nor a decrease in cardiac output, and the EEG does not show slow waves. The patient usually gains attention from such behavior and may actually have other consciously unidentified motives (2).

Aside from conversion hysteria, hyperven-

TABLE 1. *Clinical features that differentiate epileptic seizures, syncope, and pseudoseizures*

	Epileptic seizure			Syncope	Pseudoepileptic seizures
Characteristics:	Tonic–clonic: primary or secondary	Complex partial	Absence		
Components:	Tonic–clonic phases do not vary from attack to attack	Various psychomotor automatisms, but commonly similar from attack to attack	Wide range of behavior, but more simple than complex partial seizures	A common set of behavior patterns during episodes of unconsciousness	Bizarre and unusual range of behavior different from attack to attack
Posture before attack:	Any	Any	Any	Upright	Usually upright
Complaints at onset:	May have aura	May have aura	None	Sweats, pallor, pounding heartbeat	None usually
Fall:	Common	Rare	Rare	Always	Usually, but with no consequent injuries
Stereotype:	Same components and sequence from attack to attack	Same components and sequence from attack to attack	Same components and sequence from attack to attack	Same components and sequence	No stereotype
Unconsciousness or impaired and amnesic responsiveness:	Unconsciousness is present	Impaired responsiveness	Impaired responsiveness	Unconscious	Conscious
Sequence of events:	Orderly sequence of tonic and clonic phases	Orderly sequence of unresponsiveness, with arrest of motions or postures; or somatomotor signs followed by automatisms, confusion, and amnesia or bimanual–bipedal thrashing movements	Orderly sequence of sudden unresponsiveness, or altered responses with automatisms and sudden recovery	One phase consisting mainly of unconsciousness	No orderly sequence of bizarre behavior
EEG during episode:	Abnormal	Abnormal	Abnormal	Abnormal	Normal
EEG immediately after episode:	Abnormal	Abnormal	Normal	Normal	Normal
Serum prolactin levels:	Reliably increases above baseline	Reliably increases above baseline	Unknown	Unknown	Does not increase

tilation can also be mistaken for convulsive episodes. The provoking factor for hyperventilation is sometimes difficult to discover. Rapid shallow breathing is present, and the patient feels light-headed, with trembling limbs and often trembling of the whole body. Excessive loss of carbon dioxide produces paresthesias in the hands, face, and feet; carpopedal spasms may develop (2).

Hysterical faints, pseudoepileptic attacks of hyperventilation, and epileptic seizures can exist together in the same patient. The EEG and serum prolactin levels are especially useful in differentiating the two events. The EEG during and immediately after epileptic seizures is almost always abnormal. Between epileptic seizures the EEG is abnormal and shows interictal paroxysmal discharges in 40–60% of patients. The EEG is normal between, during, and after hysterical faints and pseudoepileptic attacks. Prolactin serum levels increase within 20 min of a tonic–clonic convul-

TABLE 2. *Frontal lobe epilepsies with complex partial seizures: clinical features on CCTV[a]*

I. Dorsolateral frontal lobe[b]	
1. Dorsolateral premotor cortex[c,d] (e.g., intermediate frontal gyrus)	A. Psychomotor attacks: usually no aura; starts with tonic forward extension of head, neck, and trunk as contraversive head or eye movements occur with impaired consciousness; mild clonic facial or arm movements or elevation of one arm above shoulder occur when paroxysms spread to primary cortex or supplementary motor cortex[c]
	B. Pseudoabsence: very brief lapses of consciousness lasting < 10sec with minimal automatisms; sudden in onset and cessation
2. Prefrontal or frontopolar	A. Psychic–intellectual auras, visual illusions, and hallucinations or
	B. Initial unconsciousness followed by adversive head and eye movements
	C. Frequent tonic–clonic convulsions
	D. Pseudoabsence attacks
3. Dorsolateral posterior inferior gyrus	A. Tonic or clonic oral and facial jerks; clonic seizures of arm
	B. Pseudoabsence attack
	C. Salivation, deglutition, neurovegetative manifestations during psychomotor attacks
	D. Palilalia, arrest of speech, nonfluent dysphasia
II. Mesial frontal lobe or medial frontal cortex[c]	
1. Supplementary motor	A. Psychomotor attacks: usually no aura; starts with elevation of arm, with abduction and flexion of elbow as head turns to look at hand; vocalization; elevation of lips; grimaces; hissing with impaired consciousness; late appearance of oroalimentary automatisms
	B. Ipsilateral, bilateral, or homolateral motor responses can also start psychomotor attacks
	C. Autonomic seizures: mydriasis, tachycardia, and apnea
	D. Speech arrest
	E. Secondary tonic–clonic attacks
2. Anterior cingulate cortex	A. Frequent psychic emotional auras, including fear, anger, and terror with neurovegetative signs.
	B. Psychomotor attack: starts with sudden fear, mydriasis, and epigastric discomfort, leading to impaired consciousness, bizarre arm-and-leg or ambulatory automatisms, and usually incontinence.[e] Late appearance of oroalimentary automatisms during impaired consciousness, when paroxysms spread to medial temporal lobe structures; head looks to elevated arm when discharges spread to supplementary motor area
	C. Pseudoabsence: brief impaired consciousness with minimal automatisms, but with sphincter incontinence

sion or complex partial seizure but do not change with pseudoepileptic hysterical fits (2).

Complex partial seizures from the frontal lobe are sometimes difficult to differentiaite from acute paranoid psychosis, schizophrenia, and schizophreniform psychoses. Non-convulsive frontal lobe psychomotor status can be mainly or solely characterized by psychosis with prominent paranoid features and characters of schizophrenia. Prolonged post-ictal psychosis can follow frontal lobe complex partial seizures and can be mistaken for

TABLE 2. *Continued*

III. Orbital frontal lobe[f]	
1. Anterior-orbital or mesio-orbital frontal lobe seizures	A. Rare psychoemotional or intellectual auras
	B. Psychomotor attack: sudden complex motor automatisms involving both legs, both arms, and trunk, often bizarre and frenetic,[e] which may be preceded by a loud cry; impaired consciousness and severe confusion, along with pelvic up–down movements, running movements, bipedal movements (similar to bicycling), swimming movements,[e] and karate movements, repeatedly appear as stereotyped from attack to attack mixed with staring, change of facial expression, fear, and oroalimentary automatisms in the middle or late stages of seizure
2. Posterior-orbital or temporo-orbital frontal seizures	A. Olfactory hallucinations or illusions as auras with fear or modifications of humor
	B. Neurovegetative manifestation preceding or early in the psychomotor attacks including cardiovascular, vasomotor, digestive, urinary
	C. Bizarre arm-and-leg automatisms early in the psychomotor attacks with oroalimentary automatisms, gestural automatisms, agitation and ambulation,[e] salivation, deglutition, and contraversive head–eye movements in the middle and late phases of seizure

[a]Denotes an electroclinical sequence, relatively characteristic of habitual seizures.
[b]Data taken from refs. 1–3.
[c]Previously described as Type IIA complex partial seizures (14).
[d]Together with complex partial seizures, simple partial seizures are common such as clonic jerks of the arm (when area 4 is engaged) or of the leg (when paracentral lobule is involved). Frontobasal–cingulate seizures of Wieser (8) or complex partial seizures described by Williamson et al. (15,16) and by Wada and Purves (14).
[e]Previously described as Type IIB complex partial seizures (14).
[f]Data were taken from ref. 52.

chronic schizophrenic or manic–depressive psychoses. Haloperidal may be necessary for a short period to manage the psychoses.

Frontal Lobe Seizures

Classifying Frontal Lobe Seizures

There are various reasons why frontal lobe seizures should be classified on the basis of distinct, but highly interrelated, neuroanatomical subregions and systems. It gives us insight on the origin and spread of epileptogenic discharges. Medial-to-lateral and ventral-to-dorsal subdivisions observed in the clinical manifestations of seizures parallel similar trends in subdivisions of the neuropsychologic deficits produced by frontal lobe lesions, and they also parallel behavioral correlates of regional cerebral blood flow. Anal-

ysis of cells as well as of synapses and metabolism within these defined neuroanatomical subdivisions can then be done, providing (a) targets for new modes of treatment and (b) designs for modulation of its afferent and efferent pathways. As a further dividend, with more precise diagnosis of frontal epileptogenic zones, surgical treatment can be limited to smaller resections preserving more frontal lobe functions for the patient.

Although we can theoretically differentiate the onset and spread of frontal lobe seizures rostrocaudally and mediolaterally, restricting and maintaining rigid boundaries between anatomical subcategories may not be appropriate in individual cases. The epileptogenic lesion may overlap over contiguous areas of the dorsolateral and medial or medial and orbital surfaces of the frontal lobe. Epileptogenic discharges may spread so quickly between these

TABLE 3. *Frontal lobe epilepsies with complex partial seizures: electrographic manifestations*

Interictal EEG	Ictal EEG/stereo-EEG	Route of spread
I. Dorsolateral frontal lobe 1. Dorsolateral premotor cortex[a] (such as intermediate frontal gyrus) Focal spikes or sharp waves in the frontal region or normal	• Focal flattening with low-voltage 16- to 24-Hz polyspikes that secondarily generalize or • Generalized flattening, mostly in the intermediate frontal gyrus • Generalized flattening is seen on the scalp EEG or bifrontal spikes and sharp waves or rhythmic 2- to 4-Hz waves	To the supplementary motor cortex, anteriorly to the frontal pole, thalamus, and striatum
2. Prefrontal or frontopolar	Same as above	To thalamus, striatum, and areas 6, 8, and 4
3. Posterior inferior frontal gyrus	Same as for #1 and #2	To opercular areas of motor, parietal and temporal regions and to medial temporal Ammon's horn
II. Medial premotor cortex[a] 1. Supplementary motor 1- to 3-Hz and 4- to 6-Hz irregular spike-and-wave complexes (secondary bilateral synchrony) and signs of structural damage	• Focal flattening with low-voltage 16- to 24-Hz polyspikes in the supplementary motor cortex, thereby increasing amplitude as frequency decreases to 4- to 8-Hz spikes with secondary generalization • Generalized flattening is seen on scalp EEG	To the contralateral medial hemisphere, anterior thalamus, and Ammon's horn
2. Medial frontal cortex[a] Anterior cingulate gyrus 1- to 3-Hz and 4- to 6-Hz irregular spike-wave complexes (secondary bilateral synchrony) and signs of structural damage	• Focal low-voltage 16- to 24-Hz polyspikes in the cingulate gyrus with secondary generalization and global flattening • Generalized flattening is seen on scalp EEG	To the contralateral medial hemisphere, anterior thalamus, and Ammon's horn
III. Orbital frontal cortex 1. Anterior-orbital or mesio-orbital[b] Normal or focal spikes or sharp waves in the frontal region or medial temporal region	• Focal flattening with low-voltage 16- to 24-Hz polyspikes with secondary generalization • Generalized flattening is seen on scalp EEG	To the mesiofrontal, supplementary motor, mesoparietal, and cingulate cortex and to the temporal limbic lobe
2. Posterior-orbital or temporo-orbital[b]	Same as #1	To the mesio-temporal Ammon's horn and to the limbic lobe

[a]Type IIA complex partial seizures.
[b]Type IIB complex partial seizures or frontobasal–cingulate psychomotor epilepsy.

various areas that it would be impossible to differentiate neuroanatomical areas which drive each other, such as (a) the anterior cingulate and supplementary motor areas, (b) the anterior cingulate and mesial orbital cortex, (c) the premotor, primary motor, and supplementary motor areas, and (d) the posterior orbital cortex and medial temporal structures.

Frontal lobe seizures are now classified according to Bancaud and Talairach's scheme (1) which localizes specific and dominant region and systems of the frontal lobe involved by epileptogenic zones (see Tables 2 and 3). They consist of (a) dorsolateral premotor or posterior dorsolateral frontal seizures, (b) medial frontal premotor seizures (e.g., supplementary motor or anterior cingulate), (c) anterior polar or frontopolar seizures, (d) frontal operculo-insular seizures, and (e) orbitofrontal seizures, which are, in turn, subdivided into anterior mesio-orbital and posterior orbitomedial temporal seizures. A combination of various frontal lobe regions may be involved by seizures (Tables 2 and 3). As mentioned above, it is not unusual for epileptogenic zones and lesions to occupy contiguous areas of the dorsolateral, medial, and orbital surfaces of the frontal lobe. Rarely to infrequently, temporal and frontal epileptogenic zones spread to each others' regions and fire together to produce temporofrontal seizures.

In general, tonic–clonic convulsions and simple partial seizures with somatomotor or postural signs, along with contraversive head and eye movements, are common in frontal lobe epilepsies. When psychomotor attacks appear, motor manifestations are prominent (1–5). This contrasts with the paucity of motor signs in temporal lobe seizures, where arrest of movements, staring, proptosis, and masticatory oroalimentary automatisms are more common as in amygdalar–hippocampal epilepsy (6–12). Complex partial seizures which originate from the frontal basal and anterior cingulate cortex begin with fear, bizarre vocalization, bilateral motor automatisms, bipedal movements, frenetic arm-and-leg-thrusting behavior, sexual automatisms, and running (1–4,13–17). These latter motor signs are rare in temporal lobe seizures, although fear, bizarre vocalization, and sexual automatisms can appear in temporal lobe seizures

(5–9). Oroalimentary automatisms combined with a motionless staring phase may also appear in frontal lobe seizures, but they usually occur in the middle or late stages of the attack.

Certain characteristics of oroalimentary automatisms can be valuable in differentiating frontal from temporal lobe seizures. Mastication, chewing, and smacking and licking lips are characteristic of amygdalar seizures and their temporal and subcortical connections (7–9). Swallowing, orofacial dyskinesia-like movements of mouth and lips are more suggestive of frontal opercular seizures.

Pseudoabsence attacks lasting 10–30 sec with minimal automatisms are also observed in frontal lobe seizures. Such short attacks occur frequently, often in clusters, and may be associated with sphincter incontinence. These seizures can be associated with drop attacks (1–4).

Complex partial seizures of frontal lobe origin very commonly evolve to tonic–clonic convulsion (16). Williamson et al. (17) also report their frequent evolution to complex partial status epilepticus.

Decision Flow Charts (2)

Figures 1 through 5 show decision flow charts which we have found useful in evaluating partial seizures. These flow charts *do not* constitute perfect rules that have no exemptions, since the semiology of seizures can be infinitely variable.

There are four major decision points in the reconstruction of the epileptic attack: (i) Auras: Are there warning signs and symptoms? (ii) Are somatomotor and autonomic signs present at onset? (iii) Is a lapse or impairment of consciousness present at onset? (iv) When a lapse of consciousness is present, is there an arrest reaction at the start or are automatisms or somatomotor or autonomic signs present? The onset, sequence, and rank order of clinical events during an epileptic attack provide a picture of the spatiotemporal organization of epileptogenic discharges. No one single event should be considered by itself; rather, the ensemble of clinical events should be considered as a whole (2).

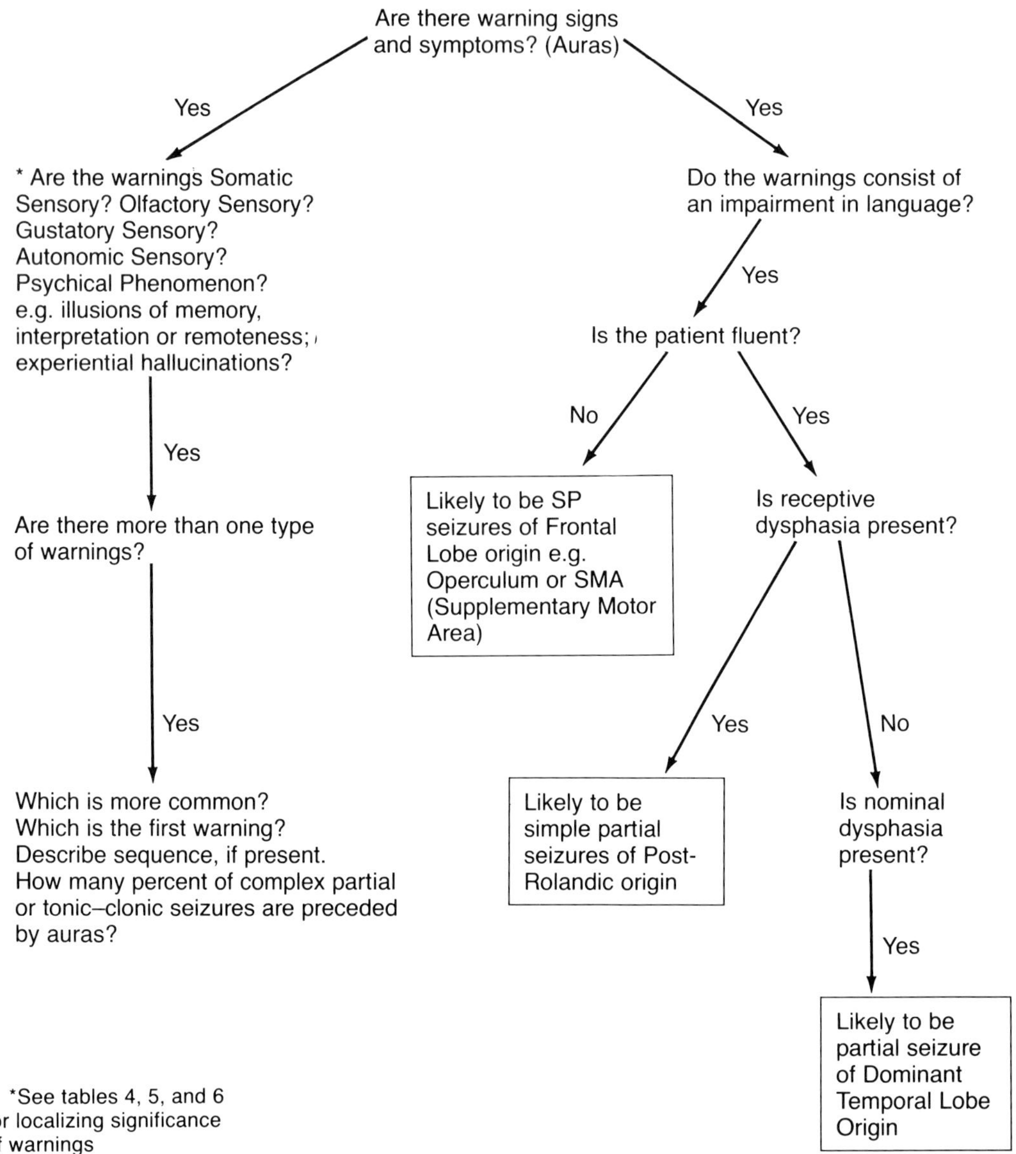

FIG. 1. Algorithm for decisions using semiology of partial epileptic seizures. Decision point 1: auras. SP, simple partial.

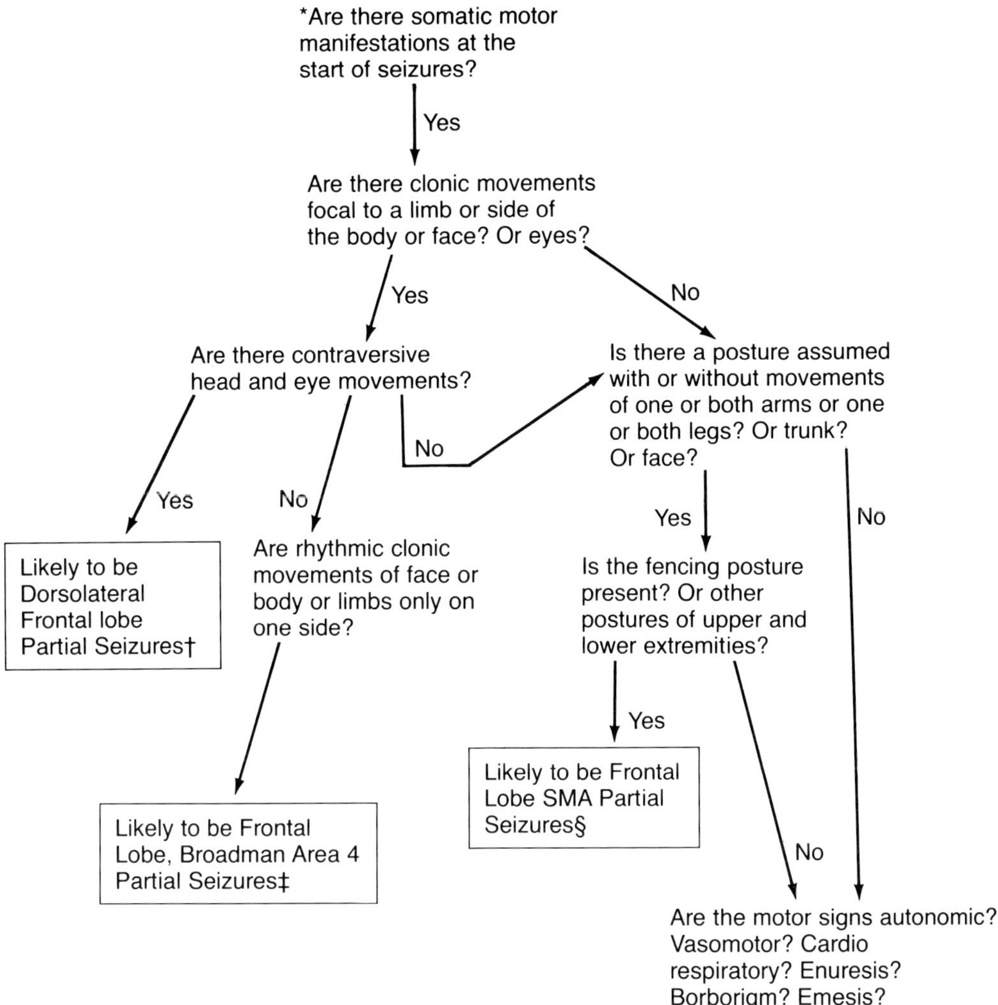

*See tables 4, 5, and 6 for localizing significance motor signs
†Can also be due to SMA or Parietal Seizures
‡Less likely to SMA or Premotor Partial Seizures
§Less likely to be Premotor Partial Seizures

FIG. 2. Algorithm for decisions using semiology of partial epileptic seizures. Decision point 2: somatic and autonomic motor signs. SMA, supplementary motor area.

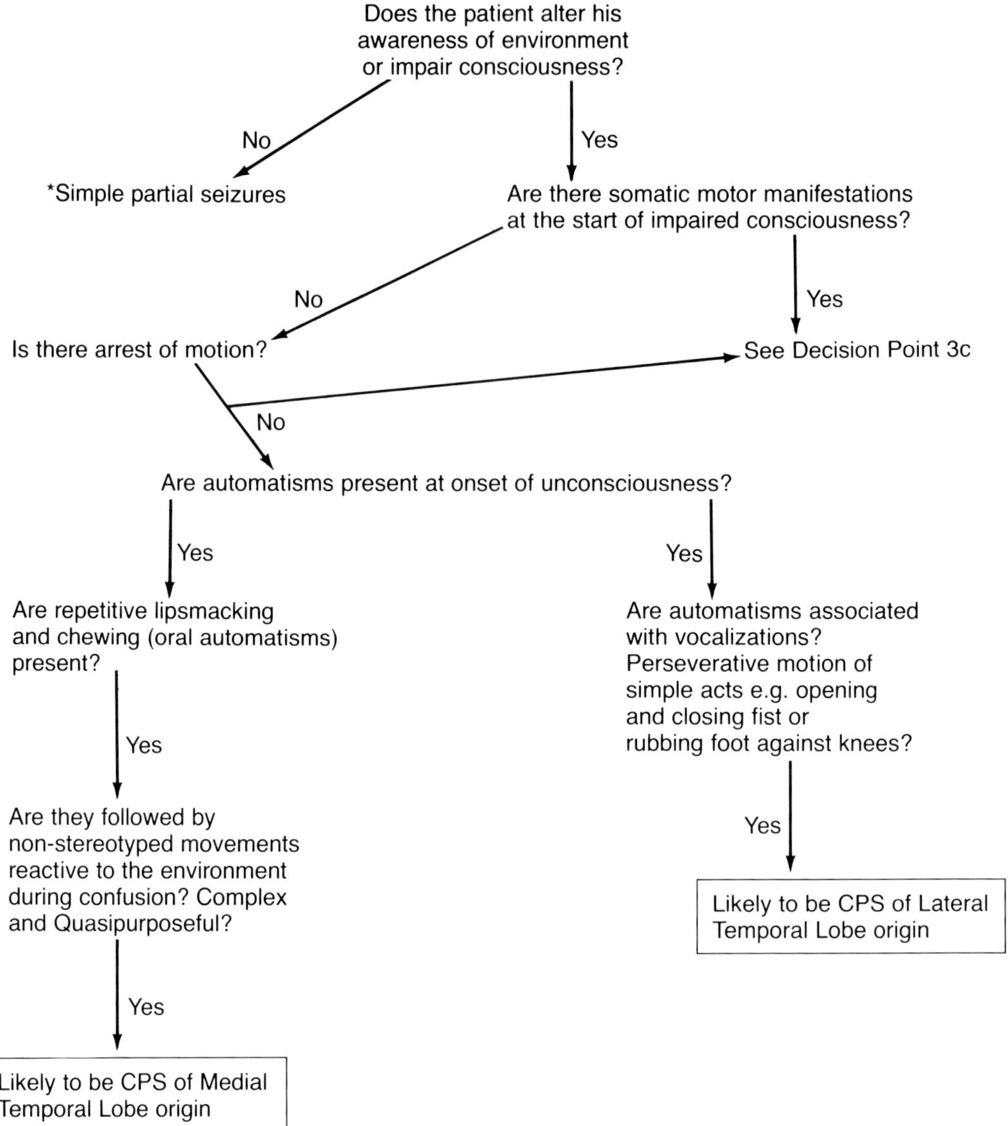

FIG. 3. Algorithm for decisions using semiology of partial epileptic seizures. Decision point 3: impaired consciousness and automatisms. Decision point 3a: arrest reaction at onset of impaired consciousness. CPS, complex partial seizure.

---

*See Tables 4, 5, and 6 for localizing significance.

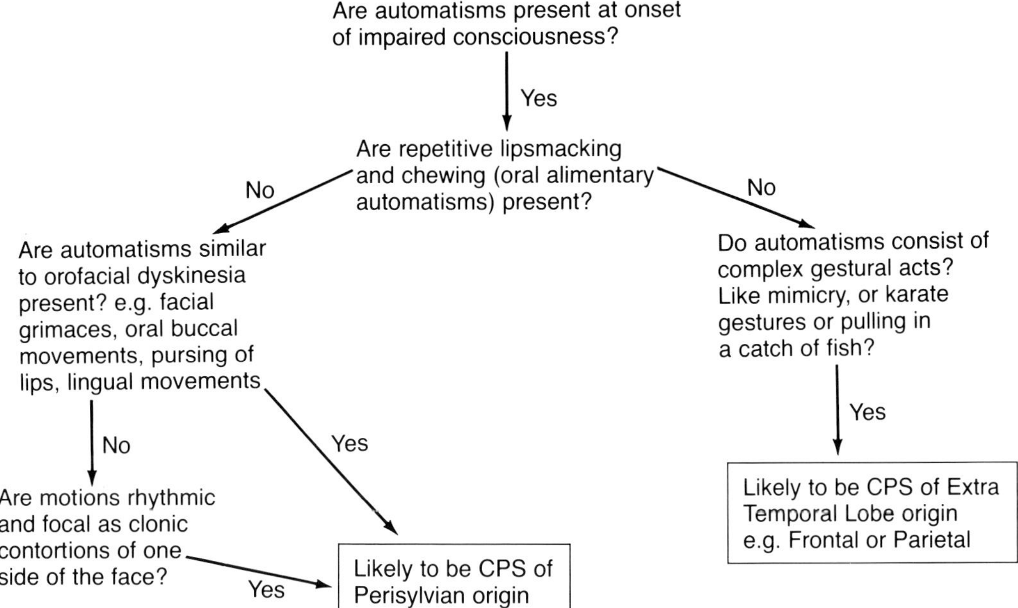

FIG. 4. Algorithm for decisions using semiology of partial epileptic seizures. Decision point 3: impaired consciousness and automatisms. Decision point 3b: automatisms. CPS, complex partial seizure.

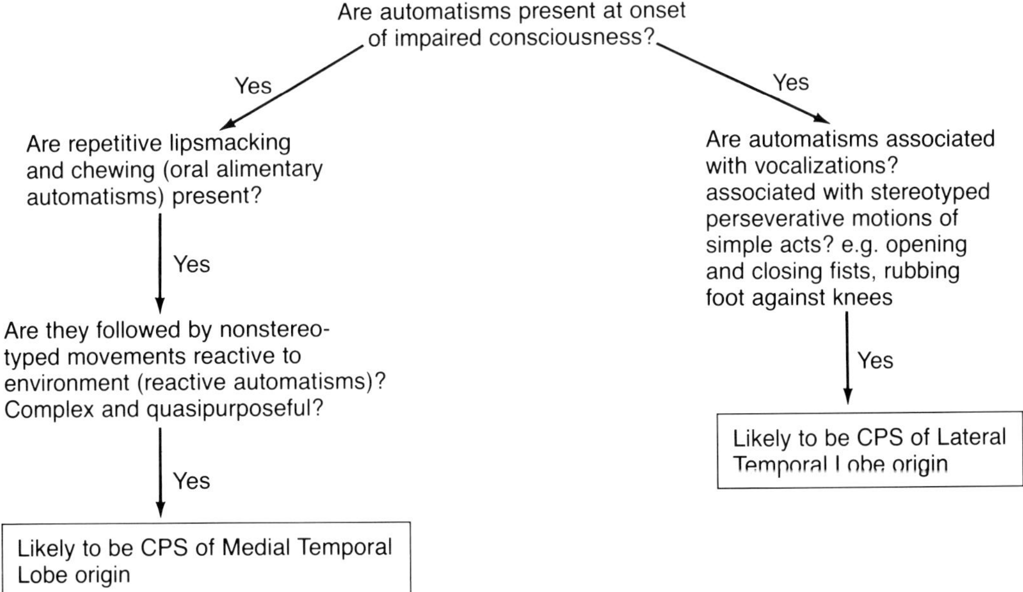

FIG. 5. Algorithm for decisions using semiology of partial epileptic seizures. Decision point 3: impaired consciousness and automatisms. Decision point 3b: automatisms. CPS, complex partial seizure.

TABLE 4. *Auras: psychical phenomena*

Clinical phenomenon	Proposed site of origin	Proof for origin	Investigators
Psychical: Intellectual aura Dreamy state; "felt as if he were saying, doing and looking at things which he had experienced before." "People seem to have strange expressions on their faces." "People and things seem to be far away."	Temporosphenoidal lobe	Clinicopathological observation	Jackson and Stewart (53, p. 535)
Forced thinking or "crowding thoughts" as intellectual aura	Deep posterior inferior frontal lobe in W.S., bifrontal in J.J., "midway from frontal pole" in T.K.	Electrocorticogram (ECoG) and relief from seizures after surgery	Penfield and Jasper (19, pp. 468–469)
Interpretive illusion a. Auditory: distance, loudness, tempo b. Visual: dimension, distances, erectness, tempo c. Comparison: familiarity, strangers, unreality d. Emotion: fear, loneliness, separation, sorrow, disgust	Lateral surface of superior temporal neocortex	Reproduction of symptoms by electrical stimulation; ECoG spikes in suspected sites of origin; relief from seizures on removal of epileptogenic zones	Penfield and Jasper (19, p. 25)
Simple auditory hallucinations	Heschl's gyrus with propagation to parietal lobe	Stereo-EEG during electrically or chemically induced seizures; relief of seizures after excision of epileptogenic zones	Bancaud (9) (220 operated temporal lobe epilepsies)
Auditory illusions	Superior temporal gyrus (including Heschl's gyrus), with propagation to limbic structures		
Visual illusions	Posterior temporal neocortex and medial temporal structures with propagation to occipital lobe		
Experiential hallucination Elements from past experience	Hippocampus, amygdala, parahippocampal gyri	Stereo-EEG during seizures; reproduction of symptoms on electrical stimulation of suspected sites	Halgren et al. (54); Gloor et al. (25); Macrae (55); Chapman (56, 57)

TABLE 4. *Continued*

Clinical phenomenon	Proposed site of origin	Proof for origin	Investigators
Psychic illusions or hallucinations or hallucinatory remembrances	External and anterior portion of superior and middle temporal gyrus (T1 and T2)	Stereo-EEG of electrically induced seizures; relief of seizures on resection of epileptogenic zones	Bancaud et al. (11) (cases: Huguette De and Etienne La)
	Middle portion of inferior temporal sulci (T4)		Bancaud et al. (11) (case: Fernand De)
	Temporal lateral neocortex and medial structures of amygdala and hippocampus		Bancaud (9)

Auras (see Fig. 1 and Tables 4 and 5)

Warning symptoms which occur immediately before the attacks and pass on into the attacks are rare to infrequent in frontal lobe seizures (1–3). Prodromes are even more rare. When auras are present, nonspecific vague complaints and nonspecific sensory complaints can be present. Psychic intellectual warnings with affective and autonomic sensory complaints can suggest the site of origin of seizure discharges. Forced thinking, forced actions, obscurity of thoughts, and alterations in the course of thoughts, such as a change in the speed of thoughts (e.g., rapid or slow conscious thoughts), suggest involvement of heteromodal frontal association cortex (1,2). These forms of psychic intellectual warnings should be differentiated from interpretive illusions, illusions of comparison and emotions, and experiential hallucinations of temporal lobe seizures (18–25). Olfactory (posterior-orbital frontal cortex) and gustatory hallucinations and illusions are rare; visual and auditory hallucinations (intermediate frontal cortex or frontoparietal operculum) are exemptions. Affective symptoms are typically unpleasant—inexpressible fear (even terror), depression of spirits, excitement, and irritability. Malaise, vague general sensations in the body, abdominal discomfort, belching, desire to defecate, thirst, and hunger are autonomic precursors, suggesting medial frontal gyrus, intermediate frontal gyrus, or oper-culo-insular involvement. An urge to urinate, conscious urination, mydriasis, eructation, palpitations and irregular heartbeats, and a conscious change in respiration can be other autonomic warnings.

The order of frequency in which these rare auras of frontal lobe seizures present themselves is not well established. The length of time they occupy varies from a few seconds to 1–2 hr, but more commonly from a few seconds to a minute. Psychic intellectual warnings exhibit relatively longer durations.

Tables 6, 7, and 8 list other auras commonly encountered in history-taking and their possible localizing significance.

Somatomotor Signs at Onset (5,10,26–28)

Figure 2 represents the second decision point and outlines the approach to the patient when somatic motor signs appear with the patient still awake and aware of his environment. Somatomotor events at the start of seizures should not make the clinician think of a temporal lobe onset. Somatomotor events at onset of seizures with or without impaired responsiveness and automatisms should suggest frontal lobe engagement by seizure discharges (1–3). Clonic contractions of orbicularis oculi or orbicularis oris or other facial muscles suggest primary motor (Brodman's area 4) involvement, but clonic jerks of the legs or hand may also mean supplementary motor area (SMA) or premotor area 6 engagement (1).

TABLE 5. *Some auras in frontal lobe seizures*

Aura	Proof	Investigators	Possible frontal lobe areas involved
Forced thinking or crowding of thoughts; forced actions	ECoG spikes in cortical sites; relief from seizures after excision	Penfield and Jasper (19, pp. 468–469)	Deep posterior inferior frontal lobe in W.S.; bifrontal in J.J.; midway from frontal pole in T.K.
A change in the speed of thoughts; obscurity of thoughts	Scalp EEG and relief from seizures after excision	Bancaud and Talairach (1)	Premotor frontal lobe; frontopolar
Olfactory and gustatory hallucinations and illusions	Electrical stimulation and ECoG	Penfield and Kristiansen (20); Bornstein (58); Lichenstein et al. (59)	Sylvian "superior operculum down in circuminsular gutter"; parietal operculum; anterior perfusated substance
	Scalp EEG and relief from seizures after excision	Bancaud et al. (11); Bancaud et al. (60); Bancaud and Talairach (1)	Posterior medial orbitofrontal cortex propagating to rhinencephalon and central and parietal operculum
Affective symptoms: inexpressible fear, terror, depression, excitement, irritability	Scalp EEG and relief from seizures after excision	St. Hilaire et al. (61); Bancaud and Talairach (1)	Anterior cingulate cortex; frontal operculo-insular cortex
Autonomic symptoms and signs: vague general sensations, belching, thirst, desire to defecate or urinate, changes in respiration and cardiac palpitations	ECoG electrical stimulation; scalp EEG; relief from seizures after excision	Penfield and Kristiansen (20); Lichenstein, et al. (59); Bancaud and Talairach (1)	Anterior cingulate; deep in Island of Reil cortex; supplementary motor area and intermediate frontal cortex

Usually, unilateral purely tonic contractions of one limb orients the physician towards the precentral frontal cortex.

Contraversive head and eye movements have usually incriminated the posterior aspect of middle frontal gyrus (Brodman's area 8), but similar changes are found when medial premotor regions are involved (5). The "fencing position" (i.e., "M2e") postures in an awake patient with speech arrest point to the supplementary motor area, but fencing posture alone or with tonic motions, lapse, and automatisms can result from both medial and dorsolateral premotor involvement (5). Salivation, pilomotor erection, and cardiorespiratory and pupillary changes can mean the presence of discharges in the frontal operculo-insular region. Penfield and Kristiansen (20), Penfield and Jasper (19), Ajmone-Marsan and Abraham (26), Ajmone-Marsan and Ralston

TABLE 6. *Other auras: special sensory phenomena*

Sensory phenomena	Proposed site of origin and engagement	Proof for origin	Investigators
Olfactory sensory			
Crude sensation of smell (e.g., burnt rubber, rotten lettuce)	Temporal sphenoidal lobe and uncus		Jackson (62)
	Olfactory bulb or uncus		Penfield and Kristiansen (20); Penfield and Jasper (19)
	Anterior perforated substance		Lichenstein et al. (59)
	Amygdala	Electrically induced after discharges	Gloor et al. (25)
	Posterior medial orbitofrontal cortex propagating to rhinencephalon and central operculum		Bancaud et al. (11); Bancaud (60)
Gustatory phenomena			
Crude sensation of taste (e.g., "the air tastes sweet," "bitter taste")	Sylvian "superior operculum down in the circuminsular gutter"		Penfield and Kristiansen (20); Penfield and Jasper (19, p. 148) (six cases)
	Parietal or central operculum; less often from basal limbic structures with propagation to operculum		Bancaud et al. (11)
	Parietal operculum		Bornstein (58)

(27), Rasmussen (28), and Bancaud et al. (11) had previously described the clinical manifestations of seizures from the intermediate frontal gyrus based chiefly on electrocorticogram (ECoG), intraoperative studies, and scalp EEG (SEEG). When epileptogenic discharges electrically occupy the intermediate frontal gyrus and Brodman's area 8 and quickly spread to area 4 or to Broca's speech area, the initial signs commonly consist of (a) subtle and very brief tonic forward or backward elevation of head, neck, and upper trunk, (b) contraversive head and eye movements (cephalotonic or clonic, oculotonic, or oculoclonic), (c) one or two mild facial clonic contractions, and (d) nonfluent dysphasia as consciousness is impaired (5,19,20,26–28). For purposes of analyses, we had previously called these psychomotor attacks "Type IIA." One must emphasize that in these attacks, motor signs can be very brief and subtle, and the entire clinical gestalt of the seizure onset may be the appearance of impaired consciousness and automatisms (14). Repeated viewing of the CCTV, however, will verify these early motor signs. Paroxysms frequently spread to the supplementary motor area so that elevation of an abducted extremity with flexed elbows can occur. Late in the sequence of events, oroalimentary automatisms (lipsmacking, pursing lips, tongue movements) occur when the amygdalar–hippocampal complex is invaded by epileptogenic discharges (5,14).

Somatomotor signs can also be manifested by the "fencing position" (i.e., "M2e") produced by the supplementary motor cortex. Penfield and co-workers (19,20) first recognized the existence of a supplementary area in the interhemispheral fissure when stimula-

TABLE 7. *Localizing value of autonomic phenomena as auras*

Clinical phenomenon	Proposed site of origin	Proof for origin	Investigators
Autonomic sensory: the epigastric aura			
Epigastric sensation	"Uncinate groups of fits" from uncinate gyrus or temporosphenoidal lobe	Clinicopathological observation	Jackson and Stewart (53, p. 539)
"Vague" or "indescribable" abdominal or thoracic sensation, sometimes called "epigastric"; or "palpitation in the precordium or epigastrium"	Either (a) deep within Sylvian fissure or within cortex of Island of Reil or (b) intermediate frontal areas, especially supplementary motor area; relief from seizures after excision of epileptogenic zones	ECoG interictal spikes in the suspected site of origin; reproduction of symptoms on electrical stimulation of (a) Sylvian area, (b) first temporal convolution, and (c) insular and circuminsular regions	Penfield and Kristiansen (20) (25 cases); Penfield and Jasper (19, p. 418) (15 cases); Lichenstein et al. (59, p. 299)
Specific abdominal sensation as belching, nausea, desire to defecate, sensation moving from epigastrium to throat	Cortex of Island of Reil	ECoG interictal spikes in the suspected site of origin; reproduction of symptoms on electrical stimulation of Island of Reil	Penfield and Rasmussen (64, p. 85)
Sensation of epigastric heaviness or pain	Ammon's horn, parahippocampal gyrus, amygdala, lateral middle temporal neocortex, posterior aspect of inferior temporal sulcus	Reproduction of symptoms on stimulation of Ammon's horn; scalp EEG during seizures; relief from seizure after removal of epileptogenic zones	Bancaud et al. (11, p. 306) (7 cases cited as Huguette De, Jean Sa, Marcel Ch, Fernand De, Sergine Lo, Antoine Mi, and Bernard Bo)
Sensation of thirst	Deep within Sylvian fissure, superior bank	ECoG of interictal spikes	Penfield and Jasper (19)
Autonomic motor			
Intestinal peristalsis ("stomach gurgling" or "gurgling of gas in abdomen")	Cortex of Island of Reil	Reproduction of symptoms on electrical stimulation of cortex of Island of Reil	Penfield and Jasper (19) (case R. Su, p. 432; case N. Ki, p. 448; case A. Br, p. 133)
Mydriasis, bilateral	Ammon's horn or amygdala	Reproduction of mydriasis on electrical stimulation during scalp EEG	Bancaud et al. (11, p. 309)

TABLE 7. *Continued*

Clinical phenomenon	Proposed site of origin	Proof for origin	Investigators
Irregular respirations; change in heart rate; pupillary change	Amygdala	Stereo-EEG during spontaneous seizures	Wieser (8, p. 198)
Mydriasis unilaterally, pallor, flushing sensation and warm feelings in the face	Amygdala	Stereo-EEG during spontaneous seizures	Swartz et al. (50)
Enuresis	Cortex of Island of Reil	ECoG of interictal spikes; relief from seizures after excision	Fiol et al. (67)
Enuresis or feeling of urination or actual urinary incontinence	Island of Reil and medial temporal lobe		Bancaud et al. (11)

tion produced vocalization, many different postures and movements, arrest or flowing of voluntary action, autonomic changes, sensations, and speech arrest. Subsequent accounts appeared in a monograph by Ajmone-Marsan and Ralston (27) and in a seizure atlas by Ajmone-Marsan and Abraham (26). Penfield and Jasper (19) described the typical posture as "slow movements of the opposite hand outward, backward and somewhat upward while the head and eyes turn toward it (as though the patient were observing what the hand was about to do)." Ajmone-Marsan and Abraham (26) described similar seizures

TABLE 8. *Localizing value of somatic sensory phenomena as auras*

Sensory phenomena	Proposed site of origin and engagement	Proof for origin	Investigators
Somatic Sensory			
Contralateral paresthesial numbness; pins and needles; tingling	Rolandic area[a]	ECoG interictal spikes; reproduction of symptoms on electrical stimulation	Penfield and Kristiansen (20)
	Amygdala		Lichtenstein et al. (59)
	Hippocampal pes and amygdala	Stereo-EEG of spontaneous seizures and of electrically induced seizures	Bancaud et al. (11)
	Hippocampal pes and amygdala	Electrically induced with or without afterdischarges	Halgren et al. (69)
	Hippocampus and amygdala	Spontaneous partial seizures	Maldonado et al. (7)

[a]"Indescribable feeling on the body or head" can sometimes be provoked by electrical stimulation in contralateral or ipsilateral extremities.

observed after metrazol stimulation and called the attacks "M2e"—"a tonic postural alteration or elevation of one arm which usually begins with flexion of the elbow followed by an abduction of the arm to approximately 90 degrees together with external rotation." These investigators hypothesized the origin and route of spread of paroxysms in these seizures (26,27). In 1965, Bancaud et al. (11) subsequently proved the actual routes of spread of paroxysms toward the cingulate cortex, the hippocampus, and frontal lobes by SEEG. Symptomatology similar to amygdalar–hippocampal seizures appeared late or in the middle of impaired consciousness. These consisted of autonomic symptoms and signs, oroalimentary automatisms, and even gestural and mimicry automatisms. Partial motor tonic seizures and urinary incontinence are also frequent (14).

Actually, only 6% of SMA seizures reported by Ajmone-Marsan and Ralston (27) consisted of M2e only or postural motions. Another 4% started with M2e, tonic facial contractions, and automatisms. Forty-five percent of seizures originating from the supplementary motor region showed either an isolated or conscious M2e, whereas 30% evolved to tonic–clonic convulsions. Eighteen percent showed tonic adversion of head and eyes along with a brief disturbance of consciousness followed by convulsions.

In 20% of patients with SMA seizures, Ajmone-Marsan and Ralston (27) observed initial automatisms mixed with postural motions (M2e), focal clonic facial jerks, and head contraversion before evolving quickly to generalized seizures. In another 4%, postural motions and tonic facial contractions preceded and led to automatisms. Ajmone-Marsan and Ralston (27) emphasized the frontal lobe origin of the epileptogenic paroxysm and contrasted these clinical sequences to motor phenomena appearing after the onset of automatisms in temporal lobe epilepsy.

Ajmone-Maran and Ralston (27) also noted that the interictal EEGs were "nonconvulsive" when seizures were characterized only by conscious M2e, whereas the interictal EEGs showed secondary bilateral synchrony when seizures progressed to unconsciousness and convulsions.

Lapses and Pseudoabsences: Impairment of Consciousness at Onset

Impairment of consciousness or a lapse at the start of seizures indicates that a complex partial seizure is present (23,24,29,30) and relates to the third decision point (Fig. 3). It may be difficult to define the exact onset of the alteration, rupture, or loss of consciousness. What is important is a direct examination of the patient during and after a seizure by verbal and nonverbal tests, assessing awareness and recent memory.

If impairment of consciousness is present, the practitioner should ask, "Is an initial arrest of motion present?" or "Are somatomotor and autonomic signs present at the start of unconsciousness? Are automatisms present at the start of impaired consciousness?" The character of the psychomotor attack during the first 10–20 sec gives the best clues as to their origin. Attacks with initial lapse of consciousness can start from the dorsolateral, medial, or orbital surfaces of the frontal lobe. Somatomotor events should be distinguished from bilateral arm and leg automatisms such as (a) bimanual bipedal or bicycling movements and (b) ambulatory or running fits.

Epilepsies in the frontopolar cortex, dorsolateral intermediate frontal gyrus, or mesial frontal cortex can also manifest as short attacks of impaired consciousness (10–20 sec in duration) with minimal automatisms suddenly appearing and ending (2–4,28). Because they appear to be like petit mal absence seizures (a form of primary generalized seizures), we call them "pseudoabsences." The ILAE classifies these seizures as complex partial seizures with impaired consciousness mainly. Such arrest of motions with impaired consciousness only or little clinical manifestation appears when epileptogenic discharges remain confined to the frontal pole and its connections to the thalamoreticular system. This was first described by Penfield and Kristiansen (20), Ajmone-Marsan and Abraham (26), and Ajmone-Marsan and Ralston (27), who demonstrated that the backward spread of seizure discharges to posterior frontal regions produced head or eyes turning, postures, and unilateral facial tonic contractions. Seizures from the anterior frontal region often start with impaired consciousness that quickly evolves to tonic–clonic convulsions (20,27).

Lapses of consciousness originating from the anterior cingulate gyrus or the frontal operculum–suprasylvian insular cortex are very difficult to differentiate from those that start in the temporal insular cortex. Because discharges spread quickly to the medial temporal pole and the posterior orbital frontal lobes, Bancaud and Talairach (1) suggest that it is more practical to consider the whole ensemble as "opercular–insular–amygdalar–orbital–hippocampal." In frontal opercular seizures, autonomic vegetative signs (mydriasis, rubefaction of face, tachycardia, piloerection, etc.) and gustatory hallucinations are frequently present at the start of seizures. Epileptogenic discharges invade the medial temporal lobe so quickly that attacks appear as if they come from the amygdala–hippocampal regions. An epigastric aura followed by an arrest reaction, masticatory automatisms, and confusion leads to gradual recovery from unconsciousness.

Mazars (31), Bancaud and co-workers (5,9, 10,32–35), Bonis (36), and Tukel and Jasper (37) deserve most of the credit for delineation of anterior cingulate epilepsy. Like epilepsies from the supplementary motor cortex, the interictal EEG may be normal or show signs of secondary bilateral synchrony (irregular, poorly formed spike-and-wave sequences firing at 1–3/sec and 4–6/sec) as described by Tukel and Jasper (37). The ictal EEG shows flattening with rhythmic polyspikes at 16–24/sec that quickly generalize (see Tables 2 and 3). Depth-electrode explorations are mandatory if cingulate epilepsy is to be recognized, since it is difficult to differentiate this from supplementary motor epilepsy. The problem is that epileptogenic paroxysms commonly spread to other areas very quickly (e.g., from the cingulate cortex to the SMA, and vice versa) and that the clinical symptoms produced by paroxysms from these two areas may be misleading. In addition, seizure discharges in the cingulate cortex frequently spread to the amygdalar–hippocampal regions and produce autonomic signs and oroalimentary automatisms in the middle and late stages of the psychomotor attacks.

Automatisms

An important consideration in the decision tree for diagnosis of partial seizures is, Are automatisms present? Are they present at onset? What are their characters? Oroalimentary? Gestural? Bizarre frenetic bimanual–bipedal? Are they stereotyped and stable from seizure to seizure? Reactive and quasi-intentional? Reactive or varying with the environment or the content of experience?

According to Quesney et al. (38), frontal lobe automatisms appear in only 4% of frontal lobe seizures. Other studies report a greater frequency and emphasize certain traits distinctive of frontal lobe automatisms. According to Penfield and Jasper (17), frontal lobe automatisms differ from temporal lobe automatisms "by a greater tendency to an invariable type of pseudovoluntary activity." Bancaud and co-workers (5,9,33) and Broglin et al. (2) describe frontal lobe automatisms as typically gestural and oriented towards the environment. Accordingly, the patient may drink a glass of water and may dress or undress. Walsh and Delgado-Escueta (14) described the bilateral arm-and-leg-thrashing automatisms similar to the reactive, bizarre, and frantic movements reported by Williamson et al. (15–17), and they also described the bimanual, bipedal, or bicycling motions described by Walsh and co-workers. In all these seizures, a large shriek and intense emotions, accompanied by fearful facial expressions, were also present.

More recently, Spencer et al. (39) emphasized sexual automatisms in psychomotor seizures of frontal lobe origin. Stoffels et al. (40,41) also reported dyspraxic or eupraxic sexual behavior (such as masturbatory movements) in anterior cingulate seizures.

In anterior cingulate epilepsy, Bancaud and co-workers (1,5,9) pointed out the interesting occurrence of sexual and genital events during automatic motions of psychomotor attacks. They reported 15 seizures in six patients whose attacks showed sexual automatisms early in the first 10 sec of the attack. Vegetative or autonomic signs and urinary incontinence were also frequently observed in these seizures.

Verbal automatisms consisting of simple

sonorous emissions or palilalic vocalizations (typically with well-formed elaborate sentences) can occur in frontal lobe seizures as described by Bonis (36) and Wieser (8).

EEG and CCTV Monitoring (1–3)

The EEG plays a decisive role in the diagnosis of epilepsy, although it is never sufficient by itself. Sphenoidal, nasopharyngeal, nasoethmoidal, supraorbital, or additional scalp electrodes can be beneficial in focalizing epileptogenic zones (1–3,38,42). Not infrequently, a single awake and sleep interictal EEG in patients with frontal lobe seizures is normal, especially when seizures originate from the mesial or orbital frontal regions. In dorsolateral frontal seizures, spikes and sharp waves may reveal a frontal focus. In mesial premotor seizures, the interictal EEG may show signs of secondary bilateral synchrony (irregular, poorly formed spike-and-wave sequences firing at 1–3 Hz and 4–6 Hz) as described by Tukel and Jasper (37). Sometimes, paroxysmal slow waves and spikes are bifrontal and do not show lateralization.

Oftentimes, attacks recorded with SEEG do not show epileptogenic discharges and instead manifest generalized flattening with low-voltage fast rhythms. Frontopolar or mesial frontal seizures may show focal, low-voltage, asynchronous, irregular 0.5- to 3-Hz spike and slow waves or rhythmic polyspikes at 16–24 Hz that quickly generalize. Depth explorations are usually necessary to differentiate the subtypes of frontal lobe seizures (3). The problem is that epileptogenic paroxysms commonly spread to other frontal areas very quickly, and that the signs and symptoms produced by spreading discharges may comprise the main ensemble of the psychomotor attack. In addition, seizure discharges frequently and quickly spread to the amygdalar–hippocampal regions, the peri-insular regions, or the lateral temporal–parietal operculum, thereby producing autonomic signs, oroalimentary automatisms, and gustatory hallucinations and causing a misdiagnosis of temporal or parietal lobe seizures.

CCTV videotaping of seizures allows the dissection and reconstruction of components of the epileptic attack, and their correlations with concomitant electrographic events are extremely helpful in differentiating frontal from extrafrontal seizures. Video–EEG monitoring has led to reclassification of seizure types (in as many as 43% of patients), has answered questions of referring physicians in 67–81% of instances (e.g., congnitive impairment, sensory perception, pseudoseizures), and has led to changes in therapy in 35% of cases. Fifty percent of patients referred for intensive monitoring involve the differentiation of pseudoepileptic seizures from epileptic attacks.

These observations on the usefulness of CCTV–EEG telemetry apply as well to frontal lobe seizures, which often have to be distinguished from psychogenic seizures. We also find CCTV–EEG monitoring of seizures useful when we cross over from polypharmacy to monotherapy and when we withdraw drug treatment after 2–5 years of successful treatment.

Identification of Underlying Causes and Trigger Factors (43–51)

Magnetic resonance imaging (MRI) and computed tomography (CT) are obligatory in all patients with frontal lobe seizures. When available, positron emission tomography (PET) is also useful. According to Swartz et al. (50), CT is abnormal in 55% of surgically treated frontal lobe epilepsy and can detect focal or regional gliosis, porencephaly, astrocytoma, and calcified granulomas. MRI is abnormal in 66% of surgically treated frontal lobe epilepsy and can also detect focal or regional atrophic processes, porencephaly, and calcified granulomas. In addition, it can identify local cicatricial gliosis, hamartomas, and low-grade gliomas undetected by, or poorly recognized on, CT scans. PET is abnormal in 66% of surgically treated frontal lobe epilepsy and can show hypometabolic zones associated with gliosis and calcified granulomas. It may be normal in low-grade astrocytoma, but it is useful in showing hypermetabolism zones of malignant gliomas.

Cerebral arteriography may be necessary to define smaller cerebral aneurysms and arteriovenous malformations. Single-photon emission computed tomography (SPECT) can show a decrease of regional cerebral blood flow in the cerebral hemisphere containing epileptogenic zones in the interictal state. Ictally, regional cerebral blood flow may increase in zones presumed to be the origin of seizures.

General Considerations

The following factors are important in deciding etiology: age at onset; birth and development history; family history; personal history; social drug habits; nature of seizures; neurologic signs; and the EEG (1–3).

Perinatal lesions, anoxia, and birth trauma without hemorrhage are observed in 25% of infants, children, and young adults with frontal lobe seizures. Postnatal head trauma causes 20% of simple partial seizures in young adults. Trauma, neoplasm, and birth injuries are the most frequent causes of frontal lobe seizures in individuals between the ages of 20 and 35 years. Neoplasms, head trauma, and cerebral infarction or hemorrhages are more common causes from 40 to 55 years of age. Cerebrovascular accidents and neoplasms are common causes when seizures start between 55 and 70 years of age (2).

Asymmetry of extremities, facial and cranial bones, may suggest cerebral hemiatrophy and an atrophic epileptogenic process. Todd's postictal hemiparesis suggests a focal process (2).

In Rasmussen's series of 346 patients from the Montreal Neurological Institute, 71% had cicatricial lesions and 29% had expansive neoplasms (28). Amongst cicatricial lesions, trauma was the most common cause (45%), followed by perinatal birth injuries, postinflammatory conditions, and diverse causes. Amongst expansive lesions, a cerebral tumor was most common; rarely, an arteriovenous malformation was present.

Specific Considerations

Seizures from Intracranial Tumors. Epileptic seizures that recur in 5–20 years may be the only symptom of a slowly growing neoplasm in the fontal lobe. Frontal lobe seizures present symptoms in 40% of brain tumors; seizures precede focal neurological signs and increased intracranial pressure in 67% of these patients. Seizures occur in 37% of glioblastomas, 70% of astrocytomas, 67% of meningiomas, and 92% of oligodendrogliomas (2).

Five to 10 percent of patients who undergo cortectomy because of drug-resistant seizures turn out to have a cerebral neoplasm. A cerebral tumor should be suspected when seizures increase in frequency, change patterns, develop status epilepticus, or develop new neurological signs or symptoms (2).

Post-traumatic Seizures. Seizures that occur within the first week of head injury are called "early post-traumatic." They occur in 4% of head-injured patients. Seizures occurring more than 1 week after head injury are called "delayed post-traumatic." Fifty percent of patients with post-traumatic epilepsy recover spontaneously within 2 years (2).

Risk factors for post-traumatic seizures are: post-traumatic amnesia of more than 24 hr, depressed skull fracture, dural tear, and focal neurological signs. In closed head injuries, brief cerebral concussion not associated with loss of consciousness rarely causes seizures. Early post-traumatic seizures are not likely to persist. Delayed post-traumatic seizures have a less favorable prognosis. Intractable drug-resistant seizures may be expected in 20–30% of cases. Onset of seizures 10 years after head injury is extremely rare (2).

Seizures From Cerebrovascular Disease. After 50 years of age, cerebrovascular diseases frequently cause seizures. Cerebrovascular arteriosclerosis without cerebral infarctions or hemorrhages rarely causes seizures. Twelve percent of patients have seizures after 6–12 months if cerebral infarction or hemorrhage is present. Only 2% of strokes develop seizures acutely; they usually present as epilepsia partialis continuans or as partial status with periodic lateralized epileptiform discharges (2).

REFERENCES

1. Bancaud J, Talairach J. Semiology of frontal lobe epileptic seizures in man. In: Chauvel P, Delgado-Escueta AV, Halgren E, Bancaud J,

eds. *Frontal lobe seizures and epilepsies.* New York: Raven Press, 1990; in press.

2. Broglin D, Delgado-Escueta AV, Walsh GO, Maldonado HM, Chauval P. Seizures and epilepsies of frontal origin: approach to the patient. In: Chauvel P, Delgado-Escueta AV, Halgren E, Bancaud J, eds. *Frontal lobe seizures and epilepsies.* New York: Raven Press, 1990; in press.

3. Delgado-Escueta AV, Swartz BE, Maldonado HM, et al. In: Wieser HG, Elger CE, eds. *Complex partial seizures of frontal lobe origin in presurgical evaluation of epileptics.* Berlin: Springer-Verlag, 1987;267–299.

4. Swartz BE, Delgado-Escueta AV. Complex partial seizures of extratemporal origin: "the evidence for." In: Wieser H, Speckmann EJ, Engel J, eds. *The epileptic focus. Current problems in epilepsy,* vol 3. London: John Libbey, 1987;137–174.

5. Chauvel P, Trottier S, Bancaud J. Somatomotor seizures from the primary motor and supplementary motor cortex. In: Chauvel P, Delgado-Escueta AV, Halgren E, Bancaud J, eds. *Frontal lobe seizures and epilepsies.* Raven Press, 1990; in press.

6. Delgado-Escueta AV, Walsh GO. Type I complex partial seizures of hippocampal origin: excellent results of anterior temporal lobectomy. *Neurology* 1985;35:143–154.

7. Maldonado HM, Delgado-Escueta AV, Rand RW, Walsh GO, Halgren E. Complex partial seizures of hippocampal and amygdalar origin. *Epilepsia* 1988;29:420–433.

8. Wieser HG. *Electroclinical features of the psychomotor seizure.* Stuttgart: Fischer (London: Butterworths), 1983.

9. Bancaud J. Epileptic attacks of temporal origin in man. *Jpn J EEG EMG* 1981;61(Suppl):71–79.

10. Bossi L, Munari C, Stoffels C, Bonis A, Bacia T. Talairach J, Bancaud J. Somatomotor manifestations in temporal lobe seizures. *Epilepsia* 1984;25:70–76.

11. Bancaud J, Talairach J, Bonis A, Schaub A, Szikla G, Morel P, Bordas-Ferer M. *La stereoelectroencephalographie dans l'epilepsie.* Paris: Masson, 1965.

12. Wieser HG, Yasargil MG. Selective amygdalohippocampectomy as a surgical treatment of mesiobasal limbic epilepsy. *Surg Neurol* 1982; 17:445–457.

13. Wada JA, Purves SJ. Oral and bimanual–bipedal activity as ictal manifestations of frontal lobe epilepsy. *Epilepsia* 1984;15(5):668.

14. Walsh GO, Delgado-Escueta AV. Type II complex partial seizures: poor results of anterior temporal lobectomy. *Neurology (Cleveland)* 34: 1–13.

15. Williamson PD, Spencer DD, Spencer SS, Novelly RA, Mattson RH. Complex partial status of frontal lobe origin: a depth electrode study. *Epilepsia* 1983;24:260.

16. Williamson PD, Spencer DD, Spencer SS, Novelly RA, Mattson RH. Complex partial seizures of frontal lobe origin. *Ann Neurol* 1985;18: 497–504.

17. Williamson PD, Spencer DD, Spencer SS, Novelly RA, Mattson RH. Complex partial status epilepticus: a depth electrode study. *Ann Neurol* 1985;18(6):647–654.

18. Hausser-Hauw C, Bancaud J. Gustatory hallucinations in epileptic seizures. *Brain* 1987; 110:339–359.

19. Penfield W, Jasper H. *Epilepsy and the functional anatomy of the human brain.* Boston: Little, Brown, 1954.

20. Penfield W, Kristiansen K. *Epileptic seizure patterns.* Springfield, IL: Charles C Thomas.

21. Penfield WP, Perot P. The brain's record of auditory and visual experience. A final summary and discussion. *Brain* 1963;86:595–696.

22. King DW, Ajmone-Marsan C. Clinical features and ictal patterns in epileptic patients with EEG temporal lobe foci. *Ann Neurol* 1977;2:138–147.

23. Feindel W, Penfield W. Localization of discharge in temporal lobe automatisms. *AMA Arch Neurol Psychiatry* 1954;72:605–630.

24. Feindel W. Temporal lobe seizures. In: Vinken PJ, Bruyn GW, eds. *The epilepsies. Handbook of clinical neurology,* vol 15. Amsterdam: North-Holland, 1974;87–106.

25. Gloor P, Olivier A, Quesney LF, Andermann F, Horowitz S. The role of the limbic system in experiential phenomena of temporal lobe epilepsy. *Ann Neurol* 1982;12:129–144.

26. Ajmone-Marsan C, Abraham K. A seizure atlas. *Electroencephalogr Clin Neurophysiol* 1960;15 (Suppl):1–215.

27. Ajmone-Marsan C, Ralston BL. *The epileptic seizure: its functional morphology and diagnostic significance.* Springfield, IL: Charles C Thomas, 1957.

28. Rasmussen T. Characteristics of a pure culture of frontal lobe epilepsy. *Epilepsia* 1983;24 (4):482–493.

29. Geier S, Bancaud J, Talairach J, et al. The seizures of frontal lobe epilepsy. *Neurology (Minneap)* 1977;27:951–958.

30. Gloor P. Physiology of the limbic system. In: Penry JK, Daly DD, eds. *Complex partial seizures and their treatment.* New York: Raven Press, 1975;27–43.

31. Mazars G. Cingulate gyrus epileptogenic foci as an origin for generalized seizures. In: Gastaut H, Jasper H, Bancaud J, Waltregny A, eds. *The physiopathogenesis of the epilepsies.* Springfield, IL: Charles C. Thomas, 1969;186–189.

32. Bancaud J. Surgery of epilepsy based on stereotactic investigations—the plan of the SEEG investigation. *Acta Neurochir (Vienna)* 1980;30 (Suppl):25–34.

33. Bancaud J, Talairach J. Macro-stereo-electroencephalography in epilepsy. In: Bancaud J, ed. *Handbook of EEG and clinical neurophysiology,* vol 10. Amsterdam: Elsevier, 1975;1013–1033.

34. Bancaud J, Talairach J, Bresson M, Morel P. Acces epileptiques induits par la stimulation du noyau amygdalien et de la corne d'Ammon. Interet de la stimulation dans la determination des epilepsies temporales chez l'homme. *Rev Neurol (Paris)* 1968;6:527–532.

35. Bancaud J, Talairach J, Morel P, Bresson M. La corne d'Ammon et le noyau amygdalien: effects cliniques et electriques de leur stimulation chez l'homme. *Rev Neurol* 1966;3:329–352.

36. Bonis A. Long term results of cortical excision based on stereotactic investigations in severe drug resistant epilepsies. *Acta Neurochir (Vienna)* 1980;30(Suppl):55–66.

37. Tukel K, Jasper H. The electroencephalogram in parasagittal lesions. *Electroencephalogr Clin Neurophysiol* 1952;4:481–494.

38. Quesney LF, Krieger C, Leitner C, Gloor P, Olivier A. Frontal lobe epilepsy: clinical and electrographic presentation. Paper presented at the XVth Epilepsy International Symposium, Washington, DC, September 26–30, 1983. Abstract, p. 177.

39. Spencer SS, Spencer DD, Williamson PD, Mattson RH. Sexual automatisms in complex partial seizures. *Neurology* 1983;33(5):527–533.

40. Stoffels C, Munari C, Bonis A, Bancaud J, Talairach J. Manifestations genitales et "sexuelles" lors des crises epileptiques partielles chez l'homme. *Rev EEG Neurophysiol* 1980;10:386–392.

41. Stoffels C, Munari C, Brunie-Lozano E, Bonis A, Bancaud J, Talairach J. Manifestations automatiques dans les crises epileptiques partielles complexes d'origine frontale. *Boll Lega Ital Epilessia* 1980;29/30:111–113.

42. Geier S, Bancaud J, Talairach J, et al. Clinical note: clinical and telestereo-EEG findings in a patient with psychomotor seizures. *Epilepsia* 1975;16:119–125.

43. Angerleri F, Provinciali L, Salvolini U. Computerized tomography in partial epilepsy. In: Canger R, Angeleri F, Penry JK, eds. *Advances in epileptology: XI Epilepsy International Symposium*. New York: Raven Press, 1980;53–64.

44. Ishida S, Yajik K, Fujiwara T, Sakuma N, Seino M, Wada YA. Correlative study of CT with EEG findings in epilepsy. *J Comput Assist Tomogr* 1978;3:71–76.

45. Jabbari B, Gunderson CH, Wippold F, Citrin C, Sherman J, Bartoszek D, Daigh JD, Mitchell MH. Magnetic resonance imaging in partial complex epilepsy. *Arch Neurol* 1986;43:869–876.

46. Kuhl D, Engel J Jr, Phelps M. Patterns of local brain metabolism determined in epilepsy by positron emission computed tomography. *Arch Neurol* 1981;38:735.

47. Mazziota JC, Engel J Jr. Advanced neuro-imaging techniques in the study of human epilepsy: PET, SPECT and NMR–CT. In: Pedley TA, Meldrum BS, eds. *Recent advances in epilepsy*. New York: Churchill Livingstone, 1985;65–100.

48. McLachlan RS, Nicholson RL, Black S, Carr T, Blume WT. Nuclear magnetic resonance imaging, a new approach to the investigation of refractory temporal lobe epilepsy. *Epilepsia* 1985;26:555–562.

49. Sperling MR, Wilson G, Engel J, Babb TL, Phelps M, Bradley WW. Magnetic resonance imaging in intractable partial epilepsy: correlative studies. *Ann Neurol* 1986;20:57–62.

50. Swartz BE, Halgren E, Delgado-Escueta AV, Blahd W, Mandelkern M, Feldstein P, Rand RW, Maldonado HM, Khonsary A. Seizure semiology, neuropsychometrics and neuroimaging correlaries in frontal lobe epilepsies. *Epilepsia* 1986;27(5):597–598.

51. Theodore WH, Dorwart R, Holmes M, Porter RJ, deChiro G. Neuroimaging in refractory partial seizures: comparison of PET, CT and MRI. *Neurology* 1986;35:750–759.

52. Munari C, Bancaud J. In: Chauvel P, Delgado-Escueta AV, Halgren E, Bancaud J, eds. *Orbital frontal seizures in frontal lobe seizures and epilepsies*. New York: Raven Press, 1990; in press.

53. Jackson JH, Stewart XY. Epileptic attacks with warning sensations of smell and with intellectual aura (dreamy state) in a patient who had symptoms pointing to gross organic disease of the right temporo-sphenoidal lobe. *Brain* 1899;22:534–549.

54. Halgren E, Walter RD, Cherlow DG, Crandall PH. Mental phenomena evoked by electrical stimulation of the human hippocampal formation and amygdala. *Brain* 1978;101:83–117.

55. Macrae D. Isolated fear. A temporal lobe aura. *Neurology* 1954;4:497–505.

56. Chapman WP, Markham CH, Rand RW, Crandall PH. Memory changes induced by stimulation of hippocampus or amygdala in epilepsy patients with implanted electrodes. *Trans Am Neurol Assoc* 1967;92:50–6.

57. Chapman WP. Depth electrode studies in patients with temporal lobe epilepsy. In: Ramey ER, O'Doherty DS, eds. In: *Electrical studies on the unanesthetized brain*. New York, Hoeber, 1960:334–50.

58. Bornstein WS. Cerebral cortical representation of taste in man and monkey. *Yale J Bio Med* 1940;12:719–736,3:133–146.

59. Lichenstein RS, Curtis M, Walker, AE. Subcortical recording in temporal lobe epilepsy. *AMA Arch Neurol* 1959;1:288–302.

60. Bancaud J. Semiologie clinique des crises epileptiques d'origine temporale. *Rev Neurol* 1987;392–400.

61. St. Hilaire et al. Clinical manifestations of the human medial frontal lobe. In: Chauvel P et al., eds. *Frontal Lobe Seizures and Epilepsies*. New York: Raven Press, 1990; in press.

62. Jackson JH, Beevor C. Case of tumour of the right temporo-sphenoral lobe bearing on the localisation of the sense of smell and on the interpretation of a particular variety of epilepsy. *Brain* 1889;12:346–357.

63. Penfield W and Rasmussen T. *The cerebral cortex of man. A clinical study of localization of function*. New York: MacMillan, 1950.

64. Foil ME et al. Ictus Emiticus: Clinical EEG and Electrocortigraphic Findings. 16th Epilepsy International, Hamburg, West Germany, Sept. 6–9, 1985.

65. Halgren E, Babb TL, Crandall Ph. Activity of human hippocampal formation and amygdala neurons during memory testing. *Electroenceph Clin Neurophysiol* 1978;45:585–601.

66. Jackson JH. On a particular variety of epilepsy ("intellectual aura"): one case with symptoms of organic brain disease. *Brain* 1899;11:179–207.
67. Munari C, Bonis A, Musolino A, Bancaud J, Buser P, Brunet P, Talairach J, Chodkiewiez JP. Amygdaloid nucleus involvement during temporal lobe seizures in man: physiopathological and surgical implications. In: Roger J, Porter RJ, eds. *Advances in epileptology: XVth Epilepsy International Symposium*. New York: Raven Press, 1984;000–000.

Advances in Neurology, Vol. 55, edited by
D. Smith, D. Treiman, and M. Trimble,
Raven Press, Ltd., New York © 1991.

21

Psychobiology of Ictal Aggression

David M. Treiman

*Neurology and Research Services, VA West Los Angeles Medical Center,
Los Angeles, California 90073; and Department of Neurology UCLA School of Medicine,
Los Angeles, California 90024*

*". . . There's glory for you!" "I don't know
what you mean by 'glory,'" Alice said. ". . .
I meant 'there's a nice knock-down argument for
you!'" "But 'glory' doesn't mean 'a nice
knock-down argument,'" Alice objected.
"When I use a word," Humpty Dumpty said
in rather a scornful tone, "it means just what
I choose it to mean—neither more nor less."*
Lewis Carroll, *Through the Looking Glass* (1)

There is an "Alice in Wonderland" quality to the history of the relationship between epilepsy and violence. Writings in psychiatric literature for at least the last 100 years have uncritically related isolated acts of violence to epilepsy (2–5). As recently as 1982, Kolb and Brodie (6) described complex partial epilepsy in the following manner: "Clinically the clouded state suggests a delirium with liberation of aggressive and self-destructive impulses. Acts of violence may be committed in the automatisms and may be of a strikingly brutal nature, the patient pursuing his crime to a most revolting extreme."

This persistent and prevailing view that there is a positive relationship between epilepsy and violence has been based on the assumption that epilepsy is more common among violent people and that violence is more common among epileptics. However, there are few data to support this assumption. Treiman (7) reviewed medical and legal issues relating to the question of epilepsy and violence and pointed out that a number of studies have shown that epilepsy is two to four times more prevalent in prison populations than in

the general population. However, there is no greater prevalence of violent or serious crimes in epileptic prisoners than in non-epileptic prisoners. Treiman (7) suggested that the increased prevalence of epilepsy among prisoners is probably a reflection of the high prevalence of epilepsy among economically deprived urban populations (from which most prisoners come) rather than a reflection of an increased frequency of criminal activity among epileptics. Treiman (7) also reviewed studies which addressed the question of whether violence is more prevalent in epileptics than in control populations. Most such studies have been biased toward intractable epilepsy populations in which there is an increased incidence of concomitant psychiatric and neurological deficits. In general, interictal violence in such populations tends to occur in young men of subnormal intelligence with character disorders, a history of early and severe epilepsy, and associated neurological deficits. When unselected populations of patients with epilepsy are studied or patients with severe psychiatric disorders or subnormal intelligence are removed from a series, there is no increased prevalence of violence. Thus Treiman (7) concluded that violent behavior is not more common in patients with epilepsy in general or in those with temporal lobe epilepsy in particular. All violence which occurs in such groups can be accounted for by other neurological or psychiatric disorders.

Although the data summarized above suggest that there is no greater incidence of interictal violence or aggressive behavior among epileptics, nor greater prevalence of epilepsy among prisoners incarcerated for violent crimes, there is still the question of whether ictal violence may occur under some circumstances. The remainder of this chapter will focus on what is known about the anatomy and physiology of possible ictal violence. In order to answer the question of whether ictal violence occurs and, if so, under what circumstances, the following questions will be considered:

1. What do we know about the nature of aggression and of violent behavior?
2. What do we know about the anatomy, physiology, and clinical presentation of ictal events?
3. What evidence is there that ictal aggression occurs?
4. If ictal aggression occurs, what are its anatomical and physiological substrates?
5. What should be the future directions of research in the consideration of the neurobiology of possible ictal aggression?

Before considering each of these individual questions, we need to define the terms "aggression" and "violence." *Aggression* is an offensive action or procedure directed toward another individual or object with the intent to control, threaten, or do harm. *Violence* is the forceful infliction of abuse or damage to another individual or object. Violence need not be the result of intentional aggression. Thus it is possible for violent behavior either to occur in the absence of aggressive intent or to be the expression of aggressive behavior.

AGGRESSION

In order to understand the psychobiology of aggression, let us first turn to animal studies where considerable attention has been focused on an understanding of aggressive behavior. Moyer (8) proposed that animal models of aggression can be classified into six types as follows:

1. *Predatory (offensive) aggression* is characterized by attack behavior that an animal directs toward its natural prey.
2. *Inter-male (competitive) aggression* is the stereotyped and ritualized attack by one male against another for purposes of establishing dominance.
3. *Fear-induced (defensive) aggression* is the attack of a threatening agent when the victim is unable to escape.
4. *Maternal aggression* is the attack of a mother toward an agent threatening its young.
5. *Irritable aggression* is an attack which is made without an attempt to escape and which is independent of the presence or absence of another modifier such as prey, young, or other males.
6. *Sex-related aggression* is aggressive behavior which is elicited by the same stimuli which elicit sexual behavior.

Identification of different types of aggressive behavior in animal models has led to an increased understanding of the anatomical substrates of such behaviors. Stimulation of a number of areas in the brain, as well as destruction of still other areas, has been associated with each of the six types of animal aggression listed above. Many such sites are located within the limbic system (especially in the amygdala and the hypothalamus). The anatomical substrates of animal aggression have been reviewed by Goldstein (9) and by Valzelli (10). Table 1 lists brain structures involved in different kinds of animal aggression as demonstrated by stimulation and by lesional studies.

The large number of anatomical sites within mammalian brains where stimulation can elicit recognizable stereotyped aggressive behavior suggests the possibility that such behavior could occur as a result of spontaneous paroxysmal abnormal electrical discharges— that is, electrical seizure activity. However, Plotnik (11) has suggested that there is an alternative interpretation of the brain-stimulation-aggression data in the experimental literature. On the one hand, stimulation of selected regions of the brain may directly elicit aggressive behavior—what Plotnik has called "primary" aggression. Such behavior could conceivably be ictal in its nature. On the other hand, aggressive behavior following electrical stimulation of the brain might not be produced directly by the electrical stimulation of that area but rather may result in a noxious

TABLE 1. *Anatomical correlates of aggression in experimental animals*[a]

Triggers	Suppressors
Predatory offensive aggression	
Anterior hypothalamus	Prefrontal cortex
Lateral hypothalamus	Ventromedial hypothalamus
Lateral preoptic nuclei	Basolateral amygdala
Ventral midbrain tegmentum	Mammillary bodies
Ventral midbrain	
Ventromedial periaqueductal gray matter	
Inter-male (competitive) aggression	
Laterobasal septal nuclei	Dorsolateral frontal lobe
Centromedial amygdala	Olfactory bulbs
Ventrolateral posterior thalamus	Dorsomedial septal nuclei
Stria terminalis	Head of caudate
Fear-induced aggression	
Centromedial amygdala	Ventromedial hypothalamus
Fimbria fornix	Septal nuclei
Stria terminalis	Basolateral amygdala
Ventrobasal thalamus	Ventral hippocampus
Maternal-protective aggression	
Hypothalamus	Septal nuclei
Ventral hippocampus	Basolateral amygdala
Irritable aggression	
Anterior hypothalamus	Frontal lobes
Ventromedial hypothalamus	Prefrontal cortex
Dorsomedial hypothalamus	Medial prepiriform cortex
Posterior hypothalamus	Ventromedial hypothalamus
Anterior cingulate gyrus	Septal nuclei
Thalamic center median	Head of caudate
Ventrobasal thalamus	Dorsomedian nucleus of thalamus
Ventral hippocampus	Stria terminalis
Ventral midbrain tegmentum	Dorsal hippocampus
Ventromedial periaqueductal gray matter	Posterior cingulate gyrus
Cerebellar fastigium	Periamygdaloid cortex
Sex-related aggression	
Medial hypothalamus	Septal nuclei
Fimbria fornix (male)	Fimbria fornix (female)
Ventral hippocampus	Cingulate gyrus
	Dorsolateral amygdala

[a]Modified from ref. 10.

or painful stimulus which, in turn, elicits an aggressive response to this stimulus. Plotnik has referred to this form of aggression as "secondary" or "pain-mediated" aggression.

Plotnik (11) proposed two strategies in order to differentiate between primary and secondary stimulation-induced aggression. In humans, he suggested, it should be possible to ask directly whether the subject perceived the stimulus as neutral or positive or negative. In animals, where it is not possible to ask the subject its perceptions, it should be possible to determine experimentally whether the animal perceives the stimulus as a positive, negative, or neutral one by observing the way the animal responds to certain situations. The question can be asked: Will the animal work to obtain stimulation (positive or rewarding), work to avoid stimulation (negative or aversive), or work to neither obtain nor avoid stimulation (neutral)?

In order to differentiate between primary

and secondary brain stimulation-induced aggression in monkeys, Plotnik et al. (12) implanted 174 electrodes into the brains of seven monkeys. The monkeys were tested as to whether they would work to obtain or avoid stimulation. Using this paradigm, 35 electrodes were defined as aversive, 22 as positive, and 117 as neutral. None of the positive or neutral brain-stimulation electrodes elicited aggression; of the 35 aversive points, 14 elicited aggression and 21 did not. The aggression which was seen was always well organized and always directed toward a submissive monkey in the social hierarchy, never against a dominant one. In these experiments the aggression always occurred after the stimulation, never simultaneously with it. Plotnik (11) interpreted the results of this study as showing that the well-directed and well-organized aggression which occurred during stimulation of some of the aversive sites was an example of secondary or pain-mediated aggression, and not an example of behavior that is primary to the stimulation of specific neurons. Electric shocks delivered to the foot or waist elicited identical well-directed aggressive responses which were also modified by social hierarchy.

Not all stimulus-induced aggressive behavior in animals is modified by the social hierarchy, however. For instance, Robinson et al. (13) reported studies in two Rhesus monkeys in which stimulation of lateral and anterior hypothalamic sites resulted in aggressive attacks against dominant animals sufficiently sustained and intense that repetitive stimulations resulted in a permanent reversal of dominance position. Robinson and his colleagues thought these attacks were examples of primary aggression because one of the three effective stimulation sites was not an aversive site (the other two yielded reliable escape performance) and because the aggressive behavior began within 5 sec of stimulus onset and continued until cessation of stimulation.

As a result of the Plotnik et al. (12) studies, Plotnik (11) proposed the following criteria for the determination that brain-stimulation-induced aggressive behavior is primary aggression: (a) Rewarding or punishing effects of brain stimulation should be studied independent of tests of aggressive response. (b) The object of the aggression should be of the same species, and the test animals should be unrestrained, freely moving animals. (c) The rank of the animal of the social hierarchy must be considered. In human studies the "high-rank" role of the physician in the social hierarchy must be recognized, and the experiment should be designed in such a way as to eliminate this potential source of bias. (d) The stimulation should be repeated until response reliability is established. (e) Only responses occurring during or immediately after stimulation should be considered to be elicited by brain stimulation as opposed to being secondary pain-induced effects. To Plotnik's criteria can be added: (f) The elicited behavior should be the same from stimulation to stimulation.

ANATOMICAL LOCALIZATION OF AGGRESSIVE BEHAVIOR IN MAN

With these criteria in mind, let us now consider what the evidence is for an anatomical localization of aggressive behavior in humans. Is it possible to identify sites at which electrical stimulation produces stereotyped aggressive behavior? Is there any evidence from ablation studies that stereotyped aggressive behavior can be eliminated or reduced by surgical destruction of specific areas of the brain?

Valzelli (10) has summarized the results of human cerebral ablation studies in controlling aggression. A number of investigators have claimed that unilateral or bilateral lesions of the amygdala abolish or reduce outbursts of destructive violence in patients who exhibit overt repetitive aggressive acts directed at self or others (14–28). Lesions of the dorsomedial thalamus (29), thalamic centromedian nucleas (30), thalamic lamella medialis (31), posteromedial hypothalamus (32–36), anterior cingulum (37), and temporal lobe (38–40) have also been said to be successful in reducing uncontrolled hostility and aggression in humans.

However, not all ablative procedures permanently alter behavior. Valenstein (41,42) reviewed postoperative results of psychosurgery ablation procedures reported in 153 articles published between 1971 and 1976. Table 2 summarizes the outcomes of 55 patients operated on for aggression, as reported by the neurosurgeons who carried out the proce-

TABLE 2. *Neurosurgeons' estimates of outcomes ablation procedures for aggression (United States 1971–1976)*[a]

Site of surgery	Excellent	Significant improvement	No change	Worse	Total
Amygdala	1	3	10		14
Thalamus	3	9	1	5	18
Hypothalamus		4			4
Multiple sites		16	3		19
Total	4 (7%)	32 (58%)	14 (26%)	5 (9%)	55

[a]Includes 14 cases of hyperactivity and two cases of body rocking (rhythmical). Adapted from ref. 42.

dures. Excellent results were achieved in four patients (7%), and significant improvement occurred in 32 (58%). Nineteen patients (35%) exhibited no significant change or became worse.

Surgical ablation of a specific area of the brain which alters behavior, however, does not prove that the site in question was the origin of the aggressive behavior, nor that the behavior could have been the manifestation of an epileptic discharge. A number of cases have been reported which have claimed that cerebral stimulation has induced aggressive behavior in humans. Because such stimulation studies provide the most direct evidence that specific anatomical sites, at least hypothetically, could be the origin of ictal aggressive behavior in humans, it may be useful to review each of these cases in somewhat more detail. Interestingly, the number of reports significantly exceeds the number of patients because several of these cases have been described multiple times in the literature. I have been able to find only eight cases where cerebral stimulation may have induced aggressive behavior in humans.

Heath et al. (43) and later King (44) reported the case of a 27-year-old schizophrenic woman who, when stimulated in the amygdala with a 5-mA current, became verbally hostile and said ". . . I'm going to hit you." When the current was lowered to 4 mA she lost her aggression, expressed remorse for her behavior, and indicated that she had no control over her feelings: "I don't know what came over me. I felt like an animal." When the 5-mA current was again applied she again became hostile. The hostility again stopped when the current was turned off. She reported no pain during the stimulation. During other treatments she developed intense fear with a desire

to run away, although the same stimulation parameters were used which had produced rage reactions.

In another case, Heath (45) reported that stimulation of the hippocampus at a rate of four per second resulted in 4-Hz spike-and-slow-wave activity in the septal region and an intense rage reaction. However, the patient was "disturbed" before the stimulation, so it is difficult to know to what extent the stimulation caused the intense rage, depersonalization, and delusions of persecution reported by Heath. Heath (46,47) has also reported intense pain accompanied by intense feelings of rage as a result of stimulation in the tegmentum of the mesencephalon and in the caudal hypothalamus.

Perhaps the most well known case of possible ictal aggression is that of Julia (22,48–51). Julia was a 22-year-old woman who had encephalitis before the age of 2 and who subsequently suffered from uncontrolled complex partial seizures associated with loss of contact with the environment and automatisms. She also had a significant behavioral disturbance, and between seizures she often had severe temper tantrums. On 12 occasions she seriously assaulted people without significant provocation, including an episode in the women's rest-room of a movie theater when she stabbed a woman in the heart after the lady brushed against her left arm while Julia was in the midst of an illusion that the left side of her body had become ugly. On another occasion she plunged a scissors blade into the lung of a nurse who did not take a prompt interest in her statement that she felt one of her running attacks coming on. Julia had an array of 20 electrodes implanted into each temporal lobe. Cerebral stimulation in the laboratory did not reproduce either her habitual seizures or any of her episodes of aggressive behavior. However, when the stimulation of the amygdala was induced by radio transmitter, and the patient was not in a laboratory situation, she exhibited a rage reaction on two occasions. While talking to the psychiatrist, she lost contact with the environment 140 sec after stimulation of the hippocampus and began beating the wall with her fists 150 sec after stimulation. On another occasion, 90 sec after stimulation of the amygdala, while she was playing a guitar and singing for the psychiatrist, she lost contact with the environment, swung her guitar past his head, and smashed it against the wall. No seizure activity was evident in the depth recordings during either episode of rage (48), although Mark et al. (49) interpreted what appears to be artifact on the electroencephalogram (EEG) of the wall-beating episode as being "a characteristic electrical seizure in the amygdala." Although this case has been described in several different reports, it is not clear how many stimulations were attempted, in what social settings, nor how often stimulation of the same site which elicited these two attacks resulted in no apparent behavioral change. The three other patients described in several of these reports (48) who also had histories of rage reactions failed to show any aggressive behavior during cerebral stimulation. Breggen (52), in a detailed discussion of each of the cases, strongly criticized the thesis presented by Mark and his colleagues that the rage reactions presented by these patients were related to epilepsy.

In Julia's two episodes of rage reaction following cerebral electrical stimulation, the rage did not occur until 1.5 and 2 min after the stimulus. Ervin et al. (53) described another patient in whom violent behavior occurred significantly longer after cerebral stimulation. The patient was a 63-year-old, mild-mannered machinist with intractable localized pain in the head and neck from terminal squamous cell carcinoma of the piriform sinus. Bilateral amygdalar electrodes were placed for chronic stimulation in an attempt to relieve the pain which had not been responsive to a number of other procedures. During the first stimulation session in the laboratory, 1.5 hr were spent testing various stimulation sites in a search for a region that might give relief to pain or cause

an elevation of mood. No change in subjective state of relief of pain was obvious from any site, but a sharp blood pressure rise occurred on stimulation of the left amygdala. The patient was returned to the ward at the end of the 90-min session. Approximately 20 min later he became wide-eyed, would not permit his nurse to come near, breathed hard, appeared extremely angry, climbed upon his bed, and attacked anyone nearby. He was incontinent and began throwing feces at anyone who came close. After a 10-min effort a group of nurses and orderlies were able to restrain him long enough to administer thorazine. He woke with total amnesia for the episode. Stimulation of the right amygdala was carried out the following day, but for a shorter period of only 20 min. On this occasion no change in the EEG, clinical state, or blood pressure was observed. However, shortly after returning to the ward he again had an attack similar to the first, but the second attack was of shorter duration. Subsequent stimulations were further limited in duration, and no episodes of this nature reoccurred.

It seems clear from the description of this episode that cerebral stimulation did not directly elicit aggressive behavior. Rather, after a prolonged session of multiple cerebral stimulations, the patient exhibited psychotic behavior which responded to thorazine. This behavior was similar to the postictal psychosis occasionally seen in epileptic patients after prolonged flurries of seizures or status epilepticus.

Hitchcock and Cairns (54) reported 18 patients who had undergone amygdalotomy because of behavioral disturbances in which abnormal aggressive behavior was featured to a greater or lesser extent. The surgical procedure involved the bilateral stereotactic placement of electrodes within the amygdalae, for the sole purpose of destroying the amygdalae by radio-frequency current. Whenever possible, the procedures were performed without premedication under local anesthesia. This was possible in nine patients; in the remaining nine patients the bilateral amygdalotomy was performed under general anesthesia because the procedure under local anesthesia was thought to be too hazardous. In six of the local anesthesia patients the effects of stimulation and coagulation were recorded in detail with the use of a tape recorder. The most significant effect of stimulation was to elicit a variety of aggressive responses ranging from coherent, appropriately directed verbal responses (speaking to the surgeon, "I feel I could get up and bite you.") to uncontrolled swearing and physically destructive behavior. Although all these patients had a history of abnormally aggressive behavior, the behavior that occurred under stimulation was never observed at other times during the evaluation. Of the six patients, two exhibited swearing, three shouted and sounded angry, and one threatened violence; in four patients a similar pattern of restless behavior was obtained, including tearing the drapes and clothes and moving hands up toward the stereotactic frame, trying forcibly to remove the frame.

Most of the patients studied by the Harvard group (49) and by Hitchcock and Cairns (54) had a history of difficult-to-manage epilepsy, along with a history of severe behavioral disturbances manifested by poor impulse control and rage reactions in response to minor provocation. In those patients for whom sufficient clinical details were available to make a judgment, there was a clear distinction between the characteristics of the patients' habitual seizures and the behavior observed during rage reactions. When bilateral removal or destruction of the amygdalae was carried out, the aggressive behavior was usually controlled, but there was little effect on the frequency or severity of the seizure disorders.

Chapman (55) studied six patients who also had both temporal lobe epilepsy and intractable assaultive behavior. Stimulation of the amygdaloid region produced afterdischarges and some of the clinical features of the patients' epileptic attacks. No aggressive or violent behavior was elicited by the cerebral stimulation. On the other hand, a large number of patients with intractable epilepsy but without a history of aggression have been subjected to cerebral stimulation without exhibiting any evidence of aggressive behavior. Sem-Jacobsen (56) implanted 3632 electrodes in 82 patients without observing aggressive behavior. Other early investigators who carried out studies of cerebral stimulation in humans, also without observing aggressive behavior, included Delgado et al. (57), Ramey and O'Doherty (58), Sheer (59), and Rand et

al. (60). More recently, as cerebral stimulation has become a routine part of evaluation of patients for possible surgical treatment of epilepsy, a large number of patients have been stimulated in various parts of the temporal lobe and in other epileptogenic structures of the brain without eliciting aggressive behavior. For example, over 200 patients have had depth-electrode implantation during the 25-year history of the UCLA Epilepsy Surgical Treatment Program, and no aggressive behavior has been elicited by cerebral stimulation designed to evaluate the duration of afterdischarges. Gloor (61,62) has also stated that at the Montreal Neurological Institute, he and his colleagues had never produced rage or anger as a response to temporal lobe stimulation in patients being evaluated for surgical treatment of epilepsy. He himself had never seen an instance of true ictal rage.

In light of this evidence, as well as in light of the large number of patients who have undergone cerebral stimulation without eliciting aggressive responses, reports of behavioral changes which are alleged to be the result of direct brain stimulation need to be evaluated with caution. Ervin et al. (53) suggested a number of potential problems with interpretation of the results of direct stimulation, which they have summarized as follows:

1. A synchronous electrical discharge is quite different from the exquisitely patterned afferent volley of physiological signals.
2. In a complex neural aggregate the electrical input may indiscriminately activate (a) excitatory and inhibitory systems, (b) afferent, efferent, and integrative systems, or (c) cholinergic and adrenergic systems.
3. The instantaneous state of cerebral organization—that is, all the other influences acting on the object structure at the time of stimulation—is unknown.
4. At best, the site stimulated is part of an integrated system, so that the stimulus is like a rock thrown in a pond—perhaps influencing by waves a distant lily pad. The stimulation of a structure says what it *can* do under certain circumstances, not necessarily what it *does* do normally.
5. Ablation is not the reciprocal of stimulation in other than very simple input and output systems.

It is particularly important to recognize that direct cerebral electrical stimulation is not the same thing as an epileptic seizure. Rather, it is the artificial introduction of a stimulus that is far more intense than the paroxysmal abnormal electrical discharge of an epileptic seizure. At best, it may demonstrate what anatomical localization within the brain *could* be associated with certain forms of stereotyped behavior. In order to evaluate the potential contribution of cerebral electrical stimulation studies to an understanding of ictal aggression, we need to consider what is known about the nature of ictal events.

NATURE OF ICTAL EVENTS

Gumnit and Leppik (63) defined a seizure as "a sudden, involuntary, time-limited alteration in behavior including change in motor activity or autonomic function, consciousness, or sensation, accompanied by an abnormal electrical discharge in the brain." Implicit in this definition is that seizures are brief intermittent spontaneous paroxysms of excessive hypersynchronous abnormal electrical activity which result in behavioral change. However, the perception of behavioral change may depend on the intensity of the evaluation. It would be difficult for an observer to ignore a generalized tonic–clonic seizure lasting several minutes. It is far more common for brief absence seizures in children to go unrecognized. There is increasing evidence that even single "interictal" spikes may be associated with transient cognitive impairment if sophisticated and sensitive test paradigms are employed (64). Are such abnormal electrical discharges seizures (albeit extremely brief) if they are associated with changes in behavior? Because all clinical seizures are associated with excessive hypersynchronous discharges of at least some neurons in the brain, does this mean that all such excessive hypersynchronous discharges of neurons are seizures, even if they are not associated with any detectable behavioral changes?

These are difficult questions to answer, and as of yet there are no unambiguous criteria to establish whether or not an event is an epileptic seizure. Rather, we are still dependent on observing a constellation of clinical and/or electrical criteria which together lead to the determination that a paroxysmal event is an epileptic seizure. Fundamental to both sets of criteria is the concept of stereotypy—that is, that the behavioral and/or electrical changes are substantially the same from event to event. Thus when we consider clinical criteria for a seizure we expect to see spontaneous, nonprovoked brief episodes of stereotyped abnormal behavior which occur independent of the psychological environment. When the seizure is associated with impairment of consciousness (which is what we expect from all seizures except for simple partial seizures, myoclonic seizure, and atonic seizures), there should be partial or complete amnesia for the event with either abrupt cessation or progressive clearing of the amnesia during the postictal phase. Behavior at the time of the event is usually primitive, nonorganized, non-goal-directed behavior which is physiologically consisent with the hypersynchronous cortical discharge. Typically, when seizures are recorded from depth electrodes at the onset, there is a high-frequency (> 60 Hz) discharge at the seizure focus which is sometimes preceded by a transient direct-current shift, sharp wave, or spike-and-wave discharge (65). Sometimes, however, there is an initial reduction in amplitude of the background and in the appearance of low-voltage high-frequency spikes which gradually decrease in frequency and increase in amplitude and then change to a spike-and-wave pattern and finally to a postictal slow pattern with gradual return to the baseline. When seizures are recorded from the scalp, typical patterns may not be seen and paroxysmal slowing may be the only EEG manifestation of the seizure. However, whether the seizures are recorded from depth electrodes or from the scalp, the morphology and location—at least at the onset—should be stereotypic from seizure to seizure.

Nine types of seizures are now recognized in the International Classification of Epileptic Seizures (66) (Table 3). Of these, myoclonic seizures, atonic seizures, and simple partial seizures are, by definition, not associated with any alteration of contact with the environment and thus are unlikely to be associated with involuntary directed aggressive behavior. Although absence seizures are

TABLE 3. *International classification of epileptic seizures*

Partial (onset) seizures
Simple partial seizure
Complex partial seizures
Partial seizures evolving to secondarily generalized
  seizures

Generalized (from onset) seizures
Absence seizures
  Atypical absence seizures
Myoclonic seizures
Clonic seizures
Tonic seizures
Tonic–clonic seizures
Atonic seizures

[a]Modified from ref. 66.

sometimes associated with mild clonic movements and other automatisms, the nature of these automatisms is that they are simple and repetitive and are never sufficiently complex to support directed aggression. Generalized tonic, clonic, and tonic–clonic seizures are manifested by repetitive convulsive movements and are not modified by the environment. Only complex partial seizures have been observed to exhibit automatic behavior of sufficient complexity that such behavior could be perceived as aggressive behavior. Thus, if directed aggression does occur as an ictal event, then the only seizure type for which it would be appropriate to classify such behavior is the complex partial seizure. For this reason, it is worthwhile to review what is known about the characteristics of complex partial seizures.

The term "complex partial seizure" is applied to a seizure in which there is an impairment of consciousness or of contact with the environment which is usually associated with automatic behavior. The onset and cessation of the complex partial seizure is usually gradual and the seizure lasts seconds to several minutes, whereas in absence seizures the duration is usually less than 15 sec. Typically, complex partial seizures begin with a motionless stare which is followed by stereotyped automatisms and then by reactive automatisms. Sometimes, however, there is no motionless stare, and the seizure begins with automatic behavior. "Stereotyped automatism" is a term that refers to automatic behavior

which is repetitive from seizure to seizure, whereas "reactive automatism" applies to automatic behavior which can be modified by the environment but for which the patient is amnestic.

The EEG of complex partial seizures may consist on unilateral or frequently bilateral low-voltage fast activity which begins focally. During the course of the seizure the amplitude gradually increases and the frequency decreases. Rhythmic spiking may be replaced by a spike-and-wave pattern which may abruptly stop and which is then followed by low-voltage slow activity that gradually returns to the interictal background activity. At times, low-voltage fast activity may not be seen at onset, but rather the seizure may be associated with paroxysmal slow waves on the EEG, particularly during surface recordings.

Delgado-Escueta et al. (67–69) have suggested that complex partial seizures can be divided into three types (Table 4). Type I complex partial seizures characteristically have mesial temporal onset, whereas Type II seizures are most commonly of extratemporal origin. Others have questioned this subclassification of complex partial seizures (70). However, there is general agreement that there is a predictable sequence of behavioral changes during the course of complex partial seizures which starts with a motionless stare and/or stereotyped automatisms that are then followed by reactive automatisms. Recognition that such a sequence of behavioral changes occurs in all complex partial seizures should allow evaluation of other paroxysmal behavioral alterations such as episodic rage to determine whether such behavioral alterations fit what is known about the natural history of complex partial seizures.

TABLE 4. *Subtypes of complex partial seizures*

Type I:	Arrest reaction and/or motionless stare Simple stereotyped automatisms Reactive automatisms
Type II:	Complex stereotyped automatisms consisting of semipurposeful motor activity Reactive automatisms
Type III:	Temporal lobe syncope

DOES ICTAL AGGRESSION OCCUR?

In any consideration of whether or not episodes of aggressive behavior are ictal, it is not enough to observe that seizures and aggression occur in the same patient or even that aggressive episodes stop after resection of an apparent seizure focus. Rather, it is essential to review a detailed second-by-second description of the alleged aggressive behavior and of the EEG in order to verify that the onset and progression of behavioral changes are correlated with EEG ictal activity.

Thirty-eight cases of possible ictal aggression or violence have been reported in the medical literature. Treiman and Delgado-Escueta (71) reviewed 29 of them in detail. In their opinion, only three of the 29 cases were strongly suggestive of a relationship between ictal epileptic attacks and violent automatisms. In 1980 an international panel of 18 epileptologists reviewed videotapes and EEGs of 33 epileptic attacks in 19 patients who were believed to have exhibited aggressive behavior during the recorded seizures (72). In the opinion of the panel, seven patients exhibited ictal aggression ranging from violence toward property to mild aggression directed toward a person. Of the remaining 12 patients, only six had pseudoseizures and six had minimal or no aggression. Five of the patients in the Delgado-Escueta series have been described in greater detail elsewhere (73–75). These five cases, along with the two reported subsequently by Wieser (76), are the only patients who are known to have clear histories of assault and whose epileptic attacks have been studied well by closed-circuit television (CCTV) and EEG. Thus there are only a few patients reported in the medical literature who have been observed to exhibit aggressive behavior and in whom there is reasonable evidence that their aggressive behavior may have been related temporally to an ictal event. Therefore, it is worthwhile to review these cases in some detail.

Two cases were described by Gunn and Fenton (77) where violent behavior may have been related to an ictal event. One was a 49-year-old alcoholic who had seizures since the age of 25. One evening, after having been drinking, he left the pub and had a seizure. He was recovering from the seizure when a policeman tried to remove him for being a nuisance. The patient lashed out and tried to hit the policeman. In the other case a 32-year-old man developed generalized convulsions at the age of 18. Two years later, while staying at his girlfriend's house, he had a generalized convulsion early in the morning. While still in a postictal confused state he violently attacked his girlfriend, as well as an elderly couple who also lived in the house. On admission to the hospital shortly thereafter, he was mentally confused and amnestic for all events following the seizure. He subsequently had a generalized tonic–clonic seizure once every 1–2 years. Each seizure was followed by a period of confusion lasting 15–60 min during which the patient appeared perplexed and frightened and, if restrained in any way, would become dangerously aggressive. Both of these cases are examples of "resistive violence" in which attempts to restrain a patient while still in a postictal confused state produces violent reactive automatisms for which the patient is completely amnestic.

Knox (78) also described six patients who exhibited resistive behavior if an attempt was made to restrain them at the end of a seizure. One patient, a 50-year-old man, had several episodes of automatisms while under observation. During these episodes he would stagger about and, if assisted, would shout "Leave me alone." On one occasion he grabbed an orderly by the throat, held him for several minutes, and yelled "I'll kill you." He kicked the doctor on another occasion. He reported that if he had a seizure at work his colleagues knew not to approach him: "It seems I don't attack them if I'm not touched."

Resistive violence has also been observed in other series of patients with complex partial seizures (67,69,79). In Ashford et al.'s (73) patient and in Treiman and Delgado-Escueta's (75) two patients, fear apparently induced automatic destruction of property, defensive kicking, and flailing. These behaviors observed on the CCTV–EEG were similar to those described in the patients' histories.

Of the 19 patients reviewed by the international panel, only one (one of Saint-Hilaire's patients) exhibited ictal aggressive acts which could have resulted in serious harm to another person. This was a mentally retarded young woman of 20 who, at the age of 3, had "a generalized infection with encephalopathy and henceforth manifested unmotivated aggressive paroxysms . . ." (74). Saint-Hilaire et al. (74) further described her history as follows:

> The aggressive outbursts happen suddenly, without any warning. She quickly moves toward a target and physically assaults it. . . . When the targets are objects, she breaks them and/or throws them. When she directs these behaviors toward humans, she will often grab the eyeglasses and break them; if a person does not wear glasses, she will direct her attack toward the face while grabbing and/or hitting.
>
> The outbursts suddenly abate and the patient declares herself tired; she "does not feel well" but her contact with the environment is restored to its usual level. These paroxysms happen many times a week despite heavy medication.

During scalp EEG observations, a secondarily generalized tonic–clonic seizure was recorded without evidence of aggressive behavior.

During depth scalp-EEG observations, several "absences" were noted during which the patient lost contact with the environment and exhibited epileptiform activity limited to the right amygdala and right temporal cortex. Stimulation of the right hippocampus only produced a local afterdischarge without behavioral change. On one occasion, stimulation of the left hippocampus was followed 95 sec later by loss of contact with the environment, irregular movements and breathing at 104 sec after the end of the electrical stimulation, and an aggressive outburst at 117 sec after the stimulation in which she rose suddenly from a prone position, attempted to grab the neuropsychologist's eyeglasses, and verbally accused him: "It's your fault, it's not right, you've done it" (74). Apparent epileptiform activity was seen in the right hippocampus throughout the 67 sec of recording; unfortunately, the entire recording from the time of the electrical stimulation and throughout the entire aggressive episode was not presented, so the time the epileptiform activity began could not be seen and was not reported in the text.

Saint Hilaire et al.'s (74) other patient was a 30-year-old bachelor sheet-metal worker who began having seizures at 6 years of age,

1 year after head trauma. During adolescence, his seizures assumed their adult pattern. They began with an aura consisting of a shiver at the level of the thorax followed by loss of consciousness. The patient then would talk or yell or insult people and spit in their faces. He remained ambulatory and was able to carry out relatively complex activities during these seizures, after which he would be amnestic.

This patient was studied with stereo-EEG. During a typical seizure the patient warned the staff that an aura was beginning at the time low-voltage fast activity could be seen in the right amygdala and right anterior temporal leads. Seven seconds later the patient whistled and struck his right thigh with his right hand at the time when the EEG frequency in the amygdala and anterior temporal cortex slowed. Twenty seconds after onset of the initial EEG change and behavioral warning, the patient yelled vulgar insults toward a nurse in the adjacent room. Insults directed toward the nurse (even though an EEG technician was closer to him) continued when, 26 sec after the onset of the seizure, rhythmic spike activity was seen not only from the amygdalar and anterior temporal leads but also from the right parahippocampal gyrus. The seizure stopped 75 sec after onset and the patient was amnestic for all events.

Wieser (76) described a boy with socially disabling behavior disorders and frequent rage attacks sometimes starting with fear and gastric sensations. There was left frontal temporal flattening on the EEG at the start of these episodes. Stereo-EEG exploration was not performed because of the severe aggressive outbursts. However, selective left amygdalohippocampectomy stopped all seizures and the rage attacks. The boy was described as being seizure-free and a calm and good student over 2.5 years of follow-up. Wieser's other patient was a 16-year-old male with "psychomotor" seizures since the age of 9; these seizures were characterized by paroxysmal speech disturbances and fits of rage leading to brawls. During his attack, he was said to abruptly raise his hand and rave or suddenly become speechless or indiscriminately attack and hit everyone around. A pneumoencephalogram showed a left temporal basal cyst communicating with the temporal horn. During stereo-EEG exploration, several rage attacks were observed and long-lasting "clonic discharges" in the left periamygdalar region were recorded which were not evident on the surface EEG. However, no data were presented regarding the exact temporal relationship between the periamygdalar discharges and the rage behavior. The patient underwent a left temporal lobectomy. The pathological specimen demonstrated a small periamygdalar capillary hemangioma. Over 4.5 years of follow-up, the patient remained seizure-free and was described as a "calm and peaceable" man.

POSSIBLE PRESENTATIONS OF ICTAL OR PERI-ICTAL VIOLENCE OR AGGRESSION

Although the evidence that directed aggression occurs as the behavioral manifestation of an ictal event is sparse (as indicated by the cases reviewed above), it is theoretically possible that such behavior could occur. In the analysis of possible cases of ictal aggression, it is worthwhile to consider five circumstances under which ictal violence or aggression may occur:

1. Primary ictal aggression—aggressive behavior which is directly stimulated by the epileptic discharge. To verify that such behavior occurs, it is important to document that the behavior in question occurs simultaneously with ictal discharges which involve the presumed site of anatomical origin of the behavior.

2. Secondary ictal aggression—aggressive behavior which is released by disinhibition of normal social controls as a result of a seizure discharge, or perhaps which occurs in response to an epileptic discharge which produces a noxious or aversive stimulus. These two possible presentations of ictal or peri-ictal aggression correspond to what Plotnik (11) has called "primary aggression" and "secondary (pain-induced) aggression" in animals stimulated with intracerebral electrodes.

3. Resistive violence—violent behavior which occurs at the end of an unequivocal well-documented seizure while the patient is still exhibiting reactive automatisms or is in a postictal confused state.

4. Violence or aggression which occurs in the context of postictal psychosis. Such aggression is not fundamentally dissimilar from the aggressive behavior seen in other patients who exhibit psychotic behavior due to other causes.

5. Nonaggressive violent automatisms—violent behavior which occurs as a stereotyped automatism but which is not directed toward a person or object and has no aggressive intent.

Most of the episodes of aggression or violence which are said to have occurred in relation to epileptic attacks are examples of resistive violence which have occurred at the end of documented complex partial or generalized tonic–clonic epileptic seizures. This is true for the two cases described by Gunn and Fenton (77), the six cases described by Knox (78) (including his one case described in detail above), and the examples reported in other series of complex partial seizures (67,69,79). In those cases where violent activity occurred at (or nearly at) the beginning of behavioral seizures, the behavior consisted of random violence and not directed aggression. For example, in Treiman and Delgado-Escueta's (75) two cases, in Ashford et al.'s (73) patient, and perhaps in one of Wieser's (76) patients, the stereotyped automatisms exhibited consisted of random flailing movements, bicycling behavior, and, in the case of Ashford et al.'s patient, whirling movements while holding onto the draperies in the room. In each case the violent behavior was not directed toward any individual and was stereotyped from seizure to seizure within the same patient. Such cases are examples of nonaggressive violent automatisms.

In the two cases described by Saint-Hilaire et al. (74), in which directed aggressive behavior appeared to be associated with ictal discharges recorded during stereo EEG, the aggressive behavior occurred after the onset of the seizure. This was true for the 20-year-old patient in whom one episode of aggressive behavior appears to have been recorded simultaneously with the scalp EEG. In this patient the aggressive outburst associated with right hippocampal activity occurred 117 sec after electrical stimulation of the left hippocampus. Furthermore, the aggressive behavior was preceded 22 sec earlier by an alteration of contact with the environment. This raises the question, Could the aggressive behavior seen in this patient have been an example of secondary ictal aggression in which the aggressive response was a reaction to a primary emotion elicited by either (a) the initial electrical stimulation of the left hippocampus or (b) what may have been a spontaneous seizure discharge in the right hippocampus starting 22 sec earlier at the time the patient lost contact with the environment? It is notable that several other seizures recorded in this patient were not associated with aggressive behavior. This raises real questions as to whether this patient's habitual aggressive behavior was indeed ictal in nature.

In Saint-Hilaire et al.'s (74) other patient the history presented suggests that the patient's habitual seizures always included episodes in which he yelled, insulted people, and spat in their faces. Again, the aggressive behavior in the example reported did not occur until 20 sec after the onset of the seizure. This also raises the question as to whether or not, if this stereotyped behavior was indeed ictal, it should be called "secondary ictal aggression" and might have been caused by a behavioral response to a noxious stimulus or emotion elicited by the initial seizure onset.

In all the cases reviewed above in which violent or aggressive behavior may have been associated with ictal activity, the exhibited behavior either (a) consisted of nonaggressive violent automatisms which were clearly stereotyped and repetitive from seizure to seizure within the same patient, (b) consisted of reactive automatisms manifested by directed aggression which always occurred after the onset of a clearly identifiable complex partial seizure which began with a typical initial loss of contact with the environment, or (c) consisted of resistive violence at the end of a complex partial or generalized tonic–clonic seizure when the patient was being restrained while still in a confused state. There are no documented cases of ictal aggression in which an organized directed attack toward another individual or object occurred as the initial or sole manifestation of an epileptic seizure and which could not otherwise be diagnosed on the basis of at least some concomitant typical features of complex partial or generalized tonic–clonic seizures.

SUMMARY

1. Aggression in animals has been classified into a number of stereotyped behavioral responses on the basis of the psychosocial environment in which it occurs. Many such responses can be either replicated or blocked by stimulation or ablation of selected sites in the brain, especially in the hypothalamus or amygdala. Stimulation of the amygdala or the hypothalamus in a limited number of humans has produced agitation, anger, or rage. Ablation of the amygdala has reduced aggression in violent patients. However, the ictal nature of episodic aggression in these patients has not been proven.

2. The diagnosis and classification of epileptic seizures is based on their characteristic clinical manifestations and electrical patterns. Independent objective markers of ictal events need to be identified. Epileptic seizures are characterized by stereotyped nondirected behavior, especially at onset. The more organized, directed, and modifiable by the environment the behavior is, the less likely it is epilepsy.

3. Ictal aggression can be classified into primary and secondary ictal aggression, resistive violence, and postictal psychosis. Few alleged cases of ictal violence or aggression fulfill criteria for ictal events; most which do are examples of resistive violence.

4. If animal models can be developed which exhibit spontaneous paroxysmal stereotypical aggression, they may be used to improve our understanding of the classification and pathophysiology of ictal aggression.

REFERENCES

1. Carroll L. Through the looking glass. In: Gasson R, ed. *The illustrated Lewis Carroll*. London: Jupiter, 1978;103–216.
2. Echeverria M. On epileptic insanity. *Am J Insanity* 1873;30:1–51.
3. Maudsley H. *Body and mind*. London: Macmillan, 1873.
4. Maudsley H. *Responsibility in mental disease*. New York: Appleton, 1874.
5. Bianchi L. *A textbook of psychiatry for physicians and medical students*. London: Baillière, Tindall & Cox, 1906.
6. Kolb LC, Brodie HKH. *Modern clinical psychiatry* 10th ed. Philadelphia: WB Saunders, 1982.

7. Treiman DM. Epilepsy and violence: medical and legal issues. *Epilepsia* 1986;27(Suppl 2):S77–S104.
8. Moyer KE. *The psychobiology of aggression.* New York: Harper & Row, 1976.
9. Goldstein M. Brain research and violent behavior: a summary and evaluation of the status of biomedical research on brain and aggressive violent behavior. *Arch Neurol* 1974;30:1–35.
10. Valzelli L. *Psychobiology of aggression and violence.* New York: Raven Press, 1981.
11. Plotnik R. Brain stimulation and aggression: monkeys, apes and humans. In; Holloway RL, ed. *Primate aggression, territoriality, and xenophobia.* New York: Academic Press, 1974;389–416.
12. Plotnik R, Mir D, Delgado JMR. Aggression, noxiousness, and brain stimulation in unrestrained Rhesus monkeys. In: Eleftheriou BE, Scott JP, eds. *The physiology of aggression and defeat.* New York: Plenum Press, 1971;143–221.
13. Robinson BW, Alexander M, Bowne G. Dominance reversal resulting from aggressive responses evoked by brain telestimulation. *Physiol Behav* 1969;4:749–752.
14. Sawa M, Ueki Y, Arita M, Harada T. Preliminary report on the amygdaloidectomy on the psychotic patients, with interpretation of oral–emotional manifestation in schizophrenics. *Folia Psychiatr Neurol Jpn* 1954;7:309–329.
15. Chatrian GE, Chapman WP. Electrographic study of the amygdaloid region with implanted electrodes in patients with temporal lobe epilepsy. In: Ramey ER, O'Doherty DS, eds. *Electrical studies on the unanesthetized brain.* New York: Paul B Hoeber, 1960;351–373.
16. Ursin H. The temporal lobe substrate of fear and anger. A review of recent stimulation and ablation studies in animals and humans. *Acta Psychiatr Neurol Scand* 1960;35:378–396.
17. Narabayashi H, Nagao T, Saito Y, Yoshida M, Nagahata M. Stereotaxic amygdalotomy for behavior disorders. *Arch Neurol* 1963;9:1–16.
18. Schwab RS, Sweet WH, Mark VH, Kjellber RN, Ervin FR. Treatment of intractable temporal lobe epilepsy by stereotactic amygdala lesions. *Trans Am Neurol Assoc* 1965;90:12–19.
19. Balasubramaniam V, Ramamurthi B. Stereotaxic amygdalotomy. *Proc Aust Assoc Neurol* 1968;5:277–278.
20. Heimburger RF, Whitlock CC, Kalsbeck JE. Stereotaxic amygdalotomy for epilepsy with aggressive behavior. *JAMA* 1966;198:741–745.
21. Narabayashi H, Uno M. Long range results of stereotaxic amygdalotomy for behavior disorders. *Confin Neurol* 1966;27:168–171.
22. Sweet WH, Ervin F, Mark VH. The relationship of violent behaviour to focal cerebral disease. In: Garattini S, Sigg EB, eds. *Aggressive behaviour.* Amsterdam: Excerpta Medica, 1969;336–352.
23. Turnbull F. Neurosurgery in the control of unmanageable affective reactions: a critical review. *Clin Neurosurg* 1969;16:218–233.
24. Balasubramaniam V, Ramamurthi B. Stereotaxic amygdalotomy in behavior disorders. *Confin Neurol* 1970;32:367–373.
25. Narabayashi H, Mizutani T. Epileptic seizures and the stereotaxic amygdalotomy. *Confin Neurol* 1970;32:289–297.
26. Vaernet K, Madsen A. Stereotaxic amygdalotomy and basofrontal tractotomy in psychotics with aggressive behaviour. *J Neurol Neurosurg Psychiatry* 1970;33:858–863.
27. Mempel E. Influence of partial amygdalectomy on the emotional disturbances and epileptic seizures. *Neurol Neurochir Pol* 1971;5:81–86.
28. Kiloh LG, Gye RS, Rushworth RG, Bell DS, White RT. Stereotactic amygdaloidotomy for aggressive behavior. *J Neurol Neurosurg Psychiatry* 1974;37:437–444.
29. Spiegel EA, Wycis HT, Freed H, Orchinik C. The central mechanism of the emotions. *Am J Psychiatry* 1951;108:426–532.
30. Andy OJ. Thalamotomy in hyperactive and aggressive behavior. *Confin Neurol* 1970;32:322–325.
31. Poblete M, Palestini M, Figueroa E, Gallardo R, Rojas J, Covarrubias MI, Doyharcabal Y. Stereotaxic thalamotomy (lamella medialis) in aggressive psychiatric patients. *Confin Neurol* 1970;32:326–331.
32. Sano K. Sedative neurosurgery: with special reference to postero-medial hypothalamotomy. *Neurol Medico-Chir* 1962;4:112–142.
33. Sano K, Yoshioka M, Ogashiwa M, Ishijima B, Ohye C. Postero-medial hypothalamotomy in the treatment of aggressive behaviors. *Confin Neurol* 1966;27:164–167.
34. Sano K, Mayanagi Y, Sedino H, Ogashiwa M, Ishijima B. Results of stimulation and destruction of the posterior hypothalamus in man. *J Neurosurg* 1970;33:689–707.
35. Kalyanaraman S. Some observations during stimulation of the human hypothalamus. *Confin Neurol* 1975;37:189–192.
36. Sramka M, Nadvornik P. Surgical complication of posterior hypothalamotomy. *Confin Neurol* 1975;37:193–194.
37. Tow PM, Whitty CWM. Personality changes after operations on the cingulate gyrus in man. *J Neurol Neurosurg Psychiatry* 1953;16:186–193.
38. Pool JL. The visceral brain of man. *J Neurosurg* 1954;11:45–63.
39. Scoville WB, Milner B. Loss of recent memory after bilateral hippocampal lesions. *J Neurol Neurosurg Psychiatry* 1957;20:11–21.
40. Terzian H. Observations on the clinical symptomatology of bilateral partial or total removal of the temporal lobes in man. In: Baldwin M, ed. *Temporal lobe epilepsy.* Springfield, IL: Charles C Thomas, 1958;510–529.
41. Valenstein ES. The practice of neurosurgery: a survey of the literature (1971–1976). In: *Appendix: Psychosurgery.* The National Commission for the Protection of Human Subjects of Biomedical and Behavioral Research. Department of Health, Education and Welfare, publication

no. (OS)77-0002. Washington, DC: US Government Printing Office, 1977;I-1-I-183.

42. Valenstein ES. Review of the literature on postoperative evaluation. In: Valenstein ES, ed. *The psychosurgery debate: scientific, legal, and ethical perspectives.* San Francisco: WH Freeman, 1980;141–163.

43. Heath RG, Monroe RR, Mickle WA. Stimulation of the amygdaloid nucleus in a schizophrenic patient. *Am J Psychiatry* 1955;111:862–863.

44. King HE. Psychological effects of excitation in the limbic system. In: Sheer DE, ed. *Electrical stimulation of the brain.* Austin, TX: University of Texas Press, 1961;477–486.

45. Heath RG. Developments toward new physiologic treatments in psychiatry. *J Neuropsychiatry* 1964;5:318–331.

46. Heath RG. Correlations between levels of psychological awareness and physiological activity in the central nervous system. *Psychosom Med* 1955;17:383–395.

47. Heath RG. Brain centers and control of behavior—man. In: Nodine JH, Moyer JH, eds. *Psychosomatic medicine: the first Hahnemann symposium.* Philadelphia: Lea & Febiger, 1962; 228–240.

48. Delgado JMR, Mark V, Sweet W, Ervin F, Weiss G, Bach-y-Rita G, Hagiwara R. Intracerebral radio stimulation and recording in completely free patients. *J Nerv Ment Dis* 1968;147:329–340.

49. March VH, Ervin FR, Sweet WH, Delgado J. Remote telemeter stimulation and recording from implanted temporal lobe electrodes. *Confin Neurol* 1969;31:86–93.

50. Mark VH, Ervin FR. *Violence and the brain.* New York: Harper & Row, 1970.

51. Mark VH, Sweet WH, Ervin FR. Deep temporal lobe stimulation and destructive lesions in episodically violent temporal lobe epileptics. In: Fields WS, Sweet WH, eds. *Neural bases of violence and aggression.* St. Louis: Warren H Green, 1975;379–391.

52. Breggin PR. Psychosurgery for the control of violence: a critical review. In: Fields WS, Sweet WH, eds. *Neural bases of violence and aggression.* St. Louis: Warren H Green, 1975;350–378.

53. Ervin FR, Mark VH, Stevens J. Behavioral and affective responses to brain stimulation in man. In: Zubin J, Shagass C, eds. *Neurobiological aspects of psychopathology.* New York: Grune & Stratton, 1969;54–65.

54. Hitchcock E, Cairns V. Amygdalotomy. *Postgrad Med J* 1973;49:894–904.

55. Chapman WP. Studies of the periamygdaloid area in relation to human behavior. In: Solomon HC, Cobb S, Penfield W, eds. *The brain and human behavior. Assoc Res Nerv Ment Dis Res Publ* 1958;36:258–277.

56. Sem-Jacobsen CW. *Depth-electrographic stimulation of the human brain and behavior.* Springfield, IL: Charles C Thomas, 1968.

57. Delgado JMR, Hamlim H, Chapman WP. Technique of intracranial electrode implacement for recording and stimulation and its possible therapeutic value in psychotic patients. *Confin Neurol* 1952;12:315–319.

58. Ramey ER, O'Doherty DS, eds. *Electrical studies on the unanesthetized brain.* New York: Paul B. Hoeber, 1960.

59. Sheer DE, ed. *Electrostimulation of the brain.* Austin, TX: University of Texas Press, 1961.

60. Rand RW, Crandall PH, Walter R. Chronic stereotactic implantation of depth-electrodes for psychomotor epilepsy. *Acta Neurochir* 1964;11: 609–630.

61. Gloor P. Discussion of B. Kaada: brain mechanisms related to aggressive behavior. In: Clemente CD, Lindsley DB, eds. *Aggression and defense: neuromechanisms and social patterns. Brain function, vol V.* Los Angeles: University of California Press, 1967;95–133.

62. Gloor P. Electrophysiological studies of the amygdala (stimulation and recording): their possible contribution to the understanding of neural mechanisms of aggression. In: Fields WS, Sweet WH, eds. *Neural bases of violence and aggression.* St. Louis: Warren H Green, 1975;5–40.

63. Gumnit RJ, Leppik IE. The epilepsies. In: Rosenberg RN, ed. *The clinical neurosciences, Section I: Neurology.* New York: Churchill Livingstone, 1983;409–440.

64. Binnie CD, Channon S, Marston DL. Behavioral correlates of interictal spikes. In: Smith DB, Treiman DM, Trimble MR, eds. *Neurobehavioral problems in epilepsy: scientific basis, insights and hypothesis. Advances in neurology,* Vol. 55. New York: Raven Press, 1991;113–126.

65. Binnie CD. Electroencephalography. In: Laidlaw J, Richens A, Oxley J, eds. *A textbook of epilepsy, 3rd ed.* Edinburgh: Churchill Livingstone, 1988;236–306.

66. Commission on Classification and Terminology of the International League Against Epilepsy. Proposal for revised clinical and electroencephalographic classification of epileptic seizures. *Epilepsia* 1981;22:489–501.

67. Delgado-Escueta AV, Kunze U, Waddell G, Boxley J, Nadel A. Lapse of consciousness and automatisms in temporal lobe epilepsy: a videotape analysis. *Neurology* 1977;27:144–155.

68. Delgado-Escueta AV, Nashold B, Freedman M, Keplinger MD, Waddell G, Miller P, Carwille S. Videotaping epileptic attacks during stereo electroencephalography. *Neurology* 1979;29:473–489.

69. Delgado-Escueta AV, Enrile-Bacsal F, Treiman DM. Complex partial seizures on closed circuit television and EEG: a study of 691 attacks in 79 patients. *Ann Neurol* 1982;11:292–300.

70. Theodore WH, Porter RJ, Penry JK. Complex partial seizures: clinical characteristics and differential diagnosis. *Neurology* 1983;33:1115–1121.

71. Treiman DM, Delgado-Escueta AV. Violence and epilepsy: a critical review. In: Pedley TA, Meldrum BS, eds. *Recent advances in epilepsy,* vol. 1. Edinburgh: Churchill Livingstone, 1983; 179–209.

72. Delgado-Escueta AV, Mattson RH, King L, Goldensohn ES, Speigel H, Madsen J, Crandall P, Deifuss F, Porter RJ. Special report. The nature of aggression during epileptic seizures. *N Engl J Med* 1981;305:711–716.

73. Ashford JW, Schulz SC, Walsh GO. Violent automatisms in a partial complex seizure. Report of a case. *Arch Neurol* 1980;37:120–122.

74. Saint-Hilaire JM, Gilbert M, Bouvier G, Barbeau A. Epilepsy and aggression: two cases with depth electrode studies. In: Robb P, ed. *Epilepsy updated: causes and treatment*. Miami: Symposia Specialist, 1980;145–176.

75. Treiman DM, Delgado-Escueta AV. Aggression during fear and fight in complex partial seizures: a CCTV–EEG analysis. *Epilepsia* 1981;22:243.

76. Wieser HG. Depth recorded limbic seizures and psychopathology. *Neurosci Biobehav Rev* 1983;7:427–440.

77. Gunn J, Fenton G. Epilepsy, automatism and crime. *Lancet* 1971;1:1173–1176.

78. Knox SJ. Epileptic automatism and violence. *Med Sci Law* 1968;8:96–104.

79. King DW, Ajmone Marsan C. Clinical features and ictal patterns in epileptic patients with EEG temporal lobe foci. *Ann Neurol* 1977;2:138–147.

Advances in Neurology, Vol. 55, edited by
D. Smith, D. Treiman, and M. Trimble,
Raven Press, Ltd., New York © 1991.

22

Ictal Amnesia and Fugue States

A. James Rowan*† and David H. Rosenbaum*

*Department of Neurology, Mt. Sinai School of Medicine, New York, New York 10029;
†The Bronx VA Medical Center, Bronx, New York 10468

Memory loss is one of the most frequently encountered complaints in the office of the epileptologist. Usually patients speak of increasing forgetfulness involving commonplace items such as appointments or what they were about to say, and they ask if their medication is to blame. Often there is no simple answer; both drugs and recurrent seizures can play a role in memory impairment. At the same time, one may consider another cause for these complaints—namely, an early stage of dementia, or depression. When patients report repeated (but discrete) periods of memory lapse, a diagnosis of recurrent seizures is entertained. A confident diagnosis of epilepsy, however, depends on a reliable observer who may, for example, describe typical complex partial seizures. Rarely does one encounter a patient with epilepsy whose *only* clinical manifestation is memory loss.

Considering that nearly all functions of the brain have a correlate in clinical seizure activity, there would appear to be no theoretical reason why a seizure cannot be represented by memory loss alone. Alternatively, amnesia could be a form of "Todd's paralysis," a functional deficit following an unobserved or subclinical seizure. In fact, in the absence of simultaneous electroencephalography (EEG) and behavioral monitoring, amnesia following such an ictus would be indistinguishable from an amnestic seizure. Since in the clinical setting it rarely has been possible to record such events in their entirety, for the purposes of this discussion we shall consider both of these conditions to be "ictal amnesia." That is, we shall define ictal amnesia as a *transient disturbance of memory function which is caused by a seizure (or by its aftereffect) and which has no other clinical manifestation.* We will not be concerned with loss of memory associated with delirium, dementia, or simple forgetfulness. Rather, we will concentrate on episodic memory loss without other evidence of cognitive dysfunction, and we will consider the differential diagnosis of such states.

Inasmuch as we are concerned with amnesia on an ictal basis, what would its theoretical characteristics be? We would expect ictal amnesia to be a recurrent, paroxysmal memory disturbance without apparent alteration of the sensorium. During the episode, the individual would appear to be relatively normal and to be able to speak clearly and carry out many of his usual activities. Personal identity would be retained. The event would be circumscribed and relatively brief, and no other clinical signs would be present. Gradual recovery to the pre-ictal state would be expected, except for a variable retrograde amnesia. It will be appreciated that this constellation of symptoms is reminiscent of transient global amnesia (TGA; see Table 1).

The syndrome of TGA was first described in 1956 by Bender (1), who referred to it as "syndrome of isolated confusion with amnesia"; in 1958 it was further elaborated by Fisher and Adams (2), who coined the term "TGA." The syndrome consists of sudden onset of profound anterograde and variable retrograde memory loss, associated with a clear sensorium and relatively normal behavior. The patient is able to converse and perform complex acts, but he may appear to be bewildered. He repeatedly asks questions which belie confusion, such as: "Where am I?

TABLE 1. *Typical characteristics of transient global amnesia*

Over age 50
Sudden onset
Anterograde memory loss
Variable retrograde memory loss
Intact immediate recall
Alert with temporal disorientation
Repeated questioning
Preserved self-identity
Duration of up to 24 hr
Full recovery
Low recurrence rate

What day is it? What is happening?" There is no loss of personal identity, and memory for remote events is relatively intact. There is no sign of associated clinical seizure activity such as automatisms. The event is prolonged, lasting up to 24 hr, average of 7–8 hr (3). The following day the patient is entirely normal and has no recollection of events during the episode. Often the episode is isolated and does not recur. However, with more widespread recognition of the syndrome, patients with repeated episodes have been described (4–6).

What is the anatomical substrate for TGA, and how might this relate to the basis of ictal amnesia? Lesions in a number of anatomical areas have been found to produce memory loss (see Table 2).

The mamillary bodies were implicated in Korsakoff's syndrome by Remy (7) in 1942. Later, Victor et al. (8) found evidence of lesions in the dorsal medial nucleus of the thalamus in patients with profound memory loss, some of whom had normal mamillary bodies. The important report of Scoville and Milner (9) in 1957 demonstrated that bilateral mesial temporal lobe lesions involving the hippocampus produced profound memory loss. Later, Mishkin (10) demonstrated in primates that lesions in the amygdala or hippocampus alone were not sufficient to produce amnesia, whereas lesions in both structures did result in memory loss. The picture was further elaborated when Warrington and Weiskrantz (11) put forth the double lesion-disconnection hypothesis, stating that involvement of two systems connecting temporal neocortex and mesial–basal frontal lobe were required for development of amnesia.

Although the preponderance of evidence implicates bilateral involvement in the development of amnesia, there have been reports of long-lasting memory loss associated with unilateral infarction of anteromedial thalamus or the mesial–temporal region of the dominant hemisphere (12).

In TGA, dysfunction of the mesial–basal regions of both temporal lobes and/or diencephalon is presumed, leaving neocortex intact. It is postulated that this is due to vascular insufficiency in the distribution of the posterior cerebral arteries (13), but the exact mechanism is not known. At least one patient has been reported, during positron emission tomography (PET), to show hypometabolism of one mesial–temporal lobe during an attack of TGA, with resolution 1 day after clinical recovery (14). Many studies have pointed out the high incidence of risk factors for cerebrovascular disease in patients with TGA (15–18). On the other hand, a subgroup of patients have had well-documented migraine (19–21). "Spreading oligemia" has been observed in classical migraine (22), and spreading depres-

TABLE 2. *Anatomic basis of amnesia*

Investigators	Comments
Remy (7)	Mamillary bodies in Korsakoff's syndrome.
Scoville and Milner (9)	Bilateral mesial–temporal lesions involving hippocampus.
Victor et al. (8)	Dorsal medial nucleus (DM) of thalamus. Five patients had mamillary body lesions without amnesia.
Squire and Moore (55)	Patient N.A.: computed tomographic evidence of damage only to DM.
Baleydier and Mauquiere (56)	Cingulate gyrus: transient amnesia.
Horel (57)	Temporal stem (connects amygdala and temporal cortex to brainstem and DM); lesions of temporal stem do not cause amnesia in rats.
Mishkin (10)	Amygdala *and* hippocampus. In primates, lesions in either structure alone are not sufficient for amnesia.

sion of Leao, thought to be its cause, has been hypothesized to cause TGA as well (23). Caplan (3) speculated that "acute arterial dyscontrol" in the territory of the posterior circulation may be the mechanism underlying most cases of TGA.

A syndrome of "Traveler's amnesia" was described in three neuroscientists who took triazolam together with alcohol in an attempt to minimize jet lag (24). The picture was similar to TGA but without bewilderment or unusual behavior. Diazepam (25) and lorazepam (26) have been implicated in other reports.

Some confusion arose from the finding of rapid inferomesial–temporal spikes during nasopharyngeal recording in some patients, but these have been found in 38% of normal individuals; this is referred to as "benign epileptiform transients of sleep" (BETS) (27). In the vast majority of cases there is no EEG abnormality. Cole et al. (28) recently and serendipitously recorded the EEG at the onset of an episode of TGA; it was normal.

Among the characteristics of TGA that would be unusual for an epileptic event is its duration. With the exception of status epilepticus, seizures are relatively brief. Furthermore, seizures are usually recurrent and are associated with an epileptiform EEG. On the other hand, seizures involving both cerebral hemispheres usually result in depression of the sensorium to a variable extent. Epileptiform activity localized to both hippocampal regions would be expected to disrupt normal function and result in memory loss similar to that seen on a vascular basis. This could happen by propagation from one temporal lobe to the other but would imply that the areas involved in the epileptic process remain quite localized and do not involve the limbic system more widely, contrary to what occurs in the case of usual complex partial seizures.

A review of the literature reveals that reports of ictal amnesia are infrequent, although there appears to be increased interest in recent years. The concept of ictal amnesia, however, is not new. The writings of John Hughlings Jackson are a treasure of prescience and elegant description in clinical epilepsy, and in 1888 he described an apparent case of ictal amnesia (29). The patient, whom he called "Z," was of unusual interest in that he was a practicing physician who suffered from grand mal and petit mal seizures and was

able to describe his symptoms with clarity and apparent insight. Jackson's (29) report, *On a Particular Variety of Epilepsy (Intellectual Aura); One Case with Symptoms of Organic Brain Disease,* contains detailed descriptions of Z's seizures, in the patient's own words. One of these seems particularly apt, conceded by Jackson to be "a very important case":

I was attending a young patient whom his mother had brought me with some history of lung symptoms. I wished to examine the chest, and asked him to undress on a couch. I thought he looked ill, but have no recollection of any intention to recommend him to take to his bed at once, or of any diagnosis. Whilst he was undressing I felt the onset of a *petit mal.* I remember taking out my stethoscope and turning away to avoid conversation. The next thing I recollect is that I was sitting at a writing-table in the same room, speaking to another person, and as my consciousness became more complete, recollected my patient, but saw he was not in the room. I was interested to ascertain what had happened, and had an opportunity an hour later of seeing him in bed, with the note of a diagnosis I had made of "pneumonia at the left base." I gathered indirectly from conversation that I had made a physical examination, written these words, and advised him to take to bed at once. I re-examined him with some curiosity, and found that my conscious diagnosis was the same as my unconscious—or perhaps I should say, unremembered—diagnosis had been. I was a good deal surprised, but not so unpleasantly as I should have thought probable.

Z died in 1894 of an overdose of chloral: at necropsy, Dr. Walter Coleman found in the left uncinate gyrus a very small cavity due to softening. Jackson and Coleman (30) described the autopsy findings in their report in *Brain* in 1898, and they also reported additional illuminating clinical details of Z's seizures. Jackson related that, when he first saw Z, he obtained a history of automatisms characterized by "modified and indistinct smacking of the tongue like a tasting movement," generally accompained by a motion of the lower jaw. Later, a "highly accomplished medical man" who had seen many of Z's attacks related that he had never noticed any such movements. "They were very slight

. . . . The noise made was only just audible." Years after Z's first visit, Jackson witnessed two of these seizures. In one, Z stopped talking, "remained standing, and made slight, very slight, just audible smacking movements of his lips." On another occasion, he stopped talking and his head bent forward. After a few seconds, he leaned over and felt about on the floor as if searching for something. Jackson later accompanied Z to his house; Z looked confused and seemed strange but, after a few minutes, appeared to be fully recovered and conversed reasonably and appropriately. The next day he recalled nothing from the time of being in Jackson's office until Jackson left him. "These post-paroxysmal actions during what we clinically call unconsciousness were as elaborate and purposive-seeming, as any of those of his normal self," Jackson relates. He also describes the notes that Z had taken with respect to the patient with pneumonia. These notes were, in fact, jumbled and confused. Thus, Z's high level of functioning during an apparent seizure turned out, after more complete information was available, to be confused and fragmented. Based on Jackson's 1898 account, it appears that Z suffered from very brief, subtle complex partial attacks, followed by a more prolonged confusional state with subsequent amnesia. After the seizure described above, the postictal confusional state merged into a phase with apparently clear sensorium for which the patient had no recall. We are again reminded of the importance of detailed observation, which remains the foundation of diagnosis in epilepsy.

Bearing in mind the tale of Z, we searched the literature for reports of seizures characterized mainly by memory loss in the absence of other cognitive deficits or a preceding clinical ictus. We were able to find eight reports on 24 patients since 1973 in which episodes of amnesia were felt by the investigators to be related to seizures (see Table 3).

Initially, cases of amnesia on an epileptic basis were included in more general discus-

TABLE 3. *Ictal amnesia*[a]

Investigators	Age/sex	Duration	Associated symptoms	EEG	Response to AEDs	Past history
Galassi et al. (39)	67 M	10–60 min	Brief LOC; automatisms	(R) T theta	"Effective"	
	70 F	10–60 min	Brief LOC; automatisms	(R) T parox theta	"Effective"	
	66 M	10–60 min	Brief LOC; automatisms	(L) T theta	"Effective"	
Miller et al. (36)	62 M	15–30 min	None	Bi-T spikes	PHT—no attacks	
	One additional patient without description					
Meador et al. (35)	47 F	15 min	Micropsia	Bi-T epileptiform	PHT—no attacks	Meningioma
Pritchard et al. (38)	65 M	10–15 min	None	Bi-T spikes	PHT—no attacks	
	64 M	60 min	None	Bi-T spikes	CBZ—one recurrence with low level	24-hr attack of amnesia
Deisenhammer (34)	11 F	10 min	None	(R) T spikes	CBZ—no attacks	
Dugan et al. (33)	82 M	3 hr	None	Bi-T spikes (? BETS)	PHT—no attacks	Bradycardia pacemaker
Gilbert (32)	67 F	4 hr	None	Bi-T spikes (? BETS)	PHT—no attacks	
Croft et al. (31)	58 F	5 hr	Difficulty dressing	Bi-T sharp	PHT—no attacks	CPS
	Six additional patients, ages 18–61, without description					
		(min to 5 hr)			all responded to AEDs	CPS and gen sz

[a]LOC, loss of consciousness; T, temporal; BETS, benign epileptiform transients of sleep; AEDs, antiepileptic drugs; PHT, phenytoin; CBZ, carbamazepine; CPS, complex partial seizures; gen sz, generalized seizures

sions of amnesia—in particular, TGA. For example, Croft et al. (31) noted that 7 of 39 patients referred for evaluation of transient amnesia were diagnosed as having an ictal basis for their symptoms (see Table 4). They based their decision on a history of (a) recognized clinical seizures in all seven (five with temporal lobe and two with idiopathic epilepsy) and (b) epileptiform EEGs in five. The investigators commented that the attacks were indistinguishable from TGA. Only one patient was described in detail. She had two amnestic attacks with repeated questioning, lasting 5 hr each, one of which was associated with inability to dress herself. The interictal EEG showed paroxysmal sharp waves and theta activity in the temporal leads. This patient also experienced episodes described as seizures in which there was sudden loss of consciousness preceded by a clutching feeling in the throat; she slumped forward and became pale, but she did not convulse. Based on the available data, a clear-cut diagnosis cannot be made in this case. The duration of the amnestic attacks and repeated questioning are consistent with TGA. The inability to dress herself, however, implies a depressed functional level which is not characteristic of TGA but which could be associated with an ictal or postictal confusional state. On the other hand, the EEG findings are not specific for epilepsy, and the episodes of loss of consciousness are more suggestive of syncope than of epilepsy.

The report by Gilbert (32) described a 67-year-old woman with a typical picture of TGA lasting some 9 hr. A diagnosis of a temporal lobe seizure was based on a sleep EEG with nasopharyngeal leads which showed independent bitemporal spike-and-wave complexes. The illustrated discharges, however, bear a close resemblance to BETS. It therefore seems likely that this patient suffered from an attack of TGA and not ictal amnesia.

Dugan et al. (33) presented a patient with a

TABLE 4. *Causes of transient loss of memory in 39 patients*

Transient global amnesia	24
Epilepsy	7
Migraine	2
Temporal lobe encephalitis	2
Psychogenic	4

[a]From ref. 31, with permission.

TGA picture with associated bradycardia. The episode lasted 3 hr, but the following day he again was found to be confused with memory difficulties. An EEG during this period demonstrated bilateral temporal spikes, possibly resembling BETS. After implantation of a cardiac pacemaker the patient remained asymptomatic for 2 months, but again he presented with symptoms of TGA. Treatment with phenytoin was begun, and the patient remained symptom-free for 8 months. Repeat EEG was normal. In view of the typical TGA symptoms and duration, and the absence of an ictal EEG during the event, the likely diagnosis in this 82-year-old man is TGA.

An 11-year-old girl who awakened with memory loss was reported by Deisenhammer (34). Her sensorium was clear, but she asked repeated questions. This episode lasted 10 min and was followed 4 and 5 weeks later by similar attacks, some occurring in the afternoon. Two hours after one of her attacks, an EEG showed high-voltage right temporal spike discharges. No further attacks occurred after treatment with carbamazepine, and an epileptic etiology was assumed. In this case the duration, attack repetition, and the EEG findings support a diagnosis of epilepsy-related amnesia. Whether the attacks were ictal or followed a subtle or unobserved seizure cannot be ascertained with certainty, but this case would seem to fit our definition of ictal amnesia.

The case reported by Meador et al. (35) sparked controversy, in part because of the title of their report: *Transient Global Amnesia and Meningioma*. Their study involved a 47-year-old woman with two brief episodes of memory loss—one self-reported and one observed. The first episode occurred on a shopping trip during which she purchased, without memory, all items on her list. It ended with return of memory registration and a feeling that she was looking through the wrong end of a telescope. The second episode consisted of a brief, spotty anterograde with circumscribed retrograde amnesia lasting several weeks. She also had reported recurrent brief episodes of simple loss of awareness for the previous 10 months. EEG showed independent bitemporal spike discharges, and a computed tomography (CT) scan of the head revealed a calcified right posterior temporal mass which proved to be a meningioma. It seems likely that these episodes were related to seizure activity. The issue of intraictal versus postictal deficit is quite interesting. If we accept micropsia as a seizure manifestation, did this patient's seizure occur after her shopping expedition, leaving in its wake a postictal retrograde amnesia?

In Miller et al.'s (36) report of 277 patients with 347 attacks of TGA, a seizure disorder was noted in eight (2.9%), two of whom were felt to have amnesic seizures. One patient was described in detail (37); he was a 62-year-old man with repeated amnestic episodes, some immediately following awakening. Attack duration was less than 30 min, and no spells typical of complex partial seizures were described. He became free of attacks after treatment with phenytoin and remained so for at least 5 years. His sleep EEG showed bilateral independent temporal spikes and sharp waves. This appears to be a case of ictal amnesia. Again, in the absence of intensive video–EEG monitoring, one cannot establish the attacks as being intraictal or postictal.

Pritchard et al. (38) described two patients with recurrent attacks of anterograde amnesia who were responsive to antiepileptic drugs. One man with rheumatic heart disease and chronic atrial fibrillation had experienced 10 "memory spells" in 4 years, one of which was described vividly: "He asked his wife to cook his favorite food, a meat and cheese tart. He devoured the food with relish and seemed normal during the meal. Fifteen minutes later, he asked his wife when she planned to serve dinner and was perplexed to learn that she had already done so." His EEG showed independent temporal spike discharges, and he became free of attacks after treatment with phenytoin. This patient's attacks qualify as ictal amnesia and, based on available data, may well have been intraictal. Pritchard's second case had a history of 24 hr of amnesia during which he worked a full day on a construction project without event. Six months later, a mealtime amnestic episode lasting 1 hr occurred. This patient's symptoms are possibly epilepsy-related, although their low frequency and the long duration of the first episode raise some doubt as to the nature of his attacks.

Recently, Gallassi et al. (39) reported on six patients with severe adult-onset memory deficit, subsequently diagnosed as complex partial epilepsy. Three had acute amnestic episodes characterized by transient antero- and retrograde amnesia which were diagnosed elsewhere as TGA. The memory disturbance followed brief losses of contact and automatisms in all three. The investigators commented on the subtle nature of the initial seizure activity and the subsequent prominence of the memory disturbance, but these clearly postictal episodes do meet our criteria for ictal amnesia. The patients also complained of interictal memory problems. Treatment with antiepileptic drugs improved both frequency of attacks and interictal memory, thus giving rise to consideration of the role of interictal epileptiform discharges in ongoing memory complaints (40,41).

To summarize, our review of these 18 cases indicates that sufficient data are available for a presumptive diagnosis in 10 (see Table 5). Of these, seven seem likely to be epilepsy-related, but only four are cases of ictal amnesia as defined earlier. In the absence of simultaneous EEG and behavioral recording, the question of whether or not such episodes can occur without a preceding subtle or subclinical seizure cannot be answered.

Although nonconvulsive status epilepticus (both absence and complex partial) usually has a clinical picture quite different from that we have discussed, the literature on the subject contains some intriguing indications that isolated memory disturbance can occur as either an ictal or postictal phenomenon. Many reports refer to a state of "epileptic fugue," but these patients are often in a "twilight state" with a greater or lesser degree of obtundation and amnesia. For example, patients with absence status may have a spectrum of impairment ranging from a subjective sensa-

TABLE 5. *Eighteen cases reported to be epileptic amnestic attacks*[a]

Transient global amnesia	3
Seizure-related amnesia	3
Ictal amnesia	4
Unclassifiable	1
Insufficient data	7
	18

[a]Probable diagnoses based on stated criteria (see text).

tion without amnesia to deep stupor. Similarly, variable degrees of amnesia are described, ranging from minimal or none to complete. Andermann and Robb (42) state that in their experience with absence status the degree of amnesia may correlate with the degree of confusion and stupor, but that in some of the attacks in which amnesia was profound, the patients were able to carry out relatively complicated activities. They describe a child who, with his family, went on a day tour while on vacation. The following day there was no recall of this outing. It is notable that his family described him as having seemed "very slow and vague." Thus, it is uncertain whether amnesia with clear sensorium occurs in absence status.

Two reports of complex partial status epilepticus are of great interest with respect to amnesia. Engle et al. (43) described an 18-year-old female with several 2-week episodes of complex partial status, characterized electrically by independently cycling bilateral temporo-occipital seizure activity. The level of consciousness fluctuated in relation to the bilaterality of discharges. At her best, when there was bilateral slowing, she was oriented to person and place and was also able to give her address and telephone number, spell, name, follow simple commands, and do simple arithmetic. Memory function at these times is not described. On two occasions, following treatment and resolution of status, she was alert and fluent with temporal disorientation and amnesia for the previous several weeks. There was severe impairment of ability to recall new information. The amnesia for the period of hospitalization remained fixed, but the short-term memory deficit resolved in a matter of weeks. This case illustrates that prolonged, reversible anterograde amnesia can be a sequel of complex partial status.

The report by Wieser (44) indicates that brief bilateral electrical discharge in the hippocampi can produce a rapidly reversible amnestic syndrome. A 22-year-old female with status epilepticus consisting of a variety of subtle and experiential seizures, as well as more typical complex partial seizures, was studied with stereo-EEG. Whenever consciousness was clouded or severe memory deficit was present (it is not clear that they ever occurred separately), there was bilateral hippocampal involvement. Most interesting was the observation that short-lasting amnesia could be experimentally induced. During long-lasting spontaneous right hippocampal discharge, electrically induced afterdischarges in the left hippocampus led to inability to recall the name of the technician and physician. When the left hippocampal discharge ceased, recall returned immediately.

A similar case involving spontaneous seizures was reported by Morrell (45), and a patient with subclinical seizures restricted to the left hippocampus was shown to have ictal deficits of short-term recall in a recent report by Bridgman et al. (46). This last case may be relevant to the frequent complaints of poor memory by patients with epilepsy, since subclinical seizures or even interictal spikes may impair memory (40,41).

This experimental evidence adds to an understanding of epilepsy-related amnesia. The memory loss may be postictal or ictal, implicating one or, more likely, both temporal lobes. We suspect that most cases of epilepsy-related amnesia are postictal in origin. Clinical observational data are, out of necessity, incomplete; subtle seizures may not be appreciated, whereas the memory loss is obvious and dramatic. If a brief seizure occurs before awakening, it is even less likely to be apparent, and the patient awakens with anterograde memory loss as the only observed manifestation.

In the differential diagnosis of episodic amnestic states, the so-called nonorganic amnesias should be considered. These fall into two broad categories: psychogenic fugue and psychogenic amnesia. Psychogenic fugue is a state of memory loss which is characterized by abrupt onset and loss of personal identity. A new identity may be assumed. According to the rigid criteria of DSM-III-R, the diagnosis cannot be made, unless there is wandering or travel (47). The episode resolves in hours to days, but there is residual anterograde loss of memory for the entire event. Paradoxically, during the fugue there is total retrograde amnesia (including loss of personal identity) without anterograde amnesia. In his admirable monograph, Janet (48) captures the essence of fugue states:

As Charcot has said, "What is most wonderful in fugues is that these individuals contrive not to be stopped by the police at the very beginning of their journey." In fact they are mad people in full delirium; nevertheless, they take railway tickets, they dine and sleep in hotels, they speak to a great number of people. We are, it is true, sometimes told they were thought a little odd, that they looked preoccupied and dreamy, but after all, they are not recognized as mad people.

Stress as a precipitant is always present, and fugue states are said to be more common in times of calamity such as war and natural disaster. Alcohol often plays a role, and such patients are nearly always depressed. Flight from suicide is thought to often underlie such episodes. In 40% there is a past history of organic amnesia (due, for example, to alcohol, trauma, or epilepsy) (49). Complicating the diagnosis is the fact that some patients are found to be malingerers.

Psychogenic amnesia, on the other hand, usually involves a circumscribed retrograde amnesia, unlike the generalized loss of memory seen in fugue (46,49). Less often, psychogenic amnesia is "continuous" and characterized by an ongoing deficit of short-term memory analogous to Korsakoff's syndrome. There is no travel or new identity. The state may be patchy or complete, usually precipitated by a profoundly disturbing or violent event, and ends abruptly, usually with complete resolution. Included in this diagnosis is "amnesia for offending" (49). Between 25% and 65% of homicides (less for other types of violent crime) are associated with amnesia surrounding the event, and in 60% of these there is amnesia only for the crime itself (50). Nearly always the memory loss is patchy or hazy, and there is no recovery during the period of psychiatric evaluation. The Minnesota Multiphasic Personality Inventory (MMPI) often shows high scores on depression, hysteria, and hypochondriasis scales. The victim usually is a close friend or relative, and a state of high arousal is often present. Alcohol abuse is also a factor. Again, psychogenic amnesia cannot reliably be distinguished from malingering.

Common features in psychogenic amnestic states include abnormal mood, extreme arousal, an unpleasant event, and alcohol. Among the hypothetical mechanisms, faulty encoding offers a plausible explanation (48). Thus, a state of extreme arousal would be expected to interfere with memory registration, as would alcohol or an intense traumatic event. Some investigators, on the other hand, feel that the amnesia represents repression of undesirable memories (51,52) which may be retrievable via hypnosis (53) or an amytal interview (54).

The differentiation between organic and nonorganic amnesia is based mainly on the following considerations. Loss of personal identity with a clear sensorium, as in fugue, does not occur in organic amnestic states. Furthermore, the anterograde amnesia of organic states does not resolve, in contrast to the spontaneous, hypnotic, or amytal restitution of memory in psychogenic syndromes. It is important to note that patients with continuous psychogenic amnesia show impaired immediate recall, whereas immediate recall is preserved in organic states. Bewilderment is not present, and there is no significant retrograde amnesia.

If ictal amnesia is indeed rare, and certainly it is rarely reported, why is this so? Its vascular analogue, TGA, is relatively common. Although there are suggestions that unilateral temporal–diencephalic dysfunction may result in memory loss without a general depression of sensorium, bilateral involvement is implicated in most cases. The answer may lie in the pathophysiology of vascular versus epileptic events. It is presumed that only the deep temporal–diencephalic structures become dysfunctional in TGA, implying a highly

TABLE 6. *Epilepsy-related amnesia: proposed criteria for diagnosis[a]*

Major criteria
1. Epileptic seizure (may be brief or subtle) immediately precedes or follows episode of amnesia.
2. Duration less than 60 min.
3. Repeated events.

Associated criteria
4. Epileptiform EEG.
5. Absence of bewilderment and repeated questioning.
6. Past history of epileptic seizures.
7. Clear response to antiepileptic drugs.

[a]Criterion 1 alone is sufficient for diagnosis, or criteria 2 and 3 *plus* one associated criterion.

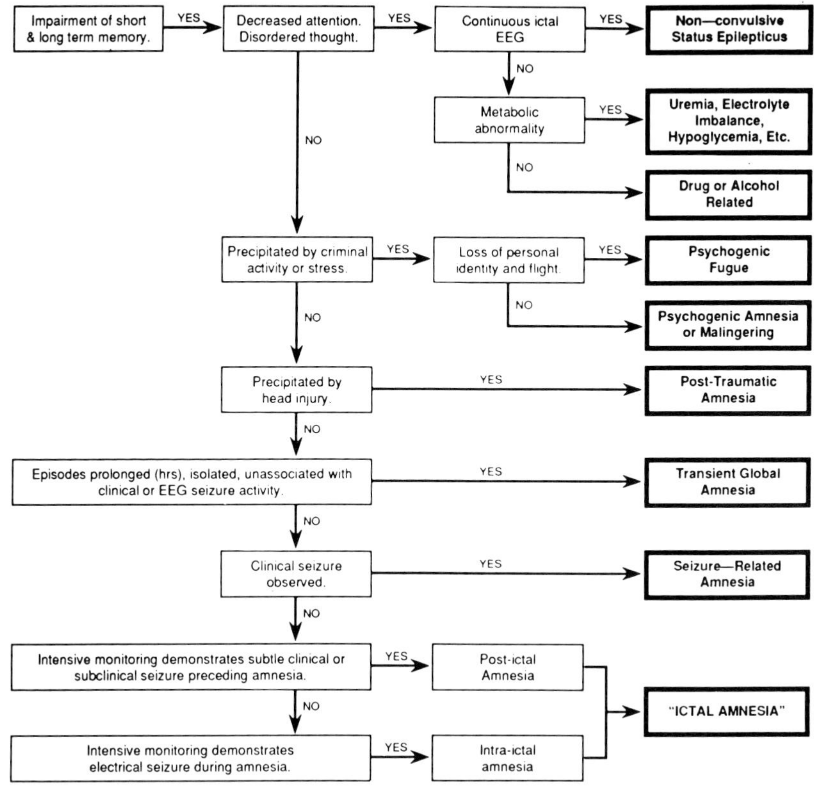

FIG. 1. Algorithm showing the differential diagnosis of episodic amnesia.

localized vascular insufficiency involving small vessels. In the case of an epileptic event, such fine localization would seem less likely. Synaptic pathways are activated by the seizure discharge which leads to more widespread involvement of nervous structures. When the seizure discharge originates in the amygdala–hippocampal complex, subsequent spread throughout the limbic system usually produces a variety of symptoms, including changes in sensorium. Thus, a seizure producing only memory loss would, out of necessity, produce either (a) limited synaptic activation or (b) inhibition which prevents spread of the discharge. Inasmuch as bilateral dysfunction is usually required for interruption of memory, ictal amnesia would result from a localized spread of the discharge to the opposite hemisphere, or from a unilateral discharge in the context of an anatomical or physiological abnormality on the opposite side. These circumstances would be expected to occur infrequently, thus providing a theoretical explanation for the rarity of ictal amnesia.

As a clinical aid, we propose major and minor criteria for the diagnosis of epilepsy-related amnesia, as listed in Table 6.

The differential diagnosis of episodic amnesia is conveniently represented by the algorithm shown in Fig. 1. Note that we use the term "ictal amnesia" to represent both post-ictal and intraictal amnesia.

REFERENCES

1. Bender MB. Syndrome of isolated episode of confusion with amnesia. *J Hillside Hosp* 1956;5:12–15.
2. Fisher CM, Adams RD. Transient global amnesia. *Trans Am Neurol Assoc* 1958;83:143–146.
3. Caplan LR. Transient global amnesia. In: Vinken P, Bruyn G, Klawans H, eds. *Handbook of clinical neurology.* Amsterdam: Elsevier, 1985; 205–218.
4. Heathfield KWG, Croft PB, Swash M. The

syndrome of transient global amnesia. *Brain* 1973;96:729–736.

5. Lou H. Repeated episodes of transient global amnesia. *Acta Neurol Scand* 1968;44:612–618.

6. Steinmetz EF, Vroom FQ. Transient global amnesia. *Neurology (Minneap)* 1972;22:1193–1200.

7. Remy M. Contribution a l'etude de la maladie de Korsakov. *Monatsschr Psychiatr Neurol* 1942;106:126–144.

8. Victor M, Adams RD, Collins GH. *The Wernicke–Korsakoff Syndrome.* Philadelphia: FA Davis, 1971.

9. Scoville WB, Milner B. Loss of recent memory after bilateral hippocampal lesions. *J Neurol Neurosurg Psychiatry* 1957;20:11–21.

10. Mishkin M. Memory in monkeys is severely impaired by combined but not by separate removal of amygdala and hippocampus. *Nature* 1978;273:297–298.

11. Warrington EK, Weiskranz L. Amnesia: a disconnection syndrome? *Neuropsychologia* 1982;20:233–248.

12. Akiguchi I, Ino T, Nabatame H, Udaka F, Matsubayashi K, Fukuyama H, Kameyama M. Acute onset amnestic syndrome with localized infarct on the dominant side—comparison between antero-medial thalamic lesion and posterior cerebral artery territory lesion. *Jpn J Med* 1987;26:15–20.

13. Benson DF, Marsden DC, Meadows JC. The amnesic syndrome of posterior temporal artery occlusion. *Acta Neurol Scand* 1974;50:133–145.

14. Volpe BT, Herscovitch P, Raichle ME, Hirst W, Gazzaniga MS. Cerebral blood flow and metabolism in human amnesia. *J Cereb Blood Flow Metab* 1983;3(Suppl 1):55–56.

15. Jensen TS, Olivarius BDF. Transient global amnesia as a manifestation of transient cerebral ischemia. *Acta Neurol Scand* 1980;61:115–124.

16. Jensen TS, Olivarius BDF. Transient global amnesia—its clinical and pathophysiologic basis and prognosis. *Acta Neurol Scand* 1981;63:220–230.

17. Matthew MT, Meyer JS. Pathogenesis and natural history of transient global amnesia. *Stroke* 1974;5:303–311.

18. Pexman JHW, Coates RK. Amnesia after femocerebral angiography. *AJNR* 1983;4:979–983.

19. Caplan LR, Chedru F, Lhermitte F, Mayman C. Transient global amnesia and migraine. *Neurology* 1981;31:1167–1170.

20. Crowell FG, Strump DA, Biller J, McHenry LC, Toole JF. The transient global amnesia–migraine connection. *Arch Neurol* 1984;4:75–79.

21. Dupuis MJM, Pierre PH, Gonsetti RE. Transient global amnesia and migraine in twin sisters. *J Neurol Neurosurg Psychiatry* 1987;50:816–824.

22. Olesen J, Larsen B, Lauritzen M. Focal hyperemia followed by spreading oligemia and impaired activation of rCBF in classic migraine. *Ann Neurol* 1981;9:344–352.

23. Olesen J, Jorgensen MB. Leao's spreading depression in the hippocampus explains transient global amnesia: a hypothesis. *Acta Neurol Scand* 1986;73:219–220.

24. Morris HH, Estes ML. Traveler's amnesia: transient global amnesia secondary to triazolam. *JAMA* 1987;258:945–946.

25. Gilbert JJ, Benson DF. Transient global amnesia. Report of two cases with definite etiologies. *J Nerv Ment Dis* 1972;154:461–464.

26. Sandyk R. Transient global amnesia induced by lorazepam. *Clin Neuropharmacol* 1985;8:297–298.

27. White JC, Langston JW, Pedley TA. Benign epileptiform transients of sleep. *Neurology* 1977;27:1061–1068.

28. Cole AJ, Gloor P, Kaplan R. Transient global amnesia: the electroencephalogram at onset. *Ann Neurol* 1987;22:771–772.

29. Jackson, JH. On a particular variety of epilepsy (intellectual aura); one case with symptoms of organic brain disease. *Brain* 1888;11:200–207.

30. Jackson JH, Coleman WS. Case of epilepsy with tasting movements and "dreamy state"—very small patch of softening in the left uncinate gyrus. *Brain* 1898;21:580–590.

31. Croft PB, Heathfield KWG, Swash M. Differential diagnosis of transient amnesia. *Br Med J* 1973;4:593–596.

32. Gilbert GJ. Transient global amnesia: manifestation of medial temporal lobe epilepsy. *Clin Electroencephalogr* 1978;9:147–152.

33. Dugan TM, Nordgren RE, O'Leary P. Transient global amnesia associated with bradycardia and temporal lobe spikes. *Cortex* 1981;17:633–638.

34. Deisenhammer E. Transient global amnesia as an epileptic manifestation. *J Neurol* 1981;225:289–292.

35. Meador KJ, Adams RJ, Flanigen HF. Transient global amnesia and meningioma. *Neurology* 1985;35:769–771.

36. Miller JW, Petersen RC, Metter EJ, Millikan CH, Yanagihara T. Transient global amnesia: clinical characteristics and prognosis. *Neurology* 1987;37:733–737.

37. Miller JW, Yanagihara T, Petersen RC, Klass DW. TGA and epilepsy: electroencephalographic distinction. *Arch Neurol* 1987;44:629–633.

38. Pritchard PB, Holmstrom VL, Roitzsch JC, Giacinto J. Epileptic amnesia attacks: benefit from antiepileptic drugs. *Neurology* 1985;35:1188–1189.

39. Gallassi R, Morreale A, Lorusso S, Pazzaglia P, Lugaresi E. Epilepsy presenting as memory disturbances. *Epilepsia* 1988;29:624–629.

40. Aarts JHP, Binnie CD, Smit AM, Wilkins AJ. Selective cognitive impairment during focal and generalized epileptiform EEG activity. *Brain* 1984;107:292–308.

41. Rausch R, Lieb JP, Crandall PH. Neuropsychological correlates of depth spike activity in epileptic patients. *Arch Neurol* 1978;35:699–705.

42. Andermann F, Robb JP. Absence status: a reappraisal following review of thirty-eight patients. *Epilepsia* 1972;13:177–187.

43. Engle J Jr, Ludwig BI, Fetell M. Prolonged complex partial status epilepticus: EEG and behavioral observations. *Neurology* 1978;28:863–869.

44. Wieser HG. Temporal lobe or psychomotor sta-

tus epilepticus. A case report. *Electroencephalogr Clin Neurophysiol* 48:558–572.

45. Morrell F. Memory loss as a Todd's paralysis. *Epilepsia* 1980;21:185.

46. Bridgman PA, Malamut BL, Sperling MR, Saykin AJ, O'Connor MJ. Memory during subclinical hippocampal seizures. *Neurology* 1989;39: 853–856.

47. American Psychiatric Association. *Diagnostic and statistical manual of mental disorders*, 3rd ed. (revised). Washington, DC: American Psychiatric Association, 1987.

48. Janet P. *The major symptoms of hysteria*. New York: Hafner, 1920;60.

49. Kopelman MD. Amnesia: organic and psychogenic. *Br J Psychiatry* 1987;150:428–442.

50. Schacter DL. Amnesia and crime. How much do we really know? *Am Psychologist* 1986;41:286–295.

51. Freud S. *Introductory lectures*. Harmondsworth: Penguin, 1915–1917.

52. Master D, Lishman WA, Smith A. Speed of recall in relation to affective tone and intensity of experience. *Psychol Med* 1983;13:325–331.

53. MacHovec FJ. Hypnosis to facilitate recall in psychogenic amnesia and fugue states: treatment variables. *Am J Clin Hypn* 1981;24:7–13.

54. Ruedrich SL, Chu CC, Wadle CV. The amytal interview in the treatment of psychogenic amnesia. *Hosp Community Psychiatry* 1985;10: 1045–1046.

55. Squire and Moore (1979)

56. Baleydier and Mauquiere (1980)

57. Horel (1978)

Advances in Neurology, Vol. 55, edited by
D. Smith, D. Treiman, and M. Trimble,
Raven Press, Ltd., New York © 1991.

23

Memory Function in Patients with Epilepsy

Pamela J. Thompson

*National Society for Epilepsy, Chalfont Centre for Epilepsy, Buckinghamshire SL9 ORJ,
England; and Institute of Neurology, Queen Square, London WC1 3BG, England*

The observation of interictal memory problems in patients with epilepsy has a long history. In the 19th century, Russell Reynolds (1) stated that "the commonest failure is loss of memory and that this, if regarded in all degrees, is more frequent than the integrity of that faculty." In 1942, when describing the nature of the memory deficits in epilepsy, Lennox (2) wrote "the patient finds it hard to recall events and names, especially those learned recently." In 1988, Loiseau et al. (3) commented that ". . . memory deficits in epileptic patients merit special attention since they seek help for these more frequently than for other mental impairments."

Self-reports of patients clearly indicate that memory problems can be a major concern that can have a significant impact on many aspects of their lives, including social functioning. One patient wrote the following about his memory: ". . . it is currently becoming quite alarming. To such an extent it is threatening my ability to continue this kind of work. Much can be done to hide the memory problems, but the difficulty of remembering names is so embarrassing and it makes socializing even more difficult." Another individual wrote of her memory: ". . . events that happen involving me which stick out in other peoples minds I have no recollection of at all much to the surprise of friends because that particular event could only have been a year ago . . . . I used to have a good memory before I developed epilepsy at the age of 14 years."

Psychometric assessment of cognitive abilities gained momentum, particularly in the latter half of the 20th century. Despite the importance of memory functioning, it is surprising that it was inadequately covered by many of the widely used test batteries such as the Wechsler Intelligence Scales and the Halstead–Reitan Battery. Research evidence, however, has accumulated which gives some support to the clinical impressions of memory disturbance in patients with epilepsy. Individuals have been reported to perform significantly less well on various memory tests than do controls without epilepsy (4–6). Some investigators, however, have found no significant differences between epilepsy patients and controls, although trends have been in the predicted direction (7–9). More support exists that the subgroups of patients who have problems with seizures originating in the temporal lobes are seemingly at greatest risk. Support that patients with temporal lobe seizures show impairments on tests of learning and memory, when compared to individuals with other types of epilepsy and control groups, come from a number of studies (10–18). However, there are investigators who have attempted to make comparisons between temporal lobe groups and other seizure types but who have reported no significant differences on the performance of memory tests (2,5–7,19,20). Inconsistent findings seem to arise when patients studied have less severe seizure disorders.

Within the group of patients with temporal lobe epilepsy, some comparisons have been made comparing those individuals with left temporal lobe foci with individuals with right temporal lobe foci. Several researchers have reported that patients with left-sided foci do less well on verbal memory tests than do those with right-sided foci, and that those with right-sided foci do less well on nonverbal memory tests than do those with left-sided foci (21–24). Other investigators have reported impairments on some tests of verbal learning and memory with left temporal lobe seizure disorders, but they have either not assessed or failed to find the converse effect with seizures originating in the right hemisphere (14,25–27). However, there are investigators who have not been able to find evidence to support such laterality effects (2, 6,10,11,20,28).

CAUSES OF MEMORY DISTURBANCE

There are many reasons why people with epilepsy may be expected to have an increased incidence of memory difficulties.

Etiology

Epilepsy can arise from a wide range of brain pathology, including head traumas, central nervous system infections and poisoning, brain tumors, vascular disease, and chronic alcoholism, to name the more frequent causes (29). These conditions can give rise to memory disturbance in the absence of epilepsy. Memory impairments in patients with epilepsy stemming from these causes would seem largely attributable to underlying brain pathology rather than to epilepsy variables. Not surprisingly, existing evidence suggests that patients with known etiology do exhibit greater memory problems than do those for whom the cause of the epilepsy is unknown (4,5).

Seizures

Seizures themselves have also been implicated as underlying memory disturbance. Most attention has been devoted to the type of seizures, and, as discussed above, people with seizures of temporal lobe origin seem at risk for memory problems. This is not surprising, given the evidence of the importance of the temporal lobes for memory functioning

which has accumulated. It is generally accepted that bilateral temporal lobe discharges result in impairment of memory; however, when assessments involve individuals with unilateral temporal lobe disturbances, the findings as already discussed have not always been clear-cut. There are many reasons for this. The origin of seizure activity in the temporal lobes is not uniform among patients. We know from research that dysfunction in different parts of the temporal lobe can give rise to various types of memory disorders (30). Whether these are detected will depend on the nature of the memory tests employed. Until recently, the assessment of memory in epilepsy has been limited and unsophisticated (31). Samples selected for study are generally biased towards more severe cases. Indeed, it is only the intractable seizure cases that are adequately investigated by electroencephalography (EEG), videotelemetry, and depth recordings to provide usually unequivocable evidence of the laterality of the focus. However, these patients are by no means representative of people with temporal lobe epilepsy in general (32). A further problem arises in those studies comparing right- versus left-sided foci, since lateralization of language and memory functions have been reported to be atypical in a significant number of patients (33). Without evidence of the cerebral dominance of these functions following procedures such as the intracarotid sodium amytal test, interpretation of studies comparing right versus left foci is problematic.

Other seizure variables have been explored, including age of onset of the disorder and duration, although these are undoubtedly interrelated with etiology and other variables. In general, the combination of early age of onset and long duration has been associated with greater memory impairment in some studies (5,22,24). As in other areas, findings have not always been consistent, and one of the larger studies of memory functioning in epilepsy undertaken by Loiseau et al. (6) has indicated that age of onset during the adolescent years might place an individual at greater risk for learning and memory difficulties.

Frequency of seizures has also been implicated, with a higher frequency of seizures having a greater disruptive influence on memory (8); however, such a relationship has not always proved significant (6,7,24). As indicated by Dodrill (34), it may be the total lifetime number of seizures (rather than seizure frequency) which is the crucial variable.

The severity of the attack may also be an important factor, but this may vary between individuals who have the same type of epilepsy and may also vary between attacks in the same individuals. It is of interest that Brittain (5) included a variable called "ictal time," which was found to be related to memory test performance; seizures of long duration are associated with poorer performance on a recognition memory test. Seizures may also become severe when they result in secondary injuries. Indeed, in our recent investigations of mental deterioration, head injury as a consequence of seizures was found to be related to severe verbal memory deficits (Mader and Thompson, *unpublished data*). However, it must always be borne in mind that seizure frequency or severity may reflect the extent and nature of any underlying brain pathology.

Seizure frequency variables are very much interwoven with such factors, and for ethical reasons it is difficult to disentangle them in patients with epilepsy. Work with animals has addressed the issue of the influence of seizure variables on learning and memory, and existing evidence suggests that the number of seizures and the severity of the attacks (measured in terms of seizure duration) are associated with memory deficits (35,36). Unfortunately, although the animal work allows considerable control of variables, it is not without problems of interpretation, such as the relationship between memory tests used in animals and those used in humans. For instance, it is impossible to test for verbal memory in animals, yet this would seem to be the dominant memory criterion in humans. In animals there is also the added problem that the procedure used to produce the seizure disorder may itself be related to memory disturbance rather than being related to the resulting seizures.

EEG Abnormality

One factor thought to influence cognitive functioning, including memory disturbance, is the occurrence of "subclinical" epileptic discharges. Evidence that such activity can influence learning and memory exists (6,37–40). It has been suggested by Hutt and Gilbert (38) that subclinical bursts of activity influence short-term working memory and leave older, established memories undisturbed. In a more recent investigation, Aarts et al. (41) report laterality effects. Discharges in the left hemisphere disturbed the registration of verbal material, whereas discharges in the right hemisphere interfered with the registration of nonverbal stimuli. Gallassi et al. (42) suggested that subclinical epileptic discharges could be responsible for interictal memory disturbances by "causing difficulty in the process of codification or consolidation of the memory trace." Other investigators have reported impairments on tests of learning and memory in association with excessive slow waves and a lower alpha index. Dodrill and Wilkus (43) reported a significant relationship between performance on a spatial memory test and a slow posterior rhythm. Bornstein et al. (18) found EEG slowing to be associated with impaired performance on verbal, but not nonverbal, memory tasks. The contribution of EEG factors such as background rhythm is not straightforward, since presumably these can be the "effect" of other variables such as underlying structural or functional brain disturbance or drug effects.

Treatment Surgery

A severe memory disorder has been observed following unilateral resection of the temporal lobe when the contralateral lobe is not intact (44). Unilateral temporal lobectomy in the presence of a healthy contralateral lobe exacerbates preexisting memory difficulties; in contrast, a resection of the dominant lobe generally impairs verbal learning and memory, and resection of the nondominant lobe generally impairs nonverbal learning and memory (45–49). Some investigators have argued that dominant lobe resections lead to greater impairments of learning and memory, but this is probably a consequence of the importance of verbal memory in our everyday lives. In addition, lack of availability of many purely nonverbal memory measures may underestimate the extent of deficits in this domain (50,51). Recent work suggests that the type and extent of the surgical resection can influence the severity of memory difficulties, with more selective techniques resulting in fewer deficits (49,52–54). One case, however, has been reported of a patient who underwent an amygdalohippocampectomy and became amnesic (55).

The impact of surgery on memory may also be influenced by postsurgical seizure relief, with patients showing more memory deficits if their seizures have not been well controlled as a consequence of the operation (47,49,56). More recently, investigators have also suggested that an improvement in memory function subserved by the contralateral temporal lobe can occur following the operation. It has been proposed that the memory functions of the unaffected hemisphere had been in some way inhibited by the seizures in the resected hemisphere. When the epileptic focus is no longer present, a release of the available cognitive abilities occurs (48,56,57). One group of investigators has reported that this phenomenon is associated with left-sided, but not right-sided, operations (58). Consensus suggests that impaired memory measured postoperatively remains fairly permanent, although some investigators—for example, Blakemore and Falconer (59)—did report some recovery 3–7 years postoperatively, with young adults showing the earliest recoveries.

Most research has focused upon the influence of temporal lobe surgery on memory test performance. Frontal lobe surgery may also impair memory, particularly where a memory task requires monitoring of temporal sequences and programming of actions (60,61); this is not surprising, given the increasing evidence of the importance of the organizational functions of this part of the brain.

Other surgical procedures have been less well investigated. Existing evidence suggests corpus callosotomy, be it complete or partial, can influence memory functioning. Some investigators have reported impairments following surgery (62,63), whereas others have observed improvements (64). In a recent study, Sass et al. (65) found no consistent change in memory functioning of patients undergoing callosotomy and suggested that variables such as preoperative language dominance may influence outcome.

Treatment: Anticonvulsant Medication

Impairments of memory in association with epilepsy were recognized long before the widespread availability of anticonvulsant medication. However, evidence has accumulated (particularly over the past decade) which suggests that anticonvulsant medication, especially if inexpertly managed, can contribute to disorders of memory, directly or indirectly via changes in concentration and processing speed (66,67). The influence of anticonvulsants on memory is most easily explored in studies using animals or "healthy" volunteers. These studies make it possible to adopt carefully controlled designs—including the use of placebos, which are generally not possible in patient groups for obvious ethical reasons.

Even allowing for carefully controlled designs, findings from work with animals have not always been conclusive. Some investigators have reported that anticonvulsants have no influence on memory (68); in contrast, other investigators have reported an improvement of memory (69), whereas others have reported detrimental effects (70). Mondadori and Classen (71) studied the effects of five anticonvulsants on learning and memory and reported four drugs as having adverse effects. Phenytoin, ethosuximide, sodium valproate, and phenobarbitone had a dose-dependent amnesic effect in experimentally induced convulsions. In contrast, carbamazepine was associated with improved memory functioning. Rowley and Gaivon (72) reported that phenytoin did not influence memory performance in animals directly. Offspring of phenytoin-treated female rats showed some impairments on tests of learning and memory, suggesting that drug effects may become transmitted to further generations. While this is a somewhat alarming finding, extrapolation to humans must be made cautiously. It does, however, highlight how complex the interactions might be. George and Mellanby (35) have suggested that the entire blame for memory difficulties cannot be due to anticonvulsants, since experimentally induced epilepsy is associated with impairments of learning and memory in the absence of anticonvulsant treatment (35).

At the National Hospital we have undertaken a series of studies which have explored the effects of five anticonvulsants—phenytoin, carbamazepine, sodium valproate, clobazam, and clonazepam—on tests of cognitive functioning, including memory (73–76). Volunteers from a homogeneous subject pool were administered anticonvulsant medication on a daily basis for 2 weeks in a crossover design with matching placebos. Psychological performance on the active drug was compared with that on the placebo. Phenytoin, clonazepam, and clobazam were associated with impairments on the tests of memory. In addition, a significant correlation was obtained between phenytoin serum concentration and individual decline in memory test performance.

Problems with interpretation of the findings do arise. Firstly, an attempt had been made to prescribe anticonvulsant doses to participants; however, the daily intake of carbamazepine (600 mg) which had the least effect on all measures may today be considered on the low side. It is not uncommon for patients with intractable seizures to be administered more than 1000 mg a day. Secondly, 2 weeks' daily intake of anticonvulsant drugs may be expected to have differing effects from those arising from more long-term administration. Finally, the influence of anticonvulsants on a healthy brain may not be the same as the effects on a seizure-prone brain.

Studies involving patients are more numerous, although findings are contradictory and confusing. Memory assessment is often limited, and it is not uncommon for digit span to be the only measure of memory employed. In general, the most dramatic effects of anticonvulsants have been reported in patients on polytherapy or with high levels of medication (77–80). Interpretation of findings is not always straightforward, as we found in our studies. We assessed patients prior to drug reduction as well as 3 and 6 months after drug reduction. Patients changing to carbamazepine showed more widespread gains on tests of memory than did patients solely undergoing a change in the number of drugs prescribed (see Fig. 1); however, the carbamazepine group also experienced a trend toward improved seizure control which was significant in the case of tonic–clonic attacks (77). Significant changes in mood were also observed in the carbamazepine group (81). Improvements observed on the memory tests could be attributable to a substitution of carbamazepine, the withdrawal of more sedating drugs, the improvement in seizure control, changes in mood, or, as seems more likely, some combination of these factors.

In investigations where comparisons were made between new referrals, effects of anticonvulsants on memory and other cognitive functions seemed less dramatic (82,83; Birbeck, *personal communication*). Furthermore, there seemed to be little difference between individual compounds. This finding is not unexpected, since any negative drug effects would be expected to be offset by improved seizure control. In studies that have followed patients being withdrawn from medication, improvements have been noted on psychological tests, including measures of memory (84).

Attention has more recently been drawn to the phenomenon of state-dependent learning. This refers to the observation that events experienced in a particular state of mind or brain may best be remembered in that state. This phenomenon has been most clearly demonstrated with alcohol and cannabis; however, some studies suggest that phenobarbitone and the benzodiazepines may have state-dependent properties. It has been argued for anticonvulsants that information learned while taking the drugs may be less easily retrievable when the drug is withdrawn (85). While this is certainly an interesting phenomenon, in epilepsy the complex situation may minimize the role of state-dependent learning. Indeed, research on the withdrawal of anticonvulsant medication suggests that those patients who successfully stop taking drugs have the best prognosis occupationally and academically. If state-dependent learning was exerting a major influence, the reverse effect might be anticipated.

Other Factors

Weiskrantz and Koella (86) have pointed out that there are many factors other than a

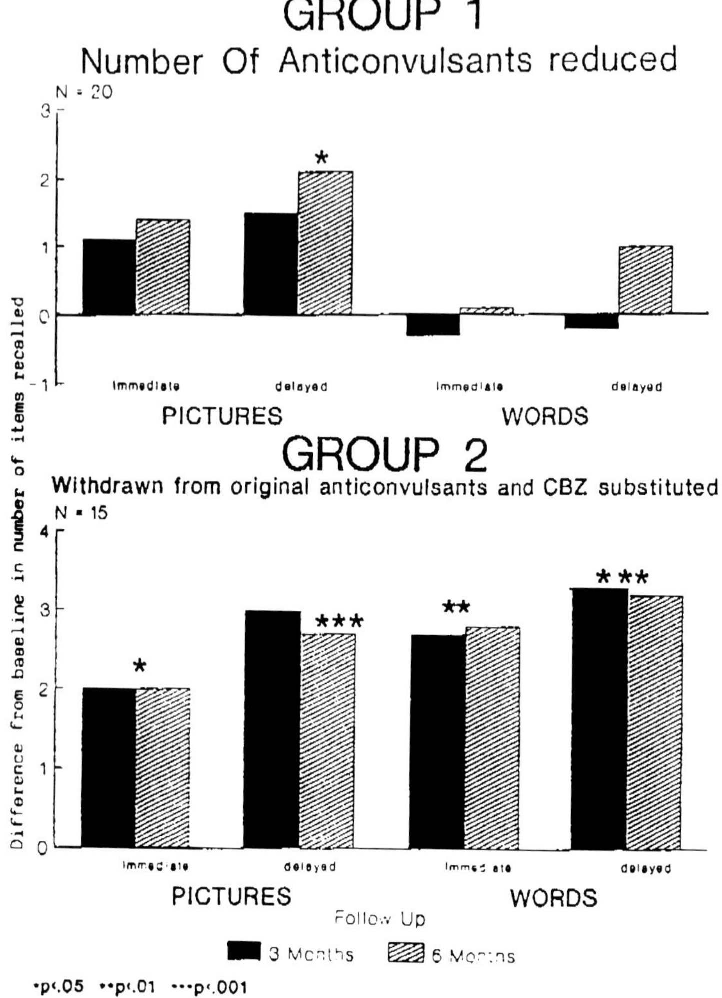

FIG. 1. Change in memory test performance of patients undergoing alterations in medications.

poor memory which may result in an individual doing badly on memory tests. They state that "it is impossible to study memory without a subject who can see or hear or attend or respond. In any single test you do not know which of these various capacities might account for the deficit." Weingartner and Thompson (87) have also drawn attention to noncognitive determinants of cognitive functioning. They point out that conditions that affect a patient's mood, ability to appreciate reinforcing events, alertness, and motivation can all influence test performance.

One factor that has received most interest has been attention. It is understood to be an important process with varying components, including alertness, selectivity, and ability to sustain concentration. Patients who have difficulty maintaining attention will have difficulty learning (88). There is some evidence that attentional difficulties can be found in at least some subgroups of patients with epilepsy (13,89,90) and that perhaps individuals with generalized seizures are most at risk. This could possibly explain why several studies have not found significant differences between patients with temporal lobe epilepsy and those with generalized epilepsy on measures of memory (3).

Another factor that can influence learning

and memory test performance is organizational skills. Aldenkamp (13) has suggested that individuals with epilepsy may have specific cognitive styles which influence their general approach to tasks. In particular, he singles out impulsive reactions and rigid thinking patterns. Both these cognitive styles would be expected to reduce an individual's ability on tests of memory. More recently, it has been suggested that perhaps language difficulties underlie or contribute to poor memory performance in at least some patient groups (91).

A person's emotional state is also important to consider. If an individual's arousal level is too low or too high, this may impair test performance. Changes in arousal level may be secondary to fatigue, possibly as a consequence of sedation, lack of sleep, anxiety, or depression. There is evidence that depression, possibly secondary to decreased motivation, may impair memory test performance, leading to forgetfulness and distortion of what is remembered (92). More recently, the possibility that mood itself may represent a state-dependent situation has been raised. According to this phenomenon, a person in a nondepressed state would be unable to recall things that had been learned while he or she was in a depressed state, and vice versa.

WHAT IS MEMORY?

An attempt to understand memory functioning in epilepsy is complicated not only by the many factors that could influence efficiency, but also by the multifaceted nature of memory itself. Often the word "memory" is used as if it were some unitary phenomenon. Certainly, patients will use the term in this way. We cannot blame them for this. How are they really expected to know of the many subsystems with different functional and structural properties that have been identified by psychologists and other researchers? (88,93) A brief mention will be given of some of the memory subsystems that have been identified, but limitations on space does not permit a detailed description of these.

"Sensory memory" is a term applied to systems which have very limited capacity and which hold information for less than a second.

The best studied of these are echoic and iconic memory—short-lived stores in the auditory and visual domains, respectively. Of slightly longer duration is "short-term memory," which refers to memory systems that are labile and transient, lasting less than a minute. Short-term memory is also referred to as "working memory" or "immediate memory." Memory lasting more than 30 sec is called "long-term memory." This has been subdivided in a variety of ways. A widely accepted division is between semantic and episodic memory. The former refers to a pool of knowledge which is shared by individuals and which is known to have a larger capacity; included in this information pool are word meanings and general knowledge. "Episodic" refers to more personal memory and has also been called "autobiographical" or "event" memory. Distinctions between memory systems have also been made on the basis of the type of information stored. The best known of these is the distinction between verbal and nonverbal memory, and evidence that these systems are structurally distinct has come from research with temporal lobectomy patients discussed earlier. Flavell and Wellman (94) have drawn attention to the concept of "meta memory," which refers to an individual's knowledge of, or awareness of, their memory or anything that is pertinent to information storage and retrieval.

Disorders of memory may be expected to occur in one or more memory systems. In addition, a disturbance could arise via a variety of mechanisms resulting from faulty encoding, faulty storage, or faulty retrieval, for example. Furthermore, there might not be a total breakdown, but there may be a reduced efficiency such that the concept of severity of memory disturbance may need to be considered. Epilepsy is a heterogeneous group of disorders, and it seems likely that a variety of different types of memory disturbances will be encountered. Many individuals may be expected to have difficulties in more than one memory system, particularly where the memory disturbance is secondary to a general effect such as impaired concentration. Epilepsy is not a static condition. For this reason the nature and severity of memory problems of a particular patient may change with time.

MEMORY ASSESSMENT: NEW APPROACHES

In recent years the assessment of memory has become more sophisticated, and these developments have increased our awareness of the existence of a variety of memory subsystems and their functional properties. However, some researchers have shown concern about the validity of using laboratory-based tests to provide information to patients as to the sorts of memory problems they might experience in their daily lives (95). For example, in most testing situations, patients are required to recall previously learned material following a prompt from the examiner. However, such prompting rarely occurs in everyday life. We have to remember not only what to do, but, sometimes more importantly, when to do it. The belief that psychological tests do not give us a complete picture of a person's memory functioning has led researchers to consider supplementary ways of assessing memory. Mayes (93) writes "the major clinical requirement is the need for tests to have clear ecological validity, reflecting the daily memory problems of patients. In response to this need, a number of subjective memory questionnaires and checklists have been devised." Psychologists utilizing this approach are generally aware of the limitations of using subjective data, but they feel that information obtained in this way, taken together with other results, can increase our understanding of memory. Studies in the field of epilepsy are few; however, existing evidence will be reviewed, and the value of this approach will hopefully be demonstrated.

An early questionnaire study was reported by Guerrant et al. (96). Three groups of patients—32 with psychomotor epilepsy, 26 with idiopathic epilepsy, and 26 with chronic illness—rated their memory. Interestingly, the patients with partial seizure disorders rated themselves as having better memory than the other groups. Broughton et al. (97) reported the findings of a study in which epilepsy patients, narcolepsy patients, and controls assessed the efficiency of their memory. Over 50% of the epilepsy group rated themselves as having memory difficulties. Many of this sample attributed memory problems to poor seizure control.

Bennett-Levy et al. (98) compared questionnaire responses of 58 post-temporal lobectomy patients with the responses of a group of individuals without epilepsy. The questionnaire consisted of 43 questions which addressed everyday memory functioning—for instance, "How is your memory for passing on messages, learning new skills, and remembering directions?" Respondents rated each item on a severity scale ranging from very good to very poor. The patient group rated their memory as being significantly poorer than that of controls on several items. Significant findings at the 1% level included memory for faces, facts about people (where met, etc.), giving messages to people, learning new skills, and remembering directions. In addition, forgetting a word in midsentence and losing the thread of a conversation were also rated as areas of difficulty for the patient group. On no items did the patient group report themselves as having better memory than the controls. Of particular interest in this study was not the complaints of poor memory (poor memory is not surprising, given that they are a postsurgical sample), but the lack of significant correlations between questionnaire responses and scores on formal memory tests which had also been completed by the participants.

A more recent, unpublished study undertaken by Easterbrook and Cull employed the same questionnaire but administered it to nonsurgical cases. Complaints of memory difficulties were less marked than in the surgical sample. The epilepsy group rated their memory as being significantly poorer than that of the control group for nine items, including remembering appointments, faces, learning new skills, and forgetting words in midsentence. However, the epilepsy group rated their memory as being significantly better than that of the control group for birthdays, numbers of houses, names of public figures, and details of shoe size. There was no relationship between complaints of poor memory and type of epilepsy (partial versus generalized). In keeping with the previous study, these researchers found that questionnaire scores did not correlate highly with performance on more traditional memory tests.

We have recently embarked on a study which adopts a questionnaire approach in the initial phase. Our investigations aim to explore further the nature and extent of memory failures experienced by patients with epilepsy in their everyday lives. The research was stimulated by the observation that some patients who complain of memory difficulties can do exceptionally well, or can fall within average limits, on tests of memory. This could be an indication of the unreliability of patient's assessments of their memory. Limited research suggests that this may sometimes be the case (16). It is possible that patients may occasionally overestimate their memory problems as a result of negative self-evaluation arising from depression, which is known to occur more frequently in epilepsy patients than in the general population (99). However, patients may also be using the term "memory" to refer to a different set of cognitive failures than those that are generally tapped by traditional memory tests.

The questionnaire employed in our study had been previously used with patients following head injury (100,101). A few modifications were made to the original questionnaire which were in keeping with suggestions made by the authors of the scale. The questionnaire contains 18 items. Sixteen refer to frequently reported memory failures such as losing belongings, forgetting names, and failing to convey messages. Two items refer to infrequent memory failures such as forgetting personal details (e.g., date of birth and address). Respondents have to rate how frequently each memory failure occurs. Frequency ratings range from "not at all" to "more than once a day." In addition, patients are also requested to rate the extent, if any, to which their memory causes them problems. Whenever possible, a similarly constructed questionnaire is completed by someone who comes into daily contact with the patient. This is usually a close relative, and for this reason we refer to this measure as the "Relative's Questionnaire."

Patients participating in this study come from a range of sources. Some are inpatients attending the National Hospitals Assessment Centre for Epilepsy; in general, these individuals have epilepsy that is more difficult to control. Outpatients attending special epilepsy clinics and patients with epilepsy managed by their general practitioners are also

being surveyed. In addition, questionnaires have also been completed by individuals without epilepsy. The majority of people participating in this initial phase of our investigation have been contacted via a postal survey. People without epilepsy are also being included in order to obtain some general information about the nature and frequency of memory complaints. An attempt will be made to match the two groups for important factors such as age, sex, and educational and occupational backgrounds. However, the main focus of the investigation ultimately will be comparisons between patient subgroups.

To date, preliminary analysis of memory questionnaire responses has been undertaken on 435 cases in the epilepsy group and on 73 cases in the non-epilepsy group. The groups are matched for age and educational background; however, at the present time there are significantly more females in the non-epilepsy group (70% versus 52%) and more unemployed people in the epilepsy group (41% versus 22%). As expected, memory complaints were more frequently reported by patients with epilepsy, and 48% acknowledge moderate or severe memory problems. In contrast, only 17% of the non-epilepsy group reported a similar degree of memory disturbance. The responses of "relatives" indicated less concern about the "subjects" memory, with 39% of the epilepsy group and 11% of the non-epilepsy group being rated as having moderate or severe memory difficulties. Significant correlations of 0.65 and 0.57 were obtained between the total score on the subject and relative questionnaires, respectively, for the epilepsy and non-epilepsy groups. Perfect agreement between the two questionnaires was not expected, since relatives would only be able to observe some of the patient's memory failures.

The five most frequently reported memory problems of the patients with epilepsy are given in Table 1. They were also among the most commonly occurring failures in the non-epilepsy group, although fewer individuals reported them as occurring on a daily basis. The most frequently noted failures by relatives were similar, although the order was slightly different. For example, "a word on the tip of the tongue" dropped to third place, perhaps because this is a failure which is less readily

TABLE 1. *The five most frequently reported daily memory failures (%)*

Type of memory failure	Epilepsy group (N = 435)	Non-epilepsy group (N = 73)
Finding that a word is on the "tip of the tongue"	43	14
Having to go back to check that you have done things	38	25
Forgetting that you were told something yesterday or a few days ago	32	14
Forgetting people's names	33	16
Losing things around the house	31	15

apparent to an observer than to the person experiencing it. The nature of some of the memory failures reported frequently by both groups might not be expected to be adequately reflected in scores on clinical tests of memory. This will be specifically explored in a later phase of our investigations; however, it could be argued that the "tip of the tongue" phenomenon might be more readily tapped by tests of naming ability and that the "going back to check" phenomenon might be more easily measured by tests of organizational skills. Indeed, others have argued that language deficits (20,91) or faulty organizational strategies (17) might partly underlie memory difficulties of patients with epilepsy.

Participants in our study also completed two rating scales of mood, namely the Hospital Anxiety and Depression Scale (102) and the Beck Depression Inventory (103). Significant correlations were obtained between complaints of memory and high levels of depression. It is possible that having a weak memory contributes to an individual's feelings of worthlessness and low self-esteem. However, as discussed earlier, being depressed may result in an inefficient memory. The relationship between memory complaints and depression deserves further consideration.

Many potential problems exist when interpreting questionnaire data (104). For instance, in our study, people volunteered to take part, and it can easily be argued that those individuals with memory problems are more likely to want to participate. Thus, complaints of memory may well have been overestimated in our survey. In addition, although participants were requested to complete subject and relative memory questionnaires separately, we cannot be sure that this occurred in all cases.

Assessment of memory efficiency in real-life situations is more problematic than the questionnaire approach. We have undertaken two studies which have attempted to do this and compare performance with scores on more standardized tests of memory. The first study measured patients memory for a medical interview. Thirty-eight patients took part, and at the time of the project they were all residents at the Chalfont Centre for Epilepsy. The age of the patients was varied (age range: 17–66 years), as was their intellectual level (I.Q. range: 70–118). As a group, they had poorly controlled seizures. The majority had partial attacks, with many experiencing secondary generalized seizures. They therefore constituted a patient sample who might be considered at risk for memory problems. The requirements of a controlled drug reduction study were explained to all participants by one investigator. This included information such as the day and time of appointments and details of tests that would be carried out. In all, 18 "bits" of information were conveyed. Immediately following this interview and again later in the day following an interval of 3–5 hr, the patients were asked (by a second investigator) to recall (as much as possible) the information the doctor had told them about the drug trial. Following spontaneous recall, standardized prompting took place. For example, to see if further information could be elicited, the patients were asked the question, "When do you have to see the doctor again?" In the same week, patients underwent a series of memory tests, including story recall, paired associates learning, recognition memory, and the Benton Visual Retention Test. Only three patients spontaneously recalled more than 50% of the interview (18 "bits" of information), although performance was improved with prompting. Information forgotten often included important details such as date and time of next appointment, requirements of blood tests, and, in particular, whether these tests had to be undertaken before morning medication or food. Inaccuracy in the recall of patients was also common. Significant correlations were obtained between only one memory test (namely, story recall) and patient's memory of the medical interview. All other correlations were in the expected direction. This study suggested that patients with difficult-to-control epilepsy may forget a significant amount of information conveyed in a medical interview. This finding is in keeping with research undertaken with other patient groups (105). This suggests that inefficient memory could result in poor compliance in this patient group, since individuals cannot adequately follow treatment instructions if they have forgotten what they have to do (106). The study also supported previous findings (discussed earlier) which indicated that traditional tests of memory may not always adequately reflect memory functions in more natural settings. Interestingly, other investigators have found that the story recall test reflects everyday memory performance (100). Generalizations from this study must, of course, be made cautiously. The population under investigation was highly selective in that they were all in a residential setting at the time of the study. During drug trials, it is generally the care staff members who are relied upon to make sure that study requirements are met. For this reason, patients may not have been particularly motivated to recall the information from the medical interview, depending on the staff to remind them of appointments, etc. In addition, a relatively large amount of information was given to each patient, and previous research suggests that recall deteriorates as information load increases (105).

In a second study, we have attempted to assess patient's ability to remember to do things at specific times of the day (simulated pill-taking) and keeping appointments. Once again we also explored the relationship between performance on these unprompted or prospective memory tests and more traditional tests of memory. Sixteen patients participated in this preliminary investigation. At the time of the study, all patients were short-term admissions to the Assessment Unit of the National Hospitals, Chalfont Centre for Epilepsy. The mean I.Q. of the group fell just below the average range, although there was a wide range of ability represented (mean I.Q. was 91; range was 72–112). Formal memory tests administered included story recall, list learning, recognition memory, and the Benton Visual Retention Test. In this study, patients were requested to remember to have a card signed by a staff member once or twice a day at a prearranged time. Staff members were not permitted to prompt the patient or to remind them of the time the card should be signed. It was originally hoped that there would be a three-time-per-day signing requirement, but this was not possible for practical reasons. The patients participating were told that the task was a test to see whether they could remember to take their pills. It was hoped that this kind of instruction would counteract the artificiality of the test by increasing motivation. In addition, patients were given two appointments per week which they had to remember to keep, unprompted by staff.

Thirteen patients repeatedly failed to have their card signed within an hour of the arranged times. Appointment-keeping was better, with only three forgetting all appointments. All patients who failed on the appointment-keeping task also failed the card-signing task. No significant correlations were found between performance on the prospective memory test and epilepsy variables or I.Q. Significant positive correlations were obtained between the card-signing test and, with the exception of one, all the clinical memory tests. Interestingly, a negative correlation was observed between a list-learning task and the card-signing task, such that a good performance on the list-learning measure was associated with a poor performance on the card-signing measure. This might be considered a spurious finding; however, it has been reported by other investigators. Wilkins and Baddeley (107) reported the findings of a study in which participants with a good memory for learning lists of words had performed rather poorly on a simulated pill-taking task. Findings such as these suggest that some conventional memory tests may be poor predictors of how well patients remember to do things without a prompt. Further studies of this nature with larger patient groups will help to improve our knowledge of the relationship between memory on traditional tests and that in everyday situations.

IMPROVING MEMORY

Much of the interest concerning memory in epilepsy has focused on reasons why there may be difficulties. Existing evidence reviewed in this chapter suggests that the causes of memory disturbance may be multifactorial. Furthermore, the factors most implicated to date—namely etiology, seizure frequency, and medication—may not always be amenable to intervention. For example, medication may be a contributory factor, but a drug reduction or change may result in reduced seizure control, which may be more undesirable than the memory problems. Little attention has been given to psychological factors that may contribute to memory problems which may be more amenable to manipulation. Strategies have been discussed in relation to other patient groups (usually individuals with severe memory impairments), and they may help to alleviate or reduce the impact of memory difficulties (108). Results of such psychological interventions have not always been dramatic; however, it could be argued that such approaches might be more successful in patients with less severe difficulties.

A variety of internal and external memory aids exist which can be used to help us remember things. It is possible that some patients with epilepsy make less use of such devices, thereby increasing the load upon their memory and increasing the risk of memory failure.

In our investigations of memory functioning in epilepsy, we are surveying our patients on their use of a variety of internal and external memory aids. Data are currently available from 672 epilepsy patients and 126 controls. Table 2 gives the most frequently reported aids and lists the percentage of individuals using them. The patient group was found to use diaries and shopping lists less frequently than did the non-epilepsy group. Of the internal aids, mental retracing and first-letter mnemonics were reported as being used significantly less often. Further analysis will be undertaken within the patient group with epilepsy. In particular, we are anxious to compare memory-aid use of patients complaining of memory problems with that of patients who are not complaining of difficulties. Interestingly, earlier pilot investigations suggested that patients with left temporal lobe foci reported less use of memory aids than did patients with other types of epilepsy. Of course, reported use of memory aids does not always mean that such strategies are used efficiently. Prevey et al. (17) demonstrated that patients with temporal lobe epilepsy, particularly those with left-sided foci, were less likely to engage in effective learning strategies than were control subjects. They suggest that "left temporal lobe subjects may not recognize the need for more active, strategic learning behaviors and therefore fail to make effective use of study time and mnemonic strategies which are available to them."

Powell et al. (109), in a study of patients being assessed for temporal lobectomy, found that the strategies employed by the patients were inefficient and that by changing the procedure required in the memory test situation, they could obtain improved results. This suggests that internal memory strategies may be taught which may have a beneficial effect on memory. Berent et al. (23), in a study of memory functioning in patients with temporal lobe epilepsy, found that patients with difficulties could improve their performance on memory

TABLE 2. *Four most frequently reported internal and external memory aids*

Memory aid	People with epilepsy, (N = 672), %	People without epilepsy (N = 126), %
External aids		
Diary	81	92[a]
Shopping list	68	76[b]
Ask for a reminder	59	54
Personal memos	59	63
Internal aids		
Mental retracing	71	84[c]
Alphabetic search	46	40
Method of loci	24	16
First-letter mnemonics	24	35[b]

[a] $p < 0.001$.
[b] $p < 0.05$.
[c] $p < 0.01$.

tests when given the opportunity to practice; in addition, they found that if the task was self-paced, the patients' memory scores also improved. Once again, this indicates that there may be psychological approaches to improve memory in people with epilepsy. More recently, Fedio et al. (48) discussed improvements in memory test performance in post-surgical cases. These investigators have attempted to explore the nature of deficits in patients, with the sole purpose of trying to alleviate them. They encouraged their patients to use mnemonic cues, and they found that patients' memories might be enhanced when appropriate retrieval cues are utilized. They did point out that performance remained significantly below that of normal subjects; nevertheless, this study does suggest that cognitive manipulation may reduce the impact of memory deficit.

Finally, in this section it is important to realize that the idea of psychological intervention is not new. In 1861, Russell Reynolds (1) suggested that the memory difficulty in epilepsy was possibly a consequence of motivational problems. He wrote: "In the epileptic here is the fault which results in defective memory, desire is too feeble," and he went on to discuss a psychological approach that might enhance memory. He suggested that "there should be regular, disciplined mental effort not only daily but hourly, of course duly graded as to time and intensity and alternated with relaxation."

CONCLUSION

Memory function in patients with epilepsy is a complicated area with many possible causes and potential manifestations. Assessment of memory is broadening, and it is hoped that this will increase our understanding. Only by describing memory problems more fully can programs be devised that will be of some practical benefit to those patients experiencing significant difficulties.

ACKNOWLEDGMENTS

This work was supported by a grant from the British Epilepsy Research Foundation.

REFERENCES

1. Russell Reynolds J. *Epilepsy: its symptoms, treatment and relation to other chronic convulsive diseases.* London: John Churchill, 1861.
2. Lennox WG. Brain injury, drugs and environment as a cause of mental decay in epilepsy. *Am J Psychiatry* 1942;99:174–180.
3. Loiseau P, Strube E, Signoret JL. Memory and epilepsy. In: Trimble MR, Reynolds EH, eds. *Epilepsy, behaviour and cognitive function.* Chichester, England: John Wiley & Sons, 1988;165–176.
4. Deutsch CP. Differences among epileptics and between epileptics and non-epileptics in terms of some learning and memory variables. *Arch Neurol Psychiatry* 1953;70:474–482.
5. Brittain H. Epilepsy and intellectual functions. In: Kulig BM, Meinardi H, Stores G, eds. *Epilepsy and behaviour.* Lisse: Swets & Zeitlinger, 1980;2–13.
6. Loiseau P, Strube E, Broustet D, Battelochi S, Gomeni C, Morselli P. Learning impairment in epileptic patients. *Epilepsia* 1983;24:183–192.
7. Scott DF, Moffatt A, Matthews A, Ettlinger G. The effect of epileptic discharges on learning and memory in patients. *Epilepsia* 1967;8:188–194.
8. Mohan V, Varma VK, Sahrey BB. Intellectual and memory functions in epileptics. *India Neurol* 1976;24:110.
9. Hunger J, Kleim J. Psychological tests by epileptic patients. *Arch Psychiatr Nervenkr* 1983;233/234:307–325.
10. Quadfasel AF, Pruyser PW. Cognitive deficits in patients with psychomotor epilepsy. *Epilepsia* 1955;4:80–90.
11. Glowinski H. Cognitive deficits in temporal lobe epilepsy: an investigation of memory functioning. *J Nerv Ment Dis* 1973;157:129–137.
12. Milberg W, Greiffenstein M, Lewis R, Rourke D. Differentiation of temporal lobe and generalised seizure patients with the WAIS. *J Consult Psychol* 1980;48:39–42.
13. Aldenkamp AP. Epilepsy and learning behaviour. In: Parsonage M, Grant RHE, Craig A, Ward AA, eds. *Advances in epileptology: XIVth epilepsy international symposium.* New York: Raven Press, 1983;221–228.
14. Mungas D, Ehlers C, Walton N, McCutchen B. Verbal learning differences in epileptic patients with left and right temporal lobe foci. *Epilepsia* 1985;26:340–345.
15. Masters DR, Thompson C, Dunn G, Lishman WA. Memory selectivity and unilateral cerebral dysfunction. *Psychol Med* 1986;16:781–788.
16. Prevey ML, Delaney RC, Mattson RH. Metamemory in temporal lobe epilepsy: self-monitoring of memory functions. *Brain Cog* 1988;7:298–311.
17. Prevey ML, Delaney RC, Mattson RH. Gist recall in temporal lobe seizure patients (a study of adaptive memory skills). *Cortex* 1988;24:301–312.

18. Bornstein RA, Pakalinis A, Drake EM, Suga JL. Effects of seizure type and waveform abnormality on memory and attention. *Arch Neurol* 1988;45:884–887.

19. Mirsky AF, Primac DW, Ajmone Marson C, Rosvold HE, Stevens JR. A comparison of the psychological test performance of patients with focal and nonfocal epilepsy. *Exp Neurol* 1960; 2:75–89.

20. Mayeux R, Brandt J, Rosen J. Interictal memory and language impairment in temporal lobe epilepsy. *Neurology* 1980;30:120–125.

21. Fedio P, Mirsky AF. Selective intellectual deficits in children with temporal lobe or centrocephalic epilepsy. *Neuropsychologia* 1969;7: 287–300.

22. Ladavas E, Umilta C, Provincali L. Hemisphere-dependent cognitive performances in epileptic patients. *Epilepsia* 1979;20:493–502.

23. Berent S, Boll TS, Giordani B. Hemispheric site of epileptogenic focus. Cognitive, perceptual and psychosocial implications for children and adults. In: Canger R, Angelini F, Penry JK, eds. *Advances in epileptology: 11th international symposium*. New York: Raven Press, 1980;185–190.

24. Delaney RC, Rosen AJ, Mattson RH, Novelly RA. Memory function in focal epilepsy: a comparison of non-surgical unilateral temporal lobe and frontal samples. *Cortex* 1980;16:103–117.

25. Perrone P, Prazzi D, Ricotta E. Neuropsychological findings in partial seizure epilepsy with a temporal EEG focus. *Boll Lega Ital Epilessia* 1984;45/46:251.

26. Masui K, Niwa SI, Anzai N. Verbal memory disturbances in left temporal lobe epileptics. *Cortex* 1984;20:361–368.

27. Hermann BR, Wyler AR, Richey ET, Rea JM. Memory function and verbal learning ability in patients with complex partial seizures of temporal lobe origin. *Epilepsia* 1987;28:547–554.

28. Delaney RC, Prevey ML, Mattson RH. Short term retention with lateralised temporal lobe epilepsy. *Cortex* 1982;22:591–600.

29. Marsden CD, Reynolds EH. Seizures in adults. In: Laidlaw J, Richens A, Oxley J, eds. *A textbook of epilepsy*. Edinburgh: Churchill Livingstone, 1988;144–182.

30. Weiskrantz L. Some aspects of memory functions and the temporal lobes *Acta Neurol Scand* 1986;74(Suppl 109):69–74.

31. Ossetin J. Methods and problems in the assessment of cognitive function in epileptic patients. In: Trimble MR, Reynolds EH, eds. *Epilepsy, behaviour and cognitive function*. Chichester, England: John Wiley & Sons, 1988;9–26.

32. Hermann BP, Whitman S. Behavioural and personality correlates of epilepsy: a review, methodological critique and conceptual model *Psychol Bull* 1984;95:451–497.

33. Powell GE, Polkey CE, Canavan AGM. Lateralisation of memory functions in epileptic patients by use of the sodium amytal (Wada) technique *J Neurol Neurosurg Psychiatry* 1987; 50:665–672.

34. Dodrill CB. Correlates of generalised tonic–clonic seizures with intellectual, neuropsychological, emotional and social function in patients with epilepsy. *Epilepsia* 1986;27:399–411.

35. George G, Mellanby J. Memory deficits in an experimental hippocampal epileptiform syndrome in rats. *Exp Neurol* 1982;75:678–689.

36. Mellanby J. A comparison of the effects of epilepsy and ageing on learning and hippocampal physiology. *Acta Neurol Scand* 1986;74(Suppl 109):123–128.

37. Wilkins RJ, Dodrill CB. Neuropsychological correlates of the electroencephalogram in epileptics. I. Topographic distribution and average rate of epileptiform activity. *Epilepsia* 1976; 17:89–100.

38. Hutt SJ, Gilbert S. Effects of evoked spike–wave discharges upon short term memory in patients with epilepsy. *Cortex* 1980;16:445–457.

39. Provinciali L, Signanno M, Giovagnoli AR. Influence of diffuse and synchronous polyspike or spike-and-wave discharges on recognition of shapes *Boll Lega Ital Epilepssia* 1984;45/46:243–245.

40. Binnie CD. Seizures, EEG discharges and cognition. In: Trimble MR, Reynolds EH, eds. *Epilepsy, behaviour and cognitive function*. Chichester, England: John Wiley & Sons, 1988;45–49.

41. Aarts JHP, Binnie CD, Smith AM, Wilkins AS. Selective cognitive impairment during focal and generalised epileptiform EEG activity. *Brain* 1984;107:293–308.

42. Gallassi R, Morneale A, Lorusso S, Pazzaglia P, Lugaresi E. Epilepsy presenting as memory disturbances. *Epilepsia* 1988;29:624–629.

43. Dodrill CB, Wilkus RJ. Neuropsychological correlates of the electroencephalogram in epileptics. II. The waking posterior rhythm and its interaction with epileptiform activity. *Epilepsia* 1976;17:101–109.

44. Penfield W, Mathieson G. An autopsy and a discussion of the role of the hippocampus in experiential recall. *Arch Neurol* 1974;31:145–154.

45. Weingartner H. Verbal learning in patients with temporal lobe lesions. *J Verb Learning Verb Behav* 1968;7:520–526.

46. Cherlow DG, Serafetinides EA. Speech and memory assessment in psychomotor epileptics. *Cortex* 1976;12:21–26.

47. Lieb JP, Rausch R, Engel J, Jann Brown W, Crandall PH. Changes in intelligence following temporal lobectomy: relationship to EEG activity, seizure relief and pathology. *Epilepsia* 1982;23:1–13.

48. Fedio P, Martin A, Browers P. The effects of focal cortical lesions on cognitive functions. In: Porter RJ, Mattson RH, Ward A, Dam M, eds. *Advances in epileptology: XVth epilepsy international symposium*. New York: Raven Press, 1984;489–498.

49. Ojeman GA, Dodrill CB. Verbal memory deficits after left temporal lobectomy for epilepsy. *J Neurosurg* 1985;62:101–107.

50. Powell GE, Polkey CE, McMillan TM. The new Maudsey series of temporal lobectomy. I. Short-term cognitive effects. *Br J Clin Psychol* 1985;24:109–124.

51. Goldstein LA, Canavan AGM, Polkey CE. Verbal and abstract designs paired associate learning after unilateral temporal lobectomy. *Cortex* 1988;24:41–51.

52. Wieser HG, Yasargil MS. Selective amygdalo-hippocompectomy as a surgical treatment for mesiobasal limbic epilepsy. *Neurochirurgia* 1982;25:39–50.

53. Nadig T, Wieser HG. Problems of learning and memory: comparison of performances before and after surgical therapy. In: Wieser HG, Elger CE, eds. *Presurgical evaluation of epileptics*. Berlin: Springer-Verlag, 1987;91–93.

54. Jones-Gotman M. Commentary: Psychological evaluation—testing hippocampal function. In: Engel J, ed. *Surgical treatment of the epilepsies*. New York: Raven Press, 1987.

55. Rausch R. Psychological evaluation. In: Engel J, ed. *Surgical treatment of the epilepsies*. New York: Raven Press, 1987;181–195.

56. Novelly RA, Augustine EA, Mattson RH, Glaser GH, Williamson PD, Spencer DD, Spencer SS. Selective memory improvement and impairment in temporal lobectomy for epilepsy. *Ann Neurol* 1984;15:64–67.

57. Nilsson LG, Christianson SA, Silfvenius H, Blom S. Pre-operative and post-operative memory testing of epileptic patients. *Acta Neurol Scand* 1984;69(Suppl 99):43–56.

58. Bornstein RA, McKean JDS, McLean DR. Effects of temporal lobectomy for treatment of epilepsy on hemispheric functions ipsilateral to surgery: preliminary findings. *Int J Neurosci* 1987;37:73–78.

59. Blakemore CB, Falconer MA. Longterm effects of anterior temporal lobectomy on certain cognitive functions. *J Neurol Neurosurg Psychiatry* 1967;30:364–367.

60. Petrides M, Milner B. Deficits in subject ordered tasks after frontal and temporal lobe lesions in man. *Neuropsychologia* 1982;20:249–262.

61. Smith ML, Milner B. Differential effects of frontal lobe lesions on cognitive estimation and spatial memory. *Neuropsychologia* 1984;22:697–705.

62. Campbell AL, Bogen JE, Smith A. Disorganisation and re-organisation of cognitive and sensori-motor functions in cerebral commissuratomy: compensatory roles of the forebrain commissures and cerebral hemispheres. *Brain* 1980;104:493–512.

63. Zaidel D, Sperry RW. Some longterm motor effects of cerebral commisurotomy in man. *Neuropsychologia* 1977;15:193–204.

64. Le Doux JE, Wilson DH, Gazzaniga MS. Manipulo-spatial aspects of cerebral lateralization: Clues to the origin of lateralization. *Neuropsychologia* 1977;15:743–750.

65. Sass KJ, Spencer DD, Spencer SS, Novelly RA, Williamson PD, Mattson RH. Corpus callosotomy for epilepsy. II. Neurologic and neuropsychological outcome. *Neurology* 1988;38:24–28.

66. Hirtz DG, Nelson KB. Cognitive effects of antiepileptic drugs. In: Pedley TA, Meldrum BS, eds. *Recent advances in epilepsy*. New York: Churchill Livingstone, 1985;161–181.

67. Trimble MR. Anticonvulsant drugs and cognitive function: a review of the literature. *Epilepsia* 1987;28(Suppl 3):S17–S45.

68. Mellanby J, Hawkins C, Wilks L. The relationship between seizures and amnesia in experimental epilepsy. *Acta Neurol Scand* 1984;69(Suppl 99):119–124.

69. Weinberger SB, Killam EK. Alterations in learning performance in the seizure prone baboon: effects of elicited seizures and chronic treatment of diazepam and phenobarbital. *Epilepsia* 1978;19:301–316.

70. Kulig BM. The evaluation of the behavioural effects of antiepileptic drugs in animals and man. In: Kulig B, Meinardi H, Stores G, eds. *Epilepsy and behaviour*. Lisse: Swets & Zeitlinger, 1980;47–61.

71. Mondadori C, Classen W. The effects of various antiepileptic drugs on E-shock-induced amnesia in mice: dissociability of effects on convulsions and effects on memory. *Acta Neurol Scand* 1984;69(Suppl 99):119–124.

72. Rowley VN, Gaivon EF. Effects of chronic administration of phenytoin on learning and offspring behaviour. *Psychopharmacology* 1977;53:259–262.

73. Thompson PJ, Huppert FA, Trimble MR. Phenytoin and cognitive functions: effects on normal volunteers and implications for epilepsy. *Br J Clin Psychol* 1981;20;155–162.

74. Thompson PJ, Trimble MR. Sodium valproate and cognitive functioning in normal volunteers. *Br J Clin Pharmacol* 1981;12:819–824.

75. Thompson PJ, Trimble MR. Clobazam and cognitive functions. Effects in healthy volunteers. In: Hindmarch I, Stonier PD, eds. *Clobazam*. London: Royal Society of Medicine, Academic Press, 1981;33–38.

76. Cull CA, Trimble MR. Cognitive sequelae of 1-4 and 1-5 benzodiazepines. *Human Psychopharmacol* 1987;2:222–229.

77. Thompson PJ, Trimble MR. Anticonvulsant drugs and cognitive functions. *Epilepsia* 1982;23:531–544.

78. Thompson PJ, Trimble MR. Anticonvulsant serum levels: relationship to impairments of cognitive functioning. *J Neurol Neurosurg Psychiatry* 1983;46:227–233.

79. Giordani B, Sackellares JC, Miller S. Improvement in neuropsychological performance in patients with refractory seizures after intensive diagnostic and therapeutic intervention. *Neurology* 1983;33:489–493.

80. Ludgate J, Keating J, O'Dwyer R, Callaghan N. An improvement in cognitive function following polypharmacy reduction in a group of epileptic patients. *Acta Neurol Scand* 1985;71:448–452.

81. Trimble MR, Thompson PJ. Anticonvulsant drugs and behaviour. In: Akimoto H, Mazamatsuri H, Seino M, Ward AA, eds. *Advances in epileptology: XIIIth epilepsy international symposium.* New York: Raven Press, 1982; 205–210.

82. Butlin AT, Wolfendale L, Danta G. Effects of anticonvulsants on memory functioning in epileptic patients. *Clin Exp Neurol* 1980;17:79–84.

83. Smith DB. Anticonvulsants, seizures and performance: the veteran's administration experience. In: Trimble MR, Reynolds EH, eds. *Epilepsy, behaviour and cognitive function.* Chichester, England: John Wiley & Sons, 1988; 67–78.

84. Gallassi R, Morneale A, Lorusso S, Procaccianti G, Lugaresi E, Baruzzi A. Carbamazepine and phenytoin comparison of cognitive effects in epileptic patients during monotherapy and withdrawal. *Arch Neurol* 1988;45:892–894.

85. Eich E. Epilepsy and state specific memory. *Acta Neurol Scand* 1986;74(Suppl 109):15–21.

86. Weiskrantz L, Koella WP. Highlights in presented papers on clinical aspects of memory functions. *Acta Neurol Scand* 1981;64(Suppl 89):75–82.

87. Weingartner H, Thompson K. Features of state-dependent cognitive dysfunctions. A framework for the analysis of learning—memory changes in seizure patients. *Acta Neurol Scand* 1986;74(Suppl 109):23–30.

88. Baddeley A. Memory theory and memory therapy. In: Wilson BA, Moffat N, eds. *Clinical management of memory problems.* Beckenham, England: Croom Helm, 1984;5–27.

89. Loiseau P, Signoret JL, Strube E. Attentional problems in adult epileptic patients. *Acta Neurol Scand* 1984;69(Suppl 99):31–34.

90. Bennett-Levy J, Stores G. The nature of cognitive dysfunction in schoolchildren with epilepsy. *Acta Neurol Scand* 1984;69(Suppl 99): 79–82.

91. Hermann BP, Wyler AR, Steenman H, Richey ET. The inter-relationship between language function and verbal learning/memory performance in patients with complex partial seizures. *Cortex* 1988;24:245–253.

92. Calev A, Korin Y, Shapira B, Kugelimass S, Lever B. Verbal and non-verbal recall by depressed and euthymic affective patients. *Psychol Med* 1986;16:789–794.

93. Mayes AR. Learning and memory disorders. *Neuropsychologia* 1986;24:25–39.

94. Flavell JH, Wellman HM. Metamemory. In: Kail RV, Hagen JW, eds. *Perspectives on the development of memory and cognition.* Hillsdale, NJ: Erlbaum, 1977.

95. Harris JE, Morris PE. Everyday memory, actions and absent mindedness. London: Academic Press, 1984.

96. Guerrant J, Anderson WW, Fischer A, Weinstein MR, Jaros JM, Deskins A. *Personality in epilepsy.* Springfield, IL: Charles C Thomas, 1962.

97. Broughton RJ, Guberman A, Roberts J. Comparison of the psychosocial effects of epilepsy and narcolepsy/cataplexy. A controlled study. *Epilepsia* 1984;25:423–433.

98. Bennett-Levy JM, Polkey CE, Powell GE. Self-report of memory skills after lobectomy: the effects of clinical variables. *Cortex* 1980; 16:543–557.

99. Robertson MM, Trimble MR, Townsend HRA. The phenomenology of depression in epilepsy. *Epilepsia* 1987;28:364–372.

100. Sunderland A, Harris JE, Baddeley AD. Do laboratory tests predict everyday memory? A neuropsychological study. *J Verb Learning Verb Behav* 1983;22:341–357.

101. Sunderland A, Harris JE. Memory failures in everyday life following severe head injury. *J Clin Neuropsychol* 1984;6:127–142.

102. Zigmond AS, Snaith RP. The Hospital Anxiety and Depression Scale. *Acta Psychiatr Scand* 1983;67:361–370.

103. Beck AT, Ward CH, Mendelson M, Mock J, Erbaugh JK. An inventory for measuring depression. *Arch Gen Psychiatry* 1961;4:561–571.

104. Hermann DJ. Questionnaires about memory. In: Harris JE, Morris PE, eds. *Everyday memory: actions and absentmindedness.* London: Academic Press, 1984;133–152.

105. Ley P. Memory for medical information. *Br J Soc Clin Psychol* 1979;18:245–255.

106. Thompson PJ. Psychological aspects of noncompliance. In: Schmidt D, Leppik I, eds. *Compliance in epilepsy (Epilepsy Res. Suppl 1)* Amsterdam: Elsevier, 1988.

107. Wilkins AJ, Baddeley AD. Remembering to recall in everyday life: an approach to absentmindedness. In: Gruneberg MM, Morris PE, Sykes RN, eds. *Practical aspects of memory.* London: Academic Press, 1978.

108. Wilson B, Moffat N. *Clinical management of memory problems.* Beckenham, England: Croom Helm, 1984.

109. Powell GE, Sutherland S, Agu GA. Serial position, rehearsal and recall in temporal lobe epilepsy. *Br J Clin Psychol* 1984;23:153–154.

Advances in Neurology, Vol. 55, edited by
D. Smith, D. Treiman, and M. Trimble,
Raven Press, Ltd., New York © 1991.

24

Memory Dysfunction in Epilepsy Patients as a Derangement of Normal Physiology

Eric Halgren,*† June Stapleton,†**
Patricia Domalski,†** Barbara E. Swartz,†**
Antonio V. Delgado-Escueta,*† Gregory O. Walsh,**
Mark Mandelkern,‡ William Blahd,‡ and
Jim Ropchan‡

*Departments of Psychiatry, Psychology, Neurology and Medicine, Brain Research Institute,
and †California Comprehensive Epilepsy Center, University of California—Los Angeles,
Los Angeles, California 90024; **Southwest Regional Epilepsy Center/Neurology, Department
of Physics, University of California-Irvine, Irvine, California 92717. ‡Nuclear
Medicine Services, Wadsworth Veterans Administration Medical Center,
West Los Angeles, California 90073*

Most of our knowledge of the anatomy and physiology of human memory has come from what has often seemed a coincidence: the critical role played by the human medial temporal lobe (MTL) in experiential memory as well as in many complex partial seizures (CPS). CPS arising in the MTL can be treated by removal of MTL structures (hippocampus, amygdala, and parahippocampal gyrus), with or without the overlying cortex, usually with excellent results (20). Postsurgical study of a single patient with epilepsy, H.M., who received a bilateral MTL removal, has led to a detailed description of the cognitive abilities that are lost, as well as preserved, in global amnesia (2–4). If a memory deficit occurs following a unilateral MTL excision, it is less severe and material-specific (5). The electrodes implanted into the MTL to localize seizure onset prior to surgical treatment have also been used to record during memory tasks. Often, clinical investigations of the MTL's role in epileptogenesis have proceeded independently (and in an unrelated theoretical framework) from investigations of MTL's role in memory, despite the fact that they are performed on the same patients and in the same structures.

We argue in this chapter that recent advances in both fields provide a starting point for their integration. We begin by reviewing the characteristics and circumstances of memory deficits in patients with epilepsy, concluding that they seem to reflect either permanent MTL damage (e.g., sclerosis), temporary dysfunction (e.g., ictal or postictal), or phasic disruption (following an epileptiform spike). We describe a neural model of human recent memory, discuss the apparent physiological manifestations of normal memory processing, and present evidence indicating that epileptogenic processes and these normal memory-related processes share the same synaptic circuits. Finally, we consider how the neurological processes developed to support associative memory may render the MTL sensitive to epileptogenic damage, how the local circuitry for autoassociative networks is prone to produce hypersynchronous discharges, and how the afferent, efferent, and modulatory connections needed for experiential memory are ideal for producing the mental and behavioral phenomena of CPS.

VARIETIES OF MEMORY LOSS IN COMPLEX PARTIAL SEIZURES

Permanent Memory Deficits

Background

Epileptic seizures may be symptomatic of a wide variety of brain dysfunction. The underlying pathology may be structural or molecular only, and it may be diffuse or focal. The original cause of the epileptogenic lesion often produces other lesions which are not epileptogenic. Thus, it is not surprising that a large sample of epilepsy patients with diverse seizure types and etiologies will, on the average, score somewhat below a normal control group on a wide variety of neuropsychological tests (6–8).

In general, the tests which show the largest and most reliable difference between normal and epileptic subjects are those which are also sensitive to other organic neurological impairments. The effects of anticonvulsants on these test measures are very difficult to determine with certainty. However, at nontoxic blood levels, anticonvulsant effects are thought by some to be minor compared to other factors influencing performance (7), but this is a subject of some controversy (9).

While on the average, patients with epilepsy score below controls on neuropsychological tests, many have normal or superior intelligence and no interictal neuropsychological deficit. Others are severely impaired. The principal factors associated with impairment are as follows: (a) a known etiology (as opposed to "idiopathic" epilepsy) (7,8); (b) early onset and long duration of the seizure disorder (10); (c) a high seizure frequency and/or a large number of total lifetime major seizures (11,12); (d) generalized tonic–clonic or CPS, rather than simple partial or petit mal only; and (e) a highly disordered electroencephalogram (EEG)—that is, frequent interictal epileptiform paroxysms with a slow posterior dominant rhythm and coexisting nonepilepti-

form transients (13–15). These factors all seem to be associated with a greater likelihood of diffuse brain damage, and thus it is not surprising that they are also associated with diffuse neuropsychological impairment.

Classical neuropsychological techniques have been applied in an attempt to detect specific deficits characteristic of the structural substrate for different seizure types, as inferred from neurophysiological and neuropathological data. In particular, CPS often start in, or primarily generalize through, limbic structures lying in the MTL. A temporal focus was originally suggested to Jackson and Colman (16) by postmortem findings in patients with "uncinate fits"; this focus has since been confirmed by well-documented studies using direct scalp EEG recordings from MTL structures simultaneously with closed-circuit television (CCTV) monitoring of ictal behavior. Postmortem studies (17) as well as histological examination of anterior temporal lobes removed as treatment for CPS have confirmed MTL sclerosis as the most frequent lesions; in addition, they have found hamartomas, arteriovenous malformations, and other lesions (18). Confirmation of the involvement of the MTL in CPS is provided by the success of anterior temporal lobectomy in eliminating the seizures of many patients (provided that MTL structures are removed) (19–23).

Although the computed tomography (CT) scan is usually normal, positron emission tomography (PET) studies indicate that the area of depressed function in many patients may extend considerably beyond the MTL. Synaptic activity and the resulting ionic fluxes use most of the energy consumed by the brain (24). Since this energy is derived almost entirely from the oxidation of glucose, measurement of the local cerebral metabolic rate for glucose ($LCMR_{Glu}$) should be a good indicator of each region's functional activity. In fact, PET has demonstrated large increases (over resting) in $LCMR_{Glu}$ in the appropriate anatomical structures in response to sensory stimulation, movement, and the performance of a cognitive task (25). In the resting state, PET has consistently indicated that the lateral temporal neocortex, as well as the MTL, is hypometabolic in patients with MTL sclerosis, even though the lateral temporal neocortex may be histologically normal (26).

It has long been noted that an interictal spike focus or an identified pathological lesion in any lobe may be associated with CPS (1). Recent anatomical work in monkeys identified pathways from association cortex of all lobes to the MTL (27,28), suggesting that in some cases the MTL, known to have a low threshold for paroxysmal activity, can be activated secondarily from a focus elsewhere. Once activated, the MTL may interfere with activity in widespread brain areas through its direct projections to the brainstem (29) as well as back to association neocortex (30,31). This sequence of electrographic events finds a parallel in the subjective and behavioral characteristics of CPS: A great variety of auras (including those suggestive of occipital, parietal, and temporal involvement) may be followed by a stereotyped loss of awareness, nonreactive automatisms, and so forth (32,33).

It is now well established that MTL damage resulting from surgery, stroke, or encephalitis may lead to a severe transmodal decrement in the patient's ability to form new memories (4,34–38). This decrement displays material-specificity corresponding to the laterality of MTL damage with respect to hemispheric speech dominance (5,38). Memory for childhood events, for information within the current span-of-attention, and for perceptuomotor skills is well-preserved, as is general linguistic and other intellectual capacities. These recent memory deficits are present presurgically in some patients with CPS. On the average, patients with probable left-hemisphere foci have decreased ability to learn word-pairs or to remember a paragraph after a delay (39,40). Those with probable right-hemisphere foci have decreased ability to reproduce a complex figure from memory (41). Less commonly noted are signs of lateral temporal lobe involvement in the dominant hemisphere (anomia) (42) or nondominant hemisphere (failure to detect picture anomalies) (43).

As would be expected, given the heterogeneity of pathological substrate for CPS, neither the PET nor the neuropsychological signs of MTL pathology are present in every patient; on the average across all patients, these deficits are rather small. Some investigators have failed to detect these deficits, possibly because they used tests (e.g., the Wechsler Adult Intelligence Scale and the original Wechsler Memory Scale) which are insensitive to the recent-memory deficits. Other difficulties in demonstrating MTL deficits arise from (a) the small number of epilepsy subjects studied and (b) the failure to include normal controls. Some patients describe generalized tonic–clonic seizures which, when they are analyzed by CCTV, are seen to actually represent secondary generalization from CPS. In any case, it is possible that even primary generalized tonic–clonic seizures may lead to hippocampal damage, due to the sensitivity of the hippocampus to metabolic and anoxic stress. Finally, the criterion used to lateralize pathology in most studies is a preponderance of interictal epileptiform spikes. However, the laterality of interictal spikes is only imperfectly correlated with laterality of spontaneous seizure onset or of structural damage (21). Thus, groups of epilepsy patients classified on the basis of clinical history or interictal spike focus are likely to be heterogeneous and overlapping in seizure type and/or true seizure focus. Therefore, comparison of memory performance across these groups may not reveal deficits which are actually present.

Incidence

A brief memory screening (BMS) battery has been developed to provide an initial assessment of recent memory functions in less than 90 min of neuropsychological testing time. It assesses verbal recent memory by testing free recall of two brief paragraphs [Logical Memory subtest of the Wechsler Memory Scale, as modified by Milner (44)] and by also testing paired-associates learning (Wechsler Memory Scale or Squire tests). It assesses nonverbal recent memory by testing free recall of a complex figure (Rey diagram). Recent memory is assessed in the context of general intelligence and cognitive functions as measured by the Wechsler Adult Intelligence Scale (WAIS), usually using the short form devised by Satz and Mogel (45). To date, the BMS battery has been administered to 61 patients with epilepsy (46), and 35 of these

TABLE 1. *Physiology of memory deficits*

	Normal memory	Verbal memory deficit	Nonverbal memory deficit	Global memory deficit	ALL
N	26	10	13	12	61
Age	35.7	37.3	42.5	47.7	39.7
	1.7	3.8	3.1	5.1	1.6
Educ.	13.1	13.1	12.3	12.6	12.9
	0.5	0.7	0.8	0.9	0.3
Age at onset	25.1	28.4	25.6	42.3	28.8
	1.7	5.9	4.1	6.6	2.0
No. seizures per month/partial	14.7	13.6	15.1	2.7	13.1
	5.7	7.5	9.2	1.6	3.6
generalized	0.7	0.6	0.0	0.2	0.5
	.3	.5	.0	.2	.2
VIQ	100.88	95.00	103.58	98.50	100.00
	2.3	3.9	5.3	6.6	2.0
PIQ	99.32	91.20	99.33	93.10	96.81
	2.5	4.1	4.7	5.1	1.9
FSIQ	100.08	92.90	101.17	96.20	98.37
	2.4	3.1	4.8	6.2	1.9
Digit span forwards	6.36	5.50	6.50	6.09	6.19
	.2	.4	.3	.3	.2
Digit span backwards	4.52	4.30	4.75	4.18	4.47
	.2	.5	.3	.4	.2
Digit symbol	7.88	6.90	6.25	6.50	7.12
	.6	.7	.6	.9	.4

showed deficits in recent memory. Ten were impaired in only verbal recent memory, 13 were impaired in only nonverbal recent memory, and 12 were impaired in both. The groups of patients with memory deficits showed no impairment in verbal, performance, or full-scale I.Q. when compared to norms or to the group of 26 patients with normal recent memory (Table 1). There were no significant differences among the four groups in terms of digit span [forwards or backwards (immediate memory)], although the lowest mean digit span forwards was in the verbal-memory-impaired group. Digit symbol was similarly impaired in all four groups, possibly due to psychomotor slowing from antiepileptic medications. In this preliminary sample, there were no differences among the four groups in terms of education, frequency of partial seizures, or frequency of generalized seizures. The global (verbal and nonverbal)-memory-

deficit group was 12 years older than the normal-memory group, although age differences did not quite reach statistical significance $[F(3,43) = 2.74, p = 0.055]$. The global-memory-deficit group had a later age at seizure onset $[F(3,32) = 4.09, p <0.02]$. In general, interictal EEG abnormalities were common in these patients (76%), whereas abnormalities on CT scan were less frequent (22%). The presence of localization of abnormalities on interictal EEG or CT scan was not predictive of the degree of memory disorder.

These results were obtained in a clinic for veterans with epilepsy. The studies reviewed by Thompson (see Chapter 23, *this volume*) indicate that memory deficits are common in less selected groups of epileptics, and that these deficits are similar to those noted in amnesia—a verbal and/or nonverbal recent memory loss with preservation of immediate and remote memory as well as of general intelligence.

Case Reports

Intensive study of individual patients further clarifies the nature of the memory loss and its relation to underlying pathology. Three cases are described. In case 1, complex status epilepticus was followed by a severe and permanent recent-memory disorder. In the other two cases, a nonverbal recent-memory disorder is associated with seizures beginning in the right MTL.

Case 1

Background. This woman suffered an episode of herpes encephalitis at the age of 21. For approximately 6 months after the acute stage of the illness, she continued to experience frequent CPS (sometimes with generalization) and several periods of complex partial status. CPS begin with a motionless stare, but focal motor signs appear within the first 10 sec. Six years after onset, occasional seizures persist, but CT, magnetic resonance imaging (MRI), and PET scans are normal.

The patient reports having had an excellent memory prior to her illness. She consistently exhibited severe retrograde amnesia of about 6 months duration. For example, she cannot remember having advanced to sargeant, nor can she recall having established a serious romantic relationship, both of which occurred some months prior to her illness. She also stated that her vocabulary was diminished but that it is now improving. In addition to her dense retrograde amnesia, she has a very poor memory for events which have occurred since her illness began. At the time of her first testing session (1 year after onset), she knew she was in Los Angeles but did not know where. She knew the month and year but was mistaken as to the date and day of the week, despite constant practicing of the place and date. She did not remember or recognize nurses or other ward personnel despite over 2 weeks of daily interactions.

The patient reports an increased volatility of emotion since her illness. When initially admitted, she showed elements of an organic psychosis which culminated in an acute paranoid episode. As a result of this episode, she was placed on a low dosage of Haldol. Currently, she is pleasant and animated, living in

the community but unable to go back to work.

Test Results. General Intelligence was in the average range on the short-form WAIS (full-scale I.Q. = 94) (45), with no marked difference between verbal and performance tests (verbal I.Q. = 93; performance I.Q. = 97). Handedness was normal "right," according to the Pin Test (Rt, mean = 47; Lt, mean = 32). Performance was in the normal range on the Formboard (Rt 5'3", Lt 4'15"; Both 2'49"; M = 6), Wechsler Memory Scale Designs (11/14), direct copy of the Rey diagram (33/36), and Digit Cancellation (1'18" with no errors). Performance on verbal tests was low: 15–19th percentile on Benton's Controlled Word Association Test (CWAT), and 5–7th percentile on Benton's Visual Naming. Remote memory for famous faces was impaired on the recall measure (2/82), but it was adequate on multiple choice (45/80). Performance was also somewhat low, but it was adequate on multiple choice tests of recent memory for public events and for TV show titles.

Recent memory was severely impaired on all tests. She could remember no content from paragraphs presented 70 min previously (logical memory). Her immediate recall of the paragraphs (a score of 6) was also somewhat below what one would expect for a person with her verbal I.Q. On three trials of paired-associates learning, she remembered 5,6,6 of the six easy pairs and 0,0,3 of the four hard pairs. On five successive presentations of the same list (A) of 15 words (AVTL), she remembered 4, 6, 5, 6, and 7. She remembered four words from the next list but then remembered none from the original list A. It is also of interest that on each of the first two recalls of list A, she gave an intrusion error from the CWAT. Nonverbal recent memory was also impaired: When she was tested on recall of the Rey diagram, her score was only 11 after a 3-min delay (compared to a score of 33 for direct copy). Also, the memory for location on the Halstead–Reitan Formboard was impaired (her score was 1).

Conclusion. This patient shows severe recent-memory deficit in the presence of preserved general intelligence and perception, characteristic of global amnesia. The 6-month retrograde amnesia revealed by her clinical history—together with grossly normal, more remote memories on formal testing—is in keeping with the depth of her anterograde amnesia. In addition to the recent-memory deficit, the test results suggest a much milder deficit in verbal processing.

Case 2

Background. This 17-year-old right-handed woman had febrile convulsions at the age of 9 months, and she has had CPS since the first grade. These seizures had been uncontrolled since age 14 despite high levels of various anticonvulsant medications. Her seizures began with a blank motionless stare, followed by grasping with the left hand, aimless wandering, and then postictal confusion. Auras, when present, could be a peculiar tingling sensation in her head, a bad overtaking force, or a bad taste. The seizure discharge began in Sp2, spreading to T4/T8 after 5–10 sec. Interictal EEGs showed spiked reversing at the right sphenoidal lead. MRI (Fig. 1) indicated increased T2 signal in the medial temporal lobe, and PET (Fig. 2) indicated decreased metabolism in the right medial and lateral temporal lobe. She was a B student in high school but complained of lethargy and word-finding problems.

Test Results (Preoperative). Overall intellectual level was low average (WAIS-R full scale I.Q. = 87), with significantly stronger verbal (verbal I.Q. = 101) than nonverbal (performance I.Q. = 73) skills. Her performance on both the Purdue Pegboard and Pin tests were well below normal, suggesting impaired motor coordination and speed, although she was consistently better with her dominant hand. On all tests of visuospatial ability (Rey Complex Figure Copy, Benton Facial Recognition, and Hooper Visual Organization), Case 2's performance was indicative of impaired visuospatial perception, as was also suggested by the WAIS-R. Her performance on the Benton Token and Visual Naming Test was normal, indicating that receptive language functioning was intact and that she was able to find appropriate verbal labels for objects. However, a borderline score on the CWAT suggested that her ability to freely generate lists of words was slightly impaired, which stands apart from her above-average vocabulary. Case 2 demonstrated an

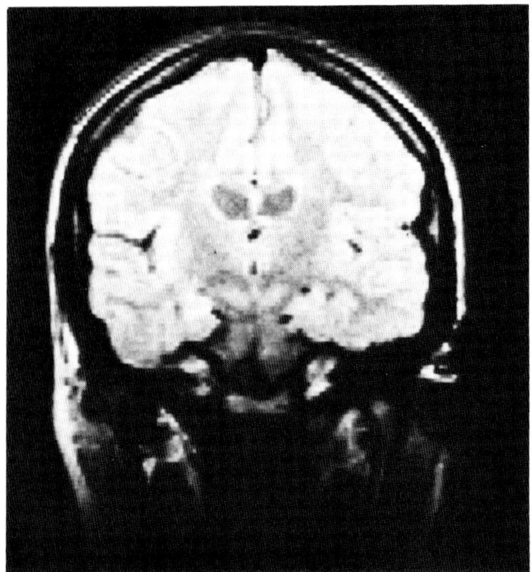

FIG. 1. MRI scan of Case 2, a woman with CPS originating in the right medial temporal lobe, where increased T2 signal is observed (leftside).

excellent ability to complete the Wisconsin Card Sorting Test, indicating that she was capable of implementing and adapting strategies based on examiner feedback. Furthermore, she was able to concisely and accurately describe the task principle verbally.

Adequate verbal paired-associate learning (WMS) and word recall [WEB: Wadsworth Memory Battery (47)] indicated adequate verbal recent memory. Immediate recall of paragraphs (logical memory) was below normal, but recall of the material after a 1-hr delay was adequate. Her ability to reconstruct the Rey Complex Figure after a 30-min delay was impaired (below 10th percentile). Further evidence of a spatial memory deficit is demonstrated on the Halstead–Reitan Tactual Performance Test. Although she was able to correctly draw eight of 10 shapes from memory, she could localize only two.

Behavioral observations, the clinical interview, and the Minnesota Multiphasic Personality Inventory (MMPI) and Washington Psychosocial Seizure Inventory (WPSI) all indicated moderate depression, centered around issues of independence. Although these issues are normal for later adolescence, they were compounded by protective parents, con-

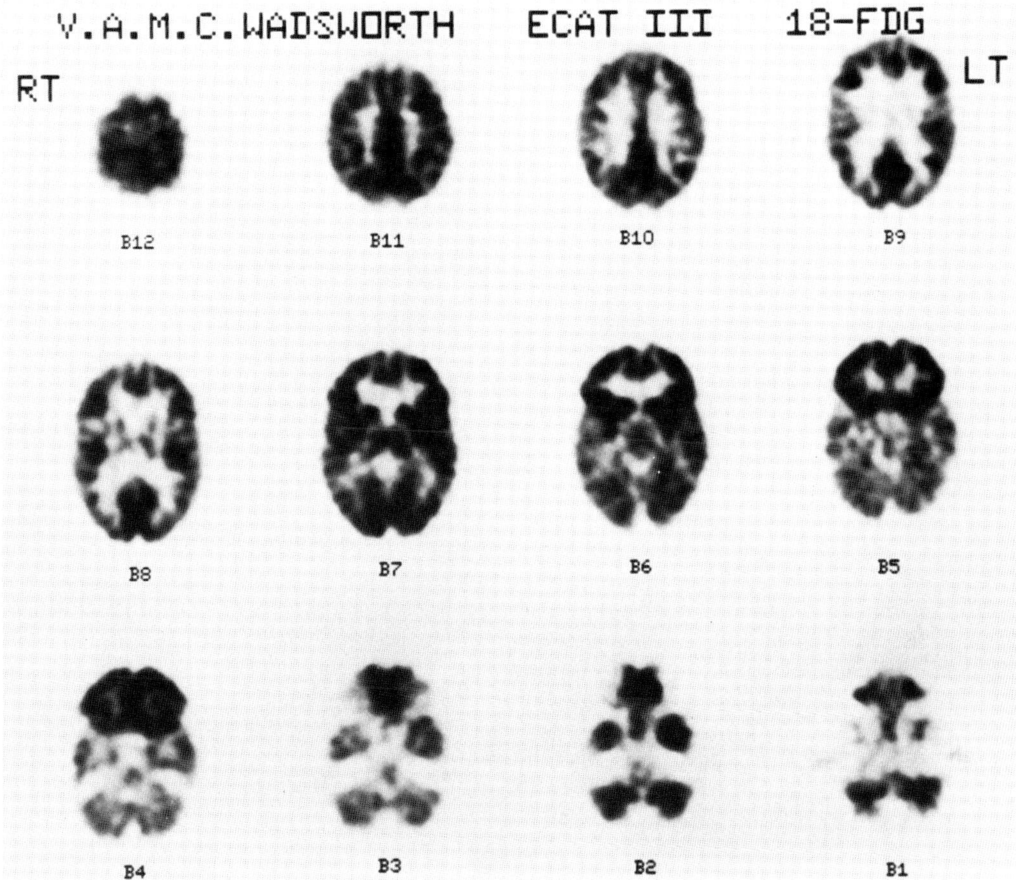

FIG. 2. PET scan of the distribution of fluorodeoxyglucose (FDG PET) in Case 2. Decreased LCMR$_{Glu}$ is seen in both medial and lateral temporal regions on the right (sections B3–B6).

stant drowsiness (presumably secondary to anticonvulsants), and an inability to drive; to make matters worse, the suburban community in which she lived did not have public transportation.

Conclusion. This patient showed moderate deficits in nonverbal recent memory, visuospatial perception, and psychomotor speed. Since the modified Wada test indicated left-hemisphere dominance for language, this implied right MTL and right temporoparietal dysfunction, compounded by high levels of anticonvulsants. After an additional 2 years of unsuccessful attempts at seizure control with different anticonvulsant regimes, a right anterior temporal lobectomy (including 4 cm of the lateral surface and the entire MTL) was performed. Postoperative pathological inves-

tigation found hippocampal sclerosis. At 1 year follow-up, psychomotor speed had dramatically improved; visuoperceptual abilities had also improved, but more moderately. Nonverbal recent memory was unchanged. The patient was attending junior college, managing a small movie theater, and maintaining an active social life. She is no longer depressed.

Case 3

Background. This 45-year-old woman began having seizures at age 23; they were characterized by brief periods of dizziness, dreaminess, and a feeling that she was "not in her body." At the time of examination, her

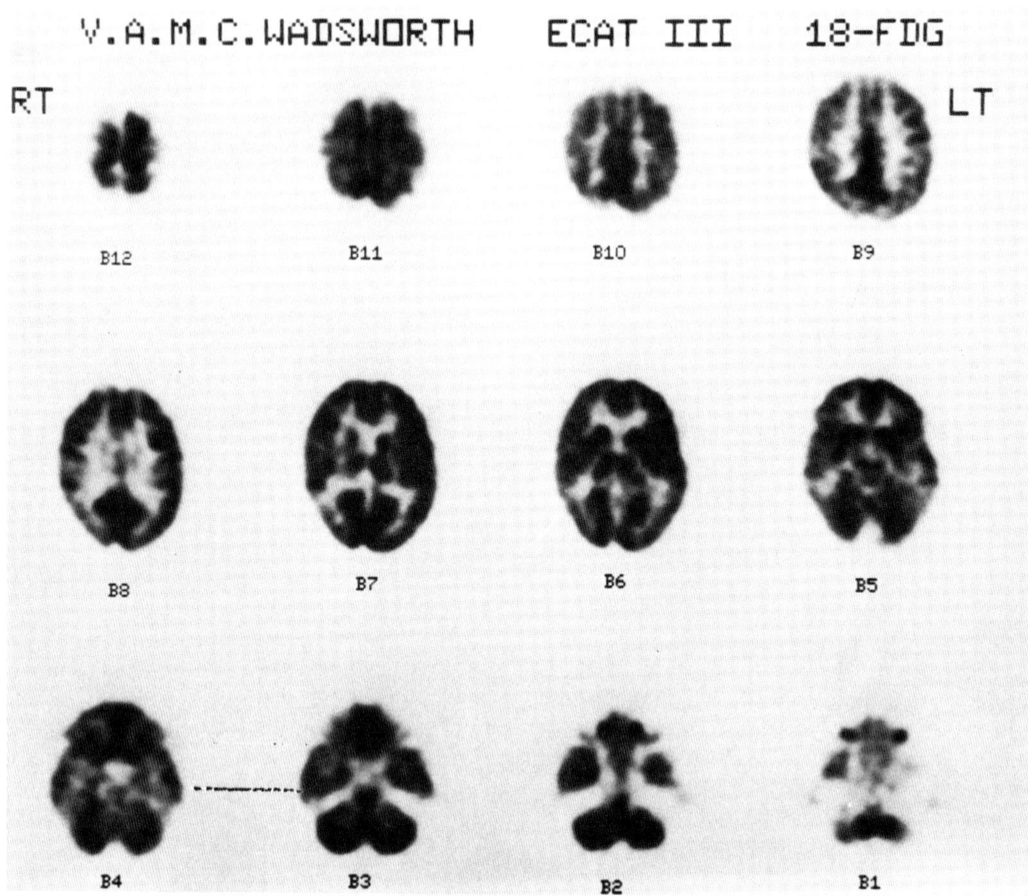

FIG. 3. FDG PET of Case 3, a patient with seizures originating in the right lateral temporo-occipital cortex in the region of the hypometabolism observed here.

seizure began with a feeling of fear and then a thought of the word "seizure." She then lost contact, pursed and smacked her lips, giggled, froze, and was confused. After returning to normal awareness, she often failed to enter events into memory (postictal transient anterograde amnesia). For example, after recovering from a seizure she went shopping with her husband for approximately a half hour. Later that day she had no recollection of what she bought, where she went, or even having gone at all, despite having acted completely normal during that time, according to her husband's report. A focal lesion in the right lateral parieto-occipital cortex was demonstrated with MRI and fluorodeoxyglucose PET (Fig. 3). Subdural strip electrodes found a right parietal discharge spreading after 3–10 sec to the right MTL (coincident with the giggle), and then diffusely. Case 3 is married and works as a music teacher in a religious preschool.

Test Results. Case 3 is right-handed and left-dominant for language, according to the modified Wada test. Full-scale (110) and performance (115) I.Q. on the WAIS-R were in the high average range, and verbal I.Q. (106) was average. Manual dexterity and psychomotor speed were normal for both hands. Performance on tests of visual perception and spatial abilities were generally normal—with the exception of the copying of the Rey diagram (score = 29), which showed impairments that were more consistent with impaired attention and fine motor control than with impaired visuospatial abilities. Language abilities such as vocabulary, word-finding, and aural comprehension were all in the average to high-average range. Although there was clinical evidence of fluctuations in attention, tests directly tapping the ability to maintain attention generally showed normal scores. Other areas of mental control, such as verbal fluency, ability to produce effective strategies, and ability to appropriately respond to feedback, were all normal. For example, she achieved six categories in the Wisconsin Card Sorting Task (which involved 85 cards), with only 13 perseverative errors.

Immediate, recent, and remote verbal memory were all in the normal range. Immediate nonverbal memory (block span = 4) was normal. Recent nonverbal memory was moderately to severely impaired. For example, recall of the Rey diagram was 5, recall of block location on the Halstead–Reitan Tactile Performance Test was 2, and recall of the location of symbols previously copied onto a page (WEB symbol location) was near-chance. These results suggest an impairment in the right medial temporal lobe. The limited psychosocial screening suggested a basically normal individual with some indication of difficulties in adjustment to her seizures.

Conclusion. This patient exhibited a transient postictal global amnesia, together with a chronic nonverbal recent-memory deficit, presumably due to spread of her seizure from a right parieto-occipital focus to the MTL. A limited resection of the seizure focus was performed, and the lesion was identified as a ganglioglioma. Postoperative neuropsychological examination revealed essentially no change from the preoperative state. However, seizures returned and the right medial temporal lobe and temporal pole were excised. She is now seizure-free.

Comment

The characteristics of the memory problems exhibited by these three patients, as well as those in our larger survey, are typical of the deficits that have been described after medial temporal lobe damage. General intelligence, as indicated by the I.Q., is preserved, as are basic language and perceptual functions. Remote memory is normal, as indicated by preserved vocabulary, general knowledge, and recognition of faces or facts that were well known many years ago. Immediate memory is also normal, according to digit and block span. In contrast, explicit (or declarative) learning of new integrations of cognitively complex materials is severely impaired. This includes deficient cued and free recall of words or stories, deficient word recognition in the verbal domain (associated with dominant MTL dysfunction), and deficient recall of diagrams or locations in the nonverbal domain (suggesting nondominant MTL dysfunction).

Patients with CPS may display verbal or nonverbal recent-memory deficits, or they may display both or neither. In some cases (e.g., Case 2 above), the memory deficit corresponds to focal MTL damage, demonstrated by neuroimaging and/or pathological examination of the surgically resected MTL. Recently, quantitative studies have found a positive correlation between MTL cell-loss and presurgical memory impairments (see Chapter 17, *this volume*). However, in other patients (e.g., Case 3 above) there is apparently no permanent MTL damage. Rather, the seizure is seen to spread to the MTL, which consequently may be chronically physiologically deranged. We shall consider this issue further in the next section, with examples of patients who have temporary memory deficits associated with temporary MTL dysfunction.

Temporary Memory Deficits

Background

By definition, the brain dysfunction in patients with epilepsy is largely transient. The simplest tasks sensitive to transient deficits are those which require simple or disjunctive reactions to sensory stimuli. When tasks of this nature are used, patients with petit mal seizures, as compared to patients with CPS, show a specific impairment (48,49). Analysis of this deficit has revealed that the transient disruptions occur during brief three-per-second spike-and-wave discharges which produce no overt behavioral signs (50–53) (intense analysis of videotapes of these episodes may reveal slight facial twitches (51)). The general methodology of these studies is to use electronic circuits to detect the spike-

and-wave discharge. This detection triggers the presentation of a stimulus to which a simple or choice reaction is required. These studies have found that: (a) production of the response was more impaired than was the reception of the stimulus; (b) complex responses may be severely impaired by paroxysms that have no apparent effect on simple responses; and (c) the complexity of the task that can be performed during spike-and-wave complexes varies between subjects, apparently in loose relationship to the extent of the cerebral involvement as reflected in the EEG.

The deleterious effects of petit mal discharges on retention in memory have been studied by first presenting a series of digits, then inducing a discharge with photic stimulation, and finally testing for recall. The recall defect is maximal if the discharge immediately follows stimulus presentation and then falls to zero after a 4-sec delay (54). The recall deficit is confined to the last two digits presented, with memory for the first two digits remaining normal (55). The opposite pattern is observed in amnesics with MTL damage, who forget the initial stimuli but remember the final stimuli in a list (56). In normal subjects, recall of the final digits is held to represent primary memory, and recall of the initial digits is considered to represent recent memory. Thus, the data suggest that petit mal discharges affect the primary memory system, whereas MTL damage impairs recent declarative memory.

An attempt to demonstrate a similar transient cognitive deficit during subclinical paroxysmal discharges in patients with partial seizures was reported by Kooi and Hovey (57,58). These investigators noted that "nonresponses" were more common during intelligence testing in epilepsy patients than in patients with other organic or functional pathology, and they also noted that these "nonresponses" were usually associated with subclinical epileptiform paroxysms. In this pioneering study, neither the seizure classification, type of interictal paroxysm, timing of the paroxysm with respect to the task, nor nature of the resulting psychological deficit were well-defined. In a more controlled study, Binnie and co-workers (59,60) found that a stimulus would tend to be lost from short-term memory if an epileptiform paroxysm had occurred during its presentation. Nonverbal

stimuli were lost if the paroxysms were lateralized to the right hemisphere, and verbal stimuli were lost if the paroxysms were lateralized to the left hemisphere (Chapter 7).

The highest degree of anatomical and temporal resolution has been reported by Shewmon and Erwin (61,62). In three patients, they found that lateralized occipital interictal spikes impaired detection of a simultaneously presented, brief (150 msec) visual stimulus in the corresponding hemifield. Spikes which extended more anteriorly tended to also produce a greater deficit when responses were made by the contralateral hand. The size of the deficit was correlated with the amplitude of the spike-and-wave complex. Interestingly, when the amplitudes of the spike and of the wave varied independently, the deficit was correlated with the wave rather than with the spike (63). Further supporting the critical role of the slow wave in disrupting neural processing was Shewmon and Erwin's finding that a deficit persisted even if stimulus presentation was delayed until the spike was over, provided that the slow wave was still present.

Longer-duration MTL paroxysmal discharges that are still too spatially restricted to produce an aura or clinical seizure have nonetheless been hypothesized to sometimes produce transient global amnesia (see Chapters 7 and 22). This syndrome is characterized by a specific deficit in recent declarative memory, accompanied by preserved language, skilled movements, and general intelligence (64,65). Although this disorder is generally considered to be due to vascular causes, patients have been reported who have repeated episodes of transient global amnesia (accompanied by temporal spike discharges) and who were cured by anticonvulsants (66–68).

In addition to preoccupying neuronal interactions with paroxysmal activity, subclinical and clinical seizures are followed by profoundly depressed neuronal activity for a period of minutes to hours. As described in the preceding section, if several seizures recur without return of full awareness (i.e., complex partial status epilepticus), then long-term, and even permanent, neuronal dysfunction may result (69). Presumably as a result of this dysfunction, in individual cases, specific anterograde and retrograde recent-memory deficits have been observed to last for weeks or months after complex partial status epilepticus (70,71).

These studies demonstrate that paroxysmal activity, from single spike-and-wave complexes to status epilepticus, can severely disrupt cognitive processing. The disrupting effects of paroxysms help explain why removal of their generators, in animals (72) or in humans (73) (see also Chapters 7 and 23), often results in improved cognitive function. However, recent memory deficits have not been demonstrated during MTL spikes, and the production of transient global amnesia by MTL paroxysms is based on circumstantial evidence. Finally, although postictal memory deficits have been described clinically since the beginning of the century, no objective or quantitative reports documenting the extent or specificity of this deficit have been published.

Postseizure Memory Deficits

A brief battery has been developed to assess the effects of a seizure on cognition and

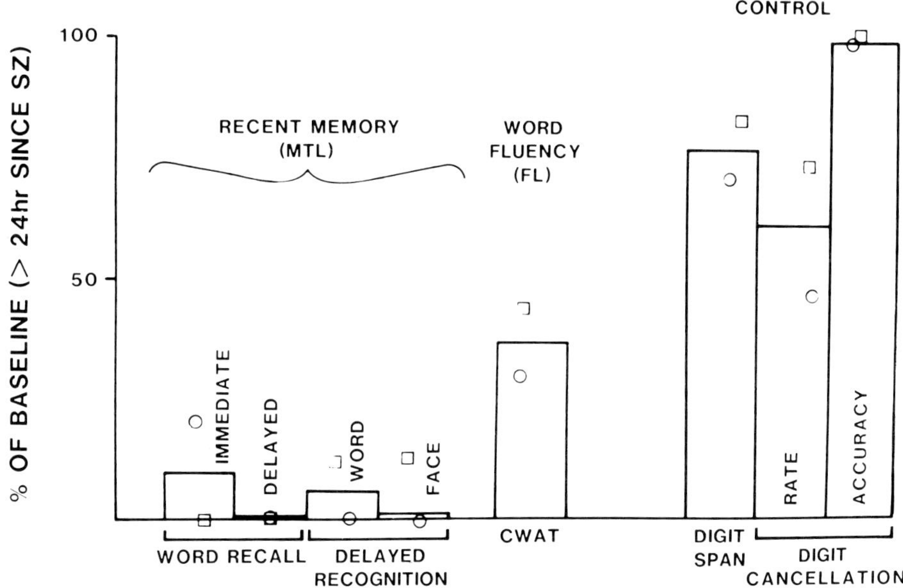

FIG. 4. The following test battery was administered: (1) present 10 low-imagery words; (2) test for immediate word recall (column 1 above); (3) present 10 faces; (4) test digit span forwards (column 6); (5) test word fluency (column 5) in timed production of words beginning with a given letter [like Benton's Controlled Word Association Test (CWAT)]; (6) test mental control using timed concellation of target digits (columns 7 and 8); (7) test delayed recall for words presented in step 1 (column 2); (8) test for "yes/no" recognition of words presented in step 1 (column 3) (~15-min delay); and (9) test delayed recognition of faces presented in step 3 (column 4). Different forms of this test battery, identical except for the stimuli used, were administered: (1) immediately postictal, as soon as verbal communication was established; (2) postictal early recovery, beginning 81 min (patient □) or 30 min (patient ○) after the first testing session began; and (3) interictal baseline, at least 24 hr after the last seizure or aura. Interictally, both patients have average intelligence. Patient □ had normal recent memory and had no known etiology for his seizures. PT ○ had depressed nonverbal recent memory, consistent with the shrapnel wound in his right medial temporal lobe (MTL). Immediately postictal, both verbal and nonverbal recent memory was severely depressed compared to baseline. Word fluency was also depressed, but less severely so, and performance on the primary memory and mental control tasks were relatively preserved. Although not illustrated in the figure, performance on all tests at the early-recovery postictal time was essentially identical to baseline performance. In other words, memory capacity was substantially or completely recovered by 30–80 min after the seizure had ended. FL, frontal lobe; SZ, seizure.

memory. It includes tests of immediate memory (Digit Span Test), verbal fluency (Controlled Word Association Test), and sustained attention (Digit Cancellation Test), as well as a new test for recent memory for words and recent memory for faces. Figure 4 illustrates the performance on this test battery by two CPS patients immediately after the postictal confusion had cleared. Postictally, both verbal and nonverbal recent memory were severely depressed compared to baseline. Verbal fluency was moderately depressed, whereas immediate memory and attention were relatively preserved. All functions had recovered by the second testing at 60–80 min postictally.

More prolonged memory deficits may occur after multiple seizures. Figure 5 illustrates the memory and general cognitive performance of three patients. In two patients, we were able to study the transient cognitive effects of an episode of prolonged or recurrent seizures from which the patient recovered. One day after the episode, one of these patients showed clear deficits on all tests, including the WAIS. The second patient showed a deficit in recent memory, both verbal and nonverbal, in the context of intact general intelligence. When tested 2 weeks later, dramatic recovery was seen and both patients had no recollection of the testing session that had occurred during the day following the episode.

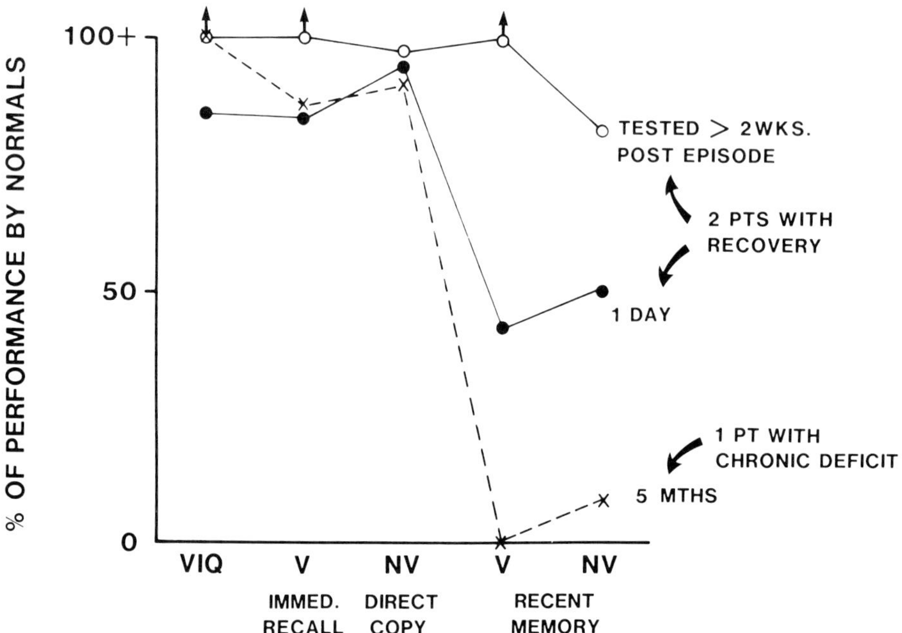

FIG. 5. Prolonged deficit with recovery (——). Two patients were tested on the day following an episode of multiple seizures (●). The same two patients were tested again 14 or 18 days after the episode (○). The verbal I.Q. (VIQ) was somewhat depressed on day 1 in one patient (15) and was normal in the other. However, by 2 weeks, both patients' VIQ had recovered to the level at which they had performed prior to the episode. Immediate recall of a paragraph was also slightly depressed on day 1, whereas direct copy of the Rey diagram was unchanged. In contrast to these weak postictal effects on general intellectual processes, performance on tests which more strongly involve recent memory (V—delayed paragraph recall; NV—delayed figure recall) were severely impaired when measured on day 1. By 2 weeks after the episode, however, recent memory performance had also recovered to normal levels. A 51-year-old, right-handed, successful salesman developed a profound and permanent anterograde amnesia [chronic deficit (– – –)] following an episode of complex partial status.

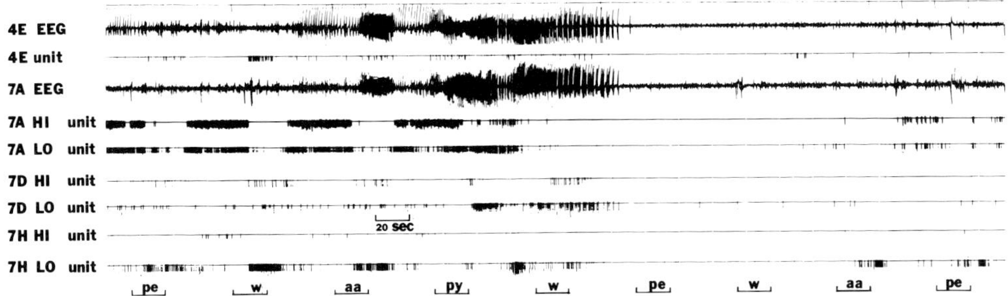

FIG. 6. Activity in one hippocampal (4E) and three amygdalar (7A, 7D, 7H) electrodes in relation to a subclinical EEG seizure which occurred during an olfactory recognition task. During the marked periods the patient sniffed from a flask containing water (w), amyl acetate (aa), pyridine (py), or phenyl ethyl alcohol (pe). The sniffing probably produced local cerebral hypoxia resulting in decreased firing by units 7A HI, 7A LO, and 7H HI, along with increased firing by units 4E, 7D, HI, and 7H LO. The displayed units represent the output of a window discrimator triggered by action potentials of a specified amplitude range. The HI units represent high-amplitude action potentials, and the LO units represent low-amplitude action potentials, each recorded with the same microelectrode. The amplitude of all accepted action potentials was at least twice the amplitude of the background activity. (From ref. 74, with permission.)

Induced Memory Deficits

Depth recordings from the human MTL often reveal seizure discharges that are accompanied by no subjective experiential phenomenon or objectively observed behavioral change (e.g., see Fig. 6). The afterdischarges (ADs) induced by electrical stimulation of the MTL resemble these subclinical seizures electrographically. In a retrospective study of 365 MTL ADs in 36 patients, 64% were accompanied by no behavioral or subjective phenomena. In particular, of these 365 MTL ADs, only 10 were found to evoke amnesia which could be detected by questions probing orientation and memory for recent events (M). Six of these 10 ADs were bilateral; the remaining four ADs were confined to the MTL opposite to that where the patient's seizures originated. Had amnesia been induced by ADs ipsilateral to seizure onset, surgery would be contraindicated. Objective memory testing during stimulation was introduced in order to increase the yield and reliability of clinically relevant information. A single-trial visually cued paired-associates paradigm, presumably sensitive to damage in either MTL (75), was used to probe recent memory. Low-current brain stimulation was delivered simultaneously to several electrode sites at 50 pulses per second during the presentation of stimulus drawings to three patients. All three experienced severe amnesia during unilateral MTL ADs induced by brain stimulation, but memory deficits were not reliably evoked by MTL stimulation in the absence of ADs (Fig. 7). Auras accompanied the AD in all three patients, but preoccupation with the auras could not account for the amnesia inasmuch as patients were able to perform mental arithmetic during auras, and no memory deficit was seen when patients experienced auras in the absence of AD.

Memory was tested during electrically triggered epileptiform spikes by requiring the delayed recognition of color slides of complex scenes presented for brief (100–200 msec) tachistoscopic exposure (76). Single-pulse stimulation synchronized with slide onset was applied to both MTLs simultaneously at increasing current levels until a significant recognition deficit was observed. Simultaneous unit and field-potential recordings at this strength indicated that local neural activity was preoccupied with responding to the electrical stimulus for about 500 msec (Fig. 8). These stimulation-evoked excitation–inhibition sequences closely resemble (in waveform and duration) spontaneous epileptiform paroxysms which have been observed in direct

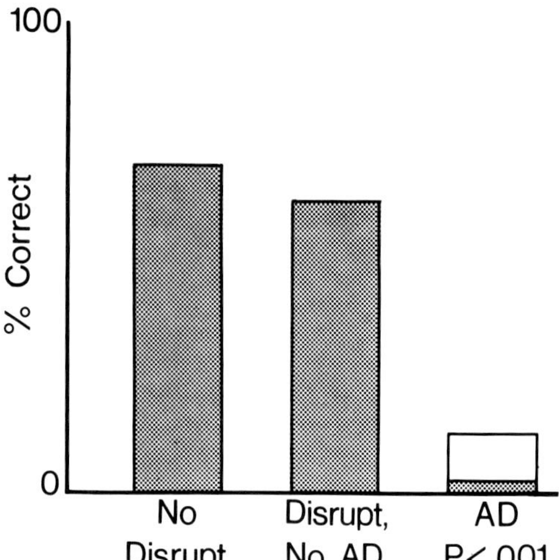

FIG. 7. Recall of response words in an image-cued paired-associates task during afterdischarges (ADs). Whereas there was a slight (nonsignificant) decline from control lists (*left bar*) to the list with stimulation which did not evoke an AD (*center bar*), ADs produced a very large decline in recall (*right bar*). All three correct recalls by patients during or after ADs were described as being "guesses" (*clear area of right bar*) (From ref. 76, with permission.)

recordings from the human MTL (77). Stimulation was then applied to each MTL in order to determine the contribution of the contralateral MTL to memory performance. In the nine patients who have been adequately tested with this paradigm, bilateral MTL disruption during both presentations of each slide greatly impaired recognition. If an equal disruption was induced but the delay between initial presentation and test for recognition was reduced to 2 sec, then no deficit was obtained, indicating that perceptual, decision, and response–execution processes were not grossly impaired.

Of these nine patients, seven had clinical evidence of a predominantly unilateral epileptogenic focus in the temporal lobe. For four of these seven patients, stimulation on the side opposite to the suspected focus produced clear memory deficits, whereas stimulation on the side of focus did not. In the other three patients, unilateral stimulation of either side was ineffective in inducing a memory deficit.

Depth recordings often reveal that interictal spiking is present bilaterally in the hippocampus, even in those patients with a clearly unilateral focal ictal onset (78). Recent studies suggest that spiking is a normal physiological activity in the nonepileptic rat hippocampus (79,84). Regardless of whether the hippocampal spikes in humans contralateral to the seizure focus represent normal or pathological activity, they provide another possible mechanism for interictal memory deficits. The above studies suggest that interictal spikes contralateral to a sclerotic or otherwise dysfunctional MTL may interfere briefly, but repeatedly, with memory formation and retrieval.

PHYSIOLOGY OF MEMORY LOSS

Normal Physiology of Human Memory

Pathways and Plasticity

As reviewed above, MTL damage impairs the conscious (or "explicit" or "declarative") recollection or recognition of recently occurring events. In the experiments described above, disruption of the MTL during memory input only, or during memory retrieval only, resulted in a memory deficit (85). Similarly, during MTL dysfunction in transient global amnesia (see above), there is a simultaneous inability to recall previously established memories (retrograde amnesia), accompanied by an inability to form new memories to be recalled after recovery from the amnesic episode (anterograde amnesia). Thus, the MTL is necessary for both the formation and retrieval of recent memories. This fact supports models in which the hippocampus contains a (perhaps imprecise) recent memory trace that is used by the association neocortex to reconstruct a recent event in its context until that event/context is abstracted and consolidated into the structure of the neocortex (86–90). Consistent with this model, the hippocampal formation receives projections from, and sends projections to, virtually all areas of posterior association cortex (91,92). Within the hippocampus itself are synapses which display a very powerful, long-lasting, and specific form of plasticity termed "long-term potentiation" (93,94). These characteristics are precisely what would be needed to link the

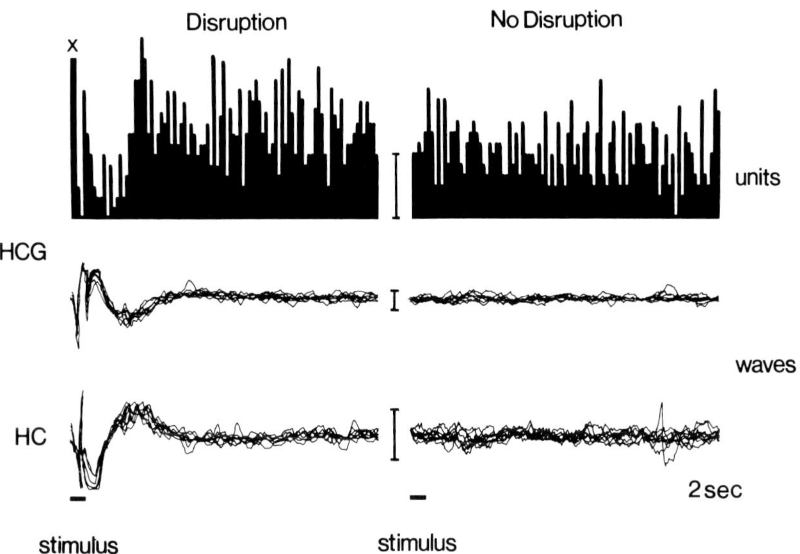

FIG. 8. Simultaneous recordings of field potential and multiple-unit activity from the left middle parahippocampal gyrus (HCG) and field potentials in the left middle hippocampus (HC) during the 100-msec exposure of the slide and the subsequent 2-sec intertrial interval. The averaged unit activity following 36 slides, along with the superimposed single-sweep field potentials following 10 slides of the test period of two different trays, is displayed. In the left histogram and traces ("disruption"), the amygdala, anterior and middle hippocampus, and middle and posterior parahippocampal gyrus were stimulated bilaterally with a single biphasic pulse at the beginning of each slide (X marks the stimulus artifact). The lack of response in the right half of the figure, which was recorded under identical task conditions but in the absence of stimulation, indicated that the response on the left is due to the electrical stimulus rather than to the slide or task. Scales indicate 5 spikes per second (units) and 200 µV (waves). (From ref. 85, with permission.)

disparate elements of highly processed neocortical input to the hippocampus within an event in order to produce an integrated associative memory trace.

Modulation and Information-Representation

The integration of these pathways and plasticity to produce memory performance can be monitored electrophysiologically. Recordings during memory tasks from depth electrodes implanted into the MTL for localization of the seizure focus have revealed large field potentials systematically related to familiarity (95). The first time a particular word or face is presented in a given task, it will evoke a large N4 (or N400) and small P3 (or P300). When the word or face is repeated, it evokes a small N4 and big P3 (96,97). N4 and P3 refer to evoked potential components, and they are each generated by the more-or-less synchronous activation of a distinct synaptic system (98). Both can be recorded at the scalp as well as in the depth, and thus they have been subjected to intensive study of their cognitive correlates in normal subjects. The N4 is evoked only by stimuli which are meaningful or potentially meaningful within a large symbolic system (e.g., words, faces, objects) (99). Once the N4 is evoked (beginning about 250 msec after the stimulus onset), its size and duration depends upon the amount and duration of processing necessary to integrate the stimulus with the ongoing cognitive context. The P3 follows the N4, and it appears to be evoked by either complex or simple stimuli, provided that the amount of processing they require is less than the amount of processing resources assigned to them (see ref. 100). Depth recordings indicate that both the N4 and P3 are generated in the MTL bilaterally and probably also in temporal, parietal, and frontal association cortices (101–104). In short, the N4/P3 appears to represent widespread cortical/MTL modulations underlying the cycle of divergent/convergent associative activation during contextual integration of cognitive stimuli (105).

The neural bases of these widespread modulations are unknown, but they are suspected to reflect the diffusely projecting cholinergic and noradrenergic triggering systems, perhaps indirectly via intrinsic GABAergic interneurons (100). These triggering systems, in turn, depend upon activation from localized antecedent cortical or limbic structures specific for each task (Fig. 9). For example, removal of the left (dominant) MTL plus overlying cortex has no significant effect on the scalp-recorded P3 potential evoked by infrequent tones (106–108). However, this same operation eliminates the P3 evoked by repeated words (96). This finding is consistent with the model presented in the previous sec-

tion. Patients with dominant MTL damage produce cortical N4/P3 sequences that show no effect of contextual trace information. Also consistent with the above model is the finding that, in the same tasks, at the time when this contextual trace information begins to influence the cortical N4/P3 sequence, human hippocampal units fire to specific words or faces (109). This information-specific firing could carry the influences of the contextual trace from the MTL to neocortex during retrieval.

Shared Circuits by Memory and Epilepsy

Because of the lack of detailed and validated neural models for human memory and epilepsy, and also because of limitations in the measurements possible in human subjects, the evidence for shared circuitry in memory and epilepsy is as yet indirect but is still suggestive of a deep and mutually revealing relationship.

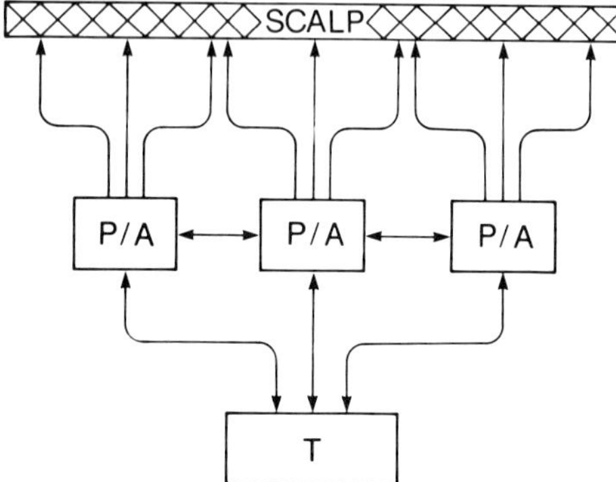

FIG. 9. Cognitive evoked-potential (EP) components recorded at the scalp seem to be generated in multiple brain structures. These structures are thus propagating generators (P) in the terminology of ref. 98. Each of these same structures may, in particular tasks, perform some computation that is necessary for the EP component to appear anywhere. In these tasks, that structure would thus be antecedent (A) to the other generators. It is likely that many cognitive EP components result from the activation of a diffusely projecting neuromodulatory trigger (T) structure that is apparently under the control of different P/A structures in different tasks. Thus, cognitive EPs may represent a mechanism whereby an individual structure can, if it is particularly competent in a given task, pace and synchronize the mode of information processing in other structures. (From ref. 126, with permission.)

Overt Mental Phenomena

Historically, the first evidence for an association between epilepsy and memory in the temporal lobe was the observation by Penfield and colleagues that the overt experiential phenomena of memory—vivid recollections (memory-based hallucinations) and intense illusions of familiarity (déjà vu)—can occur as auras in temporal lobe epilepsy (110,111). Penfield observed these phenomena during spontaneous auras as well as during auras evoked by electrical stimulation of the lateral temporal neocortex. Subsequent studies by Gloor et al. (112) (see Chapter 1), Halgren et al. (113) and Chauvel et al. (114) have supported Penfield's findings, but they suggest that an MTL/cortical circuit must be engaged in order to evoke experiential memories.

Epileptiform Activity Evoked by a Memory Task

Several factors are known to modulate the occurrence of interictal spike-and-wave complexes (SWC). Rarely, highly specific stimuli, including complex kinds of intellectual and cognitive functions, induce epileptiform dis-

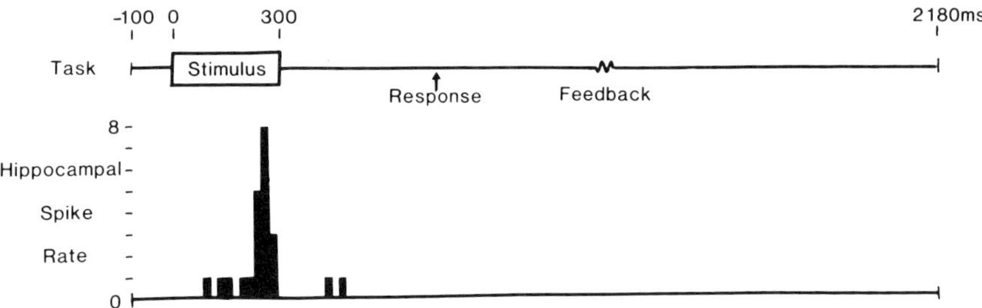

FIG. 10. Histogram of the times of occurrence of interictal spike-and-wave complexes (SWC) during a recognition memory task. Note the clustering of SWC following stimulus presentation during recognition memory. Random times of occurrence were observed during epochs of auditory oddball. Vertical scale represents rate of occurrence of SWC relative to the sampling period.

charges (115) or frank seizures (116) in susceptible subjects. During performance of a recent memory task by a patient with uncontrolled CPS and implanted electrodes, visually presented stimuli consistently evoked focal MTL interictal SWC with an average latency of 228 msec (117) (Fig. 10). The SWC were more often lateralized to the left medial temporal lobe. No consistent change in interictal spike rate was observed during performance of several other cognitive tasks during which visual or auditory stimuli were presented. Scobey and Gabor (118) produced epileptogenic foci in discrete areas of cat visual cortex by topical application of penicillin. Interictal discharges could be evoked by spots of light positioned in that portion of the visual field projecting to the visual cortex that had been made epileptogenic. This circumscribed visual field area was called the "activation field" and reflected the distribution of stimulated geniculocortical fibers projecting totally or in part to the penicillin-treated cortex. Similar activation fields may exist for epileptic foci within the MTL. It is therefore conceivable that, in some cases, interictal SWC are generated by synaptically related neuronal populations which in other circumstances are actively involved in recent memory formation and retrieval.

Interictal Slow Waves and Memory-Evoked Potentials

A large variety of epileptogenic agents evoke stereotyped interictal spike-and-wave complexes in the animal hippocampus. The interictal spike is generated by a paroxysmal depolarization shift in hippocampal pyramidal cells (119). These cells then excite interneurons that induce both "recurrent" and "surround" inhibition by increasing chloride conductance in the pyramidal cell somata (120). Recurrent inhibition is followed by a second phase of hyperpolarization, probably also due to the synaptic action of gamma-aminobutyric acid (GABA) on pyramidal cells. However, this transmission is bicuculline-insensitive, is primarily on the apical dendrites rather than being on the somata, and appears to induce an increased potassium conductance by a nonclassical mechanism (121,122). The third phase is a calcium-sensitive potassium current resulting from action potential, rather than from synaptic currents, and continuing for seconds.

We examined the MTL slow waves following interictal spikes in 16 patients with CPS (123). Ten patients displayed an interictal slow wave with characteristic morphology and depth voltage topography (Fig. 11). This "typical slow wave" (TSW) lasted 300–600 msec, was usually largest and negative in the anterior hippocampus, and was positive in the amygdala. Simultaneous recordings from ipsilateral cingulate, supplementary motor, orbitofrontal, and lateral temporal cortices, as well as from the contralateral MTL, revealed only small, apparently volume-conducted waveforms.

Although our data are limited, it appears that the TSW may be homologous to the interictal slow wave induced experimentally in animals. Like the slow wave in animals, the human TSW was accompanied by a strong in-

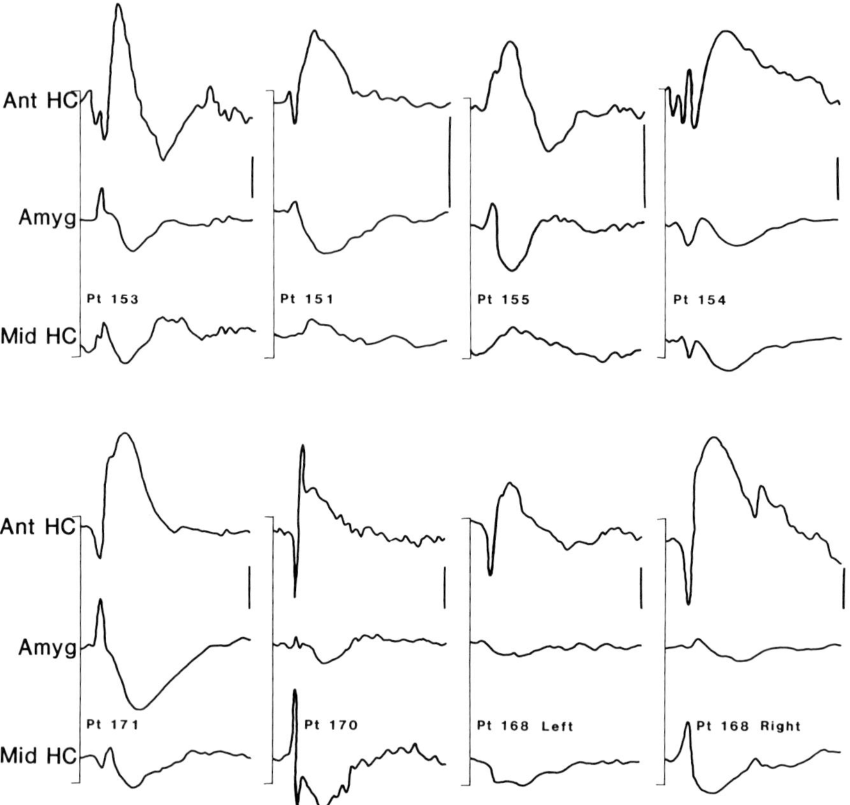

FIG. 11. Similarity of interictal spike-and-wave complexes in the right MTLs of seven patients and in both left and right MTLs (independently) of one patient (Pt 168). The interictal spike displays various morphologies, but it is usually positive (downward) in the anterior hippocampus (Ant HC) and negative in the amygdala (Amyg). The following typical wave is negative in the anterior hippocampus, positive in the amygdala, and of either polarity in the middle hippocampal formation (Mid HC). Each trace is 940 msec long. Vertical scale = 400 μV. (From ref. 123, with permission.)

hibition of MTL neuronal firing (Fig. 12). TSW voltage topography is consistent with the laminar profile thought to result from GABAergic recurrent inhibition of hippocampal pyramidal cells (124) and is also consistent with what is actually observed in the "inhibitory surround" of interictal spikes induced by topical application of penicillin to the hippocampus (125). TSW latency suggests that its major part comes from the second (bicuculline-insensitive), rather than the first (chloride conductance), component of the hyperpolarization.

The similar MTL voltage topographies of the MTL-P3 and TSW (Fig. 13) suggest that they may be generated by the same group of synapses (126,127). Generation of the MTL-

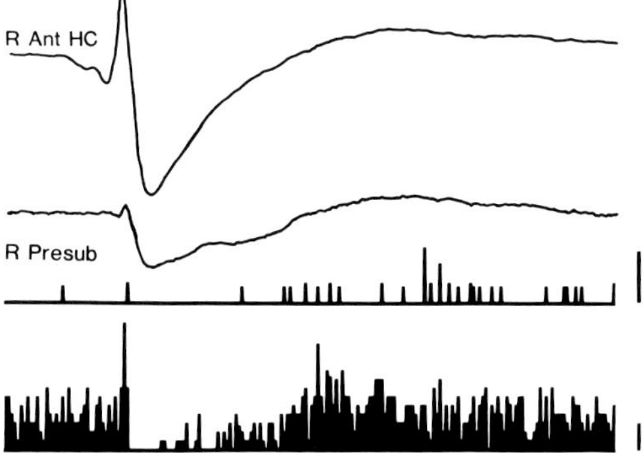

FIG. 12. Inhibition of MTL multiunit activity during TSWs. The units (recorded from the right presubiculum) show a profound inhibition following the interictal spike recorded (bipolarly) in the anterior hippocampus. Each trace is 1000 msec.

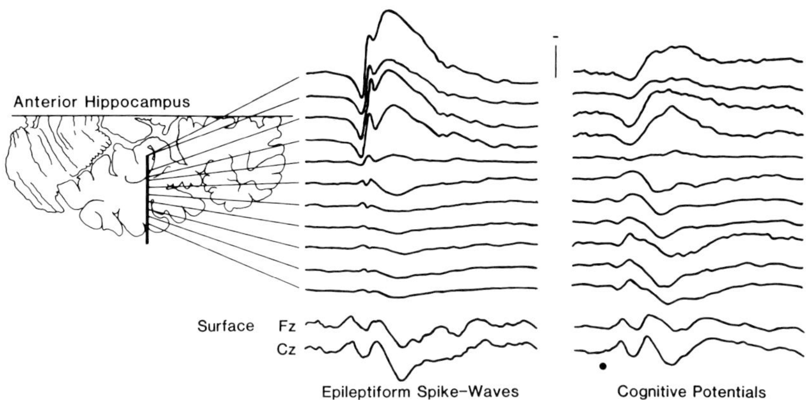

FIG. 13. Comparison of epileptiform potentials **(left tracings)** and cognitive potentials **(right tracings)**. The epileptiform potentials (TSW) are recorded from the same multilead contacts as the cognitive potentials (evoked N2/P3). Note that for contacts within the MTL, essentially identical voltage topographies (relative amplitude and reversal points) are observed for the TSW and the MTL-P3. However, at more lateral sites, the TSW falls off rapidly, whereas the P3 tends to maintain its amplitude and change its morphology. Each tracing is 1120 msec.

P3 by inhibitory synapses seems also to be consistent with both (a) its very long duration (often over 300 msec) and (b) its onset after the stimulus has been recognized and classified (128). Furthermore, while MTL unit activity in response to P3 is usually small and variable, it is, for the most part, decreased (29).

MTL Pathology and Memory-Evoked Potentials in Epileptic Patients

In our series, of 26 patients in whom P3s in the MTL have been studied, 10 show poor or absent endogenous potentials in the P3 latency range at both surface and depth, although the absence of surface P3s is highly unusual in normal subjects. Of the 16 patients with good surface P3s, 11 showed depth P3s that were probably lateralized—that is, larger in one MTL than in the other (e.g., see Fig. 14). Of these 11, six were found to have lateralized seizure onset. In all six cases, seizures began on the side of depressed MTL-P3s. These data suggest that abnormal endogenous potentials at surface or depth may reflect underlying epileptogenic pathology (130). These results have been confirmed, extended, and quantified by other depth-recording groups (131), who found an excellent correlation between laterality of the MTL seizure and uni-laterally decreased P3s in bipolar recordings in the region of the MTL. Wood et al. (132) found a positive correlation between hippocampal cell loss and the size of the locally recorded P3. In scalp recordings they found that although the scalp P3 is usually nearly symmetrical even in patients with unilaterally depressed MTL-P3s, sometimes a pronounced scalp laterality corresponding to the depth recordings is observed (104).

CONCLUSIONS: THE SIMILAR LOGIC OF SEIZURES AND MEMORIES

The evidence presented above indicates that the MTL plays a critical role in recent declarative memory as well as in complex partial epilepsy. MTL destruction produces recent-memory deficits and can cure seizures. Pathological MTL activation is observed during most CPS, and physiological MTL activation is observed during tasks engaging recent memory. The evidence further suggests that epilepsy and memory not only share the same anatomical locus in the MTL, but also use (at least to some extent) the same synaptic mechanisms, local circuitry, and distant projections. At the simplest level, the correlation of deficits in memory performance and in memory-related evoked potentials with the severity of hippocampal sclerosis suggests

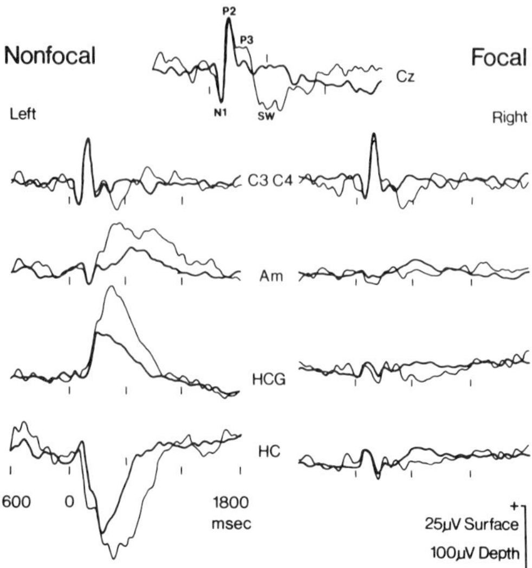

FIG. 14. Characteristic potentials recorded by electrodes in the amygdala (Am), parahippocampal gyrus (HCG), and hippocampus (HC) during an auditory oddball task with long unpredicted interstimulus intervals. Simultaneous potentials at the surface (C3, C4, Cz) show large early components N1-P2 which are identical for rare tones (*thin lines*) and frequent tones (*thick lines*). Typical of normal data also is the enhancement of P3 and SW (slow wave) to the rare tones. The limbic electrodes record only the later endogenous potentials. The polarity of these potentials inverts between the HC and the HCG (9 mm posteromedial to the HC) and the Am (26 mm anterior). Endogenous potentials are not visible in the right MTL, where this patient's seizures originated and which was noted at surgery to be sclerotic. (From ref. 130, with permission.)

that seizures hyperengage the same cells that are needed for ordinary memory.

A similar conclusion can be drawn from the temporary memory deficits that occur during and after seizures which involve the MTL. As opposed to the loss of experiential memory with epilepsy-induced MTL dysfunction, the hyperengagement of MTL circuits by epileptiform discharges can induce intense versions of these same experiential memory phenomena. Epileptiform spike-and-wave complexes are universal in patients with epilepsy and are thought, on experimental, theoretical, and surgical grounds, to trace out with phasic activation the circuits involved in actual sei-

zures (73,114,120,133). Thus, the findings that MTL spike-and-wave complexes are evoked (albeit rarely) by recent memory tasks, and that the epileptiform slow waves have the same apparent synaptic arrangement in the MTL as do memory-evoked potentials, provide converging evidence for shared circuitry between memory and epilepsy.

This sharing of circuitry appears to reflect a deeper homology between complex partial epilepsy and experiential memory. That is, the neurobiological properties and functional organization needed to implement experiential associative memory are also those that render the hippocampus susceptible to epileptogenesis. If hippocampal synapses store recent event memory, then they need to be (and are) extremely plastic. Longer-term memories are not made for all events; furthermore, they develop slowly, permitting a more controlled and less intense process. Shorter-term memories can be maintained as persisting or recirculating activity, and thus they do not require synaptic plasticity at all. This intense plasticity renders the hippocampus more metabolically active than the rest of the brain, and thus more sensitive to anoxic, hypoxic, and other insults. The proximate cause of epileptogenic damage appears to be the large calcium influx from activated N-methyl-D-aspartate receptors (134–136). The calcium influx, with its access to the cellular machinery, functions normally to permit the plasticity that event memory requires (88).

Event memory not only requires constant updating as experience unfolds, but also requires that all of the disparate elements in an event be linked together. In contrast, nonassociative memories (such as word priming) can persist for hours in amnesics with hippocampal damage, but they require only that the existing synaptic pathways be incrementally strengthened (137). Event memories require that new cell assemblies be formed, and thus that previously ineffective synaptic pathways become effective (87).

Thus, an extraordinarily large number of excitatory afferents converge on each hippocampal pyramidal cell, rendering them potentially susceptible to hypersynchronous excitation (138). In model neural circuits, autoassociation to link disparate elements is accomplished using recurrent excitatory collaterals within a neuronal pool (139–141). Such connections are present anatomically and physiologically in area CA3 of the hippocampus (142–144). Excellent quantitative functional models of CA3 indicate that these recurrent excitatory collaterals are essential for the explosive build-up of excitation that leads to, at the synaptic level, a paroxysmal depolarization shift/giant excitatory postsynaptic potential and, at the field-potential level, an epileptiform spike (145). This model has been confirmed by experiments demonstrating that experimentally induced spikes in the hippocampal system arise in CA3 (146). Thus, the need for autoassociation of diverse elements in event memory determines an internal neural circuitry that renders the hippocampus susceptible to hypersynchronous excitation, the common element of all epileptic discharge.

This combination of plasticity and recurrent excitation provides a substrate for the formation of new cell assemblies representing recent events in a single learning trial. What is to prevent such a cell assembly from being activated at a lower threshold at each successive recognition, and thus being further strengthened, and eventually entering a positive-feedback loop where its members become very strongly linked and capable of generating hypersynchronous excitation? Perhaps plasticity is inhibited to repeated events. We noted above that the MTL-P3 is larger for repeated events and may be GABAergic. GABAergic activation in the hippocampus inhibits long-term potentiation (88). Besides discouraging the formation of epileptogenic cell assemblies, this inhibitory modulation of plasticity may also limit the amount of plasticity induced by hippocampal seizures, thereby limiting the retrograde and anterograde amnesia they cause. Conversely, the malfunction of these inhibitory modulations of plasticity could provide another pathway to epileptogenesis. It is interesting to note that the apparent identity of synaptic generators for the MTL-P3 and epileptiform slow wave reflect their similar roles in inhibiting the recurrent excitation induced by the preceding MTL-N4 or interictal spike, respectively.

Finally, at the neural systems level, event memory requires the input of many different association areas that extract the various elements of an event, and it must project back to these areas to help with retrieval (86). Furthermore, given that event recall is an experiential phenomenon that redirects the contents of awareness from the external toward the internal world, these hippocampal projections should be capable of influencing conscious contents as well as the level of contact with the external world (147). These same pathways are available for an epileptic focus in widespread posterior cortical areas to gain access to the hippocampus and to the potentially hypersynchronous circuitry present there. Following epileptic "amplification" in the hippocampus, this activity can spread widely, thereby producing the plethora of auras and impaired contact that characterize CPS.

SUMMARY

Patients with CPS often display recent memory deficits. Typically, general intelligence, perceptual skills, language, remote memory, and primary memory are all normal. However, the ability to learn new combinations of cognitively complex material is deficient. This deficit may be specific for verbal material (e.g., as a difficulty with learning to recall a response word given an unrelated cue word), for nonverbal material (e.g., as a difficulty in drawing a complex figure from memory), or for both verbal and nonverbal material. Because these characteristics are typical of memory deficits after MTL damage, it is reasonable to suspect that these deficits in patients with epilepsy also reflect MTL damage.

In many cases, MTL damage is apparent from neuroimaging studies, whereas seizure semiology suggests MTL onset. In these patients, the same pathology might be the cause of both the ictus and memory deficits. In other cases, memory impairment appears to be secondary to seizures. This suggestion is supported by cases where prolonged complex partial status resulted in a permanent global amnesia. Cases with shorter-lasting memory deficits were also presented. Neuropsychological testing revealed specific recent-memory deficits that cleared 2 weeks after a flurry of CPS and 24 hr after a single seizure.

Depth recordings have demonstrated that MTL electrographic seizures can occur without subjective manifestations. When these are evoked by local electrical stimulation, a profound inability to learn new material may be observed during the afterdischarge. Similarly, artificially induced MTL spike-and-wave complexes interfere with the memory for simultaneously presented complex visual scenes.

Recent evidence suggests that all of the above phenomena may reflect the engagement by epileptiform processes of the association-cortex (AC)–MTL circuits used in normal human memory. In recent memory tasks, cognitive evoked-potential components N4 and P3 are generated in the MTL and to a lesser degree in related AC regions. The N4/P3 are strongly modulated by familiarity in recent memory. This modulation is eliminated by anterior temporal lobectomy. The typical slow wave following spontaneous MTL interictal spikes has the same MTL voltage topography, and thus probably similar synaptic generators, as the cognitive P3 potential. Furthermore, MTL spike-and-wave complexes can be evoked in recent memory tasks at a fixed latency equal to that of the N4.

In conclusion, it is suggested that specific recent memory deficits in patients with CPS may be (a) permanent, reflecting permanent MTL damage which is adjacent to or distant from the epileptogenic zone and which may result from status, (b) prolonged but not permanent, after a single seizure or many seizures, or (c) temporary, during a subclinical MTL seizure or epileptiform spike-and-wave discharge. It is possible that the AC–MTL circuits impaired in these patients may be probed noninvasively using the cognitive evoked-potential components N4/P3.

ACKNOWLEDGMENTS

This work was supported by the Veterans Administration, by the United States Public Health Service (NS18741 and CEP), and by the French Institute Nationale de la Sante et de la Recherche Medicale. Important collaborators include Michael Smith, Gary Heit, Tara O'Reilly, Richard Daims, Patrick Chauvel, and Catherine Liegeons-Chauvel.

REFERENCES

1. Ajmone-Marson C, Ralston B. *The epileptic seizure: its functional morphology and diagnostic significance*. Springfield, IL: Charles C Thomas, 1957.
2. Milner B, Teuber HL. Further analysis of the hippocampal amnesic syndrome: 14-year follow-up study of H.M. *Neuropsychologia* 1968; 6:213–234.
3. Corkin S. Lasting consequences of bilateral medial temporal lobectomy: clinical course and experimental findings in H.M. *Semin Neurol* 1984;4:249–259.
4. Scoville WB, Milner B. Loss of recent memory after bilateral hippocampal lesions. *J Neurol Neurosurg Psychiatry* 1957;20:11–21.
5. Milner B. Interhemispheric differences in the localisation of psychological processes in man. *Br Med Bull* 1971;27:272–277.
6. Dodrill CB. A neuropsychological battery for epilepsy. *Epilepsia* 1978;19:611–623.
7. Dodrill CB. In: Filskov SB, Boll TJ, eds. *Handbook of clinical neuropsychology*. New York: John Wiley & Sons, 1981;366–395.
8. Tarter RE. Intellectual and adaptive functioning in epilepsy. *Dis Nerv Sys* 1972;33:763–770.
9. Trimble MR, Thompson PJ, Huppert F. Antidepressant drugs and the seizure threshold. In: Canger R, Angelett F, Penry JK, eds. *Advances in epileptology*. New York: Raven Press, 1989; 51–57.
10. Dikmen S, Matthews CG, Harley JP. The effect of early versus late onset of major motor epilepsy upon cognitive–intellectual functions in adults. *Epilepsia* 1975;16:73–81.
11. Dikmen S, Matthews CG. Effect of major motor seizural frequency upon cognitive–intellectual functions in adults. *Epilepsia* 1977;18:21–29.
12. Seidenberg M, O'Leary DS, Berent S, Boll T. Changes in seizure frequency and test–retest scores on the Wechsler adult intelligence scale. *Epilepsia* 1981;22:75–83.
13. Dodrill CB, Wilkus RJ. Neuropsychological correlates of the electroencephalogram in epileptics. II. The waking posterior rhythm and its interaction with epileptiform activity. *Epilepsia* 1976;17:101–109.
14. Rausch R, Lieb JP, Crandall PH. Neuropsychologic correlates of depth spike activity in epileptic patients. *Arch Neurol* 1978;35:699–705.
15. Wilkus RJ, Dodrill CB. Neuropsychological correlates of the electroencephalogram in epilepsies. I. Topographic distribution and average rate of epileptiform activity. *Epilepsia* 1976;17:89–100.
16. Jackson JH, Colman WS. Case of epilepsy with tasting movements and "dreamy state"—very small patch of softening in the uncinate gyrus. *Brain* 1898;21:580–590.
17. Margerison JAN, Corsellis JAN. Epilepsy and the temporal lobes. *Brain* 1966;89:499–530.

18. Babb TL, Brown WJ. Pathological findings in epilepsy. In: Engel J, ed. *Surgical treatment of the epilepsies.* New York: Raven Press, 1987; 511–540.

19. Crandall PH. Neurosurgical management of the epilepsies. *Adv Neurol* 1975;8:265–280.

20. Delgado-Escueta AV, Walsh GO. Type I complex partial seizures of hippocampal origin: excellent results of anterior temporal lobectomy. *Arch Neurol* 1985;35:143–154.

21. Engel J Jr, Crandall PH, Rausch R. The partial epilepsies. In: Rosenberg RN, Grossman RG, Schochet S, eds. *The clinical neurosciences.* New York: Churchill Livingstone, 1989;1349–1380.

22. Jensen I. Temporal lobe surgery around the world results, complication and mortality. *Acta Neurol Scand* 1975;52:354–373.

23. Rasmussen J, Branch C. Temporal lobe epilepsy. *Postgrad Med* 1962;31:9–14.

24. Seisjo BK. *Brain energy metabolism.* New York: John Wiley & Sons, 1978.

25. Mazziotta JC, Phelps ME, Halgren E. Local cerebral glucose metabolic response to audiovisual stimulation and deprivation: studies in human subjects with positron CT. *Hum Neurobiol* 1983;2:11–23.

26. Engel J, Brown J, Kuhl D, Phelps ME, Mazziotta JC, Crandall PH. Pathological findings underlying focal temporal lobe hypometabolism in partial epilepsy. *Ann Neurol* 1982; 12:518–528.

27. Van Hoesen GW, Pandya DN. Some connections of the entorhinal and perirhinal (area 35) cortices of the rhesus monkey. I. Temporal lobe afferents. *Brain Res* 1975;95:1–24.

28. VanHoesen GW, Rosene DL, Mesulam MM. Subicular input from temporal cortex in the rhesus monkey. *Science* 1979;206:608–610.

29. Price JL. In: Ben-Ari Y, ed. *The amygdaloid complex.* Amsterdam: Elsevier, 1981;121–132.

30. Rosene DL, Van Hoesen GW. Hippocampal efferents reach widespread areas of cerebral cortex and amygdala in the rhesus monkey. *Science* 1977;198:315–317.

31. VanHoesen GW. The cortico-cortical projections of the posterior parahippocampal area in the rhesus monkey. *Anat Rec* 1980;196:195.

32. Babb TL, Halgren E, Wilson C, Engel J, Crandall P. Neuronal firing patterns during the spread of an occipital lobe seizure to the temporal lobes in man. *Electroencephalogr Clin Neurophysiol* 1981;51:104–107.

33. Bancaud J, Talairach J, Bonis A, et al. *La Stereoelectroencephalographie dans l'epilepsie.* Paris: Masson et Cie, 1965.

34. Milner B. Brain mechanisms suggested by studies of temporal lobes. In: Millikan CH, Darley FL, eds. *Brain mechanisms underlying speech and language.* New York: Grune & Stratton, 1967;122–145.

35. Milner B, Teuber HC. Alteration of perception and memory in man: reflections on methods. In: Weiskrantz L, ed. *Analysis of behavioral change.* New York: Harper & Row, 1968;269–375.

36. Penfield W, Milner B. Memory deficit produced by bilateral lesions in the hippocampal zone. *Arch Neurol Psychiatry* 1958;79:475–497.

37. Piercy MF. Experimental studies of the organic amnesic syndrome. In: Whitty CWM, Zangwill OL, eds. *Amnesia: clinical psychological and medicolegal aspects.* London: Butterworths, 1977;1–15.

38. Rozin P. The psychobiological approach to human memory. In: Rozenzweig MR, Bennett EL, eds. *Neural mechanisms of learning and memory.* Cambridge, MA: MIT Press, 1976;3–46.

39. Hermann BP, Wyler AR, Richey ET, Rea JM. Memory function and verbal learning ability in patients with complex partial seizures of temporal lobe origin. *Epilepsia* 1987;28:547–554.

40. Mungas D, Ehlers C, Walton N, McCutchen CB. Verbal learning differences in epileptic patients with left and right temporal lobe foci. *Epilepsia* 1985;26:340–345.

41. Milner B. Psychological aspects of focal epilepsy and its neurosurgical management. In: Purpura DP, Penry JK, Walter RD, eds. *Advances in neurology.* New York: Raven Press, 1975;299–231.

42. Mayeux R, Brandt J, Rosen J, Benson DF. Interictal memory and language impairment in temporal lobe epilepsy. *Neurology* 1980;30: 120–125.

43. Kolb B, Whishaw IQ. *Fundamentals of human neuropsychology,* 2nd ed. New York: Freeman, 1985.

44. Milner B. Psychological defects produced by temporal-lobe excision. *Res Publ Assoc Res Nerv Ment Dis* 1958;36:244–257.

45. Satz P, Mogel S. An abbreviation of the WAIS for clinical use. *J Clin Psychol* 1962;18:77–79.

46. Stapleton JM, Halgren E. Neuropsychological deficits associated with epilepsy: Chronic and transient dysfunction, particularly in recent memory. In: *Epilepsy international symposium abstracts,* 1983;332.

47. Copeland S, Domalski P, Halgren E. A new test with multiple forms sensitive to left and right medial temporal and frontal lobe dysfunction. Unpublished manuscript.

48. Fedio P, Mirsky AF. Selective intellectual deficits in children with temporal lobe or centrencephalic epilepsy. *Neuropsychologia* 1969;7: 287–300.

49. Mirsky AF, Primac DW, Ajmone-Marsan C, Rosvold HE, Stevens JR. A comparison of the psychological test performance of patients with focal and nonfocal epilepsy. *Exp Neurol* 1960; 2:75–89.

50. Freemon FR, Douglas EF, Penry JK. Environmental interaction and memory during petit mal (absence) seizures. *Pediatrics* 1973;51: 911–918.

51. Browne TR, Penry JK, Porter RJ, Dreifuss FE. Responsiveness before, during, and after

spike–wave paroxysms. *Neurology* 1974;24: 659–665.

52. Tizard B, Margerison JH. Psychological functions during wave–spike discharge. *Br J Clin Psychol* 1963;3:6–15.

53. Mirsky AF, VanBuren JM. On the nature of the "absence" in centrencephalic epilepsy: a study of some behavioral, electroencephalographic and autonomic factors. *Electroencephalogr Clin Neurophysiol* 1965;18:334–348.

54. Geller MR, Geller A. Brief amnestic effects of spike wave discharges. *Neurology* 1970;20: 380–381.

55. Hutt SJ, Gilbert S. Effects of evoked spike–wave discharges upon short term memory in patients with epilepsy. *Cortex* 1980;16:445–457.

56. Baddeley AD. Amnesia: a minimal model and an interpretation. In: Cermak LS, ed. *Memory and amnesia*. Hillsdale, NJ: Lawrence Erlbaum, 1982;176–189.

57. Hovey HB, Kooi KA. Transient disturbances of thought processes and epilepsy. *Arch Neurol* 1955;74:287–292.

58. Kooi KA, Hovey HB. Alterations in mental function and paroxysmal cerebral activity. *Arch Neurol Psychiatry* 1957;78:264–271.

59. Siebelink BM, Bakker DJ, Binnie CD, Kasteleijn-Nolst Trenit:e DG. Psychological effects of subclinical epileptiform EEG discharges in children. II. General intelligence tests. *Epilepsy Res* 1988;2:117–121.

60. Binnie CD, Kasteleijn-Nolst Trenit:e DG, Smit AM, Wilkins AJ. Interactions of epileptiform EEG discharges and cognition. *Epilepsy Res* 1987;1:239–245.

61. Shewmon DA, Erwin RJ. The effect of local interictal spikes on perception and reaction time. I. General considerations. *Electroencephalogr Clin Neurophysiol* 1988;69:319–337.

62. Shewmon DA, Erwin RJ. The effect of focal interictal spikes on perception and reaction time. II. Neuroanatomic specificity. *Electroencephalogr Clin Neurophysiol* 1988;69:338–352.

63. Shewmon DA, Erwin RJ. Focal spike-induced cerebral dysfunction is related to the after-coming slow wave. *Ann Neurol* 1988;23:131–137.

64. Fisher CM, Adams RD. Transient global amnesia. *Acta Neurol Scand* 1964;40:

65. Markowitsch HJ. Transient global amnesia. *Neurosci Biobehav Rev* 1983;7:35–43.

66. Gallassi R, Morreale A, Lorusso S, Pazzaglia P, Lugaresi E. Epileptic transient amnesia. *Ital J Neurol Sci* 1988;37–39.

67. Pritchard PB 3d, Holmstrom VL, Roitzsch JC, Giacinto J. Epileptic amnesic attacks: benefit from antiepileptic drugs. *Neurology* 1985;35: 1188–1189.

68. Deisenhammer E. Transient global amnesia as an epileptic manifestation. *J Neurol* 1981; 225:289–292.

69. Treiman DM, Delgado-Escueta AV. Status epilepticus. In: Thompson RA, Green JR, eds. *Critical care of neurologic and neurosurgical emergencies*. New York: Raven Press, 1980; 53–99.

70. Engel J, Ludwig BI, Fetell M. Prolonged partial complex status epilepticus: EEG and behavioral observations. *Neurology* 1978;28:863–869.

71. Treiman DM, Delgado-Escueta AV, Clark MA. Impairment of memory following complex partial status epilepticus. *Neurology* 1981;31(4 pt. 2):109.

72. Woodruff ML. Subconvulsive epileptiform discharge and behavioral impairment. *Behav Biol* 1974;11:431–458.

73. Penfield W, Jasper H. *Epilepsy and the function anatomy of the human brain*. Boston: Little, Brown, 1954.

74. Halgren E, Babb TL, Crandall PH. Post-EEG seizure depression of human limbic neurons is not determined by their response to probable hypoxia. *Epilepsia* 1977;18:89–93.

75. Halgren E, Wilson CL. Recall deficits produced by afterdischarges in the human hippocampal formation and amygdala. *Electroencephalogr Clin Neurophysiol* 1985;61:375–380.

76. Halgren E, Wilson CL, Squires NK, Engel J, Walter RD, Crandall PH. Dynamics of the human hippocampal contribution to memory. In: Seifert W, ed. *Neurobiology of the hippocampus*. London: Academic Press, 1983;529–572.

77. Babb TL, Crandall PH. Epileptogenesis of human limbic neurons in psychomotor epileptics. *Electroencephalogr Clin Neurophysiol* 1976;40: 225–245.

78. Walter RD. Tactical considerations leading to surgical treatment of limbic epilepsy. In: Brazier MAB, eds. *Epilepsy: Its Phenomena in Man*, New York: Academic Press, 1973;99–119.

79. Buzsaki G. Hippocampal sharp waves: their origin and significance. *Brain Res* 1986;398:242–252.

80. Suzuki SS, Smith GK. Spontaneous EEG spikes in the normal hippocampus. I. Behavioral correlates, laminar profiles and bilateral synchrony. *Electroencephalogr Clin Neurophysiol* 1987;67:348–359.

81. Suzuki SS, Smith GK. Spontaneous EEG spikes in the normal hippocampus. II. Relations to synchronous burst discharges. *Electroencephalogr Clin Neurophysiol* 1988;69: 532–540.

82. Suzuki SS, Smith GK. Spontaneous EEG spikes in the normal hippocampus. III. Relations to evoked potentials. *Electroencephalogr Clin Neurophysiol* 1988;69:541–549.

83. Suzuki SS, Smith GK. Spontaneous EEG spikes in the normal hippocampus. IV. Effects of medial septum and entorhinal cortex lesions. *Electroencephalogr Clin Neurophysiol* 1988;70: 73–83.

84. Suzuki SS, Smith GK. Spontaneous EEG spikes in the normal hippocampus. V. Effects of ether, urethane, pentobarbital, atropine, diazepam and bicculine. *Electroencephalogr Clin Neurophysiol* 1988;70:84–95.

85. Halgren E, Wilson CL, Stapleton JM. Human medial temporal-lobe stimulation disrupts both

formation and retrieval of recent memories. *Bran Cogn* 1985;4:287–295.

86. Halgren E. Human hippocampal and amygdala recording and stimulation: evidence for a neural model of recent memory. In: Butters N, Squire L, eds. *The neuropsychology of memory*. New York: Guilford, 1984;165–181.

87. Gardner-Medwin AR. The recall of events through the learning of associations between their parts. *Philos Trans R Soc Lond [Biol]* 1976;194:375–402.

88. Lynch G, Baudry M. Structure–function relationships in the organization of memory. In: Gazzaniga M, eds. *Perspective in memory research*. Cambridge, MA: MIT, 1988;23–91.

89. Marr D. A theory of archicortex. *Philos Trans R Soc Lond [Biol]* 1971;262:23–81.

90. Squire LR, Cohen N, Nadel L. The medial temporal lobe in memory consolidation: a new hypothesis. In: Weingartner H, Parder E, eds. *Memory consolidation*. Hillsdale, NJ: Lawrence Erlbaum, 1984;185–210.

91. Van Hoesen GW. The parahippocampal gyrus: New observations regarding its cortical connections in the monkey. *Trends Neurosci* 1982;5:345–350.

92. Amaral DG, Insausti R, Cowan WM. The entorhinal cortex of the monkey. I. Cytoarchitectonic organization. *J Comp Neurol* 1987;264:326–355.

93. McNaughton BL. Activity dependent modulation of hippocampal synaptic efficacy: some implications for memory processes. In: Seifert W, eds. *Neurobiology of the Hippocampus*, New York: Academic Press, 1983;233–252.

94. Teyler TJ, Piscenna P. Long-term potentiation as a candidate mnemonic device. *Brain Res Rev* 1984;319:15–28.

95. Smith ME, Stapleton JM, Halgren E. Human medial temporal lobe potentials evoked in memory and language tasks. *Electroencephalogr Clin Neurophysiol* 1986;63:145–159.

96. Smith ME, Halgren E. Dissociation of recognition memory components following temporal lesions. *J Exp Psychol [Learn Mem Cogn]* 1989;15:50–60.

97. Smith ME, Halgren E. Event-related potentials elicited by familiar and unfamiliar faces. In: Johnson R, Purasuraman R, Rohrbaugh JW, eds. *Current trends in event-related potential research (Electroencephalogr Clin Neurophysiol [Suppl] 40)*. Amsterdam: Elsevier, 1987;422–426.

98. Halgren E, Stapleton JM, Smith ME, Altafullah I. Generators of the human scalp P3s. In: Cracco RQ, Bodis-Wollner I, eds. *Evoked potentials*. New York: Alan R Liss, 1986;269–289.

99. Kutas M, Van Petten C. Event-related brain potential studies of language. In: Ackles PK, Jennings JR, Coles MGH, eds. *Advances in psychophysiology*. Greenwich, CT: JAI Press, 1987.

100. Halgren E. Insights from evoked potentials into the neuropsychological mechanisms of reading. In: Scheibel A, Weschsler A, eds. *Neurobiology of cognition*. New York: Guilford, 1990; 103–150.

101. Wood CC, McCarthy G, Squires NK, Vaughan HG, Woods DL. Anatomical and physiological substrates of event-related potentials. Two case studies. *Ann NY Acad Sci* 1984;425:681–721.

102. Smith ME, Halgren E, Sokolik M, et al. The intracranial voltage distribution of endogenous potentials elicited during auditory discrimination. *Electroencephalogr Clin Neurophysiol* 1990;in press.

103. Stapleton JM, Halgren E. Endogenous potentials evoked in simple cognitive tasks: depth components and task correlates. *Electroencephalogr Clin Neurophysiol* 1987;67:44–52.

104. McCarthy G, Wood CC. Intracranial recordings of endogenous ERPs in humans. *Electroencephalogr Clin Neurophysiol [Suppl]* 1987; 39:331–337.

105. Halgren E, Smith ME. Cognitive evoked potentials as modulatory processes in human memory formation and retrieval. *Hum Neurobiol* 1987;6:129–139.

106. Stapleton JM, Halgren E, Moreno KA. Endogenous potentials after anterior temporal lobectomy. *Neuropsychologia* 1987;25:549–557.

107. Wood CC, McCarthy G, Allison T, Goff WR, Williamson PD, Spencer DD. Endogenous event-related potentials following temporal lobe excisions in humans. *Soc Neurosci Abstr* 1982;8:976.

108. Johnson R Jr. Scalp-recorded P300 activity in patients following unilateral temporal lobectomy. *Brain* 1988;111:1517–1529.

109. Heit G, Smith ME, Halgren E. Neural encoding of individual words and faces by the human hippocampus and amygdala. *Nature* 1988;333: 773–775.

110. Penfield WP, Perot P. The brain's record of auditory and visual experience: a final summary and discussion. *Brain* 1963;86:595–696.

111. Mullan S, Penfield W. Illusions of comparative interpretation and emotion. *Arch Neurol Psychiatry* 1959;81:269–284.

112. Gloor P, Olivier A, Quesney LF, Andermann F, Horowitz S. The role of the limbic system in experiential phenomena of temporal lobe epilepsy. *Ann Neurol* 1982;12:129–144.

113. Halgren E, Walter RD, Cherlow DG, Crandall PH. Mental phenomena evoked by electrical stimulation of the human hippocampal formation and amygdala. *Brain* 1978,101:83–117.

114. Chauvel P, Buser P, Badier JM, Liegeois-Chauvel C, Marquis P, Bancaud J. The "epileptogenic zone" in humans: representation of intercritical events by spatio-temporal maps: intercritiques par cartes spatio-temporelles. *Rev Neurol (Paris)* 1987;143:443–450.

115. Wilkins AJ, Zifkin B, Andermann F, McGovern E. Seizures induced by thinking. *Ann Neurol* 1982;11:608–612.

116. Forster FM. *Reflex epilepsy, behavioral therapy and conditional reflexes*. Springfield, IL: Charles C Thomas, 1977.

117. Altafullah I, Halgren E. Focal medial temporal

lobe spike–wave complexes evoked by a memory task. *Epilepsia* 1988;29:8–13.

118. Scobey R, Gabor A. Properties of epileptogenic focus: activation field. *J Neurophysiol* 1977;40:1199–1213.

119. Johnston D, Brown TH. Mechanisms of neuronal burst generation. In: Schwartzkroin PA, Wheal H, eds. *Electrophysiology of epilepsy.* New York: Academic Press, 1984;277–301.

120. Wheal HV, Ashwood TJ, Lancaster B. A comparative *in vitro* study of the kainic acid lesioned and bicuculline treated hippocampus: chronic and acute models of focal epilepsy. In: Schwartzkroin PA, Wheal H, eds. *Electrophysiology of epilepsy.* New York: Academic Press, 1984;176–200.

121. Newberry NR, Nicoll RA. A bicuculline-resistant inhibitory post-synaptic potential in rat hippocampal pyramidal cells *in vitro. J Physiol (Cambridge)* 1984;438:239–254.

122. Newberry NR, Nicoll RA. Direct depolarizing action of baclofen on hippocampal pyramidal cells. *Nature* 1984;308:450–452.

123. Altafullah I, Halgren E, Stapleton JM, Crandall PH. Interictal spike–wave complexes in the human medial temporal lobe: typical topography and comparisons with cognitive potentials. *Electroencephalogr Clin Neurophysiol* 1986;63:503–516.

124. Leung LS. Potentials evoked by alvear tract in hippocampal Ca1 region of rats. II. Spatial field analysis. *J Neurophysiol* 1979;42:1571–1589.

125. Dichter M, Spencer WA. Penicillin-induced interictal discharges from the cat hippocampus. II. Mechanisms underlying origin and restriction. *J Neurophysiol* 1969;32:663.

126. Halgren E. Evoked potentials. In: Baker G, Vanderwolf C, eds. *Neuromethods.* Clifton, NJ. Humana, 1990;in press.

127. Nunez PL. *Electrical fields of the brain.* New York: Oxford University Press, 1981.

128. Desmedt JE. Scalp-recorded cerebral event-related potentials in man as point of entry into the analysis of cognitive processing. In: Schmitt FO, Worden FG, Edelmann G, Dennis SD, eds. *The organization of the cerebral cortex.* Cambridge, MA: MIT, 1981;441–473.

129. Heit G, Smith ME, Halgren E. Neuronal activity in the human medial temporal lobe during recognition memory. *Brain* 1990;in press.

130. Squires NK, Halgren E, Wilson CL, Crandall PH. Human endogenous limbic potentials: cross-modality and depth/surface comparisons in epileptic subjects. In: Gaillard AWK, Ritter W, eds. *Tutorials in ERP research: endogenous components.* Amsterdam: North-Holland, 1983;217–232.

131. Meador KJ, Loring DW, King DW, Nichols FT. The P3 evoked potential and transient global amnesia. *Arch Neurol* 1988;45:465–467.

132. Wood CC, McCarthy G, Kim JH, Spencer DD, Williamson PD. Abnormalities in temporal lobe event-related potentials predict hippocampal cell loss in temporal lobe epilepsy [Abstract]. *Soc Neurosci Abstr* 1988;14:5.

133. Pedley T. Epilepsy and the human electroencephalogram. In: Schwartzkroin P, Wheal H, eds. *Pathophysiology of epilepsy.* London: Academic Press, 1984;1–30.

134. Seisjo BK. Cell damage in the brain: a speculative synthesis. *J Cereb Blood Flow Metabol* 1981;1:155–185.

135. Olney JW, Gubareff T. Sloviter RS. "Epileptic" brain damage in rats induced by sustained electrical stimulation of the perforant path. II. Ultrastructural analysis of acute hippocampal pathology. *Brain Res Bull* 1983;10:699–712.

136. Rothman SM, Olney JW. Glutamate and the pathophysiology of hypoxic–ischemic brain damage. *Ann Neurol* 1986;19:105–111.

137. Shimamura AP. Priming effects in amnesia: evidence for a dissociable memory function. *Q J Exp Psychol* 1986;38:619–644.

138. Braitenberg V, Schuz A. Some anatomical comments on the hippocampus. In: Seifert W, eds. *Neurobiology of the hippocampus.* London: Academic Press, 1983;21–36.

139. Read W, Nenov VI, Halgren E. Inhibition controlled retrieval by an autoassociative model of hippocampal area CA3 (submitted for publication).

140. Willshaw DJ, Buneman OP, Longuet-Higgins HC. Non-holographic associative memory. *Nature* 1969;222:960–962.

141. Anderson JA. A simple neural network generating an interactive memory. *Math Biosci* 1972;14:197–220.

142. Knowles WD, Schwartzkroin PA. Local circuit synaptic interaction in hippocampal brain slices. *J Neurosci* 1981;1:318–322.

143. MacVicar BA, Dudek FE. Local synaptic circuits in rat hippocampus: interaction between pyramidal cells. *Brain Res* 1980;184:220–223.

144. Schwartzkroin PA. Regulation of excitability in hippocampal neurons. In: Isaacson RL, Pribram KH, eds. *The hippocampus,* vol 3. New York: Plenum Press, 1986.

145. Traub RD, Wong RKS. Synaptic mechanisms underlying interictal spile initiation in a hippocampal network. *Neurology* 1983;33:257–266.

146. Wong RKS, Traub RD. Synchronized burst discharge in disinhibited hippocampal slice. I. Initiation in CA2–CA3 region. *J Neurophysiol* 1983;49:442–458.

147. Halgren E. Mental phenomena induced by stimulation in the limbic system. *Hum Neurobiol* 1982;1:251–260.

148. Chauvel P, Brunet-Bourgin F, Halgren E. L'état de rêve. *Neuro-Psy* 1989;4:443–450.

Advances in Neurology, Vol. 55, edited by
D. Smith, D. Treiman, and M. Trimble,
Raven Press, Ltd., New York © 1991.

25

The Geschwind Syndrome

D. Frank Benson

Department of Neurology, UCLA School of Medicine, Los Angeles, California 90024

Little in the field of epilepsy in the past several decades has engendered such a strident degree of controversy as has the term "epileptic personality." Most epileptologists actively deny its existence, and some ardently oppose any attempt to demonstrate any personality disorder characteristic for epilepsy. A valid justification for the strength of these feelings is easy to appreciate.

For many centuries, epilepsy patients were considered untrustworthy, unwanted, and even dangerous. They were often thought to be possessed by evil (the Devil), and they were shunned and ridiculed by the general population as well as by physicians (1–4). They were forced into patterns of abnormal behavior that were easily interpreted as evidence of mental abnormality. "Epileptic personality" traits have been discussed at length by psychiatrists (5,6) and neurologists (7,8). A time-honored and robust experience placed these patients among the psychiatrically disabled.

The original anticonvulsants (bromides, barbiturates) produced a notable degree of mental dulling so that even when their seizures were controlled, they remained disabled outcasts. Only with the advent of modern anticonvulsant pharmaceuticals (particularly phenytoin) could full control of seizures be accomplished for many patients without the production of significant mental impairment; the prejudice against patients with epilepsy was strong, however, and persisted. Only through a concerted and generally successful effort to alter this image have most patients been accepted into full social rights without deprecation. Remnants of the old status remain, however; for instance, permission to drive an automobile has a totally different set of ground rules for them. The effort to remove the cloud of social ostracism from these patients is ongoing and thoroughly laudable; one of the strongest positions in this effort has been the outright denial of an "epileptic personality."

The pendulum has swung too far, however. The effort to accept the epilepsy patient as a normal citizen has fostered a strong, outspoken denial that epilepsy could be the source of any personality abnormality. The quantity and the quality of investigations on these behavior problems have been sharply curtailed, almost to the point of nonexistence. Funding for research into behavioral problems has been restricted, and even reports of observations of epileptic behavior have been limited by counterprejudice; most reports of psychiatric difficulties in these patients have met with sharp criticism. Resources available for research on interictal personality problems are virtually nonexistent. It is obvious that the conscious effort to deny existence of an epileptic interictal personality change has been successful.

Despite this background, many physicians who care for these patients recognize that some of them do have striking behavioral disabilities. Although a number of common features have been offered, more accurate descriptions, the degree of potential severity, the course of the behavioral abnormalities, and the prevalence of the behavior abnormalities among epilepsy patients remain unknown. Agreement is available on only one significant aspect: Not all epilepsy patients show personality disturbance (9–12). In fact, the incidence of various types of behavior abnormality in these patients remains virtually unknown. Whether personality changes are common or rare, whether they are related to one or to many seizure types, whether they are related to one or to a variety of anatomical foci, and whether one or several medications are more likely to be troublesome, among many other basic questions, remain unprobed. In fact, there is little solid evidence that even supports the clinical observations of a behavioral (personality) abnormality unique to epilepsy. It must be remembered, however, that lack of evidence cannot be accepted as evidence of lack.

In the past several decades, one voice that has been most effective in focusing attention on the interictal behavioral changes of the epilepsy patient has been that of Norman Geschwind (10,13). While Geschwind's writings on the topic are relatively limited, and his personal contribution was limited to the demonstration of hypergraphia as a significant sign in some epilepsy patients, his efforts to bring together the diverse observations of this disorder and to establish a cluster of salient features (a syndrome), particularly in the face of considerable opposition, warrant consideration of the term "Geschwind syndrome." Currently, this term is used in both medical and lay press, as a designation for one of the described interictal personality disturbances of epilepsy. Use of this term offers a distinct advantage. The Geschwind syndrome correctly refers to a finite, phenomenologically specific behavioral pattern; in contrast, the term "epileptic personality disorder" has a far more general connotation, suggesting that behavioral problems exist in many epilepsy patients; this consideration remains unacceptable. This presentation will focus on that cluster of clinical findings that a number of clinicians recognize as being a relatively specific complication found in some long-term epilepsy patients.

CLINICAL DESCRIPTION

Many problems other than, or in addition to, social pressures have interfered with delineation of epileptic behavioral symptomatol-

ogy. The character of what was called "epilepsy" changed significantly following the advent of the electroencephalogram (EEG) and the demonstration of many previously unrecognized seizure types, particularly the disturbance called "psychomotor," "limbic," "temporal lobe," or "complex partial" epilepsy. Only recently has characterization of behavioral disorders in epilepsy based on these new concepts and taxonomic classifications been attempted. Although abnormal behavior had been described in these patients for several millenia, these presentations provided only conglomerate descriptions of many patients, most of whom suffered intractable seizures and a variety of psychotic findings. Teasing the interictal personality disturbances from such a morass of psychiatric descriptions has not been easy and, quite honestly, has not been done.

Most formal studies of epilepsy behavioral disturbances and personality aberrations performed since the advent of modern anticonvulsants (14–17) provide a consistent picture. Modern techniques fail to demonstrate either an excess of psychiatric disorder in the epilepsy patient (12,18) or a specific epileptic personality (11,19,20). Through the 1960s the absence of particular psychiatric findings was frequently reported and a specific epileptic personality was specifically denied.

From observations made during this time (the 1960s), however, Geschwind eventually described a set of behavioral abnormalities that he had observed in patients with "temporal lobe seizure disorder" (10,13). "Behavioral change," the term proposed by Geschwind, is inexact; however, he did outline four major findings that represented what he considered a characteristic personality disorder: (i) increased concern with philosophical, moral, or religious issues; (ii) hypergraphia; (iii) hyposexuality; and (iv) irritability. Geschwind stressed the potential for a specific pathogenesis underlying these personality alterations and stated that if this were true, "this syndrome will be unique in being the only cause of major behavioral change for which a reasonably detailed pathogenesis exists" (10). On a number of occasions, Geschwind suggested that the interictal personality disorder of temporal lobe epilepsy ranked among the most characteristic of all psychiatric syndromes. He was just as absolute in his presentation of the syndrome as his contemporaries were in their denial of its existence.

One of Geschwind's students, David Bear, reviewed the medical literature seeking descriptions of psychiatric and behavioral problems of epilepsy patients reported during the previous 100 years. From this background he selected 18 features described by two or more reliable investigators; he listed these findings in three separate categories (Table 1). A forced-response questionnaire was constructed to seek the presence of these characteristics in epilepsy subjects. This questionnaire was presented to 27 patients with unilateral temporal lobe epileptogenic foci and 21 control subjects. In addition, the questionnaire was given to an independent rater, one who knew the subject well. Results from this investigation (21) demonstrated that the behavioral characteristics contained in the questionnaire occurred more often in patients with epilepsy than in the non-epilepsy population. Of more significance was a difference in the self-reports of patients which appeared to depend upon whether the right or left temporal lobe was the site of the seizure focus. Although the ratings of behavioral problems provided by the independent observers were reasonably consistent regardless of whether the seizure focus involved the right or the left temporal lobe, most patients with a left temporal lobe focus reported themselves as much less behaviorally abnormal than did those with a right-sided focus. Bear and Fedio (21) suggested that patients with a right temporal lobe focus could be considered "tarnishers," whereas those with a left temporal lobe focus were called "polishers."

The Bear–Fedio (21) study presented both a novel test vehicle and a body of solid data, but the results immediately proved difficult to use in clinical situations. The questionnaire did not separate epileptic behavior from other behavioral problems, and no control subjects with other seizure types or with psychiatric disorders had been included. Although the results have been interpreted as support for a distinct syndrome, this possibility was not even probed in this project. Rather than proving helpful, the Bear–Fedio (21) data merely added fuel to the ongoing controversy.

In a series of publications, Dietrich Blumer (a psychiatrist who has spent much of his career engaged in the study of candidates for temporal lobe epilepsy seizure surgery) presented a number of his own observations and eventually combined these into a description of the epileptic personality (9,22,23) (see Chapter 12). The major findings of the syndrome outlined by Blumer were as follows: (a) sexual changes, (b) impulsive/irritable behavior, (c) good naturedness/religiosity, (d) deepening of emotional response (viscosity), and (e) alternating moods and epileptic psychoses. While these findings were independently derived and have somewhat different emphasis, Blumer's observations are easily correlated with those of both Geschwind and Bear.

My own personal experience with behavioral problems of epilepsy patients has led to agreement with Geschwind, Bear, and Blumer, but with a slightly different characterization of the interictal personality disturbance. I have found the problem sufficiently consistent to be considered a true disorder (syndrome) with three major areas of abnormalities: (i) *circumstantiality,* a tendency to be overinclusive, involving excessive and detailed verbal output, excessive writing (hypergraphia), and a clinging, tenacious attitude (viscosity); (ii) *altered sexuality,* almost always in the direction of hyposexuality, although rare instances of homosexuality, trans-

TABLE 1. *Interictal characteristics*[a]

I. Emotionality
   Manic tendencies
   Depression
   Humorlessness
II. Altered sexuality
   Anger, hostility
   Aggression
III. Religiosity
   Nascent philosophical interest
   Augmented sense of personal destiny
   Dependence, passivity
   Paranoia
   Moralism
   Guilt
   Obsessionalism
   Circumstantiality
   Viscosity
   Hypergraphia

[a]Adapted from ref. 53, with permission.

TABLE 2. *Characteristics of the Geschwind syndrome*

I. Circumstantiality
   Overinclusive verbal output
   Hypergraphia
   Viscosity
II. Altered sexuality
   Hyposexuality
   Onset of homosexual interests (rarely)
III. Altered mental behavior
   Intense cognitive interests
   Intense emotional responses

vestism, fetishism, etc., have been reported; and (iii) *intensification of cognitive and emotional behavior,* a tendency to develop strong and deep interests in philosophic, religious, and emotional aspects of life. Table 2 presents this breakdown of the characteristics of the interictal personality disorder.

CLINICAL PHENOMENOLOGY

The first (and in most instances the most striking) characteristic of the epileptic personality is the overinclusiveness that may be manifested in a variety of manners. The most bothersome is the circumstantial, hyperdetailed, lengthy, and persistent verbal output. Gruhle (1) noted of the epilepsy patient: "It takes him a long time to get to the point, he uses expletives as well as an excessive number of polite expressions, fills in with quotations and tries to ensure himself in advance against any possible misunderstanding." The epilepsy patient wants to be certain that the listener understands, fully and without any question, all of the nuances leading to a given answer or statement. He may spend more than 10 min responding to a single question, incorporating into the response detailed background information, long narrative tales, and comprehensive explanations, but these apparent verbal wanderings usually turn out to be germane; the subject has provided a full answer. In many instances, however, the examiner does not have the time to accept so much information; the response will be interrupted during an early stage, and it often appears that the patient has produced only an unrelated rambling. It is not difficult to misdiagnose such an output as a manic flight of ideas or

even psychotic tangentiality. The patients are often insistent, sometimes crudely, in their demands that the listener hear them out, a situation that produces resentment and hostility on the part of the physician as well as the patient. The patients may actually camp in the doctors' office and/or follow them on ward rounds and other aspects of their daily activities in order to fully present their feelings; not infrequently the epilepsy patient with this personality problem will return following an interview to present additional information, to further clarify statements, or to leave a note or letter that further discusses some point raised in the previous conversation. It is this tenacious demand to present their ideas that has been termed "viscosity" or "stickiness."

A closely related phenomenon, hypergraphia, appears in some of the epilepsy patients who show circumstantial verbal output and appears to represent a circumstantial verbal output in written language form. It is limited to those patients with at least a moderate level of literacy. Many epilepsy patients with striking vocal overinclusiveness do not show hypergraphia, probably because of their background (low I.Q. or poor graphic skills). Those who do show hypergraphia may write poetry, produce novels, keep diaries or detailed logs of their daily activities, or compose essays, long discourses, or novels discussing epilepsy, medicine, or totally unrelated subjects. One patient of mine wrote three full books on the economic problems of the Middle East despite the fact that he had no immediate knowledge of economics nor of the Middle East. Letters-to-the-Editor or to mayors, governors, senators, etc., are common and may evidence both paranoia and hostility. Circumstantiality, as expressed by overinclusive verbal output, hypergraphia, and sticky personality, is a dramatically bothersome clinical feature, and its presence should alert an examiner to the possibility of an epilepsy-related personality disorder.

The second major clinical finding, altered sexuality, is now widely recognized as a significant clinical problem for some epilepsy patients. Blumer (24) reported that 35 of 50 patients with temporal lobe epilepsy showed at least some abnormality of sexual behavior; the most common finding was a chronic, global hyposexuality. Much less common were hypersexuality (this most often followed surgery or the introduction of anticonvulsant medication), ictal or postictal sexual arousal, or homosexual behavior. The chronic global hyposexuality of epilepsy represents a true loss of libido (25). Although most epilepsy patients report that they experience occasional sexual arousal, the occurrence is notably limited, often as little as one time per year. In some instances, hyposexuality is altered by appropriate seizure treatment; both anticonvulsants and surgery have produced gratifying (in fact sometimes excessive) return of sexual arousal. The relationship between the sexual alteration and the specific seizure types, age at onset, duration of the disorder, treatment for the seizures, and anatomical site of seizure focus remains unstudied. Shukla et al. (26) demonstrated that hyposexuality was far more common in temporal lobe epilepsy patients than in grand mal epilepsy patients; observations indicate that mesial temporal localization is significant (22,27), but no comprehensive study has been performed.

The third major characteristic, the alterations that affect cognitive and emotional responses, is best described as an intensification (deepening). Individual epilepsy patients with this problem express strong interest and sincere belief in cognitive entities over which they have no control. Religion, philosophy, patriotism, truth, beauty, and other abstract concepts develop an overwhelming importance. Religious conversion is common (and often recurrent). The intellectual interests tend to be serious, producing a sober, somber, humorless attitude. Ferguson et al. (28), using a novel test vehicle, demonstrated a sharp decrease in the recognition of humor in a group of temporal lobe epilepsy patients. Patients with the Geschwind syndrome tend to deal in absolutes; shades of gray (including differences of opinion) are rarely acknowledged. They believe intensely and argue insistently, although it is not uncommon to find that they have altered their belief at some future date.

A similar intensification that involves emotional behavior is not infrequent. Individuals with this problem can become excessively angry, deeply paranoid, or seriously depressed; they may act in an aggressive or vindictive manner. The intense emotional feelings may be short-lived, and if they are accompanied by verbal or physical outbursts directed against family or friends, a true remorse may be expressed. Not infrequently, however, the patient with the Geschwind syndrome may not react; rather, a grudge is slowly built up until some minor aggravation produces an intense, excessive response. Whether a relationship exists between the outbursts of intense emotion and a particular ictal or interictal state remains unstudied. Some have hypothesized a relationship between such events and a flurry of seizures (overt or covert) (22,29), but this also remains unproved lore.

When all three behavioral characteristics—circumstantiality, altered sexuality, and intensified mental state—are present in a patient, the picture is so strongly suggestive of the interictal personality disorder that seizure evaluation is indicated; and even if the initial evaluation is negative (no history of seizures, no epileptiform activity on the EEG), a therapeutic trial of anticonvulsants is warranted.

CLINICAL VARIATIONS

Some investigators have attempted to classify different epilepsy-related behaviors. Most studies have focused on involvement of either the right or the left temporal lobe as the site of the seizure focus. Differences in behavior based on left/right temporal involvement was originally championed by Flor-Henry (30, 31). He suggested that a left-hemisphere seizure focus was more likely to produce a schizophrenic-type psychotic disturbance; moreover, his data suggested some preference for affective abnormality to be associated with a right temporal lobe focus, although this was not a robust demonstration. Subsequent studies (32,33) have supported the occurrence of schizophrenic-type psychotic findings with left temporal lobe seizure focus but have provided little support for the contention that a right temporal lobe focus would lead to affective disorder.

McIntyre et al. (34) studied a small number of patients with clearly demarcated right or left temporal lobe foci utilizing a series of psychological tests designed to assess differences in cognitive style. Patients with left lateralization exhibited a more reflective style, whereas those with right-sided foci showed a tendency toward impulsive responses; a greater tendency for disturbed verbal communication was noted in the left temporal group. Whether the observations of McIntyre et al. (34), Flor-Henry (30,31), Sherwin et al., (32) Trimble (33), and others can be interpolated to the Geschwind syndrome is far from apparent. Variations in test vehicles and observed behaviors make correlation difficult.

As already noted, Bear and Fedio (21) demonstrated a striking laterality difference. Patients with right temoral lobe foci tended to rate themselves considerably less abnormal in behavior than did their close observers, and they often flatly denied many of their behavioral aberrations. Those with left temporal lobe seizure foci tended to be frank and honest, basically agreeing with the ratings given by the observers. Although this right/left differentiation has been specifically denied by some observers (11,19), none has replicated the Bear–Fedio patient/observer technique.

CRITICISMS OF THE SYNDROME

The occurrence of a personality abnormality that affects all or even a sizable number of epilepsy patients has been challenged by many investigators over the years. Among the early criticisms, Tizard (20) noted that the populations under study, the criteria for selection, and the broad, inadequate descriptions of behavior in early reports raised important questions concerning the validity of such an entity. Guerrant et al. (14) sought evidence of an epileptic behavioral abnormality (personality) through a controlled study. An extensive neurologic, psychiatric, psychologic, and electroencephalographic evaluation was administered to groups of psychomotor and grand mal seizure patients as well as to "normal" control subjects, all of whom attended the same medical clinic. No quantitative difference in the amount of either psychiatric or personality disorder was demonstrated between the three groups. The study is often criticized, however, because such a large percentage of the "normal" subjects had psychiatric abnormality that, while even greater numbers of the two epilepsy groups had problems, the difference could not reach statistical significance. Although some characteristics were noted for each group, no diagnostically significant clusters were demonstrated. Stevens (12) reported on 100 epilepsy patients from her own clinic. She divided her patients into those with temporal lobe, grand mal, and focal motor seizure patterns; the first two groups showed more psychiatric disorder than did the third group, but the difference in need for psychiatric care between the psychomotor and the grand mal patients was not significant. Stevens did note striking differences in the basic behavioral problems of the two groups, so that although no quantitative difference was demonstrated, a qualitative difference was suggested. In a clinical and social analysis of 1020 adult patients with epilepsy, Juul-Jensen (18) failed to demonstrate a specific psychopathology associated with temporal lobe or psychomotor seizures.

Formal psychological studies have also questioned the validity of a psychomotor epilepsy personality. Small et al. (15) used a number of clinical rating scales, including the Minnesota Multiphasic Personality Inventory (MMPI) (35), Wechsler Memory Scale (WMS) (36), Wechsler Adult Intelligence Scale (WAIS) (37), and others, to study 25 psychomotor and 25 nonpsychomotor epilepsy patients. No distinctions separated the two groups. Two subsequent studies by Small et al. (16,17) also failed to demonstrate personality profiles that differentiated psychomotor from nonpsychomotor patients. Mignone et al. (38) also used the MMPI and reported that neither clinical description nor MMPI profiles distinguished psychomotor epilepsy from other epilepsy. In an extensive series of studies analyzing various scales of the MMPI, Hermann and colleagues (39–42) did demonstrate some elevated scores in patients with temporal lobe epilepsy when compared to those in generalized seizure patients. The differences were neither unique nor diagnostic, however, and together with Dikmen et al. (43), he questioned whether the MMPI was a suitable instrument for probing epileptic psychopathology.

Thus, multiple studies utilizing psychologic batteries have looked at psychiatric problems in epilepsy patients, and although most have demonstrated that psychiatric abnormalities were more prevalent in the epilepsy patient than in the general population, they failed to demonstrate a specific personality disorder.

The more specific descriptions of the personality abnormalities suggested by Geschwind and colleagues, along with the rigid outline provided by Bear and Fedio in the 1970s, provided impetus for additional studies; again, most have been critical. Mungas (19) presented the Bear–Fedio Personality Inventory to approximately 150 outpatients in a Neurobehavior Clinic, including some with temporal lobe epilepsy, some with other neurologic behavioral disorders, and some with psychiatric disorders. None of the 18 traits suggested by Bear distinguished the group of temporal lobe patients from patients with either neurologic or psychiatric behavioral disorders. Mungas (19) demonstrated that most of the Bear–Fedio traits could be seen in, and accounted for by, independent psychiatric disturbances; he concluded that the traits reflected underlying personality differences and nonspecific psychopathology, not a specific behavioral syndrome.

In another sizable study, Rodin and Schmaltz (11) presented the Bear–Fedio questionnaire to 148 epilepsy patients, 18 patients attending a pain clinic, 15 psychiatric inpatients, and 40 control subjects. They found relatively robust group differences: Normal controls showed the fewest abnormal behavior traits, followed by pain patients, epilepsy patients, and patients hospitalized for psychiatric illness. They did not, however, demonstrate any difference between temporal lobe and generalized seizure patients. They attempted to replicate the independent rater technique of Bear and Fedio in a few of these patients and failed to demonstrate the polishing/tarnishing dichotomy. From these data they concluded that the inventory did not demonstrate personality traits specific for temporal lobe epilepsy, nor could it be used to distinguish between right and left temporal foci.

Thus, a sizable number of studies have been performed by competent, although not necessarily unbiased, investigators who sought a personality abnormality specific to epilepsy. Many of the early studies can be criticized for the use of inappropriate test vehicles. As an example, the MMPI was not de-signed to demonstrate the seizure personality disorder, and thus, not surprisingly, it failed in this task. Similarly, later studies featured the Bear–Fedio test, which was not designed as a diagnostic tool; as a result, these studies were also inconclusive. To date, no study either validates or invalidates the clinical observations suggesting that a unique cluster of behaviors occurs in the interictal phase of some seizure patients.

DISCUSSION

The Geschwind syndrome remains questioned and uncertain as a specific entity. It is generally agreed that the syndrome is not common, even among epilepsy patients, and it is also apparent that many of the traits can be seen in non-epilepsy behavioral disorders. Nonetheless, the combination of several otherwise uncommon findings suggests a true syndrome. This status resembles that of another clinical cluster, the Gerstmann syndrome (agraphia, acalculia, right–left disorientation, and finger agnosia), which has been proved nonexistent by appropriate biostatistical studies (44,45). None of the individual characteristics has either distinct localizing or consistent etiologic value; nonetheless, the presence of all four on a brain damage basis has substantial clinical and localizing value (46,47). Failure to support a syndrome with selected psychological/statistical techniques does not necessarily disqualify the cluster of findings from clinical use.

Several observations/interpretations in addition to the right–left difference have been offered to explain the cluster of Geschwind syndrome findings. Gastaut and co-workers (48,49) noted that certain traits present in some patients with epilepsy were the opposite of those reported in the Klüver–Bucy syndrome (50). Originally described in monkeys following bilateral anterior temporal lobectomy, the Klüver–Bucy syndrome can be recognized in humans following bilateral temporal lobe damage (51,52). Like the monkeys, patients with the Klüver–Bucy syndrome manifest hypersexuality, a constant shifting of attention, and a striking placidity. The Klüver–Bucy syndrome, clearly a result of absent anterior temporal lobe influence, contrasts sharply with the temporal lobe seizure personality traits of intense mental interest, hyposexuality, and clinging, viscous responsiveness. Table 3 outlines the differences of the two syndromes suggested by Gastaut et al. (49) and Blumer (23). Bear (53) noted this dichotomy and suggested that the epileptic personality disorder represented a sensory–limbic hyperconnection in contrast to the hypoconnection of the Klüver–Bucy syndrome. Geschwind (10) carried this proposition even further. He postulated that the phenomenon of epilepsy kindling may affect the amygdala, producing a limbic spike focus; furthermore, he hypothesized that this intermittent abnormality in the limbic system could alter perception of, and response to, environmental stimuli, thereby altering the behavior (personality). Such pathophysiologic suggestions remain entirely theoretical, and other possible explanations deserve exploration. A number have been suggested:

1. Environmental and personal psychological factors may produce the personality abnormalities; the stigma of epilepsy has not been eradicated (54,55). Many epilepsy patients are sensitive about their disorder, and it is not difficult to construct a psychodynamic explanation for a personality aberration. Some present with a "sick person" syndrome (56). Early studies (12,15,38) seriously sought pertinent underlying psychological factors, but the findings were nonspecific. Studies limited to childhood epilepsy (57,58) indicated that psychosocial factors did affect seizure frequency, and it was postulated that this early-life influence could lead to personality

problems in later years. Further studies in this direction, focused on patients showing the characteristics of the Geschwind syndrome, are warranted.

2. The age of onset itself may be of importance in development of a personality disorder. Taylor (59) demonstrated that a psychotic complication was more likely to occur in an individual with lifelong seizure disorder. Whether a similar background is true of the personality alteration remains unsettled, but anecdotal experiences demonstrate that early onset is not mandatory.

3. In a similar vein, the effect of long-term anticonvulsant medication deserves attention as a potential cause of personality aberration in epilepsy patients. Both the type of medication used and the number of years the patient has been under treatment could be factors of significance in the genesis of personality alteration. It must be recognized, however, that many patients take the same medications for many years without developing the specific characteristics of the Geschwind syndrome.

4. The socioeconomic status of the patient has been considered pertinent. Disordered personalities appear more frequent in "clinic" or teaching hospital practices than in "private" practices. In fact, many nonacademic epileptologists deny that any of their patients have the characteristics of the epileptic personality. Several possible explanations for this apparent social influence deserve consideration. Does the personality aberration prevent the patient from being work-efficient and earning sufficient income so that he or she cannot afford private medical care? Does the personality disorder indicate that the affected individual has suffered a greater degree of brain damage? Several uncontrolled studies have suggested that the private practice groups also contain patients who have behavioral abnormalities but that these problems are overlooked in the economic realities that govern the private practice.

5. It is possible that either a hereditary or a developmental abnormality may be significant, particularly if abnormality early in life is demonstrated as important in the personality disorder. Is mesial temporal sclerosis a major cause of the personality disturbance? Hematoma? Widespread cortical and/or subcortical

TABLE 3. *Differences between Klüver–Bucy syndrome and temporal hyperconnection syndrome*

Klüver–Bucy syndrome	Temporal hyperconnection syndrome
Hypersexual	Hyposexual
Hypermetamorphosis	Stickiness
Cognitive impairment	Cognitive intensification
Placidity	Emotional intensity
Structural damage to anterior temporal lobe	Seizure focus in anterior temporal lobe

damage? These are answerable questions that have yet to be explored.

6. Is there an anatomical basis for the syndrome? Differences between right temporal and left temporal lobe seizure foci have already been discussed, but whether these involve the personality or other behavioral characteristics, or even represent genuine findings, remains uncertain. Differences between medial temporal and lateral temporal location of the seizure focus may be of pertinence in the personality disorder, a hypothesis that has never been adequately explored. Similarly, anterior (rather than posterior) temporal involvement may be important. That the pathogenesis of the behavioral syndrome is not strictly based on temporal lobe damage is also possible; the personality aberration has been noted with seizure foci elsewhere in the limbic system (e.g., cingulate gyrus, insula). Conversely, both temporal and nontemporal limbic tissues can be the source of seizure activity without producing the characteristic personality alteration.

7. Finally, some investigators have suggested that an underlying (pre-morbid, inherent, intrinsic) psychiatric disorder, totally unrelated to the seizure problem, is the source of the abnormal behavior seen in some epilepsy patients. This is not illogical; psychiatric problems are common in all populations, and there is no reason that some patients with epilepsy would not also harbor an intrinsic psychiatric disorder. The presence of a distinct syndrome, however (i.e., one that does not occur in non-epilepsy subjects), makes this an unlikely explanation. If one uses the same basic care in analyzing behavioral symptomatology that is now used in classifying seizures, the tendency to lump all behavioral problems of the epilepsy patient into a "psychiatric" classification is obviously inadequate. Among the behavioral disorders, the Geschwind syndrome exists as an uncommon, but conspicuous, cluster of findings. The potential source of the Geschwind syndrome remains vague, adding to the controversy concerning its existence.

TREATMENT

If one accepts the Geschwind syndrome as a clinical entity, is there any recognized means of treating or even ameliorating the behavioral disorder? In its fully established form, the behavior of the Geschwind syndrome patient is socially unacceptable; their behavior makes family members, friends, acquaintances, medical personnel, and everyone else uncomfortable. Any improvement in their behavior would be of potential value.

Two pharmaceutical approaches have been proposed: anticonvulsants and psychotropics. Most individuals with the Geschwind syndrome have been under anticonvulsant management for many years; in most instances, this form of treatment has been successful. Many have had no overt seizures for many years, and not a few are on lower dosages of anticonvulsant than at earlier stages in their disorder. Nonetheless, careful review of the medication regime, with an eye toward improved management (either a switch to monopharmacy or change to a potentially better drug) deserves consideration. This approach can be spectacularly successful, particularly in treatment of hyposexuality (this problem has also been known to respond to appropriate seizure surgery). Unfortunately, in most instances an altered anticonvulsant regime does not alter the behavioral problem.

The second pharmaceutical avenue, psychotropic medication, is even less likely to be of help. Use of haloperidol, phenothiazine, and others of this class is not infrequent in these patients, usually without significant benefit. If schizophrenia-like symptomatology is noted, use of these drugs is indicated, but again—at least in my experience—they have provided only limited benefit.

If the patient shows deep and disturbing emotional responses such as depression, paranoia, hostility, anxiety, etc., an appropriate medication (e.g., antidepressant, antianxiety drug) can be added to the anticonvulsant regime and may help through a period of crisis. On rare occasions, electroshock therapy has been given in this situation with at least some benefit.

The most difficult aspect of the Geschwind syndrome to treat is the circumstantial, viscous personality. This state appears to be quite resistant to most anticonvulsant and psychotropic regimes. Behavioral conditioning sessions directed at increasing the epilepsy patient's awareness of his/her undesirable behavioral tendencies have been tried, but with only limited success. Unlike the patient with frontal lobe behavior who will understand the problem and the treatment but who cannot act on this knowledge, the patient with the Geschwind syndrome is unlikely to accept either criticism or advice. They are not amenable to insight psychotherapy.

In summary, treatment programs for the Geschwind syndrome are empiric and of only limited success.

SUMMARY

A characteristic personality syndrome consisting of circumstantiality (excessive verbal output, stickiness, hypergraphia), altered sexuality (usually hyposexuality), and intensified mental life (deepened cognitive and emotional responses) is present in some epilepsy patients. For identification, the term "Geschwind syndrome" has been suggested as a name for this group of behavioral phenomena. Support for, and criticism against, the existence of this syndrome as a specific personality disorder has produced more fire than substance, but the presence of an unsettled, ongoing controversy has been acknowledged (60). At present, the strongest support stems from the many clinicians who have described and attempted to manage seizure patients with these personality features. Carefully directed studies are needed to confirm or deny that the Geschwind syndrome represents a specific epilepsy/psychiatric disorder.

REFERENCES

1. Gruhle HW. Epileptische Reaktionen und epileptische Krankheiten. In: Bumke O, ed. *Handbuch der Geistenkrankheiten*, vol 8, Spezieller Teil 4. Berlin: Springer, 1930;669–728.
2. Kraepelin E. *Psychiatrie*. Leipzig: Barth, 1909.
3. Samt, P. Epileptische Irreseinformen. *Arch Psychiatr* 1876;6:110–216.
4. Schorsch G. Epilepsie: Klinik und forschung. In: Gruhle HW, Jung R, Mayer-Gross W. Müller M, eds. *Psychiatrie der Gegenwart Forschung und Praxis, Band II: Klinische Psychiatrie*. Berlin: Springer-Verlag, 1960:646–777.
5. Freud S. Dostoevsky and parricide. In: Strachey J, ed. *The standard edition of the complete works of Sigmund Freud*, vol 21. London: Hogarth Press, 1961:177–196.
6. Szondi L. *Schicksalsonalytische Therapie*. Bern: Huber, 1963.
7. Alajouanine T. Dostoevski's epilepsy. *Brain* 1963;86:209–218.
8. Geschwind N. Dostoevsky's epilepsy. In: Blumer D, ed. *Psychiatric aspects of epilepsy*. Washington, DC: American Psychiatric Press, 1984;325–334.
9. Blumer D, Benson DF. Psychiatric manifestations of epilepsy. In: Benson DF, Blumer D, eds. *Psychiatric aspects of neurologic disease*, vol 2. New York: Grune & Stratton, 1982;25–48.
10. Geschwind N. Behavioural changes in temporal lobe epilepsy. *Psychol Med* 1979;9:217–219.
11. Rodin E, Schmaltz S. The Bear–Fedio personality inventory and temporal lobe epilepsy. *Neurology* 1984;34:591–596.
12. Stevens JR. Psychiatric implications of psychomotor epilepsy. *Arch Gen Psychiatry* 1966;14:461–471.
13. Waxman SG, Geschwind N. Hypergraphia in temporal lobe epilepsy. *Neurology* 1974;24:629–638.
14. Guerrant J, Anderson WN, Fischer A, Weinstein M, Jaros RM, Deskins A. *Personality in epilepsy*. Springfield, IL: Charles C Thomas, 1962.
15. Small JG, Milstein V, Stevens JR. Are psychomotor epileptics different? A controlled study. *Arch Neurol* 1962;7:187–194.
16. Small JG, Small IF, Hayden MP. Further psychiatric investigations of patients with temporal and non-temporal lobe epilepsy. *Am J Psychiatry* 1966;123:303–310.
17. Small JG, Stevens J, Milstein V. Electroclinical correlates of emotional activation of the electroencephalogram. *J Nerv Ment Dis* 1964;138:146–155.
18. Juul-Jensen P. Epilepsy: a clinical and social analysis of 1020 adult patients with epileptic seizures. *Acta Neurol Scand* 1964;40(Suppl 5):1–148.
19. Mungas D. Interictal behavior abnormality in temporal lobe epilepsy. *Arch Gen Psychiatry* 1982;39:108–111.
20. Tizard B. The personality of epileptics: a discussion of the evidence. *Psychol Bull* 1962;59:196–210.
21. Bear DM, Fedio P. Quantitative analysis of interictal behavior in temporal lobe epilepsy. *Arch Neurol* 1977;34:454–467.
22. Blumer D, Walker AE. Sexual behavior in temporal lobe epilepsy. *Arch Neurol* 1967;16:31–43.
23. Blumer D. Temporal lobe epilepsy and its psychiatric significance. In: Benson DF, Blumer D, eds. *Psychiatric aspects of neurologic disease*. New York: Grune & Stratton, 1975;171–197.
24. Blumer D. Changes of sexual behavior related to temporal lobe disorders in man. *J Sex Res* 1970;6:173–180.
25. Gastaut H, Collomb H. Etude de comportemente sexual chez les epileptiques psychomoteurs. *Ann Med Psychol (Paris)* 1954;112:657–696.
26. Shukla GD, Srivastava ON, Katiyar BC. Sexual

disturbances in temporal lobe epilepsy: a controlled study. *Br J Psychiatry* 1979;134:288–292.

27. Blumer D. Hypersexual episodes in temporal lobe epilepsy. *Am J Psychiatry* 1970;126:1099–1106.

28. Ferguson SM, Schwartz ML, Rayport M. Perception of humor in patients with temporal lobe epilepsy—a cartoon test as an indicator of neuropsychological deficit. *Arch Gen Psychiatry* 1969;21:363–367.

29. Ounsted C, Lindsay J, Norman R. *Clinics in developmental medicine, vol 22: Biological factors in temporal lobe epilepsy*. London: William Heinemann Medical Books, 1966.

30. Flor-Henry P. Schizophrenic-like reactions and affective psychoses associated with temporal lobe epilepsy: etiological factors. *Am J Psychiatry* 1969;126:400–403.

31. Flor-Henry P. Ictal and interictal psychiatric manifestations in epilepsy: specific or non-specific? *Epilepsia* 1972;13:773–783.

32. Sherwin I, Peron-Magnan P, Bancaud J, Bonis A, Talairach J. Prevalence of psychosis in epilepsy as a function of the laterality of the epileptogenic lesion. *Arch Neurol* 1982;39:621–625.

33. Trimble MR. Personality disturbances in epilepsy. *Neurology* 1983;33:1332–1334.

34. McIntyre M, Pritchard PB, Lambrusco CT. Left and right temporal lobe epileptics: a controlled investigation of some psychological differences. *Epilepsia* 1976;17:377–386.

35. Hathaway SR, McKinley JG. *Minnesota Multiphasic Personality Inventory, edition 2*. New York: New York Psychological Corporation, 1951.

36. Wechsler D. A standardized memory scale for clinical use. *J Psychol* 1945;19:87–95.

37. Wechsler D. *The measurement and appraisal of adult intelligence*. Baltimore: Williams & Wilins, 1958.

38. Mignone RJ, Donnelly EF, Sadowsky P. Psychomotor and non-psychomotor epileptics. *Epilepsia* 1970;11:345–359.

39. Hermann BP, Schwartz MS, Karnes WE, Vahdat P. Psychopathology in epilepsy: relationship of seizure type to age at onset. *Epilepsia* 1980;21:15–23.

40. Hermann BP, Schwartz MS, Whitman S, Karnes WE. Aggression in epilepsy: seizure-type and high-risk variables. *Epilepsia* 1980;21:691–698.

41. Hermann BP, Schwartz MS, Whitman S, Karnes WE. Psychosis and epilepsy: seizure-type comparisons and high-risk variables. *J Clin Psychol* 1981;37:714–721.

42. Hermann BP, Dikmen S, Schwartz MS. Interictal psychopathology in patients with ictal fear: a quantitative investigation. *Neurology* 1982;32:7–11.

43. Dikmen S, Hermann BP, Rainwater G, Wilensky AJ. Validity of the Minnesota Multiphasic Personality Inventory (MMPI) to psychopathology in patients with epilepsy. *J Nerv Ment Dis* 1983;171:114–122.

44. Benton AL. The fiction of the "Gerstmann syndrome." *J Neurol Neurosurg Psychiatry* 1961;24:176–181.

45. Heimburger RF, Demyer W, Reitan RM. Implications of Gerstmann's syndrome. *J Neurol Neurosurg Psychiatry* 1964;27:52–57.

46. Benson DF, Geschwind N. The aphasias and related disturbances. In: Baker AB, Joynt R, eds. *Clinical neurology*, vol 1. Philadelphia: Harper & Row, 1985;ch. 1, 1–24.

47. Kirshner HS. *Behavioral neurology: a practical approach*. New York: Churchill Livingstone, 1986.

48. Gastaut H (Brazier M, translator). *The epilepsies—electroclinical correlations*. Springfield, IL: Charles C Thomas, 1954.

49. Gastaut H, Morin G, Lesevre N. Etude du comportement des epileptiques psychomoteurs dans l'intervalle de leurs crises: les troubles de l'activite globale et de la sociabilite. *Ann Med Psychol (Paris)* 1955;113:1–27.

50. Klüver H, Bucy PC. "Psychic blindness" and other symptoms following temporal lobectomy in rhesus monkeys. *Am J Physiol* 1937;119:352–353.

51. Lilly R, Cummings JL, Benson DF, Frankel M. The human Klüver-Bucy syndrome. *Neurology* 1983;33:1141–1145.

52. Terzian H, Dalle Ore G. Syndrome of Klüver–Bucy reproduced in man by bilateral removal of the temporal lobes. *Neurology* 1955;5:373–381.

53. Bear D. Temporal lobe epilepsy: a syndrome of sensory–limbic hyperconnection. *Cortex* 1979;15:357–384.

54. Dodrill CG, Batzel LW, Quisser HE, Temkin NR. An objective method for the assessment of psychological and social problems among epileptics. *Epilepsia* 1980;21:123–135.

55. Tan SY. Psychosocial functioning of epileptic patients: findings from a Canadian study. Paper presented at the 14th Epilepsy International Symposium. London, England, August 1982.

56. Stark-Adamec C, Adamec RE, Graham JM, Hicks RC, Bruun-Meyer SE. Complexities in the complex partial seizures personality controversy. *Psychiatr J Univ Ottawa* 1985;10:231–236.

57. Taylor DC, Falconer MA. Clinical, socio-economic and psychological changes after temporal lobectomy for epilepsy. *Br J Psychiatry* 1968;114:1247–1261.

58. Rutter M, Graham P, Yale W. The prevalence of psychiatric disorder in neuro-epileptic children. *Clin Dev Med* 1979;39:175–185.

59. Taylor DC. Factors influencing the occurrence of schizophrenia-like psychosis in patients with temporal lobe epilepsy. *Psychol Med* 1975;5:249–254.

60. Sorenson AS, Bolwig TG. Personality and epilepsy: new evidence for a relationship? A review. *Comp Psychiatry* 1987;28:369–383.

Advances in Neurology, Vol. 55, edited by
D. Smith, D. Treiman, and M. Trimble,
Raven Press, Ltd., New York © 1991.

26

Modern Approaches to Neuropsychological Testing

Stanley Berent

Neuropsychology Program, University of Michigan, Ann Arbor, Michigan 48109

Even though its foundations in scientific psychology and psychometric theory go back over 100 years, applied neuropsychology has a relatively short history that has been dated to the 1940s (1). In the past 40 years, applications of neuropsychological methods and procedures have progressed rapidly: They began as early experimental endeavors by about two dozen notable pioneers and gradually gained recognition as a clinical specialty that is systematically included in epilepsy and other treatment programs. It is of interest to note that of the approximately 3000–4000 members of the American Psychological Association's Division of Clinical Neuropsychology (Division 40), the majority are third- or fourth-generation neuropsychologists who have had personal contact with the "pioneers" referred to above or with the immediate students of such individuals. This may be one reason for the remarkable consistency of neuropsychological practice from one location to another, but there are other reasons as well. These will be addressed later. It can be said that neuropsychology has developed over these past decades into a bona fide specialty with its own theoretical foundations and a collection of unique methods and procedures that include neuropsychological tests and the more comprehensive neuropsychological examination in addition to other traditional procedures from the field of psychology.

Neuropsychology testing has been criticized in the past for being atheoretical (2). In fact, the neuropsychological enterprise is firmly based on several theoretical foundations. As a field, neuropsychology relates to the parent discipline of psychology. In so doing, the practitioner draws upon an extensive knowledge base that derives from diverse areas in psychology—areas such as psychobiology and social, experimental, developmental, school, and clinical psychology. A host of formal theories with relevance to epilepsy and other neurologic problems are provided by these areas. Some representative theoretical models include animal and human learning, memory, personality theory, intelligence, and, of special relevance to neuropsychology, psychometric theory. In the practice of this discipline, there is a strong commitment to the scientific method in general and to the neurosciences in particular.

It is important to note that both as a part of generic psychology and as a specialty within that larger field, neuropsychology maintains its own journals. These journals allow for the systematic archiving of information having particular relevance for members of the profession as well as for others with interest in the relationships between the brain and behavior. Other aspects of neuropsychology as a professional specialty include the presence of a professional organization, a published set of ethical guidelines, published standards for service delivery, and the availability of specialty board certification and generic licensure.

In interest and in action, neuropsychology has found areas of commonalty and compatibility with other professions. Just as the knowledge base of neuropsychology is available to other disciplines, so too are those of other specialties available to the neuropsychologist. Philosophical models accepted in the field of psychology are also likely to be the same as those accepted in other fields. The practicing neuropsychologist, like his or her neurologist colleague, for instance, is likely to subscribe to a medical model of disease. That is, they are each likely to view the signs and symptoms of disease as fitting traditional medical models of trauma, infection, and systemic disorder or as agreeing with the more recent concept of unified disease theory (3). The rapid growth of neuropsychology has sometimes led to competition between itself and other disciplines, but it is important to note that the support and encouragement given to neuropsychology by these other fields has been instrumental in its development as an applied discipline and in making neuropsychological services available to the patient.

Therefore, new developments in neuropsychological testing can only be discussed within the broader context of neuropsychology in general. The most recent development in neuropsychological testing is (a) the systematizing of its methods and (b) the evolution of these activities towards a consistent model of clinical service and academic inquiry.

THE PROCESS OF NEUROPSYCHOLOGICAL TESTING

In practice, the clinical neuropsychologist may engage in a variety of activities that are either related to the direct response to patient complaints or related to an academic end. For instance, the psychologist might be teaching, consulting to a multidisciplinary treatment team, or addressing a basic research question. It is the neuropsychological examination and the more specific activity of psychological testing, however, that is associated in the minds of most people with a neuropsychologist's role. Here and for the remainder of this chapter, the focus will be on this aspect of the neuropsychology enterprise.

In almost every professional setting, neuropsychology is expressed through a consultation model. In many instances, the model is highly formalized with specific guidelines for making referrals, the kinds of patients that can be seen, and so on. There is often a hierarchical system which may involve specially trained "test technicians" or psychometricians who administer many of the tests to patients (4). Always, there is a psychologist who maintains responsibility and authority over the program in its professional and technical aspects. This last observation is not by accident, because it is in keeping with specific ethical guidelines that have been laid down by the profession of psychology (5,6). The nature of neuropsychological practice is highly uniform in most of the world, and this is because of a variety of contingencies that are common to all programs. An example of such a contingency is the ethical consideration just noted. The aforementioned use of technicians to administer tests provides another example of this phenomenon. That is, there are several reasons why a psychologist/technician model is often employed in the testing effort (4). The use of such a model is economical because it allows one psychologist to see several patients while the "routine" portions of the testing exam are administered by the technicians. It can also be argued that "standardization" of procedures is enhanced by the use of a technician model. It is interesting to note that when one or more contingencies are varied, the consequence will be reflected in an alteration in the way a given program is expressed. For example, if the psychologist follows a "process model" of neuropsychology, the program may be less likely to employ a technician model than when a "psychological" model is used (7).

The neuropsychological process as expressed in most modern programs can be described as involving six steps (3):

1. Referral
2. Consultation phase
3. Procedure
4. Report
5. Interpretive phase
6. Follow-up

Each of the steps in this process will be described more fully in the following sections. Attention will be given to what is particularly new in neuropsychology as well, and these events will be discussed in relation to the particular step with which they are associated.

Referral

Referral questions derive from the nature of the patient complaint(s). These questions are developed through direct and effective communication between the psychologist and the referring person. The referral might be from another professional, but it might also be self-initiated by the patient or a member of the patient's family. It should be mentioned that although a major effort in neuropsychology is the standardized examination, not all referrals eventuate in testing. A referral may lead directly to treatment intervention, with psychotherapy being an example. The referral is usually initiated for clinical reasons, but, depending on the setting, it might be to initiate a protocol as part of a research project.

Consultation Phase

It is during the consultation phase that the psychologist is assessing the nature of the complaint, clarifying the complaint details, and formulating questions to be addressed in the test examination. Decisions are also being made with regard to those questions that are not amenable to testing and also with regard to alternative responses that may be available. Most often, there is a written product of the consultive interaction. Although this may initially consist of notes scribbled during a telephone conversation, these are eventually transcribed to a standard referral form. The information required to complete such a form may vary from place to place. Minimal information usually includes items such as: patient's parents', and other relevant family members' names, addresses, and telephone number; identity of referring person(s); patient's age; other demographics; and pertinent education facts. Information on special handicaps (e.g., limited vision) and/or special needs (e.g., frequent urination) is usually also noted. Referral questions are listed along with directions for whom to contact for scheduling purposes.

Procedure

The procedure in neuropsychology most often consists of an examination that employs psychological tests. The term "test" has been used carelessly at times. From the psychologists' point of view, a test, in its formal sense, is a task or set of tasks that has been studied and found to meet certain psychometric criteria. There are demands that have been formalized as "standards." These expectations have been placed (by the profession) both on the developer of such tests and on the user (8). At the very least, a test will reflect (through published research) the established "validity" of the instrument to measure what it purports to measure. Validity is a technical aspect of test development, and it is established through formal mathematical methods. As stated in the standards (8), validity is the most important consideration in test evaluation, since it refers to the ". . . appropriateness, meaningfulness, and usefulness of the specific inferences made from test scores" (ref. 8, p. 9).

"Reliability" is another aspect to be established and publicly communicated about a test. This concept basically refers to the degree to which test scores are free from errors of measurement (ref. 8, p. 19). Although the user of a test is not generally required to independently establish a test's reliability, the user does need to know to what extent the differences between forms or administrations of a particular test reflect errors of measurement as opposed to reflecting the effects of disease progression (e.g., continuation of seizures) or of another clinical event.

A test is usually "standardized." That is, there is a specified procedure for administering the test which does not vary willy-nilly. This concept of standardization has been tremendously influential in neuropsychology. On the one hand, its valuation has served as a contingency (as referred to earlier) that explains the emphasis placed on careful training and supervision of those individuals who are to administer the tests. On another level, the concept has often been extended more generally to the neuropsychology program, especially in those programs that are strongly based on a psychometric model. Such programs are likely to emphasize a standardized approach (although not as rigorously as with a specific test) in such aspects of the program as referrals, patient scheduling, formatting of written reports, and so on.

Finally, a test is "normed." That is, there is some prescribed method for relating the test scores to a theoretical or empirical distribution (ref. 8, p. 31). It should be mentioned that norms do not remove the paramount importance placed on validity and reliability issues. They simply aid in understanding what a particular score on a test means.

There are literally thousands of published psychological tests to choose from, and there are a variety of non-test procedures as well. The latter can, in light of the technical considerations just discussed, be referred to as "tasks," to distinguish them from bona fide psychological tests in the technical sense. Tasks can also be useful in the neuropsychology exam. Many automated procedures that have been introduced in recent years will fall under this rubric. Some tasks have come to be emphasized as a result of advancing knowledge about the central nervous system. Simple and choice reaction time procedures, for example, lend themselves to computerization and have become important in studies of neuropharmacology and behavior (9). The topic of automation in neuropsychology is not a simple one, and more will be said on this later.

One might now ask the question, On what basis is a given test selected to be used in a particular case? There are several factors to consider in answering such a question. The neuropsychologist must first of all consider how the test relates to the referral question(s). The technical merits of the test must next be evaluated. Finally, there are factors such as customary practice, training background, professional competencies, and other practical considerations. Each of these factors will now be discussed more fully.

Firstly, the capacity of a given instrument to generate data that will answer the referral question must be evaluated. This consideration underlies (a) the importance placed on the referral and consultation phases of the neuropsychological process and (b) the care needed in formulating questions that will be suitable for neuropsychological inquiry. "Suitability" is used here in much the same sense as it is used in any scientific inquiry.

The question posed might be as follows: Are there observable behaviors whose measurement will help answer the referral question(s)? Relevant variables become "operationally defined" according to performance on a given task. In many instances, more than one kind of data may be required in order to answer a given question. For example, a question about a patient's readiness to return to a regular classroom setting following a period of hospitalization may require test data that reflects, among other things, past school performance (e.g., reading level), general level of ability (e.g., intellect), presence or absence of cognitive dysfunction (e.g., impairment of verbal memory), and factors that may interfere with optimal performance (e.g., depression).

Secondly, the technical merits of a given test instrument, from a psychometric point of view, will be evaluated. Are the available norms suitable for comparison to the present sample? Does the test measure the theoretical construct as needed to answer the referral question? (For example, is it valid?) Will the chosen test allow for a repeat examination at a future date, or are practice effects too great to allow for such re-testing when it is needed? These are merely three questions that might be asked at this point in the process.

A third area to consider is choosing a test can be termed "convention." There are certain instruments which have been used so extensively that they have become standard components in most neuropsychological test batteries. A prime example of such a "standard" is the Wechsler Adult Intelligence Scale—Revised (WAIS-R) or its counterpart, the Wechsler Intelligence Scale for Children—Revised (WISC-R) (10). The Wechsler Intelligence Scales, in fact, have been translated into many languages and have been "normed" to many cultures. These scales are almost universally used by neuropsychologists everywhere.

A fourth consideration that enters into test selection relates to the training background of the person engaged in choosing. One could argue that there are only two factors that enter into test selection. Listed as the first and second considerations above, these factors are represented by (a) the data needed to answer a given referral question and (b) the technical merits of a given instrument. Both convention and training biases would be viewed in this case as merely extensions of the two factors just mentioned. That is, one continues to use, and continues to teach others to use, those test instruments that meet the requirements of situation and technical suitability.

There is another source of influence on test selection that is represented by the realm of what can be called practical considerations. This source is listed separately because it represents a set of extra-test considerations. In many instances, one might idealistically wish that this final type of influence not enter into decisions on test selection. Tension might arise, for example, between (a) the desires of the fiscal department of a hospital to curtail costs in delivering clinical services and (b) the clinical need as perceived by the practitioner to administer a large battery of tests to a given patient. The potential legal and ethical implications that stem from this area are many. The increase in recent years in the involvement in institution governance by the neuropsychology practitioner provides an important tool for ensuring the delivery of appropriate care while meeting institution fiscal and other administrative demands.

In the early days of applied neuropsychology, determination of brain damage, or at least dysfunction as a sign of brain damage, was felt to be of primary importance. Arguments often centered on whether function, or dysfunction, on a given task reflected a specific brain location or more generalized cerebral mediation. Controversy also surrounded the question of whether it is important to measure a number of different abilities in order to "find" the one that might be impaired, or to simply sample enough to "reveal" the results of a dysfunctional system (7). Today, neither a strict localizationist nor system point of view prevails. The brain has been accepted as an organ that has focal areas of importance for performance on specific tasks, but also one that is interactive within itself and between its various component structures and other organ systems as well. The question of presence or absence of brain damage has also undergone some evaluation over the years. Never as important to epileptology, perhaps, as it was to some other disciplines (11), the emphasis has shifted from a question of presence of

damage to requests for fuller assessment of the nature of the patient's neuropsychological functioning. It is known, for example, that among patients with chronic partial epilepsy, 70–80% will show evidence of lowered glucose metabolism (12), lowered blood flow (13), and other signs of altered brain function in the interictal state (14). Furthermore, anterior temporal lobectomies on patients with chronic complex partial seizures have revealed mesial temporal sclerosis and other structural abnormalities in 75–97% of the cases studied by pathology (13). In a patient with intractable seizures, the discovery of impairment on portions of the neuropsychology exam may be merely one more sign of underlying brain pathology, an abnormal finding to be added to others as might have resulted from computed tomography (CT), positron emission tomography (PET), electroencephalography (EEG), or magnetic resonance imaging (MRI). Indeed, one can argue that the additional positive finding would be of clinical importance, especially in a case of equivocal results on one or more studies. There is even evidence that signs of pathophysiology in some neurologic conditions are discernible on a functional level before they are on a structural level (15). I would not argue with these contentions. It has become increasingly clear, however, that the information that is derived from the neuropsychology examination is clinically valuable on levels other than the identification of a lesion. The standardized, quantitative, and sensitive nature of the neuropsychology procedures, for example, allow for baseline comparisons with test results obtained at a later time from a given patient. This test–re-test method allows for determination of progressive deterioration or even improvements in function, over time (16,17). The former consideration might be important in intractable seizure disorder where a decision about surgical intervention is eminent. The latter situation might aid in the monitoring of anticonvulsant medication effects.

Neuropsychology draws on the knowledge of the much larger field of psychology and its various specialty areas in reaching its conclusions. Many of the tests employed in the examination yield information that is of significance to the patient in terms of its implications for psychological functioning aside from presence or absence of brain dysfunction. Intelligence, for instance, is universally measured in the neuropsychology examination. As a concept, "intelligence" has been the subject of focused attention by organized psychology for over 50 years and has served as a basis for some of psychology's most sophisticated theories (18–22). Such a body of knowledge can be drawn upon to interpret results in a given test situation and to address questions that might otherwise be unanswerable. With regard to the hypothetical example posed earlier, involving a patient who is undergoing evaluation for a possible temporal lobectomy, one can ask about the presence of dysfunction, but one can query further concerning the relative nature of those impairments and their implications for the patient's everyday life. Is the patient's neurological dysfunction interfering with ability to learn new information? Has the patient suffered a decline in learning ability in comparison to estimated pre-morbid levels of function? To what extent do emotional and motivational factors contribute to the present picture of neuropsychological strengths and weaknesses? These and similar questions are addressable by the testing enterprise because of the ability to measure behavior accurately with these measures and also because of the knowledge base that supports the interpretation of their results.

The Test Battery

A neuropsychology examination typically involves the administration of a collection of tests, referred to as a "battery" (23). The tradition of using a battery was begun by the early investigators in the field who were concerned that accurate diagnosis of brain damage necessitated a large sampling of behavior (2,20,24). There are indeed a variety of sound technical metric reasons for such a point of view, and these have been reviewed elsewhere (25–28). At the same time, one can relate the nature of the procedure (including the nature of the test battery) to the demands imposed on the procedure by the referral question(s). Advances in neuroscience in the past few decades have taught us that the question of neurologic dysfunction is a complex one

that requires a comprehensive examination to address; this is because of psychometric reasons but also because of the myriad functions of the brain. When a different kind of question is posed, the nature of the behavioral data needed for its answer will also be different as will the construction of the test battery. When the question is simple, the test battery is likely to be less exhaustive than when the question is complex.

A neurologist, to illustrate the last point with a clinical example, might be treating a young epilepsy patient with an anticonvulsant medication. The patient complains that the drug is interfering with memory for things read. The neurologist refers the patient for neuropsychological testing, requesting an evaluation of the patient's memory. In response, the neuropsychologist consults with the referring person, and together they develop the questions that are relevant to the neurologist's present concern: Is the patient showing evidence of cognitive side effects from the anticonvulsant treatment? Even though the neuropsychologist will evaluate a number of behaviors (e.g., attention, intellect, affect, etc.) in order to address the basic concern with a complaint about memory, the battery of tests employed and the time spent in examination will almost certainly be far shorter than when the referral is for a comprehensive diagnostic examination.

In some ways, the idea of focused questions to the neuropsychologist, with request for examination of a more-or-less limited area of behavior, is not a new one. Some specialized examinations in particular areas such as language function have existed for a number of years (29). Nevertheless, a recent trend has been toward focused, as opposed to comprehensive, evaluations. It has here been argued that there is a theoretical basis for this shift in emphasis, but there is no doubt that economic factors have contributed to this state as well. Major legislative actions in several world governments (e.g., the introduction of "DRGs" in the United States and moves to "privatization" in England) have strongly affected the practice of medicine in general such that the controversies in neuropsychology are virtually no different than those in neurology or in other disciplines.

It is an accepted axiom in neuropsychology

that an aspect of behavior cannot be understood in isolation. In the clinical example given above, for instance, it was said that the neuropsychologist, in order to answer a question about the patient's memory, needed to evaluate aspects of behavior in addition to memory alone. The reasons behind such a strategy are, if not commonsensical, at least well known. A problem in concentration can interfere with learning and appear to the affected person as a problem with memory. Depression can result in apparent memory impairments as well (30), and impairment of attention and/or other aspects of cognition will have consequences for the individual's ability to cope with stress (4,31,32). Failure to account for such interactions could prevent a successful examination of neuropsychological function (33). One might need to know something about the patient's general level of intellectual ability to predict a level of performance in a learning task that would be reasonable for that particular individual. Certain demographic information from patient history would be needed to determine the appropriate normative data with which to compare the obtained test results. Thus, even simple referral questions will require a battery of tests which is extensive enough to satisfy the technical requirements for adequate psychometrics but which also samples the diverse areas of behavior as necessary from a psychological point of view to address the referral question(s).

Certain aspects of behavior appear to be routinely covered by the neuropsychology examination. One might argue about how to categorize these areas. For instance, some might feel that language is deserving of its own category, separate from the rest. Nevertheless, presented below is one scheme for categorizing the areas covered by the neuropsychology exam. The categories are not entirely arbitrary, since arguments can be made about the relative exclusiveness of each in addition to their interactive qualities. These areas are as follows:

1. Patient history
2. Intelligence
3. Cognition
4. Sensory and motor
5. Affect
6. Coping and adaptation

Patient History

Attempts have been made to formally standardize the patient history (34,35). Most often, however, this area of the neuropsychology examination takes place by interviewing the patient and, at times, the patient's family or acquaintances, as well as by reviewing past records (e.g., school achievement records, history of past hospitalizations, etc.). The interview is usually semistructured so that information that is known to be pertinent to neuropsychological function will be obtained, but it is open enough to allow for the report of unexpected items. In many institutional locations, an outline may be followed. There is no universally agreed upon format for this portion of the examination, although there is general agreement about techniques of the interview process (e.g., techniques of effective communication) and the major areas to be covered. The outline that I use is probably typical of many, and it is presented in the Appendix for the reader's information.

Intelligence

As mentioned earlier, intelligence has a relatively long history as a subject of psychological inquiry. This portion of the examination is almost always covered in a formal, psychometric way through the administration of psychological tests. It is well established that intelligence is multifactorial, with some factors being more susceptible to the impairing effects of damage to the brain than others (20,21). It is also accepted that general intellectual function, as measured routinely in the neuropsychological examination, is highly reflective of educational and sociocultural history. A further distinction is drawn between (a) intellectual ability as generally measured by psychological tests and (b) demands for immediate response to the environment as occurs in a cognitive act such as learning new information (4). Clinically, it is not unusual to observe a patient with an average or even superior intelligence quotient who is at the same time very poor in recalling newly acquired information. Such was the case with a 77-year-old woman seen recently in our clinic. This patient was unable to remember the simplest element of a visual reproduction task (i.e., subscale VI of the Wechsler Memory Scale) even though her general intellect was at an average level. A right-hemisphere cerebral infarct was responsible for this unhappy situation. This separation between intellectual ability and other cognitive functions has been well documented in the research literature as well as in the clinical literature, beginning with some of the earliest investigations of this sort (7).

This classification scheme is somewhat artificial even if it is based on the reality of known brain and behavior relationships. Some very important aspects of behavior are, therefore, difficult to categorize, or they have elements that place them within more than one topical area. Language function, for example, will fall under intelligence as well as cognition. Vocabulary level, to give a specific instance, is widely considered to be an aspect of general intellectual ability. Indeed, the vocabulary subtest of the WAIS-R has the highest correlation of all the WAIS-R subscales to the overall score on this test (36). On the other hand, verbal fluency is more likely to be measured during the cognitive part of the examination.

The formal measurement of academic achievement (e.g., reading level) is another important item that probably best fits within the general rubric of "intelligence." Perhaps an important factor that all behaviors under this topic, intelligence, have in common is that practice has revealed each of them to possess a different kind of susceptibility to the impairing effects of brain damage than do those abilities placed under the cognition category.

Cognition

Cognition is a complex topic, but in its simplest manifestations it includes measurement of learning, memory, attention, aspects of language, and other related behaviors. This portion of the examination often serves as the focus of the testing effort. The referral questions will influence the extensiveness with which this area is covered, but even simple questions may necessitate a relatively lengthy examination process. Certain tests have come

to be widely used in effecting this part of the examination. Halstead's battery (20) and Reitan's (24) and Boll's revisions (23) are examples of testing approaches that devote considerable attention to measurement of cognitive function. Wechsler's memory scale (21) has come to be used extensively to quantitate, as well as to make qualitative statements about, learning and memory. Still, the measurement of memory and related cognitions continues to be one of the major challenges to neuropsychology. Despite efforts to develop effective procedures in this area of neuropsychological inquiry that spans over 80 years (37), there is still a lack of a standardized approach or even consensus on an operational definition of memory.

The picture is not entirely bleak, however, Much has been learned about the complexities of cognition and about the various manifestations of processes such as learning and memory, as well as about their relationships to seizures and other aspects of neurologic function and dysfunction. It is well established, for instance, that verbal and visual learning are affected differently depending on the nature and location of a seizure focus (4). Medications and other drugs can be very specific in the aspect(s) of memory that they disrupt (16,38,39). Various forms of memory may be affected differently depending on the location of a cerebral insult or the nature of the neuropathology (40).

The case presented earlier, involving the 77-year-old woman who suffered a right-hemisphere cerebral infarct, can be used to illustrate this last point. Although this patient reflected adequate intelligence, she could earn no higher than a zero on the visual reproduction subscale of the Wechsler Memory Scale (subscale VI). At the same time, this person earned a score of 10.5 on the verbal associate learning portion (subscale VII) of the Wechsler scale, a score that reflects low but adequate learning. In fact, her performance on other portions of the overall exam were such that if the visual reproduction subscale had not been administered, the extent of her cognitive impairment might not have been known.

In addition to verbal and visual types of learning, short-term and longer-term retrieval of recently acquired information has been shown to be important as well (7). Complex problem solving, as reflected in a task such as the "categories" (23) or the "stroop" (41,42), is usually included under the topic of cognition.

Sensory and Motor

Many neurologic disorders can lead to sensory or motor symptoms, with little or no apparent involvement of other aspects of behavior (43). Motor symptoms can also interfere with adequate performance on other aspects of the neuropsychology examination. In recent work, for example, Berent and co-workers (44,45) examined a group of patients who had been diagnosed as having familial, and in some cases sporadic, olivopontocerebellar atrophy. At first and in comparison to nonaffected control participants, the patients appeared to be lower-functioning on standardized measures of intellect and cognition. These differences were found to be nonsignificant, however, when education level and motor dysfunction were statistically accounted for.

Aspects of function that are regularly attended to in this portion of the examination include motor strength, speed, and steadiness. Handedness and body-sidedness more generally can be placed here. Adequate sensation in hearing, vision, and tactile ability is also attended to, often through methods similar to those of the clinical neurologic exam. Effort is made to standardize the procedure and quantify the results whenever possible. It is in this area of the neuropsychology examination that automation and computerization has found some of its most successful applications. The automated reaction time device, for example, has been commercially available for years. Except for instances of collaborative research projects—as a multicenter anticonvulsant drug study, for example—no specific instrument or procedure has been agreed upon as an accepted standard for the field.

Affect

Here "affect" refers to the emotions of anxiety, depression, and excitement. An effort is usually made to quantify these emotions through the use of rating scales or other psychometric devices, although data from clinical interview might be used in forming conclusions. Distinctions are drawn between pathological expressions of these affects and normal variations in mood. This area of affect measurement is closely akin to the sixth category of "coping," since both have relevance to determination of psychopathology in the patient. Such determination requires more than the notation of a score on a particular rating scale. It calls for an assessment by the clinician that reflects an understanding of the test data in relation to the knowledge base referred to earlier.

Computerization has found application in this area of the neuropsychology examination as well. To date, however, the best use of such automation has been as an aid to test scoring, data reduction, profile construction, and group norming. Efforts to computerize the testing process more comprehensively than this have met with much criticism (e.g., see ref. 46 and the special series on the topic of computerized testing in the *Journal of Consulting and Clinical Psychology* 1985;53:745–838).

Coping and Adaptation

Coping and adaptation, as well as the successes and failures of these efforts, are dealt with next. Comment here requires an integration of data from all the areas to reach conclusions about such complex issues as (a) quality of the patient's life, (b) nature, extent, and kind of psychopathology when present, and (c) factors affecting considerations about treatments and prognosis. Again, the neuropsychologist must draw upon test and interview data and interpret these in light of the professional database. To give an example, it is known that there exists an intimate relationship between ability to cope with life stress and the individual's cognitive intactness and level of intellectual ability (4,7,11,31,32,42). In clinical practice, it is not unusual to have a patient referred, for example, from an extended care facility with the stated suspicion that a preexisting seizure disorder has recently worsened. The evidence used to substantiate the complaint might be lowered job or school performance, increased disruptive behavior, and withdrawal from positive social interaction. It is entirely possible that these symptoms reflect only an increase in the referred person's environmental stresses, accompanied by insufficient (though preexisting and chronic) cognitive and intellectual ability to successfully cope with these stresses.

The Report

As important as any other phase in the neuropsychology examination process is the report. A major criticism of neuropsychology testing has been that the results are made known to the referring person too late to be of clinical use. This idea of "clinical utility" has received emphasis in the neuropsychology process because criticisms such as the one above have been taken to heart. With such usefulness in mind, questions to guide the process are posed, such as the following: What can these test data tell the referring person that will aid in the clinical management of the patient? Equally as important, what is the fastest way these results can be made known?

Communication of test results increasingly occurs by way of telephone or in person and, most recently, via computer interactive mail systems. The written report becomes a vehicle for further clarification of findings and for providing additional detail from the test examination. A very important function of the written report is that it serves as a means of documentation. One of the initial reasons for direct contact between the neuropsychologist and the referring person is that it is expeditious, but it also allows for interaction between these two individuals in a way the written report cannot.

The Interpretive Phase

The interpretive phase is the fifth step in the neuropsychology testing process (3). This aspect of the enterprise may find expression in several different ways. Basically, however, it is a time when the results of the examination are acted upon in an interpretive fashion. Such action may take the form of counseling a patient and/or the patient's family with regard to the test findings and the implications

of those findings for decisions and/or other aspects of the patient's life. Questions the patient may have about the exam, the reasons behind the need for the testing, or other such issues can be addressed at this point.

Follow-up

After the interpretive phase is the follow-up phase of the process. Often, what constitutes this step is simply a note of progress that serves to document the interpretive interaction and new information or impressions as might have resulted from that interaction. At other times, more formal communication with others may be required, or perhaps further action (such as additional patient contacts) may be necessary. Repeat examinations are required in many instances, sometimes years later. The actions and documentations of those actions made at this point become very important to those future contacts.

DISCUSSION AND SUMMARY

In the preceding pages, an attempt has been made to describe the process of modern neuropsychology. A premise has been that regular forces, or contingencies as termed here, have contributed to the evolution of neuropsychology into a specialty whose programmatic expression reflects commonality across various locations. The field rests on theoretical foundations that have been carefully laid over the past 40–100 years. The value placed on these underlying theoretical considerations has found expression in the daily activities of the neuropsychologist. This represents one of the primary contingencies that has contributed to regularity in the neuropsychological approach to testing. It provides a basis for understanding how the psychologist determines which aspects of physiology and behavior to evaluate, why those aspects are more important than others that might be measured, how they are to be measured, and so on.

In its development, neuropsychology is far from complete, however. Important areas lack in standardization or even consensus as to operational definitions. Some of these areas are extremely important to patient care. Both in terms of direct delivery of care to patients and in terms of contributions to clinical and basic research, challenges exist despite the fact that neuropsychology has performed excellently in these areas to date. Standard approaches are needed, for example, to the measurement of learning and memory. A benefit of such standardization will be the compatibility of data from one center to another. Another challenge lies in learning how to incorporate the many technological advances in fields such as computerization and artificial intelligence into neuropsychological practice and research. A major difficulty here is in effecting these changes while maintaining the psychometric standards and other traditions that make neuropsychology what it is.

Trends in health-care delivery and funding must also be responded to in a manner that ensures the continuation of appropriate services to patients. The demand for examinations that are briefer than those used in the past will need to be evaluated against the increasing realization that seizure and other neurologic disorders, as well as medication and other-treatment side effects, are often very specific in the functions they impair. The importance of interactions between functional areas, as discussed earlier, will need to be addressed as well.

The latest edition of the APA standards for testing (1985) makes note of the fact that these standards are addressing a field that is evolving. In terms of the tests themselves, the standards handbook lists a number of areas that are in need of continued work. Some of the more important of these include (a) the further development of gender-specific and combined-gender norms, (b) an effective way of dealing with cultural bias in test outcome, (c) further development of computer-based test interpretation, (d) limits on validity generalizations from one test situation to another, and (e) differential predictions based on test results. These challenges will be among those that receive focused attention in the coming years. The fact that they exist is not a criticism of neuropsychology. Rather, it is a positive reflection on the state of its development.

ACKNOWLEDGMENTS

The patient history form contained in the Appendix has evolved over time. Many persons, beginning at the University of Virginia and continuing at the University of Michigan, have contributed their ideas and labors. I wish to specifically mention Thomas J. Boll, Ph.D., Bruno Giordani, Ph.D., and Shirley Lehtinen, M.A., in this regard. A note of gratitude is extended also to Mrs. Kathryn Stoddard for her assistance and to Joy Berent for her advice. This work was performed, in part, while I was a Visiting Professor at the Institute of Neurology, the National Hospital, Queen Square, London, England.

REFERENCES

1. Benton AL. Evolution of a clinical specialty. *Clin Neuropsychol* 1987;1:5–8.
2. Luria AR, Majovski LV. Basic approaches used in American and Soviet clinical neuropsychology. *Am Psychol* 1977;32:959–968.
3. Berent S, Sackellares JC. Clinical monitoring of children with epilepsy: A neurologic and neuropsychological perspective. In: Herman B, Seidenberg M, eds. *Childhood epilepsies: neuropsychological, psychosocial, and intervention aspects*. London: John Wiley & Sons, 1989;15–31.
4. Berent S. Psychological assessment in epilepsy: a case illustration. In: Kulig BM, Meinardi H, Stores G, eds. *Epilepsy and behavior*. Amsterdam: Swets & Zeitlinger, 1980;25–29.
5. American Psychological Association. Ethical principles of psychologists. *Am Psychol* 1981: 633–638.
6. American Psychological Association. *General guidelines for providers of psychological services*. Washington, DC: APA, 1987.
7. Russell EW. The psychometric foundation of clinical neuropsychology. In: Filskov SB, Boll TJ, eds. *Handbook of clinical neuropsychology*, vol 2. New York: John Wiley & Sons, 1986; 45–80.
8. American Psychological Association. *Standards for education and psychological testing*. Washington, DC: APA, 1985.
9. Cull CA, Trimble MR. Automated testing and psychopharmacology. In: Hindmaroh I, Storier P, eds. *Human psychopharmacology*, vol 1. New York: John Wiley & Sons, 1987;113–153.
10. Wechsler D. *Manual for the Wechsler intelligence scale for children—revised*, New York: New York Psychological Corporation, 1974.
11. Berent S. Psychopathology and other behavioral considerations for the clinical neuropsychologist. In: Filskov S, Boll TJ, eds. *Handbook of clinical neuropsychology*, vol 2. New York: John Wiley & Sons, 1986;279–304.
12. Engel J Jr, Kuhl DE, Phelps ME. Patterns of human local cerebral glucose metabolism during epileptic seizures. *Science* 1982;218:64–66.

13. Siegel GJ, Abou-Khalil B, Sackellares JC. Imaging of regional cerebral metabolism and blood flow in epilepsy. In: Sen AK, Lee T, eds. *Receptors and ligands in neurological disorders*. Cambridge, England: Cambridge University Press, 1988;211–234.

14. Abou-Khalil B, Siegel GJ, Sackellares JC, Gilman S, Hichwa R, Marshall R. Positron emission tomography studies of cerebral glucose metabolism in chronic partial epilepsy. *Ann Neurol* 1987;22:480–486.

15. Young AB, Penney JB, Starosta-Rubinstein S, et al. PET scan investigations of Huntington's disease: cerebral metabolic correlates of neurologic features and functional decline. *Ann Neurol* 1986;20:296–303.

16. Berent S, Sackellares JC, Giordani B, Wagner JG, Donofrio PD, Abou-Khalil B. Zonisamide (CI-912) and cognition: results from preliminary study. *Epilepsia* 1987;28:61–67.

17. Thompson PJ, Trimble MR. Further studies on anticonvulsant drugs and seizures. In: Karl-Axel M, ed. *Second workshop on memory functions*. Copenhagen: Munksgaard, 1981;51–57.

18. Hebb DO. Clinical evidence concerning the nature of normal adult test performance. *Psychol Bull* 1941;38:593.

19. Cattell RB. The measurement of adult intelligence. *Psychol Bull* 1943;40:153–193.

20. Halstead WC. *Brain and intelligence*. Chicago: University of Chicago Press, 1947.

21. Wechsler D. A standardized memory scale for clinical use. *J Psychol* 1945;19:87–95.

22. Matarazzo JD. *Wechsler's measurement and appraisal of adult intelligence*, 5th ed. New York: Oxford University Press, 1972.

23. Boll TJ. The Halstead–Reitan neuropsychology battery. In: Filskov SB, Boll TJ, eds. *Handbook of clinical neuropsychology*, vol 1. New York: John Wiley & Sons, 1981;577–608.

24. Reitan RM. Investigation of the validity of Halstead's measures of biological intelligence. *Arch Neurol Psychiatry* 1955;73:28–35.

25. Lezak MD. *Neuropsychological assessment*, 2nd ed. New York: Oxford University Press, 1983.

26. Filskov SB, Boll TJ, eds. *Handbook of clinical neuropsychology*, vol 1. New York: John Wiley & Sons, 1981.

27. Filskov SB, Boll TJ, eds. *Handbook of clinical neuropsychology*, vol 2. New York: John Wiley & Sons, 1986.

28. Anastasi A. *Psychological testing*, 6th ed. New York: Macmillian, 1988.

29. Goodglass H, Kaplan E. *The assessment of aphasia and related disorders*, 2nd ed. Philadelphia: Lea & Febiger, 1983.

30. Albert MS, Moss MB. *Geriatric Neuropsychology*. New York: The Guilford Press, 1988;158–161.

31. Dodrill CB. Psychological consequences of epilepsy. In: Filskov SB, Boll TJ, eds. *Handbook of clinical neuropsychology*, vol 2. New York: John Wiley & Sons, 1986;338–363.

32. Trimble MR. Psychiatric aspects of epilepsy. *Psychiatr Dev* 1987;4:285–300.

33. Goodglass H. The assessment of language after brain damage. In: Filskov SB, Boll TJ, eds. *Handbook of clinical neuropsychology*, vol 2. New York: John Wiley & Sons, 1986;172–197.

34. Endicott J, Spitzer RL. A diagnostic interview: the schedule for affective disorders and schizophrenia. *Arch Gen Psychiatry* 1978;35:837–844.

35. Spitzer RL, Endicott J. *Schedule for affective disorders and schizophrenia (SADS)*, 3rd ed. New York: Biometrics Research Institute, 1978.

36. Wechsler D. *Wechsler adult intelligence scale—revised*. New York: New York Psychological Corporation, 1981.

37. Erickson RC, Scott ML. Clinical memory testing: a review. *Psychol Bull* 1977;84:1130–1149.

38. MacLeod CM, Dekaban AS, Hunt E. Memory impairment in epileptic patients: selective effects of phenobarbitone concentration. *Science* 1978;202:1102–1104.

39. Trimble MR, Richens A. Psychotropic effects of anticonvulsant drugs. In: Burrows GD, Werry JS, eds. *Advances in human psychopharmacology, II*. 1981.

40. Weingartner H, Grafman J, Boutelle W, Kaye W, Martin PR. Forms of memory failure. *Science* 1983;221:380–382.

41. Stroop JR. Studies of interference in serial verbal reaction. *J Exp Psychol* 1975;18:643–662.

42. Koss E, Ober BA, Dilis DC, Friedland RP. The stroop color-word test: indication of dementia severity. *Int J Neurosci* 1984;24:53–61.

43. Gilman S, Newman S. *Manter and Gatz's essentials of clinical neuroanatomy and neurophysiology*, 7th ed. Philadelphia: FA Davis, 1987.

44. Berent S, Giordani B, Gilman S, et al. A quantitative analysis of cognitive, intellectual, and emotional function in olivopontocerebellar atrophy. *Neurology* 1988;38:285.

45. Gilman S, Markel DS, Koeppe RA, et al. Cerebellar and brain stem hypometabolism in olivopontocerebellar atrophy detected with positron emission tomography. *Ann Neurol* 1988;23:223–230.

46. Adams KM. Concepts and methods in the design of automata for neuropsychological test interpretation. In: Filskov SB, Boll TJ, eds. *Handbook of clinical neuropsychology*, vol 2. New York: John Wiley & Sons, 1986;561–576.

APPENDIX

Neuropsychological Patient History

I. Identifying Data   Date: ______________________

Name of Patient ________________________________ Telephone: ______________________

Address ____

Age ______ DOB ____________ SEX ______ Race ________ Reg. # (or S.S. #): ____________

Dept ______________________________ Marital Status: S   M   Sep.   D   W   (yrs? ________)

Outpatient/Inpatient ________ (ward) Referred by: ______________________________________

Education ______________________________ Religion ____________________________

(College attended ______________________________ Major ____________________________)

Occupation: Present ______________________________ Previous: ____________________________

Height ______________ Weight ______________ lbs. ____________________________________

II. History of Present Problem:
Tell me in your own words why you think you were referred for his testing.

____

____

What questions are you hoping we will be able to answer with these tests? ____________________

____

When did your problem begin? (Stroke, seizure, whatever) ______________________________

____

What medications are you taking now? ____

____

Have you in the past or presently had any problems with:

1) Loss of consciousness ____

2) Memory ____

3) Numbness or tingling in limbs (paralysis) ____

4) Vision ____

5) Hearing ____

6) Other sensory changes (taste, smell, touch) ____

7) Learning problems while in school (specifically: reading, spelling, writing, arithmetic, drawing) ______

____

____

8) Work problems (if working) ____

9) Coordination difficulties or change ____

10) Abnormally high fever ____

11) Seizures (type, duration, frequency) _______________________________

12) Allergies (to meds) ____

13) Head trauma ____

14) Broken bones ____

15) Injuries to arms, hands &/or fingers ______________________________

16) Headaches ____

17) Do you think your personality has changed in the past few years? Explain how.

____

____

Have you had any of the following:

Polio ___________ Meningitis ___________ Huntington's Chorea ___________

Diabetes ___________ Encephalitis ___________ High Blood Pressure ___________

Fainting ___________ Syphilis or ___________ Rheumatic or ___________

              Gonorrhea ___________ Scarlet Fever ___________

Other medical problems which are a part of your history: _______________________

____

____

Other hospitalizations (give date, reason): ____________________________________

____

Have you ever had shock treatments? ___________ When? ___________________________

What medications have you used previously (taken for at least a month)? ___________

____

III. Family History

Members of household: ____

Handedness:	Family Member	Age	Health Problems	Yrs of Educ.	Occupation
R L	1. Spouse or significant Other				
	2. Patient's Mother				
	3. Patient's Father				
	4. Patient's Children				
	(a)				
	(b)				
	(c)				
	(d)				
	(e)				

Handedness:	Family Member	Age	Health Problems	Yrs of Educ.	Occupation
	In order of birth:				
	5. Patient's Siblings				
	(a)				
	(b)				
	(c)				
	(d)				
	(e)				
	(f)				
	(g)				
	(h)				

Is there any history of emotional or neurological problems in your family? (Alcoholism, psychiatric hospitalizations, neurological problems)

____

IV. Social History

Smoking Yes _______ No _______ _________ pkg/day $\times$ _______ years

Drinking Yes _______ No _______ If yes, amount: ___________________________________

Drugs (yes or no to the following:)

    Sleeping Pills ____________

    Phenobarb   ____________

    Marijuana   ____________

    Morphine   ____________

    Heroin   ____________

    Others   ____

V. Additional Information:

____

____

____

____

Advances in Neurology, Vol. 55, edited by
D. Smith, D. Treiman, and M. Trimble,
Raven Press, Ltd., New York © 1991.

27

Neurobiological, Psychosocial, and Pharmacological Factors Underlying Interictal Psychopathology in Epilepsy

Bruce P. Hermann*† and Steve Whitman‡

*EpiCare Center, Baptist Memorial Hospital, Memphis, Tennessee 38103; †Semmes-Murphy
Clinic, Memphis, Tennessee; Department of Psychiatry, University of Tennessee,
Memphis, Tennessee 38146; and ‡Center for Urban Affairs and Policy Research, Northwestern
University, Evanston, Illinois 60201

Epilepsy, in a very effective and efficient manner, mounts a multidimensional assault on the quality of patients' lives. Some individuals succumb to this attack and subsequently exhibit a variety of maladaptive behaviors and characteristics. Others, however, manage to overcome epilepsy's negative effects and subsequently lead full and productive lives. It is important that the major dimensions of epilepsy's influence be clearly recognized, since effective treatment and prevention of the neurobehavioral problems associated with epilepsy will depend on our coming to terms with the multifaceted aspects of this neurological disorder.

Although a bewildering array of variables have been shown or suggested to be involved in the determination of emotional and behavioral problems in epilepsy, we have previously suggested that most potential risk factors can be organized into a simple conceptual model.

This model is entirely dependent on the observations of previous investigators who have pointed out the many factors which may affect the patient with epilepsy. Perhaps the major contribution of the approach to be presented is that it points out one way in which these previous observations can be formulated in order to empirically address the problem of psychopathology in epilepsy in a comprehensive manner.

In this chapter we will briefly review the characteristics of this model and subsequently examine its utility in predicting behavioral and emotional problems in adults and children with epilepsy. In doing so, we will emphasize the *psychosocial* predictors of psychiatric distress, since most of the other chapters in this volume discuss biological predictors of problem behavior.

A CONCEPTUAL MODEL

Prior to addressing the predictors of psychopathology in epilepsy, we must first define what we mean by the term "psychopathology." In order to do this we will refer to the literature and point to the specific interictal behaviors of most interest to researchers in this field. It has been previously suggested that the dependent measures/behaviors of major interest fall into six categories: (i) aggression, (ii) sexual dysfunction (primarily hyposexuality), (iii) affective disorders (primarily depression), (iv) schizophrenia-like psychosis, (v) changes in personality and behavior, and (vi) a heterogeneous category, general psychopathology, which is characterized by a diversity of assessment methods designed to detect the presence of significant psychiatric distress (1). Studies in this latter category have used measures such as the General Health Questionnaire, standardized personality and behavioral measures [e.g., the Minnesota Multiphasic Personality Inventory (MMPI)], or other indices reflective of emotional disorder (e.g., admission to a mental health center).

With regard to each of these six behavioral areas there have been numerous investigations which have attempted to identify the overall rate of problem behavior and/or determine whether these behaviors occurred more often in epilepsy patients than in healthy controls and other illness groups. However, within the context of the generalities that emerge from these investigations, there is the expected variability at the individual level. Simply put, some individuals with epilepsy exhibit significant interictal psychopathology, whereas some do not. As would therefore be expected, there have been many investigations which have attempted to identify the factors which predispose patients with epilepsy to a particular behavior problem of interest. The identification of these so-called "risk factors" is a crucial venture, since it represents the first stage in the effort to develop meaningful treatment and prevention programs.

What adds confusion to the literature is the fact that there is only a mild-to-moderate degree of consistency in the pool of potential risk factors which have been empirically investigated, both within and between specific behavior problem areas. Furthermore, many reasonable risk factors have been suggested but have never been empirically evaluated.

In the attempt to impose some order upon this state of affairs, we have suggested that most potential risk factors can be classified into three groups which reflect the major dimensions of epilepsy: neurological, psychosocial, and medication-related (1,2). We will briefly review each of these categories, identify examples of potential risk factors, and then examine some of the specifics involved in using this multietiological model to predict interictal psychopathology in epilepsy.[1]

---

[1] In previous publications (1,2) we have provided detailed literature reviews pertaining to the relationship between specific neurological, psychosocial, and medication variables with measures of psychopathology. In the material to follow, such analyses will not be re-presented. The interested reader can consult these existing references.

Neurobiological Factors

Many neurobiological and neurophysiological variables define the parameters of an individual's epilepsy (Table 1). For instance, when attempting to understand the characteristics of a patient's epilepsy, there needs to be consideration of the etiology, the age at onset of the epilepsy, the number of years that the patient has had the disorder, the specific classification of the patient's seizure type or types, and the degree of seizure control which has been achieved. Information is also needed as to the interictal and ictal electroencephalographic (EEG) characteristics, results of imaging studies [magnetic resonance imaging (MRI) and computed tomography (CT) scans], phenomenological characteristics of the seizures, and the neuropsychological correlates of the epilepsy. Additional potentially important (but perhaps less discussed) factors would include disruptions and alterations in the efficiency of cerebral metabolism [as revealed by positron emission tomography (PET) scan], alterations in specific neurotransmitter systems, and disruptions in other basic neurobiological mechanisms. As noted, these and other variables constitute the so-called neurobiological spectrum of epilepsy. A considerable amount of research to date has centered around the relationship between particular psychosocial problems (e.g., psychopathology) and select subsets of these neurobiological factors, the hope being that the results might simultaneously yield information pertaining to the organic precursors of psychopathology, as well as identifying groups of patients with epilepsy at increased psychiatric risk.

Pharmacological Factors

The treatment of epilepsy rests primarily on the administration of anticonvulsant medications. Significant advances have resulted in the development of new anticonvulsant medications which are especially effective for particular seizure types and which produce fewer adverse side effects. These medications, as well as some of the older, well-established drugs, clearly improve seizure control in a majority of patients. However, some characteristics of these medications, or their usage,

TABLE 1. *Potential multietiological risk factors*

Neurobiological	Psychosocial	Medication
Age at onset	Locus of control	Monotherapy versus polytherapy
Duration of disorder	Fear of seizures	Presence/absence of barbiturate
Seizure type	Adjustment to epilepsy	medications
Seizure control	Parental overprotection	Folate deficiency
Ictal/interictal EEG	Perceived stigma	Hormonal/endocrine effects
characteristics	Perceived	Medication-induced alterations in
Presence/absence of	discrimination	monoamine metabolism
structural damage	Stressful life events	Medication-induced alterations in cerebral
Phenomenological aspects of	Financial stress	metabolism
the seizures	Employment status	
Neuropsychological function	Social support	
Efficiency of cerebral		
metabolism		
Alterations in neurotransmitter		
systems		

are relevant to our discussion of risk factors for psychiatric problems (Table 1).

From the clinical standpoint, perhaps the most common problem is the inappropriate use of anticonvulsants. Unfortunately, one sees a substantial number of individuals who have been placed on three, four, and even five medications, occasionally in conjunction with a stimulant medication which has been prescribed to counter the sedating effect of the anticonvulsants. This practice of polytherapy is counter to the prevailing suggested modern medical practice of monotherapy whenever possible, utilizing the most efficacious drug (with the fewest side effects) for the patient's particular seizure type (3).

In addition to the number of medications that are used, specific consideration needs to be given to the particular anticonvulsant which is prescribed. Some very effective, safe, and well-established drugs can predispose some individuals to significant psychological and social problems. Perhaps the best-known example concerns the drug phenobarbital. This barbiturate anticonvulsant may cause paradoxical hyperactivity in children and may also predispose susceptible individuals to significant depression (4,5). There has been a recent report indicating that the use of phenobarbital in children with epilepsy is associated with depression in cases where there is a familial history of psychopathology (6).

The effects of the anticonvulsant medications can be somewhat insidious. Theodore et al. (7,8) at the National Institutes of Health have reported interesting findings concerning the effects of drug withdrawal on cerebral metabolism as measured by PET. When phenobarbital was removed, cerebral metabolism increased by 37%. When phenytoin was removed there was a rise of about 14%, and when carbamazepine was removed there was a rise of about 10%. Therefore, anticonvulsant drugs clearly affect cerebral metabolism, and this can be noted on PET studies. At present it is not clear exactly what a global rise in cerebral metabolism means in terms of psychiatric status, but it would be reasonable to suggest that such improvements in brain function may be associated with improvements in psychological function.

Finally, anticonvulsant medications can have other broad and systemic effects which may directly or indirectly impact upon the adequacy of behavioral and/or social functioning. An extended discussion of the mechanisms whereby anticonvulsants exert such effects is beyond the scope of this chapter. However, it should be noted that Reynolds (4,9,10) has suggested that anticonvulsants can adversely affect mental functioning by (a) causing neuropathological changes in the central nervous system, (b) inducing folate deficiency, (c) altering monoamine metabolism, and/or (d) affecting hormonal or endocrine functioning.

Psychosocial Factors

This is a broad rubric which refers to the many ways in which epilepsy might impact upon the patient with epilepsy, both directly and indirectly. A very heterogeneous group of considerations are involved, and only a few investigators have attempted to bring some order to this literature.

In 1960 Lennox (11) presented his model of the psychosocial impact of epilepsy. He referred to five major considerations: (i) the canker of secrecy, (ii) educational problems, (iii) the roadblock of employment, (iv) law, and (v) war. Through this schema he tried to indicate that society oftentimes had sanctions against epilepsy victims [e.g., reluctance to employ people with epilepsy; unreasonable legal restrictions in many areas (a so-called literature of indignation)], that epilepsy itself could contribute, in part, to the development of significant difficulties (e.g., academic underachievement), and that the development of epilepsy could be the result of social policy (e.g., war). Lennox stressed that once epilepsy was acquired, attention needed to be devoted to determining the ways in which the neurological and social features of epilepsy contributed to problems in living, as well as the ways in which people were hindered in their socioemotional development and attainment by society's, and their own, adverse reactions to epilepsy. Through the identification of the above, Lennox hoped that many of the psychosocial problems associated with epilepsy could be prevented.

A major contemporary contribution to the understanding of the psychosocial ramifications of epilepsy was provided by the National Commission for the Control of Epilepsy and Its Consequences (12). This group offered a definitive account of the economic, social, and personal costs of epilepsy in the United States. It rightly had a major impact on the subsequent development of comprehensive epilepsy centers in the U.S., and their final report provides a contemporary review of the psychosocial complications of the epilepsies.

More recent reviews of the psychosocial consequences of epilepsy have been colored by assessment methodology. For instance, Levin et al. (13) recently reviewed the literature pertaining to the psychosocial dimensions of epilepsy utilizing the framework of the Washington Psychosocial Seizure Inventory (WPSI) (14). The WPSI is a self-report questionnaire designed to assess the psychosocial problems associated with epilepsy. Table 2 shows the major dimensions of psychosocial impact assessed by the WPSI and also shows examples of some of the relevant research findings noted by Levin et al. As can be seen, a substantial number of psychosocial problems have been found to be associated with epilepsy.

Thompson and Oxley (15), in an investigation of the socioeconomic accompaniments of drug-resistant epilepsy, utilized the Social

TABLE 2. *Some psychosocial problems associated with epilepsy as reviewed by Levin et al. (13)*

Family background and adjustment
Overprotection; rejection; overindulgence; alterations in family activities and interactions; decreased parental expectations; poor compliance with medical management; familial maladjustment; increased stress, guilt, and concealment; jealousy in siblings

Emotional adjustment
Anxiety; depression; low self-esteem; anger; violence; increased psychiatric distress; suicide; psychosis; schizophrenia-like illness; personality change; sexual dysfunction; hysteria; paranoia; epileptic personality; stress; mood disorders; manic states; fear

Interpersonal adjustment
Low marital rates; social isolation; social withdrawal; adverse reactions of others to epilepsy; attitudes of others toward the person with epilepsy

Vocational adjustment
Unemployment; underemployment; employment discrimination; unhappiness with vocational situation

Financial status
Lowered income; dependence on federal subsidy; financial burdens of epilepsy

Adjustment to seizures
Perceived and/or real stigma and discrimination; fear of seizures; lack of understanding of epilepsy; nonacceptance of epilepsy by patient; nondisclosure; embarrassment; dread of seizure occurrence

Medicine and medical management
Patient and physician relationship; physician's knowledge of epilepsy and ability to communicate; compliance with treatment program

Problems Questionnaire (SPQ) to examine patients' level of satisfaction with various aspects of their lives, including employment, finances, housing, social activities, relatives, marriage/relationships, and legal matters. It is instructive to examine the proportion of patients with epilepsy ($N = 92$) reporting significant areas of social difficulty on the SPQ. The specific areas of social concern, along with the proportion of patients reporting difficulties, were as follows: work (71%), housing (29%), finance (37%), social activities (73%), relatives (28%), marriage/relationships (51%), and legal matters (3%).

Clearly, a wide variety of problems in living are associated with epilepsy, particularly in patients with more severe cases.

Summary

Overall, epilepsy's influence can be represented by at least three dimensions: neurological, psychosocial, and medication-related. Each dimension is represented by many specific factors; some of these are known to be of importance, whereas others are only suspected of having pernicious effects. Table 1 provides only some of the variables which might reasonably fall under each dimension. It would be reasonable to expect that individuals with epilepsy would vary widely in their vulnerability to these three dimensions. Some individuals may be wracked by the neurological factors underlying their epilepsy; other may be handicapped by their own reactions to the disorder, as well as by the reactions of society; and others are perhaps most hampered by the inappropriate treatment of their epilepsy. The majority of patients would most likely have varying combinations of these three dimensions.

What is the combined influence of neurological, social, and medication factors on patients' emotional and behavioral status? It is to this issue that we now turn.

THE CASE OF PSYCHOPATHOLOGY

There has long been an interest in the relationship between epilepsy and a variety of emotional and behavioral problems. A wide variety of theories, both reasonable and unreasonable, have been proposed to account

for interictal psychopathology in epilepsy (16). The most recent phase of research in this area was initiated by Gibbs et al. in 1948 (17) when they suggested that patients with psychomotor seizures with an anterior temporal lobe spike focus (known as "complex partial seizures of temporal lobe origin" in the current nomenclature) were particularly likely to manifest a variety of psychiatric disorders when compared to patients with other epilepsies. Since that publication, interest in the relationship between so-called temporal lobe epilepsy and psychopathology has been intense, and the controversy sustained. Furthermore, interest in other biological factors has been raised (e.g., the relationship between laterality of a temporal lobe lesion and specific psychiatric disorders; the relationship between seizure control and psychiatric status).

Interestingly, while it is true that our knowledge of the social consequences of the epilepsies has been long-standing and that our interest in epilepsy–psychopathology relationships has existed for many centuries, there has been a striking and curious lack of intermingling of these two interests. It would appear reasonable to suggest that the stigma, discrimination, unemployment, financial stress, social exclusion, and other social factors which are known to be associated with epilepsy might contribute to the development and maintenance of some psychopathologies (e.g., depression) but not others (e.g., schizophrenia-like illnesses). Unfortunately, there is virtually no database pertaining to the relationship of social factors to psychopathology in patients with epilepsy, a fact which has recently been demonstrated (18).

It is the purpose of the remainder of this chapter to investigate the utility of the model of epilepsy presented earlier to predict psychiatric distress in children and adults with epilepsy. A particular interest of ours was the relationship between social factors and psychopathology, given the limited amount of previous research. However, these social factors were examined within the context of a multietiological model.

We will first present the results of an investigation into the correlates of psychopathology in a large sample of adults with epilepsy, followed by an investigation of social competence and psychopathology in children with epilepsy, aged 6–16.

Predictors of Psychopathology in Adults with Epilepsy

The goal of this study was to specifically investigate the relationship between psychosocial factors and psychiatric distress in epilepsy within the context of the multietiological model described earlier. We will provide the details of our methodology immediately below, followed by a review of the implications of these results for the epilepsy–psychopathology literature.

Subjects

The subject pool represented referrals to the inpatient monitoring units of the Baptist Memorial Hospital Epilepsy Center. Patients were referred to the center for assessment of suitability for focal resection of their epileptogenic lesion, for further diagnostic evaluation because of an unacceptable degree of seizure control, or for reasons concerning differential diagnosis.

The specific sample investigated here consisted of 102 epilepsy patients whose diagnosis was confirmed by continuous (24 hr) closed-circuit television (CCTV)–EEG monitoring with scalp and/or sphenoidal and/or subdural strip electrodes. Monitoring was typically carried out until several spontaneous seizures were recorded. The sample comprised a consecutive series of inpatient evaluations with the exception that we did not include patients who were mentally retarded [Wechsler Adult Intelligence Scale—Revised (WAIS-R) Full-Scale I.Q. less than 70] or who had a significant reading disability (below the 5th percentile on the Reading Scale of the Wide Range Achievement Test—Revised). Table 3 provides characteristics of the final sample.

Since a primary aim of the present study was to determine the multietiological correlates of psychopathology, three sets of predictor variables were investigated (Table 4): neurobiological, psychosocial, and medication variables. These factors will be overviewed below.

Neurobiological Variables

Seven traditional neurobiological variables which are among those commonly considered

TABLE 3. *Subject characteristics*

Average age (years):	31.2 (9.3)[a]
Average education (years):	12.7 (2.3)
Average I.Q.:	89.8 (10.97)
Gender:	45 males
	57 females
Seizure type:	Partial (*N* = 97)
	8 simple partial
	90 complex partial
	55 secondarily generalized
	Generalized (*N* = 5)
	2 absence
	4 tonic–clonic
	4 other
Average age at onset (years):	14.9 (11.1)
Average duration (years):	16.3 (10.6)
Number of seizure types:	1 = 40
	2 = 59
	3 = 3
Secondarily generalized seizures in addition to simple and/or complex partial seizures?	
	yes = 55
	no = 42
	unknown = 5
Structural abnormality underlying the epilepsy?	
	yes = 15
	no = 87
Medication	55 monotherapy
	46 polytherapy
	1 none
Taking barbiturate medications?	
	yes = 14
	no = 88

[a]Standard deviation is given in parentheses.

to play some role in the etiology of psychopathology and epilepsy were included for evaluation. These seven variables were coded from patient charts by a board-certified neurosurgeon with special expertise in epilepsy while blinded to all the behavioral and psychological data. These predictor variables included: (a) age at onset of recurrent seizures, (b) duration of disorder, (c) lateralization of unilateral temporal lobe seizure onset using scalp and/or sphenoidal and/or subdural strip electrodes, (d) seizure type [partial seizures (simple, complex, and/or secondarily generalized) versus primary generalized seizures],

TABLE 4. *Multietiological predictor variables*

Neurobiological	Psychosocial	Medication
Age at onset	Perceived stigma	Monotherapy versus
Duration of epilepsy	Perceived limitations	polytherapy
Laterality of seizure onset	Adjustment to seizures	Presence/absence of barbiturate
Seizure type	Vocational adjustment	medications
Etiology	Financial status	
Presence/absence of secondarily	Life-event changes	
generalized seizures	Social support	
Number of different seizure types	Locus of control	

(e) presence versus absence of a structural lesion believed to underlie the patient's epilepsy (e.g., tumor, cyst), (f) presence/absence of secondarily generalized seizures in addition to simple and/or complex partial seizures, and (g) the number of different seizure types experienced by the patient. It should be noted that we did not analyze the frequency of seizures. Most patients were presented to our center because of an unacceptable degree of seizure control, and the distribution of this variable was therefore relatively truncated. We sought to index the severity of the patients' epilepsy through other variables (i.e., number of different seizure types, presence/ absence of secondarily generalized seizures).

Psychosocial Variables

As reviewed above, a wide variety of social and psychological constructs have been hypothesized to be among the determinants of psychopathology in epilepsy. Variables selected for inclusion in this study were those which could be assessed with self-report instruments of adequate reliability and validity and/or which could be measured via questionnaires specifically designed to assess psychosocial problems in patients with epilepsy. The following eight variables were included for evaluation.

Perceived Stigma and Perceived Limitations

These variables were assessed by two scales developed via the factor analysis of the responses of 445 adults with epilepsy to a 21-item questionnaire inquiring about their attitudes and experiences with epilepsy (19). Factor analyses were performed on the total group of 445 subjects as well as on several subgroups of subjects, and the same factors consistently emerged from the analyses.

The Perceived Stigma Scale consists of six items to which subjects respond on a four-point scale reflecting their degree of agreement. The scale specifically assesses the extent to which people with epilepsy feel that they are victims of prejudice because of their epilepsy. The coefficient of internal reliability was high ($\alpha = 0.75$).

The Perceived Limitations Scale consists of five items which are the statements or expressions of constraints that may be imposed by the disorder. Their underlying theme is the sense of vulnerability to the physical consequences of the disorder. The coefficient of internal reliability was again high ($\alpha = 0.80$).

Adjustment to Seizures, Vocational Adjustment, and Financial Status

These three areas of psychosocial concern were assessed by the WPSI (14).

The Adjustment to Seizures Scale of the WPSI consists of 15 items which inquire into whether the person with epilepsy resents having epilepsy, feels less worthwhile because of the epilepsy, is embarrassed about the diagnosis and/or seizures, and feels accepted by others.

The Vocational Adjustment Scale of the WPSI consists of 13 items which assess whether epilepsy is interfering with the person's ability to obtain a job or whether it is interfering with the degree of satisfaction with current vocational situation, and it also assesses whether or not there appears to be a need for vocational counseling services.

The Financial Status Scale of the WPSI

consists of seven items which assess whether the individual has significant financial problems and whether he or she worries a great deal about financial difficulties.

For each scale, increasing scores reflect increasing seriousness of impairment and concern.

Life Event Changes

Assessment of the number of stressful life events occurring during the past 6 months was carried out via the Life Experiences Survey (LES) (20). The LES consists of 47 life-event changes which can be rated on a six-point Likert scale according to the desirability/undesirability of the events. The LES items were originally chosen to represent life changes frequently experienced by individuals in the general population. An acceptable degree of test–retest reliability has been demonstrated, as has the fact that the LES scores are not associated with measures of social desirability (20). For this investigation we used the absolute number of life-event changes which occurred during the past year as the predictor index from the LES.

Social Support

The Social Support Questionnaire (SSQ) (21) is a 27-item survey which assesses two major aspects of social support: (i) the *amount* of social support available to the individual and (ii) his/her *satisfaction* with the available support. The subject is asked to list the people whom he/she can turn to and rely on in a variety of situations, and then he/she is asked to describe the satisfaction with the support rendered.

Factor analyses of the SSQ have supported the notion of two social support indices (number, satisfaction). Coefficients of internal reliability are uniformly high ($\alpha > 0.95$), and scores do not correlate with measures of social desirability (21).

For the purposes of this investigation we utilized the number of individuals available to provide social support (SSN) as the measure of interest derived from the SSQ. The higher the score, the more social support available to the patient.

Locus of Control

In order to assess each patient's locus of control we utilized Rotter's (22) Internal/External Control of Reinforcement Scale. Although this scale has been widely utilized, some concerns have been raised regarding its factor structure, scale format, and correlation with social desirability measures. Based on Askanasy's (23) findings (i.e., the scales most likely tap a unitary construct, and there is no significant correlation between social desirability and total score on Rotter's scale), we relied on the scoring procedures originally described by Rotter, with higher scores indicating a more external locus of control.

Medication Factors

Only two medication variables were utilized because at the time of CCTV–EEG monitoring the patients were on markedly reduced levels of their anticonvulsant medications, or the medications were withdrawn altogether. Therefore, we examined the patient's most recent (preadmission) medication schedule and determined (a) whether the patient was on a program of monotherapy or polytherapy and (b) whether his/her anticonvulsant program included any barbiturate medications.

Dependent Measures

In order to provide an overview of the psychological status of this sample, two dependent measures were utilized: (i) the Center for Epidemiological Studies in Depression scale (CES-D) (24), a self-report measure of depression; and (ii) the Emotional Adjustment Scale from Dodrill et al.'s (14) WPSI, a self-report measure of emotional status which has recently been shown to correlate with MMPI profile elevations (25). Each dependent measure was treated as a continuous variable, with increasing scores indicating increasing psychopathology.[1]

---

[1] An analysis and extended discussion of the depression findings have been presented in *Journal of Epilepsy*, 1989;231–237.

TABLE 5. *Significant predictors of elevated CES-D scores*

Variable	r	p
Adjustment to epilepsy	0.46	< 0.01
Financial status	0.36	< 0.01
Perceived stigma	0.32	< 0.01
Locus of control	0.28	< 0.01
Life-event changes	0.22	< 0.05
Vocational adjustment	0.21	< 0.05
Social support	−0.21	< 0.05

Data Analyses

First, Pearson correlation coefficients were computed between each of the continuous neurobiological, psychosocial, and medication variables and between each of the two dependent measures. Dichotomous predictor variables were analyzed via Student's t test. A subsequent intercorrelation matrix of the predictor variables revealed that there was substantial intercorrelation. Therefore, in order to identify *independent* (nonredundant) predictors of psychopathology, those variables which showed a significant relationship ($p < 0.05$) with each dependent measure were subsequently entered into a stepwise multiple regression analysis for that outcome variable.

Results

Tables 5 and 6 show the predictor variables that exhibited a significant ($p < 0.05$) relationship with each dependent measure, and Tables 7 and 8 list the results of the multiple regression analyses.

Increased depression scores (CES-D) (Ta-

TABLE 6. *Significant predictors of elevated WPSI for the emotional adjustment scores*

Variable	r	p
Adjustment to epilepsy	0.59	< 0.001
Vocational adjustment	0.33	< 0.001
Financial status	0.32	0.001
Perceived stigma	0.28	< 0.005
Locus of control	0.26	< 0.005
Social support	−0.25	< 0.01
Age	0.22	< 0.05
Life-event changes	0.19	< 0.05
Perceived limitations	0.18	< 0.05

TABLE 7. *Results of the regression analysis for CES-D*

Significant variables	p
Stressful life events	0.01
Adjustment to epilepsy	0.002
Financial status	0.007
Gender	0.003

ble 5) were associated with increased perceived stigma, lower social support, an increased number of stressful life events during the past year, poor adjustment to epilepsy, vocational difficulties, financial stress, an external locus of control, and female gender. Four of the seven variables remained statistically significant when entered into a stepwise multiple regression analysis (Table 7). Specifically, increased depression was associated with an increased number of stressful life events during the past 6 months, poor adjustment to epilepsy, financial stress, and female gender. The multiple correlation ($R = 0.58$) indicated that these four variables accounted for about 34% of the variance in the CES-D scores. Two remaining variables just missed reaching conventional levels of statistical significance in the regression model: lower social support ($p = 0.06$) and an external locus of control ($p = 0.07$).

For the WPSI Emotional Adjustment Scale the following variables were associated with increased (problem) scores (Table 6): increased perceived stigma, increased number of life-event changes, poor adjustment to epilepsy, vocational problems, financial stress, external locus of control, decreased social support, increased perceived limitations, and younger chronological age. Two variables remained significant when all were entered into a stepwise regression analysis (Table 8): poor adjustment to epilepsy and an external locus of control.

TABLE 8. *Results of the regression analysis for WPSI Emotional Adjustment Scale*

Significant variables	p
Adjustment to epilepsy	0.001
Locus of control	0.045

Comment

Three general observations can be made based on the findings reviewed above. First, it is clear that psychosocial factors bear a strong relationship to the measures of psychopathology utilized in this investigation. Because the approach of this study was correlational in nature, cause–effect relationships cannot be made. What is clear is that it appears as if psychosocial factors constitute an important dimension in understanding psychiatric distress in epilepsy and that well-controlled, *prospective* studies are now needed to identify causal relationships. Such investigations in the general population have identified several similar factors (e.g., life-event changes, financial stress, locus of control) as being causal in the etiology of depression (26,27). Whether they are similarly causal among patients with epilepsy remains to be determined.

Second, the results of the regression analyses indicated that two factors are particularly powerful: financial status and adjustment to epilepsy. The former variable has long been suggested as an important variable in the adjustment of people with epilepsy, whereas financial status has rarely been mentioned. It should also be pointed out that the regression analyses, while highly significant, were modest in their explanatory power, suggesting that much remains to be uncovered in the future.

Third, the biological and medication variables were surprisingly poor predictors of interictal psychopathology. This may be due, in part, to the nature of the population under investigation—namely, patients with poorly controlled seizures, the majority of whom were surgical candidates. Perhaps in a more representative population of patients with epilepsy, with more variability in the severity of their epilepsy, significant relationships may be detected. As will be seen in the study of children with epilepsy that follows, this was indeed the case. Finally, medication variables were assessed to a minimal extent because the patients were withdrawn from their anticonvulsants during their inpatient monitoring. Again, evaluation of a more representative outpatient population with a better diversity of pharmacological indicators will increase the yield of significant predictors.

We will now briefly turn to a similar, but more limited, investigation of a large sample of children with epilepsy. These results will similarly reinforce the utility of a multietiological model but, unlike the results obtained during the investigation with adults, will point to the power of several biological variables.

Social Competence in Children with Epilepsy

This investigation deals with a large sample of children with epilepsy (aged 6–16 years) and will attempt to identify the predictors of overall behavioral adjustment and social competence. Most research in the area has attempted to identify the correlates of behavioral and social deficiencies, but here we will additionally attempt to use our model to predict behavioral and social *competence* in the pediatric population. The main results of the social competence analyses have been published elsewhere (28), but the psychopathology analyses are presented here for the first time.

Subjects

The subject pool consisted of children with epilepsy between the ages of 6 and 16 who were attending a special epilepsy clinic at the University of Illinois Medical Center. Chil-

TABLE 9. *Multietiological predictor variables*

Neurobiological	Psychosocial	Medication
Age at onset	Parents' marital status	Monotherapy versus polytherapy
Duration of disorder	Family income	Drug type
Seizure type		Number of drug categories
EEG pattern		
Seizure control		
Etiology		

dren excluded from the regular school system because of mental handicap (i.e., those placed in educationally mentally handicapped or trainable mentally handicapped settings) were excluded from consideration for this investigation. However, children attending alternative schools because of behavioral dysfunction were included in the subject pool as were children who attended special learning disorder classes as part of their regular educational programming.

The final sample consisted of 183 consecutively referred children with epilepsy, excluding families who were Spanish-speaking only.

TABLE 10. *Average values or proportions for the independent variables, grouped by hypothesis (N = 183)*

Biological variables	
Average age at onset	6.3 years
Average duration of disorder	5.1 years
Seizure type	
Partial	53%
Primary generalized	40%
Partial and primary generalized (mixed)	7%
EEG pattern	
Corticoreticular	33%
Focal	43%
Mixed	12%
Other	12%
Seizure control	
Good	30%
Fair	30%
Poor	40%
Etiology	
Symptomatic	21%
Idiopathic	68%
Unknown	11%
Psychosocial variables	
Parents' marital status	
Married	57%
Divorced or separated	34%
Other	8%
Average median family income	$17,835
Medication variables	
Number	
Monotherapy	49%
Polytherapy	37%
None	14%
Drug class[a]	
Barbiturates	53%
Succinimides	14%
Hydantoin	43%
Valproic acid	18%
Carbamazepine	12%
Other	14%
Number of drug categories	
0	14%
1	49%
2	26%
3	8%
4	3%

[a]Percentages are based on the number of children on medication (*N* = 157), and they add to more than 100% because several children were taking more than one type of medication.

Predictor Variables

The variables identified in Table 9 represent the potential predictor variables of interest for this study. Previous publications from our group will allow the interested reader to obtain more detailed information about the methodology and operational definitions of each potential predictor variable (29). Table 10 provides summary information regarding the characteristics of the sample, grouped according to each of the predictor variables.

Dependent Measure

The behavior and social competence of each child was assessed by means of an interview with the child's mother or guardian using the Child Behavior Checklist (CBCL) (28,30). This behavioral assessment inventory was designed to record, in a standardized format, the behavioral problems and social competence of children aged 6–16 years. The CBCL consists of 20 social competence and 118 behavioral problem items.

For the purposes of this investigation we utilized the CBCL summary measures of Total Behavioral Problems and Total Social Competence. The latter represents a composite measure reflecting the amount and quality of the child's participation in sports, hobbies, games, activities, organizations, and friendships as well as school performance and social interaction. Raw scores are converted to standardized T scores ($\bar{x} = 50$, SD = 10). Higher scores indicate increasing social competence, whereas lower scores indicate less adequate social competence. The former measure is a summary index of the extent and frequency of behavioral problems exhibited by the child. Raw scores are similarly converted to standardized T scores, with high scores indicating more behavioral problems.

Data Analysis

Data analysis was similar to that previously described. First, simple Pearson correlation coefficients were computed between each of the predictor variables and the measures of Total Social Competence and Total Behavioral Problems. Because there is intercorrelation among the potential predictor variables, those factors showing a significant relationship with each dependent measure were then entered into a stepwise multiple regression analysis so that independent (nonredundant) predictors of each dependent variable could be identified.

Results

Tables 11 and 12 present the variables that were significantly associated with social competence and psychopathology, their Pearson correlation coefficients, and levels of statistical significance. As can be seen, increased social competence (Table 11) was associated with an intact parental marriage, good seizure control, higher family income, later age at onset of epilepsy, a shorter duration of epilepsy, and not experiencing multiple seizure types. Interestingly, monotherapy ($p = 0.087$) was positively associated with increasing social competence, and polytherapy ($p = 0.051$) was negatively associated, but these relationships just missed conventional levels of statistical significance. It is also worth noting that of those variables that did reach statistical significance, the correlations were not high and explained the relatively small proportions of the variance. Because there was intercorrelation among the identified significant predictor variables, they were subsequently entered

TABLE 11. *Statistically significant Pearson correlations between Total Social Competence and potential predictor variables*

Variable	r	p
Good seizure control	0.21	0.003
Intact parental marriage	0.20	0.004
Higher family income	0.18	0.007
Shorter duration of disorder	0.17	0.013
Later age at onset	0.17	0.013
Single seizure type	0.12	0.049

TABLE 12. *Statistically significant Pearson correlations between Total Behavior Problems and potential predictor variables*

Variable	r	p
Inadequate seizure control	0.38	< 0.01
Divorced/separated parents	0.32	< 0.01
Symptomatic etiology	0.17	< 0.05

into a stepwise multiple regression analysis; the resultant multiple R was 0.39, indicating that 15% of the variance was accounted for by the predictor variables. Four significant ($p < 0.05$) variables associated with increased social competence were identified: good seizure control, an intact parental marriage, shorter duration of epilepsy, and higher family income.

An increased number of behavior problems (Table 12) was significantly associated with poor seizure control, divorced/separated parents, and epilepsy of symptomatic etiology. When these three variables were entered into a stepwise regression analysis the multiple R was 0.52, and all three variables remained highly statistically significant ($p < 0.01$).

Comment

The results of this investigation demonstrated that it is possible to identify multietiological predictors of overall social competence and behavior problems in children with epilepsy. Neurobiological (good seizure control and shorter duration of epilepsy) and psychosocial (intact parental marriage and higher family income) variables were associated with increased social competence in children with epilepsy. Behavior problems were similarly associated with both biological (poor seizure control, symptomatic etiology) and social (divorced/separated parents) factors. These findings are intuitively appealing. They suggest that a multidisciplinary approach to children with epilepsy is indicated, stressing both (a) up-to-date, modern medical management in order to bring seizures under the best control possible and (b) the need for attention to the welfare and well-being of the family unit. Finally, as was found to be the case in the study of adults, socioeconomic considerations are extremely relevant.

CONCLUSION

As we stated at the outset of this chapter, epilepsy mounts a multidisciplinary assault on the quality of patients' lives. We have suggested that this assault could be characterized by three dimensions (neurobiological, psychosocial, medication-related), with each dimension being represented by many specific variables. Examples of relevant variables were provided in Table 1.

To some degree we have been able to show how these three dimensions are associated with measures of interictal psychopathology and social competence in adults and children with epilepsy. Although these findings are of interest, significant methodological problems remain. For instance, casuality patterns are yet to be determined, and significant amounts of variance remain unaccounted for, suggesting that powerful predictor variables remain to be identified.

The model that has been suggested, along with the empirical approach that has been utilized, is only one of many potential avenues to untangling the etiology of interictal psychopathology in epilepsy. It is the multietiological orientation to the problem, rather than the specifics of the model, which is key at present.

An open-minded and comprehensive approach to identifying the determinants of a broad range of specific behavior problems may lead to the detection of greater relative loading of one particular dimension (e.g., neurobiological) to a particular psychopathology (e.g., schizophrenic-like illness), whereas other dimensions (e.g., psychosocial) may be of greater etiological importance to other psychopathologies (e.g., depression). The investment of research time and monies should be well worth the effort because meaningful treatment and prevention programs will result.

ACKNOWLEDGMENTS

We sincerely thank Angie Braddock for typing and processing this manuscript. We also thank Dr. Roger Vanderzwagg, Health Services Research, Baptist Memorial Hospital, for analyzing portions of the data presented in this manuscript.

REFERENCES

1. Hermann BP, Whitman S. Behavioral and personality correlates of epilepsy: a review, methodological critique, and conceptual model. *Psychol Bull* 1984;95:451–497.
2. Hermann BP, Whitman S. Psychopathology in epilepsy: a multietiological model. In: Whitman S, Hermann BP, eds. *Psychopathology in epilepsy: social factors.* New York: Oxford University Press, 1986;5–37.
3. Porter R. *Epilepsy: 100 elementary principles.* Philadelphia: WB Saunders, 1984.
4. Reynolds EH. Biological factors in psychological disorders associated with epilepsy. In: Reynolds EH, Trimble MR, eds. *Psychiatry and epilepsy.* Edinburgh: Churchill Livingstone, 1981; 264–290.
5. Trimble MR, Reynolds EH. Anticonvulsant drugs and mental symptoms: a review. *Psychol Med* 1976;6:169–178.
6. Brendt DA, Crumrine PK, Varma RR, et al. Phenobarbital treatment and major depressive disorder in children with epilepsy. *Pediatrics* 1987; 80:909–917.
7. Theodore WH, DiChiro G, Margolin R, Fishbein D, Porter RJ, Brooks RA. Barbiturates reduce human cerebral glucose metabolism. *Neurology* 1986;36:60–64.
8. Theodore WH, Bairamian D, Newmark ME, DiChiro G, Porter RJ, Larson S, Fishbein D. Effect of phenytoin on human cerebral glucose metabolism. *J Cereb Blood Flow* 1986;6:315–320.
9. Reynolds EH. Anticonvulsant drugs, folic acid metabolism, fit frequency and psychiatric illness. *Psychiatr Neurol Neurochir* 1971;74:167–174.
10. Reynolds EH. Anticonvulsants and mental symptoms. In: Sandler M, ed. *Psychopharmacology of anticonvulsants.* New York: Oxford University Press, 1982.
11. Lennox WG. *Epilepsy and related disorders,* vol. 2. Boston: Little, Brown, 1960.
12. National Commission for the Control of Epilepsy and Its Consequences. *Plan for nationwide action on epilepsy, 1978.* DHEW publication No. NIH 78-276. Washington, DC: National Institute of Health, 1978.
13. Levin R, Banks S, Berg B. Psychosocial dimension of epilepsy: a review of the literature. *Epilepsia* 1988;29:805–816.
14. Dodrill CB, Batzell LW, Quiesser HR, Temkin NR. An objective method for the assessment of psychological and social problems among epileptics. *Epilepsia* 1980;21:123–135.
15. Thompson PJ, Oxley J. Socioeconomic accompaniments of severe epilepsy. *Epilepsia* 1988;29 (Suppl 1):S9–S18.
16. Guerrant J, Anderson WW, Fischer A, Weinstein MR, Jaros JM, Deskins A. *Personality in epilepsy.* Springfield, IL: Charles C Thomas, 1962.
17. Gibbs EL, Giggs FA, Fuster B. Psychomotor epilepsy. *Arch Neurol Psychiatry* 1948;60:331–339.

18. Whitman S, Hermann BP. The architecture of research in the epilepsy—psychopathology literature. *Epilepsy Res* 1989;3:93–99.
19. Ryan R, Kempner K, Emlen AC. The stigma of epilepsy as a self-concept. *Epilepsia* 1980;21:433–444.
20. Sarason IG, Johnson JH, Siegel JM. Assessing the impact of life changes: development of the Life Experiences Survey. *J Consult Clin Psychol* 1978;46:932–946.
21. Sarason IG, Levine HM, Basham RB, Sarason BR. Assessing social support: the Social Support Questionnaire. *J Pers Soc Psychol* 1983;44:127–139.
22. Rotter JB. Generalized expectancies for internal versus external control of reinforcement. *Psychol Monogr* 1966;80.
23. Askanasy NM. Rotter's Internal–External Scale: confirmatory factor analysis and correlation with social desirability for alternative scale formats. *J Pers Soc Psychol* 1985;48:1328–1341.
24. Radloff LS. The CES-D Scale: a self-report depression scale for research in the general population. *Appl Psychol Measurement* 1977;1:385–401.
25. Warner M, Dodrill CB. Economical screening of emotional status using the WPSI. *J Epilepsy* 1990;in press.
26. Kaplan GA, Roberts RE, Camacho TC, Coyne JC. Psychosocial predictors of depression. *Am J Epidemiol* 1987;125:206–220.
27. Lewinsohn PM, Hoberman HM, Rosenbaum M. A prospective study of risk factors for unipolar depression. *J Abnorm Psychol* 1988;97:251–264.
28. Achenback TM, Edelbrock CS. *Manual for the Child Behavior Checklist and Revised Behavior Checklist*. Burlington, VT: University of Vermont, 1983.
29. Hermann BP, Whitman S, Hughes JR, Melyn M, Dell J. Multietiological determinants of psychopathology and social competence in children with epilepsy. *Epilepsy Res* 1988;2:51–60.
30. Achenbach TM, Edelbrock CS. Behavioral problems and social competencies reported by parents of normal and disturbed children aged four through sixteen. *Monogr Soc Res Child Dev* 1981;46:1–82.

Advances in Neurology, Vol. 55, edited by
D. Smith, D. Treiman, and M. Trimble,
Raven Press, Ltd., New York © 1991.

28

Emotional Effects on Seizure Occurrence

Richard H. Mattson

Department of Veterans Affairs, VA Medical Center, West Haven, Connecticut 06516

A variety of environmental factors appear to modify brain excitability, thereby affecting the likelihood of seizure occurrence. These modulators include sleep deprivation, alcohol abuse, menstrual or diurnal cyclic changes, and, infrequently, specific sensory stimulation (1–8). Frequently, patients and families identify emotional stress as a likely reason for an increase in the frequency of seizures. Gowers (3) noted that 30% of seizures could be attributed to such stressors, although it is not entirely clear how he separated hysteroepilepsy (presumably pseudoseizures) from epileptic seizures worsened by psychological factors. In an extensive survey, Servit et al. (9) found that patients and neurologists frequently found "neurotigenic" stress to be the most common reason for increased frequency or exacerbation of seizures.

In a more recent study, Temkin and Davis (10) followed 12 patients for a 3-month period and recorded both emotional state and seizure activity. A highly significant association was found between daily "hassles" and occurrence of seizures. They noted that the history did not clearly indicate a close minute-to-minute temporal relationship between emotional stress and seizures. Webster and Mawer (11) studied 18 patients with chronic epilepsy and found a definite association between life events and seizure frequency, especially in those with partial seizures. Documentation that emotional stress could elicit seizures was provided by studies carried out by Feldman and Paul (12). They showed videotapes to patients related to areas of personal emotional vulnerability and observed the triggering of seizures. Interestingly, replaying the tape of

the seizures to the patient provided some insight as to the provoking material and resulted in some ability to ameliorate the seizures. Fenwick (see Chapter 11, *this volume;* also see refs. 13 and 14) also has suggested that true epileptic seizures may be "psychogenic," a term indicating that true epileptic seizures could be induced by psychological factors, either self-induced or occurring sporadically. A number of other induced seizures associated with cognitive activity are properly thought to be psychologically induced but not necessarily associated with any particular emotional stress. These cognitively induced seizures have been documented in a laboratory setting by a number of investigators (13). Fenwick has theorized that in relevant areas of cortex having hyperexcitable epileptic foci, normal stimuli involving psychological processes may activate the seizures in these areas. He suggested that such psychological precipitation is analogous to seizures of primary sensory type such as those located in sensory cortex and triggered by somatic stimulation in appropriate areas of the body.

Although many anecdotal case reports have indicated an association between emotional stress and seizures, few studies have been carried out to document the frequency of such factors in a general population of patients with epilepsy, except as mentioned above. In particular, the mechanism whereby emotional stress might elicit seizures has been incompletely defined. Although the concept of activation of specific neural networks has been proposed, clinical studies have not been carried out to substantiate such a theory.

CLINICAL SURVEY

Because sufficient information was not available regarding the frequency of occurrence, as well as regarding possible mechanisms, we carried out studies in a large series of patients followed over the course of 2 years at the clinics in the Yale New Haven Hospital and the VA Medical Center, West Haven. Patients underwent a detailed survey of factors that might induce or precipitate seizures. The patients were asked about an extensive number of factors, including missed medication, emotional stress, sleep deprivation, menstrual cyclic effects, alcohol or other drug use, diurnal variations, and specific triggering mechanisms such as light, sound, touch, etc. The period of observations included the preceding 2 years. Patients were asked to indicate whether their seizures occurred more frequently in association with these factors than would be expected by chance alone. Specific anecdotes were obtained, and the reports were reviewed with other family members and available medical records. The association was then graded as "none," "possible," or "probable." The relationship between seizures and emotional stress was specifically classified into separate seizure subgroups: simple partial (focal), complex partial (psychomotor), or generalized.

One hundred and seventy-seven patients completed the detailed survey of precipitating or modulating factors associated with occur-

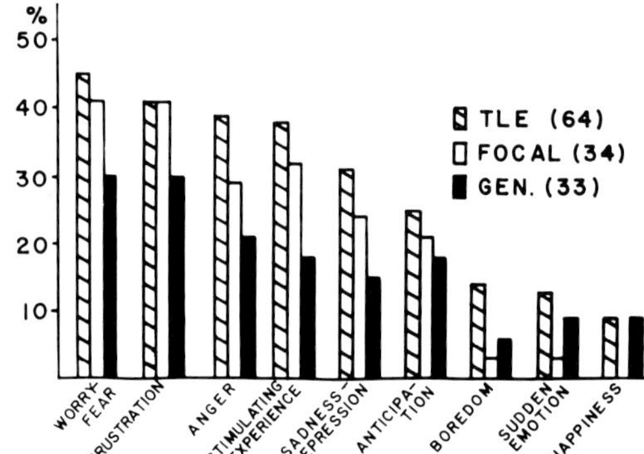

FIG. 2. Association of specific emotional state with seizure recurrence by seizure type.

rence of seizures. Missed medication was the most common reported cause of recurrence, but the second most frequently reported factor was emotional stress. Fifty-eight percent of the patients indicated that their attacks occurred more frequently during these times. (Fig. 1). Although some patients noted a close temporal relationship between stress and seizures, most patients often did not report an immediate effect. The association was sometimes noted over a period of days or even weeks of life events, rather than minutes or hours. At times, some patients even noted that the seizures occurred immediately following the cessation of emotionally stressful life events. The effects of different types of psychological stresses and seizure types were compared (Fig. 2). Worry, frustration, anger, and stimulating experiences were most commonly reported to be associated with worsening of seizures, and such effects were more frequently reported in the patient group having complex partial [temporal lobe epilepsy (TLE)] seizures than in those with generalized (GEN) or simple partial (focal) seizures. These differences did not reach levels of statistical significance.

CLINICAL NEUROPHYSIOLOGICAL PATIENT STUDY

A subgroup of six patients who closely associated stress with seizure occurrence was studied with calendars of life events to document possible correlations. This group was

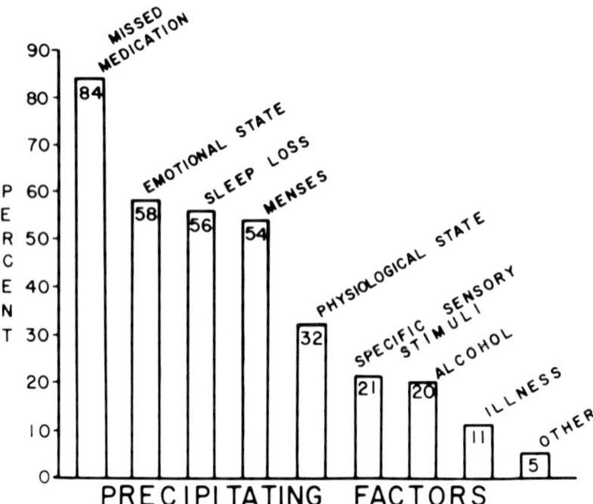

FIG. 1. Frequency of association of various factors with exacerbation.

then studied on the research ward and/or in the clinical neurophysiology lab to determine a possible mechanism of action.

For patients observed on the ward, a standard rating for affective, cognitive, motor, and more complex behavior was completed by the nursing staff. All patients had standard blood tests, including those for antiepileptic drug levels and cortisol levels; these tests were performed in the morning and afternoon. Polygraphic recordings were carried out in the laboratory for documentation of the number of seizures occurring spontaneously as well as to count the number of paroxysmal bursts of spikes or spike-and-waves and determine the total length of paroxysmal activity per unit time during a 4-hr recording. Because preliminary evidence suggested that hyperventilation was playing a significant role in seizures of four patients, a detailed study was carried out to include stressful, structured interviews with simultaneous closed-circuit video monitoring and electrographic recording of epileptiform activity. An electromyogram also was connected to the extremity involved in one patient's partial seizures. The polygraphic recording monitored hyperventilation with a pneumograph, and end-tidal CO_2 analysis was performed on blood from the nasopharynx using a Beckman CO_2 analyzer. Periodic arterial blood gas determinations were obtained for correlation with the other physiologic measures. A tachograph displayed changes in heart rate. In addition, on other occasions these four patients had an intravenous infusion of 10 mg of hydrocortisone during the clinical polygraphic studies. Blood samples measured cortisol samples over the next 4 hr.

At least three possible mechanisms for emotionally induced seizures were observed in these patients and will be illustrated by case reports.

A 21-year-old man had a lifelong history of partial and occasional secondarily generalized seizures which were incompletely controlled. Seemingly independent of his epilepsy, the patient had episodes of significant thought disorder with paranoid delusions requiring hospitalization on several occasions. His history indicated that the seizures were more frequent at the times of his psychiatric exacerbations. Both the patient and the family

agreed that the emotional problems preceded the seizures, although the relationship became difficult to define after a few days of both seizures and psychosis. Hospitalization and observation during one of the psychotic episodes showed prominent epileptiform activity that differed from his usual electroencephalogram (EEG), which was of borderline normal type. Observation and further history in the hospital made clear that the patient's paranoia and delusions caused agitation and profound sleeplessness. After remission of his psychotic phase, and normalization of his EEG, purposeful sleep deprivation again elicited the electrographic abnormality without recurrent agitation and thought disorder (Fig. 3). These findings suggested that the emotional disturbance led to sleep deprivation, which, at least in part, caused EEG activation and increased seizure frequency.

A 23-year-old white woman had a lifelong history of partial and secondarily generalized seizures. Partially disabled, she lived at home with her family and received considerable special attention. Her father had also become ill (with cardiac disease), which required attention to be focused on him from time to time. When this occurred, the patient's seizures often exacerbated. On admission to the hospital and with improvement in her depression, the seizures significantly improved. During psychiatric treatment the patient admitted that at the times of stress she would take the antiepileptic drug medication given to her by her mother and put it in her mouth but shortly thereafter would purposely spit it into the toilet. After 1 or 2 days her seizures commonly exacerbated. In this case, emotional stress led to noncompliance with medication, resulting in secondary seizure exacerbation.

Four other patients had seizure exacerbation under psychological stress, and there was reason to suspect hyperventilation as a significant mechanism. In all four patients, hyperventilation in the laboratory activated partial or generalized electrographic epileptiform abnormalities. On occasion, anxiety induced overbreathing and led to increased seizures. One patient was studied in detail in order to understand the mechanisms.

A 31-year-old white woman underwent extensive repeated clinical and neurophysiologic

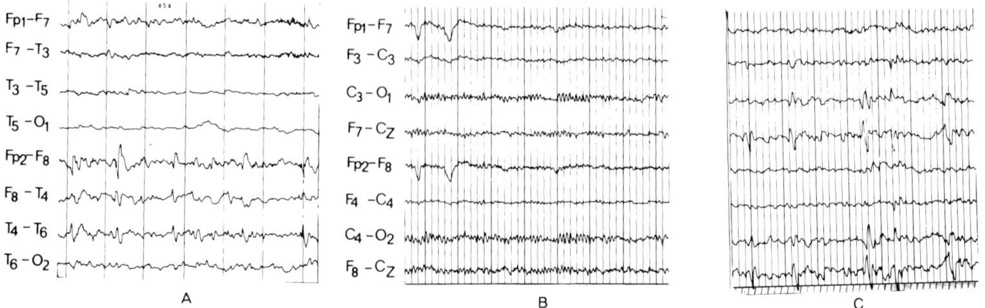

FIG. 3. A: Altered EEG showing right temporal spikes during psychosis and during seizure exacerbation. **B:** Normalization of the EEG during remission of seizures and psychosis. **C:** EEG abnormality reproduced following sleep deprivation.

studies to document an association between stress and seizures. She had a lifelong history of partial seizures of traumatic origin. These began with sensory motor attacks progressing at times to complex partial seizures. She also had episodes of anxiety and depression and described a feeling of being unable to "catch her breath" during periods of anxiety and agitation which particularly occurred during family arguments. The family strongly concurred with the patient's observation of the association.

The combination of seizures and psychiatric problems led to her admission to the Clinical Research Unit. Daily ratings of her psychological status were made by the nursing staff; in addition, the patient kept a diary of daily events, with specific tabulation of frequency and timing of her seizures. Finally, she had daily EEGs performed, with quantitation of paroxysmal activity twice daily. Antiepileptic drug levels and twice-daily cortisol levels were monitored.

No relationship could be detected between daily scores of depression, anxiety, or other measures of stress and the occurrence of paroxysmal activity measured in the laboratory. No relationship was found between (a) cortisol levels on days of high scores for ratings of emotional upset and (b) cortisol levels on days of seizure occurrence. In contrast to these overall daily assessments, the professional staff observed an increase in seizures during stressful group therapy meetings.

Because the patient reported difficulty "catching her breath" during periods of anxi-

ety and stress, the response to hyperventilation was evaluated polygraphically in the laboratory setting with closed-circuit video monitoring. Hyperventilation carried out on request of the staff resulted in a marked build-up in left-sided spike-and-wave activity which became more generalized and which progressed to focal motor movements of the right hand (Fig. 4). This paroxysmal response decreased after completion of the voluntary overbreathing. Some minutes later the patient often began to hyperventilate involuntarily. This could be aborted if one of the investigators entered the room and distracted her with innocuous conversation. She was unaware of the fact that she involuntarily hyperventilated on these occasions, but she often had seizures in series. These were associated with anxiety and "a fearful feeling." The build-up of paroxysmal activity and focal seizures could be promptly aborted by rebreathing a mixture of 95% O_2 and 5% CO_2 (Fig. 5). Although attempts to provoke seizures by seemingly stressful interviews failed to show increased abnormalities, spontaneous increased activation with hyperventilation and increased epileptiform activity on the EEG accompanied the appearance of unfamiliar personnel or new procedures in the laboratory. Finally, a family meeting was carried out in the laboratory which led to arguments, dissension, and evolution of one of the patient's seizures. Despite the altercation among the family members and apparent anger and agitation on the part of the patient, neither hyperventilation nor increased seizure activity was observed

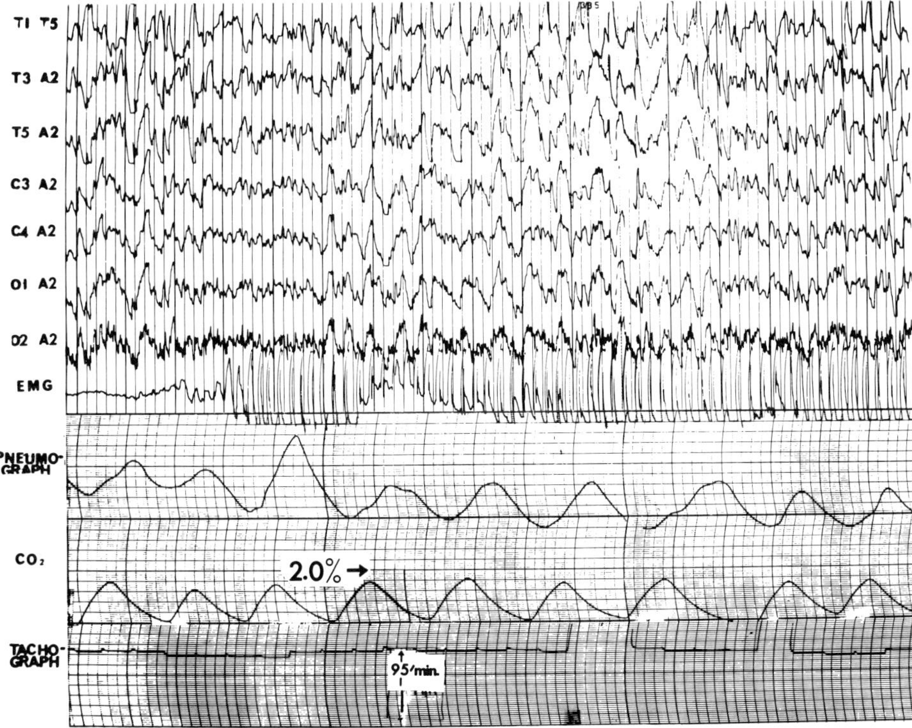

FIG. 4. Polygraphic recording of hyperventilation-induced partial seizure. The rapid breathing was associated with decrease end-tidal CO_2, rhythmic spike-and-wave discharge, focal motor seizures (EMG), and tachycardia.

initially. Approximately 15 min later into the meeting with seemingly no greater stress, but at a time when the patient was being criticized, involuntary overbreathing gradually increased and culminated in an overt seizure with findings essentially the same as shown in Fig. 5.

Another patient showed similar activity with anxiety-provoked hyperventilation, but this individual also had other factors involved in seizure precipitation which acted by other mechanisms.

A 40-year-old white man with inclusion body encephalitis suffered from cortical blindness, mild organic brain syndrome, and myoclonic seizures. Ward observations documented that during times of frustration and anxiety, the frequency of his seizures greatly increased. At these times, his seizures also could be triggered by an unexpected touch of his arm shortly after awakening. This was re-

producible if the stimulus occurred less than every 2–3 sec. Rhythmic tapping at a more rapid rate failed to elicit myoclonic seizures. During polygraphic study in the laboratory, hyperventilation significantly increased isolated poly-spike-and-wave discharges with bilateral myoclonic jerks. Seemingly stressful interviews failed to elicit either hyperventilation, increased electroencephalographic abnormality, or overt seizures. On the other hand, on several different occasions when equipment was malfunctioning and he detected anxiety and frustration of the investigators, he also became obviously anxious and had both involuntary overbreathing and an increase in seizures. At these times, his susceptibility to reflex myoclonic jerks by touching his arm was similarly more active. In addition, the jerks could also be sometimes triggered by suddenly clapping or calling out his name, especially if unexpected. Although this

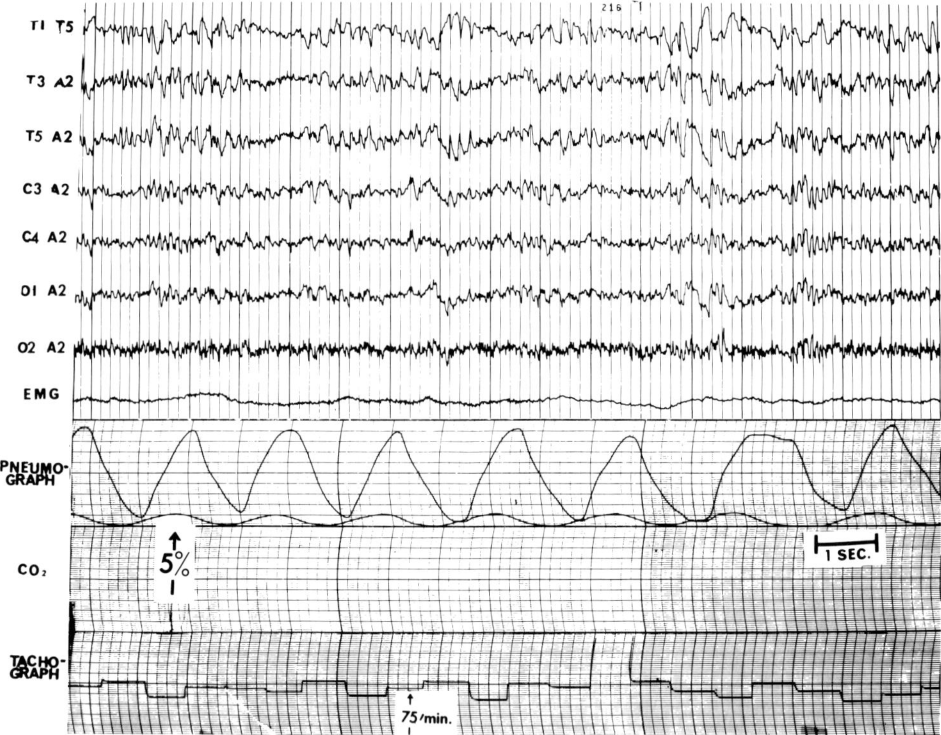

FIG. 5. Clearing of electrographic and clinical activity recorded in Fig. 4 following rapid rebreathing of a mixture of 95% O_2 and 5% CO_2.

patient's seizures were commonly noted to be exacerbated by anxiety, a major diurnal pattern also was noted. Both spontaneous and elicited seizures occurred most frequently shortly after awakening in the morning.

In addition to the polygraphic studies with stressful interview, four of the six patients were given 10 mg of hydrocortisol, resulting in an increase to levels 2–10 times that of normal blood. No clinical or electrographic changes were seen over a 4-hr course.

COMMENTS

The effect of emotional or psychologic factors on the frequency of seizures was studied in several ways. First, a detailed survey was carried out in a group of epileptic patients, and a strong relationship was reported by patients and families. This often occurred when stress was present over a period of days or weeks rather than from minute to minute.

These findings are consistent with other studies dating back to observations of Gowers (3), and they have been expanded by a review of Servit et al. (9). Recent reports by Feldman and Paul (12), Temkin and Davis (10), and Webster and Mawer (11) provide further evidence of an association between emotional stress and seizures.

In addition, our study suggested that certain types of emotional stressors such as worry, anxiety, frustration, and anger were most likely to be reported as aggravating factors. This seemed to be somewhat more apparent with patients having complex partial seizures than with those having generalized or simple partial attacks. Studies such as ours and those of other investigators are limited by lack of evidence that such events are truly related and not simply a spontaneous occurrence. Some "logical" explanation may be sought by the patient and family. This effort to find some plausible reason for seizure exacerbation may lead to a tendency to ignore the fact that many seizures occur without emotional stresses. A few studies have attempted to demonstrate by statistical measure that stressful life events may correlate with worsening of seizures (10,11). Stevens (14) noted an increase in electroencephalographic abnormalities during stressful interview, but she did not clearly provoke seizures by this mechanism. Most other psychologically triggered seizures which have been studied and documented involved specific cognitive tasks such as reading, calculating, etc., but did not clearly have an emotional content (8; also see Chapter 11, *this volume*). Six patients in our studies were evaluated in great detail. We found that fairly reproducible mechanisms played a role in exacerbation of seizures. In one patient the emotional stress interfered with his ability to sleep. We were able to reproduce both epileptiform activity and seizure occurrence using the activating technique of sleep deprivation, even at a time when he was not under emotional stress. In his case it seemed that the seizures were aggravated by sleep deprivation which was caused by cyclic cognitive/affective disturbance. Sleep deprivation has been reported by numerous investigators to be an activating or facilitating factor in seizure occurrence (4–15). Because disruption of sleep commonly accompanies a variety of emotional disturbances (particularly worry and depression), it is not surprising that some exacerbation can be attributed to this mechanism.

Missed medication proved to be the primary reason for occurrence of seizures in one of the six patients. The purposeful manipulation of blood levels to bring on seizures is probably not a common occurrence, but denial of illness, preoccupation, and anger all increase the likelihood that a less-than-optimal drug regimen will be followed (16). Indeed, our survey suggested that the most potent factor in seizure exacerbation was missed medication. In four patients, anxiety led to overbreathing with a subsequent increase in epileptiform activity as well as seizures. In one patient studied in great detail, evidence was persuasive that the hyperventilation induced changes in CO_2, which, in turn, probably decreased cerebral circulation. The importance of hyperventilation and changes in blood gases was demonstrated by failure to

see activation at times of emotional stress if hyperventilation did not occur. The ability to reproduce the attacks by hyperventilation in the absence of emotional distress, along with the ability to abort the increased excitability by rebreathing 95% O_2 and 5% CO_2, supports the evidence for the pathophysiological mechanism.

These studies provide no evidence to indicate whether seizures are aggravated by emotional stresses frequently or only under isolated conditions. Similarly, we are not able to say which mechanisms operate in patients when emotional stress is associated with altered seizure susceptibility, nor are we able to say whether multiple factors may converge to lower the threshold. Our cases demonstrate that secondary noncompliance with antiepileptic drug medication, sleep deprivation, and hyperventilation alone or together may be the mechanism by which cerebral excitability is altered. Although not studied in this group of patients, other drug use such as antidepressants or neuroleptics at times of psychological stress might also contribute to altering the seizure threshold. The tendency for people to drink excessive amounts of alcohol at times of stress, or to use other drugs such as cocaine, might also contribute to these emotionally related seizure increases.

The mechanisms that have been discussed all bring about changes in general brain excitability and can be thought of as modulating factors. It is less clear whether emotional stimuli can specifically trigger seizures by neural reflex mechanisms. Groups of patients are well identified whose seizures, usually of myoclonic type, can be triggered by startle (see Chapter 11, *this volume*). This need not have an emotional element.

Although the evidence seems persuasive that a patient's emotional state may influence the occurrence of seizures, opposite effects are sometimes reported. In such instances, seizures do not occur during the time of anxiety, but rather at a time later in the day or in the week when the patient is relaxing and his stresses have eased. It may be that these emotional stresses have an alerting or desynchronizing effect, whereas later relaxation allows synchronization of epileptiform activity as occurs in drowsiness.

Although available evidence supports the

idea that emotional factors may alter seizure susceptibility, the close interrelationship between psychological stresses and occurrence of apparent seizures should raise the question of the differential diagnosis. Convulsive syncope is a common alternative diagnosis and should certainly be considered when attacks occur only under certain circumstances, such as when a patient is undergoing treatment in the dentist's office chair, giving blood, etc. Nonepileptic attacks (pseudoseizures, hysterical seizures) also need to be considered even in patients with well-documented epilepsy.

SUMMARY AND CONCLUSIONS

Emotional factors can alter the likelihood of seizure occurrence, and they usually increase the frequency of attacks. Our case studies showed that such activation is brought about through missed medication, sleep deprivation, and hyperventilation. Less well documented is the possibility that increased excitability and seizures may be due to direct neuronal activation of limbic circuits, although such a mechanism would be quite plausible.

REFERENCES

1. Aird RB. The importance of seizure-inducing factors in the control of refractory forms of epilepsy. *Epilepsia* 1983;24:567–583.
2. Gastaut H, Tassinari CA. Triggering mechanisms in epilepsy, the electroclinical point of view. *Epilepsia* 1966;7:85–238.
3. Gowers WR. *Epilepsy and other chronic convulsive diseases*. William Wood & Co., 1885.
4. Mattson RH, Pratt KD, Calverly JR. Electroencephalograms of epileptics following sleep deprivation. *Arch Neurol* 1965;13:310–315.
5. Mattson RH. Selection of antiepileptic drug therapy. In: Levy RH, Dreifuss FE, Mattson RH, Meldrum B, Penry JK, eds. *Antiepileptic drugs*, 3rd ed. New York: Raven Press, 1989; 103–225.
6. Mattson RH, Cramer JA. Epilepsy, sex hormones and antiepileptic drugs. *Epilepsia* (suppl) 1985;26(1):S40–S51.
7. Mattson RH, Fay L, Sturman J, Cramer JA, Mattson EM. The effects of alcohol on seizures in patients with epilepsy. In: Porter RJ, Mattson RH, Cramer JA, Diamond I, eds. *Alcohol and seizures: basic mechanisms and clinical concepts*. Philadelphia: FA Davis, 1990; in press.
8. Symonds C. Excitation and inhibition in epilepsy. *Brain* 1959;82:133–146.
9. Servit Z, et al. Reflex influences in the pathogenesis of epilepsy in light of clinical statistics. In: *Reflex mechanisms in the genesis of epilepsy*. Amsterdam: Elsevier, 1963;107–114.
10. Temkin NR, Davis GR. Stress as a risk factor among adults with epilepsy. *Epilepsia* 1984;25 (4):450–456.
11. Webster A, Mawer GE. Seizure frequency and major life events in epilepsy. *Epilepsia* 1989;30 (2):162–167.
12. Feldman RG, Paul NI. Identity of emotional triggers in epilepsy. *J Nerv Ment Dis* 1976;162: 345.
13. Daube JR. Sensory precipitated seizures: a review. *J Nerv Ment Dis* 1966;141:524–539.
14. Stevens JR. The emotional activation of the electroencephalogram in patients with convulsive disorders. *J Nerv Ment Dis* 1959;128:339.
15. Bennet DR, Mattson RH, Ziter FA, Calverly JR, Liske EA, Pratt KL. Sleep deprivation: neurologic and EEG effects. *Aerospace Med* 1964;35: 888.
16. Leppik I, Schmidt D, eds. *Compliance in epilepsy. Epilepsy Research*, Suppl 1. Amsterdam: Elsevier, 1988;111–117.

Advances in Neurology, Vol. 55, edited by
D. Smith, D. Treiman, and M. Trimble,
Raven Press, Ltd., New York © 1991.

29

Legal Implications of Behavioral Changes in Epilepsy

John Gunn

Department of Forensic Psychiatry, Institute of Psychiatry, London SE5 8AF, England

PRISONERS WITH EPILEPSY

A previous paper has reviewed some of the issues relating to the law and epilepsy (1), including the disproportionate number of people with epilepsy who seem to be sent to prison. My British survey in the 1960s suggested that at least seven, and probably eight or nine, sentenced prisoners in every 1000 suffer from epilepsy. This suggestion has been made to appear low by an Illinois survey (2), which found that the prevalence in that state was 21 per 1000. There is no ready explanation for this discrepancy, and unfortunately our most recent prison epidemiological survey in England is not yet complete, although early indications suggest that that British figure will be much the same as before or a little higher.

There is, therefore, plenty of scope for a transatlantic comparative study to examine this difference more extensively. Such a study would need to concentrate primarily on sociological, criminological, and attitudinal issues, since the British and American studies were in agreement that there is no particular type of offense which seems to be especially related to epilepsy; notably there is no special relationship between violent crime and epilepsy (2,3).

To recap the British survey, one or two tables may be helpful. A spot census of all epilepsy patients and all doubtful epilepsy patients was made throughout the prisons of England and Wales. These patients were visited, interviewed, and examined, together

with the next case in the file at the prison concerned. Originally there were 192 cases of prisoners with epilepsy and 192 controls. However, after examination it was clear that only 158 were actually suffering from epilepsy, and 12 of the control cases doubtfully had epilepsy, definitely had epilepsy, or had recovered from epilepsy, leaving 180 non-epilepsy cases. Table 1 shows that the prisoners did not differ in terms of their current offense; Table 2 shows that the offenses did not relate to type of epilepsy; and Table 3 shows that, when rated for degree of violence in the current offense, the groups did not differ. The survey also showed that the groups did not differ in terms of previous convictions. Of course, none of this is to say that there are *no* associations between behavior and epilepsy. Such a proposition would be absurd. There are, for example, the phenomena of epileptic automatisms, and very rarely this disorder may lead to serious antisocial consequences (4). We know also that there is an increased rate of road accidents in those people with epilepsy who are allowed to drive (5), although the increased rates may not be much different from those in other chronic diseases such as diabetes (6,7). What the statistics seem to show is that simplistic notions about people with epilepsy being more aggressive (or more violent) than other people are erroneous. However, there seem to be a few mechanisms which may link epilepsy and antisocial behavior in particular cases:

1. A direct relationship exists such that the antisocial act is part of the seizure itself. One

TABLE 1. *Current offenses*

Crimes	Epileptics	Controls
Property	105 (66%)	108 (60%)
Violence	23 (15%)	40 (22%)
Sex	14 (9%)	12 (7%)
Other	16 (10%)	20 (11%)
Totals:	158	180

$\chi^2 = 3.81$ (3 df): not significant

TABLE 3. *Degrees of violence compared*

Degree of violence	Epileptics	Controls
0	123 (81%)	124 (77%)
1	3 (9%)	5 (15%)
2	10	19
3	15 (10%)	14 (9%)
Unratable	7	18
Totals:	151	162

$\chi^2 = 2.93$ (2 df, amalgamating 1 and 2):
not significant

or two cases like this were found in the British prison survey, but they are unusual.

2. Both abnormal behavior and epilepsy may be related to brain malfunction, even though the abnormal behavior is not a phenomenon of epilepsy in itself. For example, cases can be found in which disinhibited antisocial behavior is probably related to serious head injury, and concomitant seizures are also related to the brain injury.

3. Low self-esteem may lead to a variety of antisocial behaviors. Epilepsy itself, combined with the rejection suffered by some people with epilepsy, may lead to low self-esteem.

4. Epilepsy may lead to mood changes and/ or psychotic states. Such abnormal mental states may be the basis of antisocial behavior.

5. Poor environments seem to be the linking factor in quite a number of cases. Children reared in financially and emotionally impoverished households are, for a whole variety of reasons, more likely to suffer illness, including illness of the brain, and are also more likely to be antisocial in their struggle for survival.

TABLE 2. *Property and violent offenders by diagnosis*

Diagnosis	Property	Violence	Total
Subcortical	15 (79%)	4 (21%)	19
Temporal	34 (83%)	7 (17%)	41
Other focal	22 (82%)	5 (19%)	27
NK	34 (83%)	7 (17%)	41
Totals:	105	23	128

$\chi^2 = 0.17$ (3 df): not significant

6. An interesting group of patients develop head injuries and epilepsy as a result of their antisocial behavior, rather than the other way around. "Tearaways," reckless drivers, and boys who fight and use weapons are all quite obviously at greater risk for head injury and epilepsy.

Whitman et al. (2) suggested that there are two major explanations for an increased prevalence of epilepsy in U.S. prisons: (i) the detrimental effects of epilepsy on socioeconomic status and (ii) an increased prevalence of epilepsy in the communities from which prisoners are disproportionately drawn. In another paper (8) they state quite boldly that "poor people have more epilepsy" and conclude that "the elevated prevalence of epilepsy in prison . . . is . . . an accurate reflection of an elevated prevalence rate among poor people." Data from the British prison survey partially supported this view (9). Each man was asked about the size of his childhood sibship (including half-siblings, foster siblings, and adoptive siblings who lived in the household for 12 months or more) and whether the home in which he spent the longest part of his childhood included a bathroom, or if at any stage the man had had to share a bed with another person for a month or more. (Any man who had spent more than 15 years of his childhood in an institution was put into a separate category.) It turned out that the men came predominantly from large families, with approximately 10% of each group belonging to a sibship of 10 or more children (Table 4). In a national survey of children born during the first week of March 1946, Douglas and Blomfield (10) found that the number of

TABLE 4. *Number of siblings*

Number of siblings	Epileptics	Controls
0 or 1	25 (16%)	32 (18%)
2, 3, or 4	65 (41%)	74 (41%)
5, 6, 7, or 8	46 (29%)	57 (32%)
9 or more	17 (11%)	15 (8%)
NK	5	2
Totals:	158	180
Mean	4.50	4.10
SD	3.26	2.85

$t = 1.18$ (329 df): not significant

British homes containing three or more children varied according to social class: Only 27% of professional homes, 40% of skilled manual workers' homes, and 43% of unskilled homes. The British prison survey found that 64% of control homes and 68% of epilepsy homes contained three or more children during the prisoners' childhood. These data suggest that both epilepsy and control prisoners are coming from larger families than are their general population counterparts, which in turn may indicate a relative but equal impoverishment for the two groups. The data on bathrooms and bedrooms could initially seem to tell the same story (Table 5), but there the matter is a little more confusing, since the figures shown are in fact quite close to those obtained by Douglas and Blomfield (10), who found that 43% of all families were without a bathroom in 1948, and that 26% of all 4-year-old children in 1950 shared a bed. However, direct comparisons are not possible because the prisoners are younger than the national

TABLE 5. *Childhood home*

Features	Epileptics	Controls
Bath and bed	73 (46%)	89 (49%)
Shared bed, had bath	17 (11%)	20 (11%)
Own bed, no bath	25 (16%)	26 (14%)
Shared bed, no bath	30 (19%)	33 (18%)
Institution	10 (6%)	11 (6%)
NK	3	1
Totals:	158	180

$\chi^2 = 0.31$ (4 df): not significant

survey children and should be expected therefore to have grown up in slightly better conditions.

Thus, the relationship between the epilepsy rate in prisons and poverty may be complex, but the obvious implication remains: Preventive medicine in this branch of neurology has a good deal to do with obtaining effective socioeconomic improvements for the disadvantaged groups in our societies.

Factors which we were not able to examine but which would need to be examined to comment further on the British–American discrepancy in imprisonment rates of people with epilepsy are as follows: sentencing policies, provisions for noncustodial penal control, patterns of sheltered accommodation in the community, and the availability of hospital beds for patients with brain injury and/or behavior disorders. It may be, for example, that as the availability of such beds decreases in Britain because of government policy, the number of people with epilepsy who end up in prison will actually rise. It will certainly be interesting to see if there has been a rise between 1966, the date of the earlier survey, and 1988.

Whatever the result, it is clear that prisons contain substantial numbers of people with epilepsy. Part of the clinical task is to reduce that number.

ATTITUDES TOWARDS EPILEPSY

Social attitudes determine legal developments, and here there are signs of improvement. An earlier paper (1) discussed attitudes in terms of the history of epilepsy and the discriminatory laws that had been passed against epilepsy patients. It also reported some Gallop Poll surveys (one of them commissioned by us) which suggested quite clearly that attitudes towards people with epilepsy are improving. In the past 10 years these improvements seem to have continued. Schmidt and Wilder (11), commenting on American aspects of epilepsy and the law, tell us that the last law limiting the right of persons with epilepsy to marry in the United States was repealed in 1982. It is gratifying to read in that paper that every state in the United States now has legislation which enables well-controlled patients to drive legally. The United Kingdom also has legislation which permits such driving (see below).

Clear examples of the way in which attitudes towards people with epilepsy have improved are also seen within the prisoner world. In Great Britain, regulations about the restrictions on people with epilepsy to wear normal clothing, to be housed in ordinary prison location, and to undertake prison work have relaxed. They have not entirely disappeared, but there are significant improvements. Finally it has been more than 10 years now since I set up a hostel for ex-prisoners with epilepsy near our hospital in south London. The hostel has been very successful, but the number of epilepsy patients leaving prison and requiring specialized accommodation because nobody else would take them has dropped to the point where we are now no longer specializing in that group. Our intake in the hostel these days is a mixed range of patients with both neurological and psychiatric disorders. It is encouraging that aftercare organizations no longer discriminate against people with epilepsy.

EPILEPSY AND DRIVING

Schmidt and Wilder (11) tell us that, in general, most states in the United States require that an epilepsy patient be seizure-free for only a period of 1 year before a driving license is granted. In the United Kingdom the effect of a fairly complicated piece of law is to grant driving licenses to those with a history of epilepsy who, on the basis of medical evidence, have been free from attacks for at least 2 years or have had them only while asleep for at least 3 years, with or without treatment (12). However, it seems that in nine states the law requires the attending physician to report patients to licensing authorities, whereas in the United Kingdom this is not an absolute requirement and is left to the conscience and judgment of the individual doctor.

As Fenwick (5) pointed out, advising a seizure patient about driving is a complex business because in addition to the risk of seizures, there is also the possibility of drowsiness due to medication. Furthermore, there are other coexisting medical and social prob-

lems; for example, some patients are mentally handicapped, and others drink heavily. In Great Britain we also have an absolute rule that anyone who has had a seizure after the age of 5 years is automatically barred from ever driving a heavy goods vehicle, driving a public service vehicle, or holding an airline pilot's license.

EPILEPSY AND INSANITY

Not everyone may agree about the improvements in attitudes towards people with epilepsy. In 1988, Fenwick (5) reviewed some of the legal issues relating to epilepsy. He echoed an earlier point that patients with epilepsy have been discriminated against for centuries (1). He went on to say, "This is certainly true as regards the law." He was referring to a recent British development in which the seizure is now to be called a disease of the mind, and he said, "It is unreasonable that patients with epilepsy should have to carry the additional burden that whenever they have a seizure they are, in law, insane, even though this will not be formally recognized unless they offend during a seizure." He concluded that "The law on automatism as it now stands is illogical, leads to much hardship and suffering, and so clearly needs revision."

Fenwick (5) was referring to the case of Regina versus Sullivan, and the patient was one of Dr. Fenwick's at the Maudsley Hospital. Why was he so cross? These are the outline facts quoted from Fenwick (5) in 1988:

> Sullivan, a man of previous good character, was a patient who suffered partial complex seizures with occasional secondary generalizations from the age of 8. He had had two severe head injuries which have resulted in widespread brain damage and some degree of personality change. His major attacks ceased in 1979, and only the partial complex seizures remained. These seizures spread rapidly and bilaterally into both amygdala and hippocampal structures, so that Sullivan had no memory for the seizure or events immediately after the seizure. During a partial complex seizure, Sullivan attacked and seriously injured an elderly neighbor. The seizure and the attack were witnessed, and both prosecution and de-

fense accepted that there was no medical doubt that the assault took place during an epilepsy automatism.

Mr. Sullivan was advised to plead not guilty to the charges on grounds of noninsane automatism. However, the trial judge ruled that this plea was not available because if the patient carried out the act during a seizure, then he must plead not guilty on grounds of insanity. Now if this plea had succeeded, then the court would have had to send him to the hospital under the English Criminal Procedure (Insanity) Act, where he would have been held as a detained patient under a restriction order, which means that his doctors could not release him without the consent of either the Home Secretary or a special Mental Health Review Tribunal chaired by a judge. This seemed a daunting prospect to Mr. Sullivan and his advisors, and so very wisely he pleaded guilty.

Dr. Pamela Taylor (13) was also involved in this case and she, too, has written about it. She sums up the dilemma faced by the defendant:

> We told him that the judge was prepared to consider him not guilty by reason of insanity. "But I am not insane," said PS. We advised him, because of the consequences of this, to plead guilty. "But I am not guilty," said PS. Even the eloquent counsel paused, then PS spoke again: "But you are three intelligent, educated people—I'll do whatever you say."

Perhaps it is not surprising that everybody was upset that this man had to plead guilty to an act which he could not remember and which he probably could not control, nor is it a surprise that it went to the Court of Appeal. Nevertheless, the court confirmed the original decision, although they allowed it to go to the House of Lords, where the decision was also confirmed, thus enshrining in English law that a criminal act perpetrated during a seizure is an *insane* act and not one that is subject to the total acquittal of automatism.

There is an age-old tradition in Anglo-Saxon common law, that a guilty deed requires two components: an act which is in breach of the law, and a guilty mind intending the act to be carried out. Yet, like many traditions, this one is not very close to practical reality. For example, there are a growing number of offenses which are called crimes of absolute liability, so that in English law it is no defense to say, "I did not intend to drive faster than the speed limit, officer." The fact that you were driving faster than the speed limit is in itself sufficient for conviction. Similarly, if an English shopkeeper sells certain types of defective goods (e.g., a loaf of bread with a dead mouse in it), he is in breach of the criminal law, even though he did not intend anyone to have a bad loaf and indeed did not know that any loaves in his shop were defective. Such cases of absolute liability are mainly confined to minor offenses, but they are quite a large proportion of the total number of cases going through the criminal courts.

In all other cases the prosecution theoretically has to prove that the accused had a guilty mind—that is, that he intended to break the law. In practice, it would seem, no matter what the law books say, that if the defendant wishes to plead nonintention, then the onus of proof is on him rather than the other way around, because he has to find an acceptable excuse. For example, a depressed man or woman who takes something from a shop while preoccupied with miserable painful thoughts, and who shows poor concentration, will find it very hard to convince a court that he did not intend to steal the goods he took without paying.

The traditional excuses against a guilty mind include accident, provocation, duress, legal infancy, and insanity. For insanity it is quite explicit that the burden of proof rests with the defense. In Great Britain, until 1800, all of these defenses (including insanity) could lead to an absolute acquittal. In 1800, however, James Hadfield, who was a French wars veteran and who had had severe brain damage which led to a severe mental illness, shot at King George III but was unsuccessful in his attempt. Hadfield was tried for attempted treason, which carried the death penalty. In his psychotic way, he was hoping that he would be found guilty so that he could be executed. This would then be a form of suicide which would be acceptable to God. Most people at that time would have had their wishes granted, but Hadfield was fortunate in having a remarkably good defense lawyer. He was acquitted on grounds of insanity. Now this was a full acquittal, and to avoid the slightest chance of such "innocent" people wandering the streets again, Parliament rushed through a special bill saying that people who were found not guilty by reason of insanity should in fact be detained in hospital at His Majesty's pleasure. This same law, in updated form, exists in the United Kingdom today so that an insanity acquittal leads to indefinite detention in the hospital, the very issue which caused consternation in the Sullivan case. The really interesting thing about the 1800 law, however, is that some mental arguments were excluded from this new regulation. If the defendant could show that he was behaving automatically in a state of unconsciousness, perhaps sleepwalking, then he would be acquitted because of his "noninsane automatism" and he would go scot-free, just as if it had been proved that he had had an accident.

It is this latter point which has given rise to increasing controversy in recent years and which has been the subject of much judicial interference over the past decade or two; this is because judges have tried to include more people, who they presumably regard as dangerous, under the insanity umbrella, since it does have restrictions attached to it. Insanity is, of course, defined in legal terms by the McNaughten Rules. To demonstrate insanity, it has to be shown that at the time of the act, the accused person was laboring under such a defect of reason, from disease of the mind, so as not to know the nature and quality of the act he was doing, or if he did know it, that he did not know he was doing something wrong. The important points to note in this definition are the emphasis on cognition and the fact that it is a *legal* description of insanity—it makes no pretense to be a medical diagnosis and certainly does not equate to psychosis. It is also easy to see how the rules could be used positively in a case of epilepsy, provided that the mental disturbances are called "defects of reason" and provided that epilepsy is accepted as a disease of the mind. Here is a big factor in the argument. Some would want to say that epilepsy is a disease of the brain and not of the mind. Very convenient for some purposes, but with increasing knowledge, as Freud had predicted, it does become ever

more difficult to sustain a Cartesian view of human mental functions.

The case which is of crucial importance here is the Bratty case. In 1961 Mr. Bratty was charged with killing a girl whom he had taken for a ride in his car. He alleged that at the time of the killing a blackness came over him, and he just did not know what he was doing. It was suggested that he might be subject to attacks of psychomotor epilepsy. At his trial the defense asked the jury either to acquit the accused on a plea of automatism, to find him guilty of manslaughter, or to find him not guilty by reason of insanity. The judge instructed the jury to discount the plea for automatism on the ground that there was no evidence to support it. Bratty was convicted of murder, and on appeal the judge's direction on the matter of automatism was upheld; the case, just like the Sullivan case, went to the House of Lords, where again the appeal was rejected. In the House of Lords, Lord Denning made an important statement about the distinction between (a) insanity defined as a disease of the mind and (b) noninsane automatism. He said: "It seems to me that any mental disorder which has manifest itself in violence and is prone to recur is a disease of the mind. At any rate it is the sort of disease for which a person should be detained in hospital, rather than be given an unqualified acquittal."

To say the least, this is a pragmatic definition and it illustrates three points. First, British judges are in the business of trying to establish social order and control, and they make up rules which are aimed in that direction. Second, mental concepts such as mind, intent, responsibility, insanity, and so on, are not the prerogative of the relatively new profession of psychiatry; instead, they belong to mankind as a whole. They are older than psychiatry, older than medicine itself, and they are very much the province of the lawyer, who has the power to provide his own definitions. Third, a person who is violent is to be regarded either as being responsible for his actions or as being subject to the laws and rules relating to mental disorder.

Since the Bratty case, two important judgments, besides the Sullivan case, have modified and yet reinforced Denning's judgment.

In 1973 the Court of Appeal reinterpreted the Denning judgment by saying that a disease of the mind did not include transitory malfunction caused by the application to the body of some external factor, and they were considering a case in which automatism during an episode of hypoglycemia caused by an overdose of insulin was said to have occurred (R versus Quick & Paddison, 1973). The second case was R versus Hennesy (1989), in which a diabetic claimed automatism for a criminal act of taking and driving a car away, on the grounds that he was a diabetic and hyperglycemic. The trial judge ruled that if the defendant wanted to plead a mental excuse he would have to do so under the McNaughten Rules and thus plead insanity. The defendant changed his plea to one of guilty. The ruling was upheld by the Court of Appeal.

Fenwick (5) regarded the Bratty case as an unsatisfactory foundation for a change in the law because when he read the papers he found that there was very little medical evidence that the act committed by Mr. Bratty was in fact committed during a seizure. However, the House of Lords in the Sullivan case were not concerned with such medical niceties; instead, they were concerned with matters of general principle and reaffirmed in effect the previous view that if you are violent because of something that goes wrong in your head, something that could go wrong again, then you must be covered by the rules relating to insanity and subject to hospital care and Home Office restrictions—in some ways a modern, non-Cartesian view of man.

THE LAW IN PRACTICE

The indignation that this case has raised is entirely understandable. There was apparent injustice—injustice which bemused Mr. Sullivan at his own trial. Nevertheless, the injustice which has been perpetrated is small, and in my view it does not offset the general improvement in attitudes, mentioned earlier. Furthermore, just to be provocative, the general direction of this particular legal trend is one I endorse.

In Great Britain, and perhaps everywhere in the world, the law is becoming more prag-

matic. For the vast majority of mentally abnormal offenders, whatever their illness, the questions addressed by the court are as follows: "Have we got the right person?" "Did he or she carry out the illegal act?" "Is this act worthy of punishment?" "Is it likely to happen again?" "Is medical treatment required?" The traditional view of carefully framed logic with questions of responsibility argued out in front of reasonable men is largely myth. It is a useful myth because it forms a theoretical backdrop to reality, but it has little relationship to what actually goes on in a court.

In 1986, for example, the English courts found 384,000 people guilty of indictable or serious offenses, 1,066,000 guilty of motoring offenses and 444,000 guilty of other nonindictable (minor) offenses, making a total of 1,894,000 convictions (14). In addition, 15 were found unfit to plead (equivalent to incompetent to plead in the United States), one was found not guilty by reason of insanity, and no one was found not guilty by reason of noninsane automatism (14,15). Of the 1.9 million convicted people, almost 43,000 were sent to prison, another 40,000 were put on probation, 1.6 million were fined, and approximately 700 or 800 were put on hospital orders under the Mental Health Act. These 700 or 800 patients put on hospital orders had initially been found guilty and were sent to the hospital in lieu of prison. So in 1986, a not atypical year, only one individual was totally excused of a criminal conviction on psychiatric grounds (Table 6). Of the 501 people convicted of homicide that year, 78 were found guilty of manslaughter by reason of diminished responsibility and three were found guilty of infanticide also using psychiatric factors.

TABLE 6. *Convictions in 1986— England and Wales*

384,000	Indictable offenses
1,066,000	Motoring offenses
444,000	Summary offenses
1,894,000	Total number of convictions
15	Unfit to plead
1	Insane
0	Automatism

What all this means in simple terms is that of the millions of people tramping through British courts each year, only a handful are actually let off because of psychiatric factors. Some 80 people have their homicide charges reduced to manslaughter on psychiatric grounds, but nevertheless they are found guilty, and about 800 are sent off to the hospital (most of them with no further legal controls) because of their mental disorder. Thousands of other mentally abnormal people are dealt with in some other way. Our own research suggests that 1% of our prison population (some 200–300 prisoners) are actually psychotic, and up to one-third of our prisoners require some kind of psychiatric help (16).

Whenever figures of this kind are presented in the United States, eyebrows are raised. American skeptics are invited to undertake a careful examination of the legal process in their own state. What is usually found in the United States is that although a few more insanity acquittals do happen than in the United Kingdom, and many more people are deemed incompetent, the majority of patients suffering from psychosis and other mental illnesses are nevertheless found guilty. The most poignant reminder of this has been given by Lewis et al. (17), who looked at 15 death-row inmates (13 men and 2 women) in five different U.S. states. Thirteen of the 15 had exhausted all avenues of appeal and were close to death. Obviously, none of them had been found not guilty by reason of insanity nor had been found guilty but insane, nor were they otherwise excused on psychiatric grounds. In clinical terms, however, they *all* had significant pathology: One patient had auditory hallucinations and believed that Christ had made him commit the murder; another felt controlled by outside forces; yet another thought his victim was trying to poison him; and so on. Of particular relevance to this discussion is that two patients had a history of seizures, and more than half of them showed neurological abnormalities on examination or computed tomography (CT) scan. These investigators do not tell us anything about the socioeconomic or ethnic backgrounds of the prisoners, but it would not be surprising if the condemned persons differed on these social parameters from other people charged

with murder who escaped the death penalty. This study tells us that forensic psychiatry and the law in action do not necessarily protect sick people from the rigors of punishment, even when that punishment is as extreme as the death penalty.

For historic and indeed for practical reasons, the criminal hearing is divided into three phases: a pretrial phase, when the preliminaries, including issues of fitness to plead or competence, are dealt with; a trial phase, during which the basic questions about the right person are dealt with; and a sentencing phase, in which punishment, disposal, treatment, and prevention are addressed, often in some detail. In spite of the fact that we traditionally regard responsibility and intention as exclusively a matter for the middle phase (i.e., the trial), such matters in practice do spread across all three phases. Responsibility particularly spreads into the sentencing phase and becomes imputability. Questions of insanity, as well as of diminution of responsibility by psychiatric factors, are now very rarely dealt with in the trial phase. Indeed in Great Britain the only cases in which they are dealt with during the trial are the relatively small number of homicide cases which go through the courts each year. In such cases they are only dealt with in the trial phase for technical reasons concerning mandatory sentencing. Thus if a highly abnormal, clearly "mad" schizophrenic assaults someone, steals something, sets fire to a building, or in any other way breaks the law, then the chances are that his or her trial will be concerned with factual matters; furthermore, if the right person has been apprehended, the chances are that he or she will be found guilty and then dealt with in the sentencing phase by a consideration of need and mitigation. In Great Britain the likeliest disposal for such a patient would be a hospital order in which the patient is handed over to doctors for treatment. We also have an arrangement in Great Britain that should the offense be a minor one and dealt with in a magistrate's court, then it is possible for the magistrate to quash the conviction in retrospect, to avoid stigmatizing the patient's character with a criminal conviction. This is only done in selected cases and is not available to a higher court. One simple but useful modification which could be made to our existing law would be to allow the higher court to have a similar power.

So, if Mr. Sullivan had been schizophrenic instead of epileptic and had assaulted his neighbor in a similar way, there would have been no question of an automatism or other type of acquittal defense being raised. He would have been found guilty and given some sort of medical disposal. What actually happened to Mr. Sullivan? He too was found guilty and he too was given a medical disposal, a probation order with a condition of medical treatment.

THE POSITION IN THE UNITED STATES

In 1986 Treiman (18) undertook a very extensive review of the relationship between epilepsy and violence (see Chapter 21). In that review he summarized 75 U.S. cases in which epilepsy had been used as a legal defense against criminal charges over an unspecified long period of time. Forty-five of the cases involved murder, 11 manslaughter, 10 assault or battery, 6 robbery, and 3 others. In only one of the 75 was the defense used successfully:

> Robert H. Torsney was a New York City policeman. On Thanksgiving night, 1966, he and five fellow officers were called to a Brooklyn housing project to settle a domestic dispute, which they did peacefully. As Torsney walked back to his car he passed a group of teenage boys. One of them, 15-year-old Randolf Evans, asked, "Did you come from apartment 7-D?" The officer had not, but Torsney replied, "You're damn right I did," pulled his gun, and, without further provocation, shot Evans in the head.

At his trial, Torsney claimed that he had a psychomotor seizure at the time of the shooting and he was found not guilty by reason of insanity and ordered into a State Hospital. Five weeks later an examining physician said he had never shown any signs of epilepsy. Six months later he was released as not mentally disordered or brain damaged.

What a beautiful example of the law in action! Those who are not used to courts will be appalled. Treiman very reasonably goes on to set down sensible medical criteria necessary for making a diagnosis of epilepsy in someone charged with a crime. Unfortunately, however, the problem is that courts may or may not decide to use sensible medical criteria. It is lawyers who set the rules in court, not doctors. It could well be that in Torsney's case the jury would have excused him one way or another no matter what the doctors said, just as in the notorious British Yorkshire Ripper case the jury convicted the accused of murder in the face of unanimous medical evidence of schizophrenia, which should have reduced the charge to manslaughter.

DISCRIMINATION

Why do I actually approve of the trend in British law which denied Mr. Sullivan an acquittal? First, I believe that it is a form of unwarranted medical discrimination to have a law which distinguishes between (a) patients who have a brain illness creating seizures and (b) patients who have a brain illness creating other forms of abnormal behavior. Of course, people with epilepsy are not psychotic when they have a seizure, whereas schizophrenics may be psychotic when they have an outburst; furthermore, epilepsy patients may not be conscious when they are lashing out, whereas schizophrenics are. These are medical facts which are valid and interesting, but they are facts on a different axis from the one which is of primary interest in these cases. The point here is that if Mr. X, a schizophrenic, attacks his neighbor in the middle of an episode of florid psychosis, then he, body and brain, requires medical attention and perhaps some social control. When a biological entity called Mr. Y who has epilepsy carries out an act of aggression in a seizure, he is in exactly the same position. To argue a distinction between such people is to take a Cartesian philosophical stance about the mind in the machine which disappeared from science some time ago.

The second reason I am happy about the trend is as follows: It lifts most of the medical debate out of the trial, thereby eliminating the potential misuse of medical evidence, but it leaves plenty of scope for the experts to put their arguments to the court in the sentencing phase of the hearing. In Great Britain, this means that the adversarial confrontation is over and that a balanced discussion can take place between the judge (who will decide what to do with the accused) and one or more doctors. I realize that in some states the jury also has a role in sentencing, but I do not believe that this detracts from the general point that removing the medical evidence from the trial as much as possible improves the quality of interaction between court and doctor.

The important issue for the epilepsy patient, and for the schizophrenic patient alike, is that public and lawyers are increasingly educated about the nature of brain disease, its possible complications, and its treatment and prognosis. If widespread understanding can come about, then the law can be used as a means of providing benefits to both patients and public. There is a long way to go because much of the law remains, and probably will always remain, concerned with actually doing harm to selected individuals. Nevertheless, there is some hope that with the increasing sophistication of lawyers, patients with brain diseases and psychological disorders will eventually find themselves largely exempt from most of such harm.

Mr. Sullivan was given a probation order with a condition of treatment. What that means is that the state provides him free of charge with an outpatient medical service and a skilled social worker. His only restraint is that he has to use these services. Not many would regard the outcome as illiberal. Unfortunately, however, he does also have to bear the stigma of a criminal conviction. One or two simple reforms to British law would avoid stigmatizing every patient in this way. If Mr. Sullivan had been tried in a magistrate's court, the magistrate could have nullified or quashed the conviction at the sentencing stage. This simple device is used infrequently, but it is available to prevent the kind of injustice worried about here, and it would not be difficult to extend this power to higher courts.

Law and medicine inhabit rather different worlds and use different concepts and philosophies. Inevitably, however, there is interaction between the two. One of the doctor's tasks is to improve matters for his patients by focusing firmly on medical and social issues.

Certainly the law can be a useful ally, and when it can it should be used. Struggle with the law is, however, rarely worth it; lawyers always win on their own territory, because they write the rules of the game! Medicine can achieve a great deal by investing in science and in the provision of services.

As far as the epilepsy population is concerned, several developments are required. We need much more information about the socioeconomic correlates of epilepsy. We need better and more frequent provision of specialist services for the small but important group of patients who have both epilepsy and behavior disorder—an unpopular, unattractive group of patients, but a needy one nevertheless. Above all, we need specialized inpatient services, both (a) the acute investigative type of service and (b) long-term facilities for those unable to manage even in sheltered accommodation. With a general program of social and medical improvements, legal questions would be increasingly focused on practical matters such as disposal and treatment.

CONCLUSION

More people with epilepsy end up in prison than would be expected by chance. This is probably less related to neurological and psychological factors than it is to socioeconomic ones. There may be fewer people with epilepsy going to prison in the United Kingdom than in the United States. This needs further study.

Attitudes towards people with epilepsy are, in general, improving. They are less ostracized, and special laws against them are falling into disuse. The patients with the best seizure control are being allowed to drive. Nevertheless, there is still some debate, in the United Kingdom at least, as to whether legal attitudes towards people with epilepsy have fundamentally improved. Some would see this in the fact that this patient has been deprived of a special loophole in the criminal law and now has to jump the same hurdles as other patients with brain disorder. On the other hand, this development may mark the beginning with regard to closing the gap in attitudes towards epilepsy and other brain dysfunctions. However, there is further progress yet to be made for the whole wide range of brain-damaged people. Physicians, researchers, and epidemiologists need to draw attention to the marked social correlates of brain disorder and to seek improvements in conditions for deprived people, and they also need to champion social improvements as an important aspect of prevention in this field.

Medicolegal specialists need to keep a close lookout for discriminatory tactics on the part of the law; equally important, however, they need to maximize the use of the laws available to ensure that brain-damaged people are protected from penal measures which aim to do further harm, and they need to fight hard for a medically apposite disposal in each and every case. Above all, we all need to ensure that adequate services are available for these people so that courts can be encouraged to look at caring and rehabilitative disposals in a realistic and practical sense.

REFERENCES

1. Gunn J. Medico-legal aspects of epilepsy. In: Reynolds E, Trimble M, eds. *Epilepsy and psychiatry.* Edinburgh: Churchill Livingstone, 1981;165–174.
2. Whitman S, Coleman TE, Patmon C, Desai BT, Cohen R, King LN. Epilepsy in prison: elevated prevalence and no relationship to violence. *Neurology* 1984;34:775–782.
3. Gunn J. *Epileptics in prison.* London: Academic Press, 1977.
4. Gunn J, Fenton G. Epilepsy, automatism and crime. *Lancet* 1971;1:1173–1176.
5. Fenwick P. Epilepsy and the law. In: Pedley TA, Meldrum BS, eds. *Recent advances in epilepsy.* Edinburgh: Churchill Livingstone, 1988;241–251.
6. Crancer A, McMurray L. Accident and violation rates of Washington's medically restricted drivers. *JAMA* 1968;205:272–276.
7. Waller JA. Chronic medical conditions and traffic safety. *N Engl J Med* 1965;273:1413–1420.
8. Whitman S, Coleman T, Berg B, King L, Desai B. Epidemiological insights into the socioeconomic correlates of epilepsy. In: Hermann BP, ed. *A multidisciplinary handbook of epilepsy.* Springfield, IL: Charles C Thomas, 1980;243–271.
9. Gunn J. *Epileptics in prison, an epidemiological and a control study.* MD thesis, University of Birmingham, 1969.
10. Douglas JWB, Blomfield JM. *Children under fire.* London: Allen & Irwin, 1958.
11. Schmidt RP, Wilder BJ. Epilepsy and the law: a commentary from the United States perspective. In: Pedley TA, Meldrum BS, eds. *Recent advances in epilepsy.* Edinburgh: Churchill Livingstone,
12. Fits and fitness to drive. *Br Med J* 1976;1:1235–1236.
13. Taylor P. Epilepsy and insanity. In: Fenwick P, Fenwick E, eds. *Epilepsy and the law.* Royal Society of Medicine International Congress and Symposium Series No. 81. London: Royal Society of Medicine, 1985;15–22.
14. Home Office. *Criminal statistics—England & Wales 1986.* London: HMSO, 1987.
15. Home Office. Statistics of mentally disordered offenders, England and Wales 1985 and 1986. *Home Office Stat Bull* 1988;28/88.
16. Gunn J, Robertson G, Dell S, Way C. *Psychiatric aspects of imprisonment.* London: Academic Press, 1978.
17. Lewis DO, Pincus JH, Feldman F, Jackson L, Bard B. Psychiatric, neurological, and psychoeducational characteristics of 15 death row inmates in the United States. *Am J Psychiatry* 1986;143:838–845.
18. Treiman DM. Epilepsy and violence: medical and legal issues. *Epilepsia* 1986;27(Suppl 2):77–104.

CASES CITED

Bratty versus Attorney General for Northern Ireland. *All Engl Law Rep* 1961;3:523–539.
R versus Quick & Paddison. *All Engl Law Rep* 1973;3:347. Also in: Smith JC, & Hogan B, eds. *Criminal Law, Cases and Materials,* 3rd ed. London: Butterworths, 1986;193–196.
R versus Hennesy. *Times Law Rep,* January 31, 1989.

Subject Index

A

Absence seizure
  carbamazepine, 261
  clonazepam, 261
  ethosuximide, 261
  ethotoin, 261
  mephenytoin, 261
  metharbital, 261
  methsuximide, 261
  paramethadione, 261
  phenacemide, 261
  phenobarbital, 261
  phensuximide, 261
  phenytoin, 261
  primidone, 261
  trimethadione, 261
  valproate, 261
Abstract concept, intensification, 415
Acetazolamide, affective illness, 255
Adaptation, neuropsychological testing, 431–432
Adenosine, 40
S-Adenosylmethionine
  folate cycle, 53
  folic acid, 54–55
  methylation, 53
Affect, 9–17
  neuropsychological testing, 431
Affective illness
  acetazolamide, 255
  alprazolam, 253–255
  antiepileptic drugs, 239–270
    anticonvulsant differential, 245–250
    combination therapy, 245–250
  benzodiazepine-active anticonvulsant, 253–255
  chlorazepate, 253–255
  clobazam, 253–255
  clonazepam, 253–255
  diazepam, 253–255
  ethosuximide, 256
  GABA agonist, 255
  kindling, 262–268
  lorazepam, 253–255
  paradoxical normalization, 131
  phenytoin, 255
  psychosensory symptoms, 249
  valproate, 250–253
Aggression, 11
  amygdalotomy, 346–347
  anatomical correlates, 343
  anatomical localization, 344–348
    ablative procedures, 344–345

    cerebral ablation studies, 344
  animal models, 342
  cerebral stimulation, 345–346, 347–348
  fear-induced, 342
  inter-male, 342
  interictal disturbance, 103–106
  irritable, 342
  maternal, 342
  nature of ictal events, 348–349
  predatory, 342
  primary ictal, 352
  sex-related, 342
  social hierarchy, 344
  types, 342
Alprazolam, affective illness, 253–255
Alternative psychosis, paradoxical normalization,
    clinical appearances, 129–130
gamma-Aminobutyric acid
  depression, 55–56
  folic acid, 55–56
  interictal psychiatric disorder, 50–52
  seizure, 55–56
gamma-Aminobutyric acid agonist, affective
    illness, 255
Amnesia, 24. *See also* specific type.
  anatomic basis, 358
  complex partial status epilepticus, 363
  differential diagnosis, 363
  differential diagnosis algorithm, 365
  mamillary body, 358
  organic vs. nonorganic, 364
  temporal lobe seizure, 23, 24–25
  Todd's paralysis, 357
  triazolam, 359
Amygdala-kindled seizure
  carbamazepine, 262
  clonazepam, 262
  diazepam, 262
  electroconvulsive seizure, 240, 242, 243, 244
  ethosuximide, 262
  methsuximide, 262
  phenobarbital, 262
  phenytoin, 262
  sodium valproate, 262
Amygdalotomy, aggression, 346–347
Anatomical localization, aggression, 344–348
    ablative procedures, 344–345
    cerebral ablation studies, 344
Anger, 21
Anticonvulsant, behavioral effects, 213
Anticonvulsant rhythm, epilepsy, 177–179

Antiepileptic drugs
  affective illness, 239–270
    anticonvulsant differential, 245–250
    combination therapy, 245–250
  behavioral effects, 213–221
    drug effects study critique, 217–221
  central nervous system development
    animal studies, 229–231
    child, 225–235
    human studies, 225–229
    in vitro studies, 231–234
  cognitive effects, 197–209
  fetus, 225–229
  head circumference, 225–227
  manic-depressive illness, 240–270
  mechanism of psychotropic efficacy, 256–260
  memory, 372–373
  mood change, 190–192
  neuron, 225–235
  paradoxical normalization, 133–136
    time element, 134
Antiepileptic drugs, polypharmacy, 201
Anxiety, 9–11
  seizure occurrence, 456–457
Assaultive behavior, temporal lobe epilepsy, 347
Auditory hallucination, 3
Aura, frontal lobe seizure, 328–331
  localizing value of autonomic phenomena,
    332–338
  localizing value of somatic sensory phenomena,
    333
  psychical phenomena, 328–329
  special sensory phenomena, 331
Autobiographic memory, 375
Automatism, 25–27
  frontal lobe seizure, 335–336
  memory, 172
  nonaggressive violent, 352
  temporal lobe seizure, 23, 24–25
  time course, 172

B

Baclofen, 258
Barbiturate
  behavioral effects, 214–217
  cognitive effects, 197
Behavior
  contingent negative variation, 165
  cortical excitation, 165
  defined, 1
  phenobarbital, 198–199
  phenytoin, 198–199
  seizure, 172
  temporal lobe surgery, 279–290
Behavioral change
  corpus callosotomy, 293–298
    historical background, 293–294
    lateralized cerebral deficits, 297–298

    memory deficits, 297
    neurological observations, 294–297
  legal issues, 461–471
Behavioral effects
  anticonvulsant, 213
  antiepileptic drugs, 213–221
    drug effects study critique, 217–221
  barbiturate, 214–217
  benzodiazepine, 213, 214–217
  carbamazepine, 214–217
  phenytoin, 214–217
  valproic acid, 214–217
Behavioral treatment, seizure, 163–179
Benign epileptiform transients of sleep, 359
Benzodiazepine
  behavioral effects, 213, 214–217
  cognitive effects, 208
Benzodiazepine-active anticonvulsant, affective
    illness, 253–255
Biofeedback, epilepsy, 177–179
Biological antagonism, interictal psychiatric
    disorder, 48–50
Bipolar illness, valproate, 254
Brain injury
  psychosis, 80
  schizophrenia, 80
Brain weight, phenobarbitol, 229–231

C

Capsular neuramnidase, 69–70
Carbamazepine, 49
  absence seizure, 261
  amygdala-kindled seizure, 262
  behavioral effects, 214–217
  biochemical effects, 256, 257
  cognitive effects, 204–207
  complex partial seizure, 261
  depression, 244–245
    prophylaxis, 245
  dysrhythmic syndrome, 263
  fetus, 227
  kindling, 262–268
  limbic kindling, 239
  limbic substrate, 260–262
  mania, 240–244, 246–247, 248, 252
    prophylaxis, 245, 251
  memory, 372–373
  mood change, 191
  paroxysmal syndrome, 263
  psychosensory symptoms, 249
  psychotropic effects, 191, 239
  time course, 256, 257
  tolerance, 266–268
Carbamazepine congener
  depression, 244–245
    prophylaxis, 245
  mania, 240–244, 246–247, 248, 252
    prophylaxis, 245, 251

Central nervous system development,
    antiepileptic drugs
  animal studies, 229–231
  human studies, 225–229
  in vitro studies, 231–234
Cerebral cortex, 2
Cerebral electrical stimulation, rage reaction,
    345–346
Cerebral stimulation, aggression, 345–346,
    347–348
Cerebrospinal fluid monoamine metabolite,
    interictal psychiatric disorder, 47–48
Cerebrovascular disease, frontal lobe seizure, 337
Cerebrum, 2
Child
  antiepileptic drugs, central nervous system
      development, 225–235
  epilepsy
    behavioral consequences, 153–162
    eating, 157
    ictal-speech automatism, 159
    learning, 159–160
    outline findings, 155–156
    parameters, 155–156
    patient referral, 154–155
    patient sources, 154–155
    psychopathology, 86
    psychosocial vocabulary, 153–162
    relating, 160
    sleep, 156–157
    social impact, 153
    socializing, 160
    speech, 158–159
    thinking, 159
    voiding, 157–158
    walking, 158
    working, 160–161
  social competence, 448–450
Chlorazepate, affective illness, 253–255
Choice reaction time, transitory cognitive
    impairment, 114
Circumstantiality, 414
Clobazam
  affective illness, 253–255
  cognitive effects, 208
Clonazepam
  absence seizure, 261
  affective illness, 253–255
  amygdala-kindled seizure, 262
  cognitive effects, 208
  complex partial seizure, 261
Cognition, neuropsychological testing, 430–431
Cognitive activity, EEG discharge, 121
Cognitive deficit, epilepsy, 117–119
Cognitive effects
  antiepileptic drugs, 197–209
  barbiturate, 197
  benzodiazepine, 208

  carbamazepine, 204–207
  clobazam, 208
  clonazepam, 208
  diazepam, 208
  ethosuximide, 208
  phenobarbital, 197, 198–201
    attention, 200
    I.Q. fall, 200–201
    memory, 200
    short-term memory, 200
  phenytoin, 197, 201–204
    carbamazepine, 202–203
    motor speed, 204
    reaction time, 204
    serum levels, 202–203
  primidone, 208
  temporal lobe surgery, 280–287
  valproate, 201, 207–208
Color perception, 3
Complex partial epilepsy, memory, 386–398
  incidence, 387
  permanent memory deficits, 386–393
  temporary memory deficits, 393–398
Complex partial seizure
  carbamazepine, 261
  clonazepam, 261
  cortical dysgenesis, 59–75
  defined, 349
  environment, 172
  ethotoin, 261
  frontal lobe epilepsy
    decision flow charts, 323–327
    electrographic manifestations, 322
  frontal lobe seizure, clinical features, 320–321
  mephenytoin, 261
  metharbital, 261
  methsuximide, 261
  paramethadione, 261
  phenacemide, 261
  phenobarbital, 261
  phenytoin, 261
  primidone, 261
  psychosis, 81
  subtypes, 349
  temporal lobe dysgenesis, 59–75
    birthing history, 66, 67
    capillary tree, 67
    capsular neuramnidase, 69–70
    cerebral glucose, 67
    degenerating neurons, 66
    dendritic change, 63–66
    developmental malformations, 62
    early onset, 66
    family seizure history, 66
    glioma, 61–62
    hamartoma, 61–62
    heterotopia, 61–62
    hippocampal cell loss, 61

Complex partial seizure, temporal lobe dysgenesis
    (*contd.*)
    hippocampal sclerosis, 61
    hippocampus dendrites, 64–66
    historical overview, 61
    mesiotemporal sclerosis, 66, 68
    microvascular changes, 62–63
    neuroembryogenesis, 68
    neuropathological substrate, 61
    oxygen, 67
    phagocytes, 66
  trimethadione, 261
  valproate, 261
Complex partial status epilepticus, amnesia, 363
Complex partial status of frontal lobe origin,
    26–27
Complex partial status of temporal lobe origin,
    26–27
Confusional state, 25–27
Consciousness, 21–25
Contingent negative variation, behavior, 165
Coping, neuropsychological testing, 431–432
Cornu Ammonis, development, 60
Corpus callosotomy, behavioral change, 293–298
    historical background, 293–294
    lateralized cerebral deficits, 297–298
    memory deficits, 297
    neurological observations, 294–297
    Cortical dysgenesis, complex partial seizure,
        59–75
    Cortical excitation, behavior, 165
    Cyclic nucleotide, 40

D
Defensive rage
    anatomical substrates, 104
    stimulation-induced, 104–105
Déjà vu, 8–9, 10
Dentate gyrus, development, 60
2-Deoxyglucose method, seizure, 36–37
Depersonalization, paradoxical normalization,
    131
Depression, 99
    gamma-aminobutyric acid, 55–56
    carbamazepine, 244–245
        prophylaxis, 245
    carbamazepine congener, 244–245
        prophylaxis, 245
    epilepsy, 89–90, 186–194
    psychosis, 89–90
    seizure, 55–56
    vigabatrin, 50–51
Derealization, paradoxical normalization, 131
Desensitization, epilepsy, 174–176
Diazepam
    affective illness, 253–255
    amygdala-kindled seizure, 262
    cognitive effects, 208

Dilantin encephalopathy, 202
Dopamine, 92
    epilepsy, 50, 51
    psychosis, 50, 51
Down's syndrome, 154
Driving, epilepsy, 464
Dynorphin, 39
Dysphasia, 30, 31
Dysphoric state, paradoxical normalization, 131
Dysrhythmic syndrome, carbamazepine, 263
Dysthymic pain disorder, mental change, 188

E
EEG
    frontal lobe seizure, 336
    interictal discharges, 113
    larval discharges, 113
    paradoxical normalization, 128–129
        epileptiform discharges, 129
    subclinical discharges, 113
EEG discharge
    cognitive activity, 121
    transitory cognitive impairment, 121
Electrical brain stimulation, transitory cognitive
        impairment, 119–121
    cortex, 119
    depth electrode, 120
    foramen ovale, 120
    functional effect specificity, 119–120
    subcortical structures, 119
    temporal lobe, 120
Electroconvulsive seizure, amygdala kindling,
        240, 242, 243, 244
Electroconvulsive therapy, as anticonvulsant,
        240, 241
Emotion, seizure occurrence, 453–460
Emotional distress, 21
Endocrine, 41–42
Energy consumption, seizure, 35
Energy metabolism, 35–38
Enkephalin, 39
Environment, complex partial seizure, 172
Epilepsy
    administrative label, 154
    anticonvulsant rhythm, 177–179
    biofeedback, 177–179
    child
        behavioral consequences, 153–162
        eating, 157
        ictal-speech automatism, 159
        learning, 159–160
        outline findings, 155–156
        parameters, 155–156
        patient referral, 154–155
        patient sources, 154–155
        psychopathology, 86
        psychosocial vocabulary, 153–162
        relating, 160

sleep, 156–157
social impact, 153
socializing, 160
speech, 158–159
thinking, 159
voiding, 157–158
walking, 158
working, 160–161
cognitive deficit, 117–119
depression, 89–90, 186–194
desensitization, 174–176
dopamine, 50, 51
driving, 464
incidence, 317
insanity, 464–467
interictal disturbance
  aggression, 103–106
  depression, 99, 102
  direct effects of underlying lesions, 99–100
  hamartoma, 100
  ictal events, 100
  neurobiological evidence, 97–107
  neurobiological factors, 98–100
  neuroendocrine system, 101–102
  pharmacological effects, 98–99
  psychosis, 103
  recurrent seizures, 101
  schizophrenia, 103
  secondary epileptogenesis, 102
  sleep, 98
interictal psychosis, 143–151
  classification, 144–146
  historical aspects, 143
  laterality, 149–150
  mechanisms, 150–151
manic-depressive psychosis, 89
memory, 369–381, 385–406
  anticonvulsant medication, 372–373
  assessment, 376–380
  attention, 374
  Beck Depression Inventory, 378
  causes, 370–371
  complex partial seizures, 385–387
  EEG abnormality, 371
  emotional state, 375
  epileptiform activity evoked by memory task,
    400–403
  Hospital Anxiety and Depression Scale, 8
  induced memory deficits, 397–398
  medial temporal lobe, 385–387
  overt mental phenomena, 400
  physiology, 398–403
  postseizure deficits, 395–396
  questionnaire approach, 376–377
  real-life situation assessment, 378–380
  shared circuits, 400–403
  surgery, 371–372
  treatment, 371–375

mood change
  anticonvulsant, 190–192
  ictal, 185–187
  interictal, 187–189
  peri-ictal, 185–187
mood disorder, 185–194
  treatment, 192–193
neurobehavioral disorder, 317–337
  mood changes, 190
nonspecific EEG biofeedback, 178–179
paradoxical normalization, 132–133, 137
prisoner, 461–463
  environment, 462
  prevalence, 461
  property offense, 462
  violence, 462
psychiatric symptoms, 83
psychological methods for treatment, 172–177
psychopathology
  adjustment, 445–446
  conceptual model, 439–443
  financial status, 445–446
  life event changes, 446
  locus of control, 446
  medication factors, 446
  multietiological predictor variables, 448
  multietiological risk factors, 441
  neurobiological factors, 440
  neurobiological variables, 444–445
  perceived limitations, 445
  perceived stigma, 445
  pharmacological factors, 440–441
  predictors, 444–448
  psychosocial factors, 441–443
  psychosocial variables, 445–446
  social competence in children, 448–450
  social support, 446
  vocational adjustment, 445–446
psychophysiological methods for treatment,
  177–179
psychosensory symptoms, 249
psychosis, 50, 51, 81–86, 84, 87
  affinity between, 146–149
  antagonism between, 146
  association, 144
  phenomenology, 148–149
  prevalence, 146–147
  risk factors, 147–148
psychotherapy, 176–177
punishment program, 174
relaxation, 174–176
relief avoidance, 174
reward management, 173–174
schizophrenia, 86–88
  biological antagonism between, 50
self-control strategies, 174–176
social attitudes, 463–464
suicide, 89

Epilepsy (*contd.*)
  temporal lobe surgery, 279–290
  violence, 341
Epileptic fugue, 362
Epileptic personality, 411
Epileptic seizure. *See also* Seizure.
  differential diagnosis, 319
  international classification, 348–349
Epileptiform EEG abnormality disappearance,
    acute behavioral symptomatology, 127–141
Episodic memory, 375
Ethosuximide
  absence seizure, 261
  affective illness, 256
  amygdala-kindled seizure, 262
  cognitive effects, 208
  memory, 372–373
  paradoxical normalization, 133
Ethotoin
  absence seizure, 261
  complex partial seizure, 261
Event memory, 375
Excitatory amino acid neurotransmitter, 38

F
Fear, 9, 12–13, 21
Fetus
  antiepileptic drugs, 225–229
  carbamazepine, 227
Fluorodeoxyglucose, 37
Folate cycle
  S-adenosylmethionine, 53
  methylation, 53
Folic acid
  S-adenosylmethionine, 54–55
  gamma-aminobutyric acid, 55–56
  interictal psychiatric disorder, 52–54
  seizure, 55–56
"Folie epileptique," 143
Forced normalization, 127–141
Free fatty acid, 40–41
Frontal lobe epilepsy, complex partial seizure
  decision flow charts, 323–327
  electrographic manifestations, 322
Frontal lobe seizure
  aura, 328–331
    localizing value of autonomic phenomena,
      332–338
    localizing value of somatic sensory
      phenomena, 333
    psychical phenomena, 328–329
    special sensory phenomena, 331
  automatism, 335–336
  causes, 336–337
  cerebrovascular disease, 337
  classification, 321–323
  complex partial seizure, clinical features,
    320–321

diagnosis, 318–321
EEG, 336
hyperventilation, 319
hysterical faint, 318–321
impairment of consciousness at onset, 334–335
incidence, 317
intracranial tumor, 337
lapse, 334–335
neurobehavioral disorder, 317–337
post-traumatic, 337
pseudoabsence, 334–335
psychosis, 318–321
somatomotor sign, 329–334
syncope, 318–321
trauma, 337
trigger factor, 336–337
Fugue state, 357–365
  status epilepticus, 362

G
Ganglioglioma, transient postictal global amnesia,
    391–393
Gene expression, seizure, 35
Geschwind syndrome, 411–420
  characteristics, 414
  clinical description, 412–414
  clinical phenomenology, 414–415
  criticisms, 416–417
  interictal characteristics, 413
  Klüver-Bucy syndrome, 417–418
  temporal hyperconnection syndrome, 417–418
  treatment, 419–420
  variations, 415–416
Glioma, 61–62
Global amnesia, temporal lobe surgery, 281–282
Glucose metabolism, seizure, 35
Grand mal epilepsy, psychiatric symptoms, 85
Guilt, 9–11

H
Hallucination, 3
  left temporal lobe, 4
  subjectively experienced phenomenology, 3
Halstead-Reitan battery, transitory cognitive
    impairment, 114
Hamartoma, 61–62, 100
Head circumference, antiepileptic drug, 225–227
Herpes encephalitis, memory, 389–390
Heterotopia, 61–62
Hippocampal cell loss, 61–62
Hippocampal-dentate complex, 71
Hippocampal fissure, development, 60
Hippocampal sclerosis, 61–62
Hippocampal-subicular complex, migration along
    radial glial stalks, 70–71
Hippocampus
  development, 60
  structural anomaly, 72–73

Hunger, 17
Hypergraphia, 414
Hyperventilation
  frontal lobe seizure, 319
  seizure occurrence, 456–457
Hypochondriacal state, paradoxical
      normalization, 130–131
Hyposexuality, 413–415
Hysterical faint, frontal lobe seizure, 318–321
Hysterical state, paradoxical normalization,
      130–131

I

Ictal aggression
  evidence for, 350–351
  nature, 348–349
  postictal psychosis, 352
  presentations, 352–353
  primary, 352
  psychobiology, 341–353
  secondary, 352
Ictal amnesia, 357–365
  characteristics, 357
  defined, 357
Ictal behavior
  neurobiological substrate, 1–42
    affect, 9–17
    aggression, 11
    amnesia, 24
    anatomical substrates, 1–2
    anxiety, 9–11
    automatism, 25–27
    confusional state, 25–27
    consciousness, 21–25
    defined, 1
    dysphasia, 30, 31
    experiential phenomena, 17–21
    fear, 9, 12–13
    guilt, 9–11
    hunger, 17
    laughter, 11–16
    memory, 8–9
    neurophysiological mechanisms, 2
    perception, 2–8
    seizure discharge effect, 2
    sexual behavior, 14–16
    speech, 30–31
    thirst, 17
    unresponsiveness, 24
    violence, 11
  neurochemical substrate, 35–42
    adenosine, 40
    brain creatine concentration, 35
    cerebral blood flow, 36
    cerebral lactate, 35
    cyclic nucleotide, 40
    dynorphin, 39
    endocrine, 41–42

energy metabolism, 35–38
    enkephalin, 39
    excitatory amino acid neurotransmitter, 38
    fluorodeoxyglucose, 37
    free fatty acid, 40–41
    glucose, 35
    inhibitory amino acid neurotransmitter, 38
    ionic changes, 37–38
    metabolic change behavioral significance, 42
    monoamine, 39
    neurotensin, 39
    neurotransmitter metabolism, 38–41
    oxygen, 35
    peptide, 39–40
    prostaglandin, 40–41
    protein synthesis, 41–42
    second messenger system, 40–41
    substance P, 39
Ictal manifestations, temporal lobe epilepsy
    frequency, 302–304
    seizure discharge location, 302–304
Illusion, 2
Immediate memory, 375
Infection, psychosis, 80
Inhibitory amino acid neurotransmitter, 38
Insanity, epilepsy, 464–467
Intelligence, neuropsychological testing, 429–430
Intensification, 415
Interictal behavior, metabolic basis, 47
Interictal defensive reactivity, 104
Interictal disturbance
  aggression, 103–106
  epilepsy
    aggression, 103–106
    depression, 99, 102
    direct effects of underlying lesions, 99–100
    hamartoma, 100
    ictal events, 100
    neurobiological evidence, 97–107
    neurobiological factors, 98–100
    neuroendocrine system, 101–102
    pharmacological effects, 98–99
    psychosis, 103
    recurrent seizures, 101
    schizophrenia, 103
    secondary epileptogenesis, 102
    sleep, 98
Interictal psychiatric disorder
  gamma-aminobutyric acid, 50–52
  biological antagonism, 48–50
  cerebrospinal fluid monoamine metabolite,
      47–48
  folic acid, 52–54
  neurochemical aspects, 47–56
Interictal psychosis, epilepsy, 143–151
  classification, 144–146
  historical aspects, 143
  laterality, 149–150

Interictal psychosis, epilepsy (*contd.*)
  mechanisms, 150–151
Interictal spike, behavioral correlates, 113–123
Intracarotid sodium amobarbital procedure,
    temporal lobe surgery, 281
Intracranial tumor, frontal lobe seizure, 337
Ionic distribution, seizure, 35
Isocortex, association areas, 2

K
Kindling
  affective illness, 262–268
  carbamazepine, 262–268
  pharmacology, 265
Klüver-Bucy syndrome
  Geschwind syndrome, 417–418
  temporal hyperconnection syndrome, 417–418

L
Lapse, frontal lobe seizure, 334–335
Laughter, 11–16
Left amygdala, seizure, 4, 6–7
Left hippocampus, seizure, 4, 6–7
Left parahippocampal gyrus, seizure, 4, 6–7
Left temporal lobe, hallucination, 4
Legal issues, 461–471
Limbic kindling, carbamazepine, 239
Limbic substrate, carbamazepine, 260–262
Limbic system, simple focal seizure, types, 133
Long-term memory, 375
Lorazepam, affective illness, 253–255

M
Macropsia, 2–3
Mamillary body
  amnesia, 358
  transient global amnesia, 358
Mania
  carbamazepine, 240–244, 246–247, 248, 252
    prophylaxis, 245, 251
  carbamazepine congener, 240–244, 246–247,
      248, 252
    prophylaxis, 245, 251
  neuroleptic, 248
  valproate, 252
Manic-depressive illness, antiepileptic drugs,
    240–270
Manic-depressive psychosis, epilepsy, 89
Memory, 21. *See also* specific type.
  automatism, 172
  carbamazepine, 372–373
  complex partial epilepsy, 386–398
    incidence, 387
    permanent memory deficits, 386–393
    temporary memory deficits, 393–398
  epilepsy, 369–381, 385–406
    anticonvulsant medication, 372–373
    assessment, 376–380

    attention, 374
    Beck Depression Inventory, 378
    causes, 370–371
    complex partial seizures, 385–387
    EEG abnormality, 371
    emotional state, 375
    epileptiform activity evoked by memory task,
        400–403
    Hospital Anxiety and Depression Scale, 378
    induced memory deficits, 397–398
    medial temporal lobe, 385–387
    overt mental phenomena, 400
    physiology, 398–403
    postseizure deficits, 395–396
    questionnaire approach, 376–377
    real-life situation assessment, 378–380
    shared circuits, 400–403
    surgery, 371–372
    treatment, 371–375
  ethosuximide, 372–373
  herpes encephalitis, 389–390
  improving, 380–381
  loss, 357
    causes, 361
  nature, 375
  normal physiology, 398–400
    information–representation, 399–400
    modulation, 399–400
    pathways, 398–399
    plasticity, 398–399
  phenobarbitone, 372–373
  phenytoin, 372–373
  seizure, 370–371
  sodium valproate, 372–373
  temporal lobe epilepsy, 369–370
Memory aid, 380
Memory flashback, 9
Memory recording, interference, 9
Meningioma, transient global amnesia, 361
Mental change, dysthymic pain disorder, 188
Mephenytoin
  absence seizure, 261
  complex partial seizure, 261
Mesial temporal sclerosis, 68
Mesuximide
  paradoxical normalization, 132, 133
  psychosis, 132, 133
Meta memory, 375
Metharbital
  absence seizure, 261
  complex partial seizure, 261
Methsuximide
  absence seizure, 261
  amygdala-kindled seizure, 262
  complex partial seizure, 261
Methylation
  S-adenosylmethionine, 53
  folate cycle, 53

Micropsia, 2–3
Mnemonic phenomena, 8
Monoamine, 39, 47–48
Monoamine precursor, 48
Mood change
  antiepileptic drug, 190–192
  carbamazepine, 191
  epilepsy
    anticonvulsant, 190–192
    ictal, 185–187
    interictal, 187–189
    peri-ictal, 185–187
  phenobarbital, 191
  phenytoin, 191
  temporal lobe epilepsy, 188–189
Mood disorder, epilepsy, 185–194
  treatment, 192–193
Motion illusion, 2–3
Motor ability, neuropsychological testing, 431
Multiple-squeak response, 104

N

Neurobehavioral disorder
  epilepsy, 317–337
  frontal lobe seizure, 317–337
Neurobiological substrate, ictal behavior, 1–42
  affect, 9–17
  aggression, 11
  amnesia, 24
  anatomical substrates, 1–2
  anxiety, 9–11
  automatism, 25–27
  confusional state, 25–27
  consciousness, 21–25
  defined, 1
  dysphasia, 30, 31
  experiential phenomena, 17–21
  fear, 9, 12–13
  guilt, 9–11
  hunger, 17
  laughter, 11–16
  memory, 8–9
  neurophysiological mechanisms, 2
  perception, 2–8
  seizure discharge effect, 2
  sexual behavior, 14–16
  speech, 30–31
  thirst, 17
  unresponsiveness, 24
  violence, 11
Neurochemical substrate, ictal behavior, 35–42
  adenosine, 40
  brain creatine concentration, 35
  cerebral blood flow, 36
  cerebral lactate, 35
  cyclic nucleotide, 40
  dynorphin, 39
  endocrine, 41–42

energy metabolism, 35–38
  enkephalin, 39
  excitatory amino acid neurotransmitter, 38
  fluorodeoxyglucose, 37
  free fatty acid, 40–41
  glucose, 35
  inhibitory amino acid neurotransmitter, 38
  ionic changes, 37–38
  metabolic change behavioral significance, 42
  monoamine, 39
  neurotensin, 39
  neurotransmitter metabolism, 38–41
  oxygen, 35
  peptide, 39–40
  prostaglandin, 40–41
  protein synthesis, 41–42
  second messenger system, 40–41
  substance P, 39
Neuroembryogenesis, 68
Neuroleptic, mania, 248
Neuron
  anticonvulsant effects, 225–235
  antiepileptic drug, 225–235
Neuropsychological testing, 423–437
  adaptation, 431–432
  affect, 431
  cognition, 430–431
  coping, 431–432
  follow-up, 432
  intelligence, 429–430
  interpretive phase, 432
  motor ability, 431
  normed, 426
  patient history, 429, 435–437
  philosophical models, 424
  process, 424–432
  reliability, 425
  report, 432
  sensory ability, 431
  test battery, 428–429
  test selection, 426–427
  theoretical foundations, 423
  validity, 425
Neurotensin, 39
Neurotransmitter seizure, 35
Neurotransmitter metabolism, 38–41
Night terror, 157
Nightmare, 157
Nonverbal memory, 375
Nonverbal recent memory, 390–391
Nuclear schizophrenia, 88

O

Oxazolidine, paradoxical normalization, 133

P

Paradoxical normalization, 127–141
  affective disorder, 131

Paradoxical normalization (*contd.*)
  alternative psychosis, clinical appearances,
      129–130
  antiepileptic drug, 133–136
    time element, 134
  depersonalization, 131
  derealization, 131
  dysphoric state, 131
  EEG, 128–129
    epileptiform discharges, 129
  epidemiology, 132–133
  epilepsy, 132–133, 137
  ethosuximide, 133
  hypochondriacal state, 130–131
  hysterical state, 130–131
  mechanisms, 137–139
  mesuximide, 132, 133
  oxazolidine, 133
  pathogenesis, 137
  praepsychotische verstimmung, 130
  prepsychotic dysphoria, 130
  psychosocial factors, 136–137
  related syndromes, 130–132
  twilight state, 131
  valproic acid, 134
  vocationally disintegrated, 136
Paramethadione
  absence seizure, 261
  complex partial seizure, 261
Paroxysmal syndrome, carbamazepine, 263
Partial epileptic seizure, semiology, 324–327
Peptide, 39–40
Perceptual hallucination, 20, 21
Perceptual illusion, 3, 20, 21
Peri-ictal aggression, presentations, 352–353
Periaqueductal gray region, 104
Personality effects, temporal lobe surgery, 287
Petit mal status, 26–29
Pharmacology
  illness course, 264–266
  kindling, 265
Phenacemide
  absence seizure, 261
  complex partial seizure, 261
Phenobarbital
  absence seizure, 261
  amygdala-kindled seizure, 262
  behavior, 198–199
  brain weight, 229–231
  cognitive effects, 197, 198–201
    attention, 200
    I.Q. fall, 200–201
    memory, 200
    short-term memory, 200
  complex partial seizure, 261
  mood change, 191
  tolerance, 199–200
Phenobarbitone, memory, 372–373

Phensuximide, absence seizure, 261
Phenytoin
  absence seizure, 261
  affective illness, 255
  amygdala-kindled seizure, 262
  behavior, 198–199
  behavioral effects, 214–217
  cognitive effects, 197, 201–204
    carbamazepine, 202–203
    motor speed, 204
    reaction time, 204
    serum levels, 202–203
  complex partial seizure, 261
  memory, 372–373
  mood change, 191
Post-temporal lobectomy psychosis, 90–91
Postictal aggression, 104
Postictal psychosis, ictal aggression, 352
Praepsychotische verstimmung, paradoxical
      normalization, 130
Predatory attack
  anatomical substrates, 104
  stimulation-induced, 104–105
Prepsychotic dysphoria, paradoxical
      normalization, 130
Prescience illusion, 9, 10
Primary psychogenic epileptic seizure, 166–168
Primidone
  absence seizure, 261
  cognitive effects, 208
  complex partial seizure, 261
Prisoner, epilepsy, 461–463
  environment, 462
  prevalence, 461
  property offense, 462
  violence, 462
Prostaglandin, 40–41
Protein synthesis, 41–42
Pseudoabsence, frontal lobe seizure, 334–335
Pseudoseizure, differential diagnosis, 319
Psychogenic amnesia, 363–364
Psychogenic epileptic seizure, 166–168
Psychogenic fugue, 363–364
Psychomotor epilepsy
  psychiatric findings, 83
  psychosis, 81
Psychomotor seizure
  electroclinical features, 302–312
  stereoelectroencephalographically recorded,
      302–312
Psychomotor speed, 390–391
Psychopathology, epilepsy
  adjustment, 445–446
  conceptual model, 439–443
  financial status, 445–446
  life event changes, 446
  locus of control, 446
  medication factors, 446

multietiological predictor variables, 448
multietiological risk factors, 441
neurobiological factors, 440
neurobiological variables, 444–445
perceived limitations, 445
perceived stigma, 445
pharmacological factors, 440–441
predictors, 444–448
psychosocial factors, 441–443
psychosocial variables, 445–446
social competence in children, 448–450
social support, 446
vocational adjustment, 445–446
Psychosis
  associated heredodegenerative disorders, 81
  brain injury, 80
  classified, 79
  complex partial seizure, 81
  defined, 79
  depression, 89–90
  dopamine, 50, 51
  epilepsy, 50, 51, 81–86, 84, 87
    affinity between, 146–149
    antagonism between, 146
    association, 144
    phenomenology, 148–149
    prevalence, 146–147
    risk factors, 147–148
  frontal lobe seizure, 318–321
  infection, 80
  mesuximide, 132, 133
  psychomotor epilepsy, 81
  schizophrenia, 87
    electroencephalography, 88–89
  temporal lobe, depth electrode study, 90
  temporal lobe epilepsy, 81, 84
  tumor, 80–81
Psychosocial effects, temporal lobe surgery,
    287–288
Psychotherapy, epilepsy, 176–177
Punishment program, epilepsy, 174

R

Rage reaction, cerebral electrical stimulation,
    345–346
Reactive automatism, defined, 349
Relaxation, epilepsy, 174–176
Relief avoidance, epilepsy, 174
Resistive violence, 350, 352
Retrohippocampal formation, 71
Reward management, epilepsy, 173–174
Right temporal lobe seizure, visual hallucination,
    4, 5

S

Schizoaffective illness, valproate, 254
Schizophrenia
  anatomic studies, 91–93

brain injury, 80
  as disorder of embryogenesis, 68–71
  epilepsy, 86–88
    biological antagonism between, 50
  psychosis, 87
    electroencephalography, 88–89
  temporal lobe epilepsy, 70
    anterior temporal cortex, 73
    behavioral symptoms, 73
    early onset, 73
    genetic components, 72
    hippocampus cellular alterations, 72
    hippocampus structural anomalies, 72–73
    incidence, 72
    psychological symptoms, 73
    similarities, 71–73
  ventricular dilatation, 90–92
Second messenger system, 40–41
  seizure, 35
Secondary psychogenic epileptic seizure, 168
Seizure. *See also* specific type.
  gamma-aminobutyric acid, 55–56
  behavior, 172
  behavioral treatment, 163–179
  2-deoxyglucose method, 36–37
  depression, 55–56
  energy consumption, 35
  evocation, 163–179
    mechanism of spread, 165–166
    terminology, 165
  folic acid, 55–56
  gene expression, 35
  genesis, 163–164
  glucose metabolism, 35
  indirect primary inhibition, 170–171
  inhibition, 163–179
  ionic distribution, 35
  left amygdala, 4, 6–7
  left hippocampus, 4, 6–7
  left parahippocampal gyrus, 4, 6–7
  memory, 370–371
  neurotransmitter, 35
  primary inhibition, 169–171
  second messenger system, 35
  secondary inhibition, 171–172
  situations, 168
Seizure disorder, transient global amnesia, 362
Seizure occurrence
  anxiety, 456–457
  emotion, 453–460
  hyperventilation, 456–457
  stress, 453–460
Semantic memory, 375
Sensory ability, neuropsychological testing, 431
Sensory memory, 375
Sexual behavior, 14–16
Sexuality, altered, 413–416
Short-term memory, 375

Signal Detection Task, transitory cognitive
    impairment, 114
Simple focal seizure, limbic system, types, 133
Simple Motor Task, transitory cognitive
    impairment, 114
Simple Reaction Time, transitory cognitive
    impairment, 114
Sleep, 98
  childhood epilepsy, 156–157
Sodium valproate
  amygdala-kindled seizure, 262
  memory, 372–373
Somatomotor sign, frontal lobe seizure, 329–334
Speech, 30–31
Spike-and-wave seizure, 164
Status epilepticus, fugue state, 362
Stereoscopic vision, 3
Stereotyped automatism, defined, 349
Stress, seizure occurrence, 453–460
Subclinical discharge
  defined, 113
  nature, 114–115
  timing, 114–115
Subicular complex, development, 60
Subiculum, development, 60
Substance P, 39
Suicide, epilepsy, 89
Syncope
  differential diagnosis, 319
  frontal lobe seizure, 318–321

T
Temporal hyperconnection syndrome
  Geschwind syndrome, 417–418
  Klüver-Bucy syndrome, 417–418
Temporal lobe
  defined, 79
  limbic structures, 2
  psychosis, depth electrode study, 90
Temporal lobe dysgenesis, complex partial
    seizure, 59–75
  birthing history, 66, 67
  capillary tree, 67
  capsular neuramnidase, 69–70
  cerebral glucose, 67
  degenerating neurons, 66
  dendritic change, 63–66
  developmental malformations, 62
  early onset, 66
  family seizure history, 66
  glioma, 61–62
  hamartoma, 61–62
  heterotopia, 61–62
  hippocampal cell loss, 61
  hippocampal sclerosis, 61
  hippocampus dendrites, 64–66
  historical overview, 61
  mesiotemporal sclerosis, 66, 68

  microvascular changes, 62–63
  neuroembryogenesis, 68
  neuropathological substrate, 61
  oxygen, 67
  phagocytes, 66
Temporal lobe epilepsy
  ascending epigastric aura, 301
  assaultive behavior, 347
  ictal manifestations, 301–312
    bilateral, 306–310
    frequency, 302–304
    ictal discharge spread, 304
    ictal symptoms spread, 304
    intracerebral electrical stimulation, 311
    seizure discharge location, 302–304
    seizure spread to opposite hemisphere,
        306–310
    symptom-site correlation, 304–306
  memory, 369–370
  mental change, 188
  mood change, 188–189
  psychosis, 81, 84
  schizophrenia, 70
    anterior temporal cortex, 73
    behavioral symptoms, 73
    early onset, 73
    genetic components, 72
    hippocampus cellular alterations, 72
    hippocampus structural anomalies, 72–73
    incidence, 72
    psychological symptoms, 73
    similarities, 71–73
  symptom catalogues, 301
  temporal lobectomy, mental state, 91
Temporal lobe seizure
  amnesia, 23, 24–25
  automatism, 23, 24–25
Temporal lobe surgery
  anatomical substrates, 284–286
  behavior, 279–290
  cognitive effects, 280–287
  confrontational naming, 284
  cross-center behavior comparisons, 280
  epilepsy, 279–290
  global amnesia, 281–282
  intracarotid sodium amobarbital procedure, 281
  left (language-dominant) temporal lobe changes,
      283, 285
  memory changes, 282–283
  new memories, 282–283
  optimal outcome prediction, 288–290
  organizational learning, 284
  personality effects, 287
  psychosocial effects, 287–288
  right temporal lobe changes, 286–287
  rote-verbal learning, 283–284
  semantic learning, 284
  standardized resections, 279–280

surgical boundary variation, 280
    verbal memory, 283
Temporal lobectomy, temporal lobe epilepsy,
    mental state, 91
Tests of attention and recall, transitory cognitive
    impairment, 114
"Thinking epilepsy," 168
Thirst, 17
Todd's paralysis, amnesia, 357
Transient global amnesia, 357–365
    anatomical substrate, 358
    characteristics, 357–358
    duration, 359
    mamillary body, 358
    meningioma, 361
    seizure disorder, 362
Transient postictal global amnesia, ganglioglioma,
    391–393
Transitory cognitive impairment, 113
    Choice Reaction Time, 114
    cognitive deficit nature, 115
    cognitive deficit specificity, 116–117
    cognitive deficits in epilepsy, 117–119
    detection, 115–116
    driving automobile, 122
    EEG discharge, 121
    electrical brain stimulation, 119–121
        cortex, 119
        depth electrode, 120
        foramen ovale, 120
        functional effect specificity, 119–120
        subcortical structures, 119
        temporal lobe, 120
    Halstead-Reitan battery, 114
    practical implications, 121–123
    psychosocial functioning, 122
    Signal Detection Task, 114
    Simple Motor Task, 114
    Simple Reaction Time, 114
    subclinical discharge, 121–122
    tests, 114
    Tests of Attention and Recall, 114
    treatment, 123
    Wechsler battery, 114

Trauma, frontal lobe seizure, 337
Traveler's amnesia, 359
Triazolam, amnesia, 359
Trigger factor, frontal lobe seizure, 336–337
Trimethadione
    absence seizure, 261
    complex partial seizure, 261
Tryptophan, 48–49
Tumor, psychosis, 80–81
Twilight state, 362
    paradoxical normalization, 131

U
Unresponsiveness, 24

V
Valproate
    absence seizure, 261
    affective illness, 250–253
    bipolar illness, 254
    cognitive effects, 201, 207–208
    complex partial seizure, 261
    mania, 252
    schizoaffective illness, 254
Valproic acid
    behavioral effects, 214–217
    paradoxical normalization, 134
Ventricular dilatation, schizophrenia, 90–92
Verbal memory, 375
Vigabatrin, depression, 50–51
Violence, 11
    epilepsy, 341
    resistive, 350, 352
Viscosity, 414
Visual hallucination, 4
    right temporal lobe seizure, 4, 5
Visuospatial perception, 390–391

W
Wechsler battery, transitory cognitive
    impairment, 114
Working memory, 375